The Polymerase Chain Reaction

Kary B. Mullis
François Ferré
Richard A. Gibbs
Editors

Foreword by James D. Watson

With 112 Illustrations

Birkhäuser
Boston • Basel • Berlin

Kary B. Mullis
La Jolla, CA 92037
USA

François Ferré
The Immune Response Corporation
5935 Darwin Court
Carlsbad, CA 92008
USA

Richard A. Gibbs
Institute for Molecular Genetics
Baylor College of Medicine
One Baylor Plaza
Houston, TX 77030
USA

Printed on acid-free paper.

© 1994 Birkhäuser Boston

Birkhäuser

ISBN 0-8176-3607-2 (hardcover)   ISBN 0-8176-3750-8 (softcover)
ISBN 3-7643-3607-2 (hardcover)   ISBN 3-7643-3750-8 (softcover)

Typeset by Sherman Typography, York, PA.
Printed and bound by The Maple Press Company, York, PA.
Printed in the United States of America.

9 8 7 6 5 4 3

Cover illustration: Based on a photograph taken by Kary Mullis in a museum in Cologne. "The mosaic had been taken from Italy by the Germans. I think it was from Pompeii. I saw a similar design still intact in its original location in Herculaneum but had no camera that day. Vesuvius covered both cities in 79 A.D. I would guess that the structure of DNA was probably worked out about two thousand years before Watson was born and therefore nineteen hundred and eighty-eight years before Crick. The Romans, however, seemed to think that atoms were square, and most likely the significance of the structure did escape their notice. Of course, this was long before Avery."

The Polymerase Chain Reaction

From the Reviews–

"The editors have tapped many of the leaders in PCR innovation to explore their particular twists on the technique and to discuss its impact on their fields. The resulting chapters provide thorough examinations of basic and advanced PCR techniques, with a satisfying balance between theoretical analyses and observed results, and often include the type of anecdotal advice not found in journal articles. Mullis's preface has the stream-of-consciousness style of a newsy letter, and he introduces many of the authors with colorful, good-natured similes and personal anecdotes that amuse and add depth to the following chapters. Mullis tells a good story as he recounts his invention of PCR in 1983 and the subsequent patent travails."

— **SCIENCE**

"PCR The Polymerase Chain Reaction is not just a manual of techniques, but represents the considered experience of practitioners, some familiar with the use of PCR and some interested in extending its application to new areas...A chapter on nonbiological applications, using PCR as a product tag, was unique and extraordinary. Some contributions, such as one on infectious diseases, and another on genetics, plants and PCR, incorporate large numbers of publications and applications in their respective fields...Overall, it is a useful book and, for a variety of reasons, is unique among books in this field. I am delighted to have a copy."

— **Trends in BioTechnology**

Foreword

James D. Watson

When, in late March of 1953, Francis Crick and I came to write the first *Nature* paper describing the double helical structure of the DNA molecule, Francis had wanted to include a lengthy discussion of the genetic implications of a molecule whose structure we had divined from a minimum of experimental data and on theoretical arguments based on physical principles. But I felt that this might be tempting fate, given that we had not yet seen the detailed evidence from King's College. Nevertheless, we reached a compromise and decided to include a sentence that pointed to the biological significance of the molecule's key feature—the complementary pairing of the bases. "It has not escaped our notice," Francis wrote, "that the specific pairing that we have postulated immediately suggests a possible copying mechanism for the genetic material."

By May, when we were writing the second *Nature* paper, I was more confident that the proposed structure was at the very least substantially correct, so that this second paper contains a discussion of molecular self-duplication using templates or molds. We pointed out that, as a consequence of base pairing, a DNA molecule has two chains that are complementary to each other. Each chain could then act ". . . as a template for the formation on itself of a new companion chain, so that eventually we shall have *two* pairs of chains, where we only had one before" and, moreover, ". . . the sequence of pairs of bases will have been duplicated exactly." The process of DNA replication of necessity *doubles* the numbers of DNA strands present and does so precisely as regards sequence. At that time, of course, we could offer no biochemical evidence as to how this process might be carried out. We recognized that the strands would have to be unwound and that this would be difficult to achieve without everything getting tangled, but our conviction that the structure was correct made us confident that evolution had found a solution to this problem. Another question we raised was whether an enzyme was required, once nucleotides had found their complements in the original chain, to join them, speculating that the template chain might itself act as the equivalent of an enzyme.

Over the next few years, experiments were carried out that confirmed our general scheme, so that by 1956 the decision to hold a Symposium entitled *The Chemical Basis of Heredity* was not only possible but made sense. At that meeting, Max Delbruck and Gunther Stent presented theoretical arguments showing the possibility of unwinding DNA, although we had to wait until the late 1970s before the proteins that carry out unwinding were isolated. One consequence of unwinding and replication as we envisaged it was that DNA replication should be semiconservative, and this was demonstrated convincingly by Mat Meselson and Frank Stahl in 1958. Also reported at the 1956 meeting were the first results of Arthur Kornberg, who was beginning to dissect the biochemical pathways that carry out DNA replication. While DNA polymerase I was later shown not to be the enzyme responsible for DNA replication in *E. coli*, the demonstration that what was thought to be an immensely complex process could be analyzed by a simplified *in vitro* system, marked a turning point in studying DNA replication.

Quite apart from its importance in DNA replication, base pairing came quickly to play an important technical role when it was realized that base pairing confirmed *specificity* on the interactions between the separated strands of a DNA molecule. This was demonstrated experimentally in the late 1950s, when Julius Marmur and Paul Doty were able to denature DNA and, on cooling the solutions slowly, recover molecules that were double stranded by physical and biological criteria. When hybrid DNA molecules were made by using DNA strands from different organisms, the degree of reassociation depended on how closely related were the organisms from which the DNA came. A little later, Sol Spiegelman with Ben Hall and Alex Rich independently showed that RNA and DNA strands would hybridize. Following the development of cloning in the early 1970s, hybridization became a powerful method for detecting sought-after sequences, especially with the development of Ed Southern's convenient technique. The critical importance of the specificity conferred by nucleotide sequence was exemplified in the 1980s when oligonucleotides, synthesized to be complementary to known sequences, began to be used as probes, so-called allele-specific oligonucleotides (ASOs). Thus in 1983, Savio Woo's laboratory reported the diagnosis of emphysema cased by mutations in α-1 antitrypsin by using oligonucleotides specific for the normal and mutant forms of the gene.

So by 1986, we could use *in vitro* systems to synthesize DNA with high efficiency, and because both DNA sequencing and oligonucleotide synthesis had become routine, we knew that oligonucleotides could be used as primers to direct the synthesis of specific sequences. But it was only through a phone call from Mike Botchan that I learned that these various elements had been combined in a simple fashion with extraordinary results. In early 1986, I was in the last stages of planning that year's Cold Spring Harbor Laboratory Symposium on Quantitative Biology, *The Molecular Biology of Homo Sapiens*. It was the 51st Symposium and it seemed right to begin our second 50 years with a subject that had changed out of all recognition in recent years and a topic of special interest to us all. Mike told me of Kary Mullis and the exciting work going on at Cetus, and I resolved to invite him to present his work at the Symposium. Although a paper had been published in *Science* in December of 1985, this was the first occasion on which the polymerase chain reaction was described in a public meeting. Kary's presentation was all that I had been led to expect and the excitement that it aroused was palpable, although my main recollection is his suggestion that because "G" and "C" are hard to distinguish in printouts of sequence, "guanosine" should be changed to "wuanosine," "G" and "W" being easier to tell apart. This suggestion had the additional benefit, Kary claimed, of producing W–C base pairs, thus giving me a base, Francis already having his.

By 1987, although only a handful of papers using PCR had been published, its potential was evident and we decided to devote a Banbury Center meeting to the myriad novel applications being developed. The meeting, held in December 1988, demonstrated that the polymerase chain reaction now ranked with cloning and DNA sequencing as an indispensable tool in the molecular biologist's armamentarium. And not only has it become an indispensable tool, but PCR has provided new ways to approach a problem. For example, cloning of genes for olfactory receptors was achieved by using conserved sequences of G-protein-coupled, seven segment trans-membrane receptors as primers for polymerase chain reactions performed on olfactory cells. It is estimated that these receptors constitute a new multigene family with several hundred members.

The field in which PCR has had the most extraordinary impact is human genetics. One beneficiary is the Human Genome Project, and indeed all the projects that are looking to complete the mapping and sequencing of the genomes of *Drosophila*, *C. elegans*, the mouse, *Arabidopsis*, and so on. It seems to me that the immensity of what has to be done would overwhelm us if we did not have the power of the polymerase chain reaction to assist us. How slow progress would be without direct sequencing, mapping using microsatellite repeats, and sequence tagged sites. It is perhaps no coincidence that one of the first public discussions of the proposal to map and sequence the human genome took place at the same Symposium where PCR was presented. But in a quite remarkable way for an esoteric technique, PCR has had an impact far beyond the confines of the research laboratory. The first paper on PCR dealt with the diagnosis of sickle cell anemia, and the rapid implementation of DNA-based diagnosis has continued to depend on and further exploit the simplicity and specificity of PCR in detecting mutations. The simplicity of the reaction will ensure the development of diagnostic tests that can be used to screen populations, and its specificity will be used to search for multiple mutations in a single reaction by using sets of primers.

All this has not been achieved without difficulties of a kind that we could well do without. Research scientists have been able to use PCR freely, but companies developing diagnostic tests have been hampered by uncertainties in what licensing restrictions they might be subject to, and clinical geneticists have been concerned that royalty fees will make the costs of PCR-based tests prohibitive. I had warned that this situation was not likely to be acceptable to a Congress concerned with health care costs or to a public seeking better health care. One year ago, Roche began to enforce strictly its patent for heat stable *Taq* polymerase, raising concerns that scientists pursuing research that uses large quantities of the enzyme will be unable to buy what is needed. However, first steps toward devising a more acceptable pricing policy are the very recent decisions by Roche to offer discounts to very large scale users (with extra reductions for designated genome centers) and to license two other companies to sell the enzyme. These are welcome moves, but the danger remains that with federal funding becoming increasingly scarce, a highly successful and desirable human genome research program and its medical applications may be delayed.

It is a pleasure to be able to end on a happy note. Even as I write this, Kary Mullis is at the Nobel Prize ceremony in Stockholm, sharing the 1993 Prize for Chemistry with Mike Smith, developer of methods for site-directed mutagenesis. Thus PCR and mutagenesis join with DNA sequencing as techniques that have transformed the way scientists work, and prove once again that the golden age of molecular biology is far from over.

Preface

The polymerase chain reaction (PCR) has been employed extensively in the medical and biological sciences since it was formally introduced at the Cold Spring Harbor 51st Symposium on Quantitative Biology (Mullis et al., 1986) and it has repeatedly resulted in three complaints. The first is that PCR has made DNA research boring. Projects that formerly required some subtle deduction, clever manipulation, special insight, or good fortune are now within easy reach of anyone willing to assemble a few reagents and a cycler, and follow a well-worn routine.

The second has arisen as a minor lament from professional molecular biologists who on seeing for the first time the simplicity of PCR openly regret that they failed to stumble on it themselves. For the former the solution is obviously to do things using PCR that were next to impossible before and are now conceivable but difficult. As for the second, I can answer with an old Bob Dylan refrain, "Can I help it, if I'm lucky?" The third complaint comes from the medical diagnostics community and will be the subject of further comment presently.

Indeed, PCR has to a surprising extent transformed the way we do molecular biology. It has become an integral part of the DNA laboratory, and one that we would rather not do without even if it does make things at times a little like work. The computer seemed to wander into the world and from there into the biology laboratories just when the explosion of available DNA and protein sequence information would have put an otherwise uncomfortable strain on the limited number of graduate students and computationally inclined monks that could have been exploited for the task of organizing and analyzing this new kind of information. Curiously in the same almost too timely way PCR was discovered beside a buckeye tree near Highway 128 in Mendocino County (Mullis, 1990), just when the time was ripe for it to accelerate the assault on the awesome complexity of information in the macromolecular archives of life on earth.

Roger Penrose, in *The Emperor's New Mind* (Penrose, 1989), proposes that in the case of certain inventions, "where much more comes out of the structure than is put into it in the first place," or in the case of "an engineering innovation with a beautiful economy, where a great deal is achieved in the scope of the application of some simple, unexpected idea, (the invention) might appropriately be described as a discovery rather than an invention.''

I entertained thoughts like this about PCR, toying between discovery and invention, and as its uses and variations multiplied far beyond my grasp and it became in the households I visited not only a household noun but also a household verb, I settled on discovery. I was amused to come across the idea in the context of Penrose's chapter on mathematical truth with its implication that certain things may or may not be invented, but others were there already, and given time, would be discovered.

On the other hand now and then I read that PCR caused a revolution in molecular biology. Specifically, I know of two kinds of revolution in molecular biology. There is the kind where a band of angry, young, well-armed molecular biologists, having formented their plans in the chill, rarefied air of the UCLA winter symposia, meeting clandestinely on the slopes during the morning talks, and later in the darker corners of the bar while the poster sessions wind down, converge in the Spring on Bethesda, assault rifles and ugly unpatriotic slides on hand, to settle once and for all the issue of NIH post-doc stipends.

Then there is the other kind, referred to as a paradigm shift, or a retreat to the drawing board, when disappointing data can no longer be hidden or explained by old notions. New concepts become fashionable and new paragraphs have to be written for introductions to papers and grants. Usually there are a number of powerful elders in important places that have to retire or die before things get rolling. Like for instance, Maddox, who is aging at the same rate as everybody else, or Dan, who may take a little longer. It could happen here.

But I do not recall either kind of revolution here on account of PCR. New paragraphs and grants. But assault rifles? No. Paradigmatic shifts? I do not think so. It was just business as usual exploring genes. Things went faster and easier and the range of possibility expanded. Nobody had to die for PCR to be accepted. It was just a new tool. That it came out of the organic chemistry lab of a biotechnology company was interesting but not shocking. Things had begun to flow from industry to academia already to some degree. And chemistry had been gnawing at biology all century.

Being a simple little thing PCR tends to work its was into many studies. Everyone thinks of their own little twist to put on it to make it work for their own particular problem. If in any way at all, that is the way PCR has been remarkable. As the inventor, I like taking credit for all the adaptations, but this is getting a little ridiculous. Far too much has been done with it now to think that anyone, even the intrepid authors assembled here by François, Richard, and me, can really definitively describe it, much less take credit for it. There are too many papers out there, and like technical papers tend to be when there are a lot of them all in one stack and they aren't yours, become so tedious that no one would live through reading them all anyhow! This book hopefully will relieve the reader of some of this burden.

We have tried to find some people who have read a lot of them and have something unusual to offer from their own experience, and in the limited sense at least that the authors selected are the only people who have experienced having chapters in this book, we succeeded. That was a relief.

We have tried to organize the book in a somewhat logical fashion. There are two very distinct things that the polymerase chain reaction does. It generates a particular discrete DNA molecule that was not present to begin with, and it amplifies DNA molecules selectively. The first of these functions includes the search, cut-and-paste, and append operations that support the analogy often made between PCR and a word processor.

The latter, amplifier function is a separate matter. We might have tried to divide the book along those lines, but alas, one never does one without the other, and both seem necessary in almost every application. It is part of the magic of PCR.

So we planned a set of chapters largely devoted to methodology and another set oriented to particular areas where PCR has been applied. There is a lot of overlap. Few strictly methodological people are working with DNA.

A refreshing exception is Carl Wittwer, from, strangely enough, the Pathology Department at Utah Medical School. I would have thought, Chemical Engineering at Cal Tech, but I knew otherwise. If I were you, I would read his paper, or have someone more technically competent explain it. Carl has thought about PCR in a way that very few others have, and his thoughts are crisp and practical. I have always known that a good physicochemical description of PCR would be very useful, but deriving one was over my head. Others have tried but not succeeded.

Gavin Dollinger has written an interesting chapter. He claims that "There are at least three reasons for wanting to tag a commercial object with a submicroscopic label." He fails to remind the reader directly of the scene in *Blade Runner* where Harrison Ford discovers the source of a fish scale he found in the apartment of a "replicant." The Chinese seller of fish who has what looks like a scanning electron microscope on the counter beside her cash register examines the submicron label on the scale and reports "No, Mr. Dekker, this not fish, this reptile; it artificial." PCR machines are cheaper than SEMs and the labels would be smaller. Gavin has written a good chapter, but he missed this key reference, and did not speculate on how long it might have taken to make this identification if the scale had been tagged with DNA. With the advent of scanning probe microscopes this may not be a theatrical issue.

Craig Tuerk describes something called SELEX that is a potential winner in the race to achieve the best rational process for creating high affinity binding agents for anything at all. There is a lot of competition in this area because this capacity is central to not only diagnostics, but therapeutics. The way Craig goes about it is also interesting from the point of view of the evolutionary theorist. He is in the running with Affymax, Selectide, a host of others, and those attempting epitope expression on the surface of lambda phage.

The Editors' Award for the chapter with the most intriguing name goes to Svante Pääbo. He has moved to Munich and he prefers old bones to new ones, preserved brains to currently active ones. He has been on TV a lot. We do not know what will become of him or the nice German lady he is sure to marry someday.

The award for the chapter produced on shortest notice goes to Skip Garner. I was under the impression for many months that Skip was warned that we wanted a chapter from him about the same time as we warned Perucho, McClelland, Heller, and Tullis all of whom, and François, live near La Jolla and are frequent guests in my house. So we do not know whose fault it was, but Skip started late. Skip is one of the smartest people I know. He began his career trying to control nuclear fusion. Somebody pointed him to it, and he said sure, no problem. Then somebody said, how about biology, again, no problem. Skip notices how easy it is to do things, and he is a valuable asset during a weekend in the country. I'm planning to read his chapter.

Manuel Perucho, the man from La Mancha, should get some award for listing over 200 references only two of which bear his name, while including at least one citation to two of the three editors of this book. Manuel, how about Gibbs? Using McClelland's AP-PCR method on his colorectal tumor samples, he is sticking his neck out by looking at his experimental results without fear of what they declare. The article establishes the author's scholastic base in case someone might think him insensitive to convention; it is worth reading and lending to your friends to read.

A couple of years ago I went down to Louisiana to see Jeff Chamberlain get married. Jeff was in Tom Caskey's department at Baylor. In the 1960s Tom and I, and Tom's wife, went to the same high school in Columbia, South Carolina. I did not know Tom then; he left Dreher High School the year I arrived, but I met him about 20 years later at Cold Spring Harbor. It was 1986. I liked him right away. Sound of his voice maybe, but it could have been the quality of his curiosity. Hard to know. It took a couple of years before we diciphered our mutual origins. Our moms lived down the street from each other. Tom's chapter explains, for his mother's sake what he has been doing in Texas all this time. Jerry Lewis might go for it. Howard Hughes did. But Tom's mom is concerned that he has been too long away from home. Tom has this feeling that if something beneficial for public health is possible, then it should be done right away and that his post-docs ought to be doing it. In spite of how ridiculous it might sound it has worked more than it hasn't. They work nights in Houston.

Of the folks in Tom's lab, Jeff Chamberlain was one of my favorites. The wedding was in Lake Charles and the bride was a woman of striking beauty with a name like a boy. Joel. Her dad was an absolutely charming southern doctor who raised horses and peacocks on the edge of a bayou in Lake Charles. Marrying somebody who loves her dad, is a good way to insure that you'll be taken good care of. The sins of the father are often visited on the husband, and if they are few, the husband gets a good deal. The Catholic priest who administered the vows probably was unaware of this and delivered a fairly lengthy social worker kind of wedding chat that could have been entitled "Can This Marriage Be Saved." I got sleepy. A lot of modern clergymen seem to succumb to this temptation, citing statistics about broken homes and such right in front of the bride.

Nonetheless, it seems like Jeff has done alright. He is now in Michigan and is still living happily with Joel. His chapter in this book describes a really satisfying adaptation of PCR in which nine different amplifications are done simultaneously. It is not satisfying for the supply side people who would prefer the one-reaction, one-tube, one-shot-of-polymerase philosophy, but for the people who entertain nightmares concerning all the different genes that really could be checked in a newborn baby or a fetus, and for Jerry Lewis, who is happy to know that those crazy scientists have found a way to detect Duchenne Muscular Dystrophy before the boy is even out of the womb, multiplex PCR is really a neat trick. It was not easy, and Jeff explains how it happened in his chapter.

We all wish him and Joel a happy life together, but more than that, those of us who love this book have to thank Joel and Jeff for bringing Richard Gibbs and me together in Lake Charles that weekend. In fact I was in the back of a cab riding home from one of the more rowdy functions of the wedding with Richard Gibbs, when he slipped in some conversation about a book he had agreed to edit for Birkhäuser and then he flattered me, I think, and asked me to help him, and I was too naive to say no.

What a mistake. Books are no fun. You can never finish your part on schedule and you feel guilty for a long time until you finally do; and then you feel like you could have done a lot better job if you hadn't been rushed. There's no way you are going to come out of it feeling good. Maybe when you see it on your bookshelf. But then you read your chapter.

A few months later back in La Jolla, after letting Richard take advantage of me like that, I had the good sense to flatter François Ferré one night and convince him to become the third editor. In the jargon of the publishers, and by then Richard and I,

François was to be the working editor. And François did work! On the other hand Gibbs is from Australia, where you cannot remember anything much, even if you did make some promises once, because it is so far away by the time you get somewhere it does not matter. And blood is rushing to your head all the time from being upside down.

I didn't work on the book because I was busy.

So the book being actually published is because of François. And he is the person who failed to catch all the mistakes, and Gibbs and I trusted him to find them! I met his father once. He wears good boots, and makes good wine and rules over a bit of France near Poitiers where his family has lived for a long time and that contains a crumbling castle from the thirteenth century. The man would have been in the wrong century in any century. He is a dear, as is his son. What is it about François that would make you want to introduce him as your friend to your fiancé or your mother is hard to describe. It is not that he does not see the need to compromise. That could be a cold trait and François is warm like an orange hearth at Christmas with a big dog lying over it. He is not frantic. He is noble in the very best sense. Read his excellent chapter on quantitation written with his colleagues at Immune Response Corp. All this won't come out in his chapter. He's a professional.

Michael McClelland was the off-duty birdwatcher who cleverly thought up the technique of AP-PCR. That is what he called it, Arbitrarily Primed PCR. It was easy to do but hard to interpret. Michael prefers sitting in his office to standing in his lab and has always been a theoretician. It is well suited to Michael's style and he has exploited it gallantly. The technique has attracted a number of other practitioners and a plethora of new names. The ultimate status of the new names coincides with the likelihood that no one who independently named it did so after they had a fair chance to know that Michael had already. This contradicts the logic of the most plausible supposition that such a technique would not have been discovered twice, but it does not in itself question the honor of the gentlemen who gave it its second and third names. The fourth and fifth names are in some doubt. That AP-PCR just next door to Michael's lab stands for Absolutely Preposterous PCR sets one to thinking that it probably happened only once.

Rick Tullis, who resembles Santa Claus, and whose name has a nice ring to it, has provided us with an intriguing chapter. In his first paragraph, if I follow his logic correctly, I believe he states that "radioactivity" might be included in the category of "nonradioactive detection." I think he might be showing off his ultrapedantic capabilities just to see if anyone notices.

But he taught me how to ski, and how to play Donkey Kong, both at the same UCLA Symposium in Squaw Valley in 1981. The alternative would have been for us to go to the meetings and listen to the news from Michael Bishop, Harold Varmus and the rest of the troops out on the cancer front, and there was a big storm coming in, the slopes were about to be closed, some people were about to be killed in an avalanche, Jennifer Barnett was on her way up from Berkeley right in front of the storm. I was about to get down K-2 after only one week of ski instruction. So what the hell, Tullis is a joy, let him have his pedantry!

At the end of the book there are two chapters on nonscientific issues, one by Ellen Daniell, who followed PCR from Cetus to Roche, and one by me, who flew the coop early but came back for the trial.

Which brings us to the third complaint I mentioned at the start of this Preface. This was the very real complaint of the medical diagnostics community during the years between 1986 and 1992 concerning the restrictive commercial policies of the Cetus Corporation, which were perceived to be limiting the widespread practical applications of PCR. Jim Watson, who has endearingly not established his reputation in the world by remaining silent when his social sensitivities were aroused (see Foreword), put it rather bluntly to me in private during a gathering of genome enthusiasts at UCLA. I agreed with him completely and would quote him directly, but to challenge the reader's imagination will paraphrase his comments into my own sentiments on the subject. The relevance of all this is only historical since Cetus is now out of the picture. In July 1991 Hoffmann-La Roche bought the PCR Division from Cetus and what remained of the old Whale was folded into Chiron. How Hoffmann-La Roche will handle the brokering or commercial development of PCR remains to be seen.

An enlightened commercial policy for licensing the polymerase chain reaction, given an awareness of its almost universal utility in DNA diagnostics and worldwide interest in its immediate applications, would recognize that no lasting purpose could be served by arrangements to restrict access in any way to this new technology.

In my opinion a reasonable percentage of gross revenues from any company interested in applying PCR in the diagnostics marketplace, would have been an acceptable and expected mechanism whereby Cetus could have accomplished the corporate goals of its stockholders. The immediate results of the restrictive policies adopted by Cetus with regard to the use of PCR for detecting infectious diseases were adverse sentiment from within the diagnostics industry, words of advice from Jim Watson, and needless expenditure of research funds by government agencies and private companies to find a substitute for PCR. These funds could have rather supported development of practical PCR applications on which Cetus could have drawn royalties. But then something happened that ironically rewarded Cetus for its contrary position.

In the summer of 1989, in reaction to being denied access to PCR by Cetus, who had promised it all to Roche, DuPont challenged the validity of two Cetus PCR patents, the primary one being US 4,868,202 (Mullis, 1987) in a civil suit in the Northern California District federal court and also filed for patent reexamination with the Office of Patents and Trade Marks. All of this cost Cetus millions of dollars and a lengthy diversion for its managers, lawyers and scientists. But once the lawsuit was settled and the '202 was thoroughly validated, the very high profile of the battle that had been fought in the PTO and federal court had so enhanced the perceived value of PCR that Cetus was able to command a higher price for that fancy little piece of paper than had ever before been payed for a US Patent. Hoffmann-La Roche paid Cetus $300,000,000. DuPont had done Cetus a favor. Our last chapter is my summary of this trial.

Kary Mullis
La Jolla, CA

References

Mullis K, Falcoma F, Scharf S, Snikl R, Horn G, Erlich H (1986): Specific amplification of DNA in vitro: the polymerase chain reaction. *Cold Spring Harbor Symp Quant Biol* 51:260.

Mullis K (1987): US Patent 4,683,202 Process for amplifying nucleic acid sequences.

Mullis K (1990): The unusual origin of the polymerase chain reaction. *Sci Am* 262:56.

Penrose R (1989): *The Emperor's New Mind: Concerning Computers, Minds, and the Laws of Physics.* Oxford: Oxford University Press.

Contents

Contributors

W. French Anderson University of Southern California School of Medicine, NOR 614, Norris Cancer Center, 1441 Eastlake Avenue, Los Angeles, California 90033, USA

Bjorn Andersson Institute for Molecular Genetics, Baylor College of Medicine, One Baylor Plaza, Houston, Texas 77030, USA

Salvatore J. Arrigo Department of Microbiology and Immunology, Medical University of South Carolina, 171 Ashley Avenue, Charleston, South Carolina 29425, USA

Peter Bitterman Division of Pulmonary Medicine, Department of Medicine, University of Minnesota, Box B2, Mayo Memorial Building, 420 Delaware Street SE, Minneapolis, Minnesota 55455, USA

Veronique Boyer The Immune Response Corporation, 5935 Darwin Court, Carlsbad, California 92008, USA

Bruce Budowle Forensic Science Research and Training Center, Laboratory Division, FBI Academy, Quantico, Virginia 22135, USA

Eric Buxton The Immune Response Corporation, 5935 Darwin Court, Carlsbad, California 92008, USA

C. Thomas Caskey Howard Hughes Medical Institute, Baylor College of Medicine, One Baylor Plaza, Houston, Texas 77030, USA

Joel R. Chamberlain Program in Cellular and Molecular Biology, University of Michigan Medical School, Ann Arbor, Michigan 48109, USA

Jeffrey S. Chamberlain Department of Human Genetics, Center for Genome Technology and Genetic Disease, University of Michigan Medical School, Ann Arbor, Michigan 48109, USA

D. Stephen Charnock-Jones Department of Obstetrics and Gynecology, University of Cambridge, The Rosie Maternity Hospital, Hills Road, Cambridge CB2 2SW, United Kingdom

Jamel Chelly ICRF Human Genetics Laboratory, Institute of Molecular Medicine, John Radcliffe Hospital, Headington, Oxford OX3 9DU, United Kingdom

Michael L. Cleary Laboratory of Experimental Oncology, Department of Pathology, Stanford University School of Medicine, Stanford, California 94305, USA

Donald M. Coen Department of Biological Chemistry and Molecular Pharmacology, Harvard Medical School, 250 Longwood Avenue, Boston, Massachusetts 02115, USA

Catherine T. Comey Forensic Research and Training Center, Laboratory Division, FBI Academy, Quantico, Virginia 22135, USA

Luc d'Auriol CNRS UPR 41, Centre Hayem Hôpital Saint Louis, 75010 Paris, France

Ellen Daniell Director of Licensing, Roche Molecular Systems, Inc., 1145 Atlantic Avenue, Alameda, California 94501, USA

Gavin Dollinger Chiron Corporation, 4560 Horton Street, Emeryville, California 94608-2916, USA

Janet Embretson Department of Microbiology, University of Minnesota, Box 196, 1460 Mayo Memorial Building, 420 Delaware Street, SE, Minneapolis, Minnesota 55455-0312, USA

François Ferré The Immune Response Corporation, 5935 Darwin Court, Carlsbad, California 92008, USA

Michael A. Frohman Department of Pharmacology, School of Medicine, SUNY at Stony Brook, Stony Brook, New York 11794-8651, USA

H.R. Garner General Atomics Corporation, P.O. Box 85608, San Diego, California 92186-9784, USA

Richard A. Gibbs Institute for Molecular Genetics, Baylor College of Medicine, One Baylor Plaza, Houston, Texas 77030, USA

Larry Gold Department of Molecular, Cellular, and Developmental Biology, University of Colorado, Boulder, Colorado 80309, USA, and Nexagen, Inc., 2860 Wilderness Place, Suite 200, Boulder, Colorado 80301, USA

Stacey Griffin The Immune Response Corporation, 5935 Darwin Court, Carlsbad, California 92008, USA

Ashley T. Haase Department of Microbiology, University of Minnesota, 1460 Mayo Memorial Building, 420 Delaware Street, SE, Minneapolis, Minnesota 55455-0312, USA

Oliva Handt Zoological Institute, University of Munich, Postfach 20 21 36, D-80021 Munich, Germany

Kenshi Hayashi Division of Genome Analysis, Institute of Genetic Information, Kyushu University, Maidashi 3-1-1, Higashi-Ku, Fukuoka 812, Japan

Michael J. Heller Nanotronics, Inc., 3347 Industrial Court, San Diego, California 92121, USA

Gerald Z. Hertz Department of Molecular, Cellular, and Developmental Biology, University of Colorado, Boulder, Colorado 80309, USA

Manfred N. Hochmeister Department of Forensic Medicine, Institut für Rechtsmedizin, University of Bern, Bern, Switzerland

Rhonda J. Honeycutt California Institute of Biological Research, 11099 North Torrey Pines Road, Suite 300, La Jolla, California 92037, USA

Matthias Höss Zoological Institute, University of Munich, Postfach 20 21 36, D-80021 Munich, Germany

Stephen P. Hunger Laboratory of Experimental Oncology, Department of Pathology, Stanford University School of Medicine, Stanford, California 94305, USA

Edward Jablonski Syngene, Inc., 3252 Holiday Court, La Jolla, California 92037, USA

Axel Kahn Laboratorie de Recherches en Génétique et Pathologie Moléculaire, Unité 129 INSERM, Institut Cochin de Génétique Moléculaire, 24 rue du Faubourg St. Jacques, 75014 Paris, France

Sheela MacDougal-Waugh Nexagen, Inc., 2860 Wilderness Place, Suite 200, Boulder, Colorado 80301, USA

Annie Marchese The Immune Response Corporation, 5935 Darwin Court, Carlsbad, California 92008, USA

W. John Martin Department of Pathology, University of Southern California, Box 463, 1200 North State Street, Los Angeles, California 90033, USA

Michael McClelland California Institute of Biological Research, 11099 North Torrey Pines Road, La Jolla, California 92037, USA

Sherrol H. McDonough Gen-Probe, Inc., 9880 Campus Point Drive, San Diego, California 92121, USA

Didier Montarras Unité de Biochimie, Institut Pasteur, 25 rue du Roux, 75015 Paris, France

Richard A. Morgan Clinical Gene Therapy Branch, National Center for Human Genome Research, 9000 Rockville Pike, Building 49, Room 2676, Bethesda, Maryland 20892, USA. Former Affiliation: Molecular Hematology Branch, National Heart, Lung, and Blood Institute, National Institutes of Health, Building 10, Room 7D-18, Bethesda Maryland 20892, USA

Kary B. Mullis La Jolla, California 92037, USA

Norman C. Nelson Gen-Probe, Inc., 9880 Campus Point Drive, San Diego, California 92121, USA

Christian C. Oste Bioanalytical Systems Group, Beckman Instruments, Inc., P.O. Box 2500, 2500 Harbor Boulevard, Fullerton, California 92634-3100, USA

Svante Pääbo Zoological Institute, University of Munich, Postfach 20 21 36, D-80021 Munich, Germany

Manuel Perucho California Institute of Biological Research, 11099 North Torrey Pines Road, Suite 300, La Jolla, California 92037, USA

Patrick Pezzoli The Immune Response Corporation, 5935 Darwin Court, Carlsbad, California 92008, USA

Christian Pinset Unité de Biochimie, Institut Pasteur, 25 rue du Roux, 75015 Paris, France

Matthias Platzer Max-Dulbrück-Centre for Molecular Medicine (MDC), Robert-Rössle-Straße 10, 13125 Berlin-Buch, Germany

Gudrun B. Reed Associated Regional and University Pathologists, 500 Chipeta Way, Salt Lake City, Utah 84108, USA

Ernest Retzel Department of Microbiology, University of Minnesota, 1460 Mayo Memorial Building, 420 Delaware Street, SE, Minneapolis, Minnesota 55455-0312, USA

Kirk M. Ririe Idaho Technology, 149 Chestnut Street, Idaho Falls, Idaho 83402, USA

James M. Robertson Applied Biosystems Division, Perkin-Elmer Corporation, 850 Lincoln Centre Drive, Foster City, California 94404, USA

André Rosenthal Institute of Molecular Biotechnology, Department of Genome Analysis, P.O. Box 100813, 07708 Jena, Germany

Belinda J.F. Rossiter Institute for Molecular Genetics, Baylor College of Medicine, One Baylor Plaza, Houston, Texas 77030, USA

Antti Sajantila National Public Health Institute, Department of Forensic Medicine, University of Helsinki, Helsinki, Finland

Darryl Shibata LAC/USC Medical Center, 1200 North State Street, Room 2428, Los Angeles, California 90033, USA

François Sigaux Laboratoire d'Hematologie Moléculaire, Centre Hayem Hôpital Saint Louis, Paris, France

Bruno W.S. Sobral California Institute of Biological Research, 11099 North Torrey Pines Road, Suite 300, La Jolla, California 92037, USA

Steve S. Sommer Department of Biochemistry and Molecular Biology, Guggenheim 15, Mayo Clinic/Foundation, Rochester, Minnesota 55905, USA

Dominic G. Spinella The Immune Response Corporation, 5935 Darwin Court, Carlsbad, California, 92008, USA. Current Affiliation: Cytogen Corporation, 307 College Road East, CN 5307, Princeton, New Jersey 08540-5309, USA

Katherine Staskus Department of Microbiology, University of Minnesota, 1460 Mayo Memorial Building, 420 Delaware Street, SE, Minneapolis, Minnesota 55455-0312, USA

Eugene Tu Nanotronics, Inc., 3347 Industrial Court, Suite A, San Diego, California 92121, USA

Craig Tuerk 327E Lappin Hall, Morehead State University, Morehead Kentucky 40351, USA

Richard H. Tullis Synthetic Genetics, Inc., 10455 Roselle Street, San Diego, California 92121, USA

Erica L. Vielhaber Department of Biochemistry and Molecular Biology, Guggenheim 15, Mayo Clinic/Foundation, Rochester, Minnesota 55905, USA

James D. Watson Cold Spring Harbor Laboratory, Box 100, Cold Spring Harbor, New York 11724, USA

John Welsh California Institute of Biological Research, 11099 North Torrey Pines Road, La Jolla, California 92037, USA

Carl T. Wittwer Department of Pathology, School of Medicine, University of Utah, 50 North Medical Drive, Salt Lake City, Utah 84132, USA

PART ONE
Methodology

SECTION I
Basic Methodology

1

Manipulation of DNA by PCR

Kenshi Hayashi

Introduction

The advent of polymerase chain reaction (PCR) has greatly accelerated the progress of studies on the genomic structure of various organisms, and any region in even highly complex genomes can be specifically amplified in a few hours by the technique, if the flanking nucleotide sequences are known (Saiki et al., 1988). Virtually any DNA sequence can also be engineered by "copying and pasting" with PCR as a replacement for conventional recombinant DNA technology where DNA is manipulated by "cutting and pasting" using restriction endonucleases and ligase (Frohman and Martin, 1989). PCR therefore overcomes problems associated with the often limited availability of sites for the restriction endonucleases. PCR can be started from even a single molecule of DNA, and as a consequence many conventional analytical fractionation techniques are now effectively many times more sensitive than before.

This chapter contains a brief review of some basic PCR principles and a detailed examination of some recently developed PCR-based techniques.

General Considerations

Flexibility of Primer Design

The most common use of PCR is for selective amplification of a unique region, from a highly complex template such as mammalian genomic DNA. The specificity of amplification depends on the design of primer sequences. A range of 20–24 nucleotide-long primers is most frequently used because this length is usually selective enough to specify a single site in a genome of high complexity, such as the human genome. However, longer primers and annealing at a higher temperature can make PCR amplification more selective. The melting temperature (T_m) of 40mer oligonucleotide is estimated to be 15°C higher than that of 20mer oligonucleotide of similar base composition (Sambrook et al., 1989). Thus, using 40–45mer primers and annealing at 72°C, an optimal temperature for chain elongation by the *Taq* DNA polymerase, the PCR should be the most selective under generally employed buffer conditions, as far as the chain length of primers is concerned.

Various computer software programs, both commercial and public, are currently available

The Polymerase Chain Reaction
K.B. Mullis, F. Ferré, R.A. Gibbs, editors
© 1994 Birkhäuser Boston

for selecting primer sequences in defined regions. While these programs can often be convenient and helpful, without complete knowledge of the entire sequence of the genome being studied, even the best program is not perfect.

In a reaction that lacks a perfectly matched primer–template combination, amplification beginning from the site that contains some mismatch yields products with the terminal sequences replaced by those of the primers. This flexibility of primer design has greatly increased the versatility of PCR.

Fidelity of Amplification

DNA polymerase makes errors at a low but finite rate that varies depending on the enzyme, condition of the reaction, and the sequence (Eckert and Kunkel, 1991). For example, the errors produced by *Taq* DNA polymerase are primarily single-base substitutions. The rate can be higher than 10^{-3} per nucleotide at high Mg^{2+} and high nucleotide concentrations, and less than 10^{-6} per nucleotide under other conditions. Other enzymes with proof reading activity, such as *Vent* polymerase, are believed to produce errors much less frequently than the *Taq* DNA polymerase (Eckert and Kunkel, 1991).

During the PCR, amplification products serve as templates for the subsequent cycles. Therefore, sequence changes caused by errors of the DNA polymerase are "inherited." Since there is no selection based on the functional significance of sequence information, these sequence changes can accumulate. Consequently, a significant percentage of the amplified fragments may carry "mutations."

The percentage of fragments with a correct sequence after PCR can be mathematically estimated, assuming a random distribution of errors, and that both mutated and correct sequences are amplified at the same efficiency (Krawczak et al., 1989; Hayashi, 1991). If amplification proceeds with an efficiency of k, then the amount of old (O, present at the beginning of the cycle) and new (N, synthesized during the cycle) strands at the end of each cycle have the following relationship:

$$O = 1/(k + 1)$$
$$N = k/(k + 1)$$
$$0 < k < 1$$

The probability of producing fragments without error (p) in one cycle of amplification is given by the probability of no-hit in a Poisson distribution.

$$p = \exp(-mL)$$

where m is the error rate of the polymerase per nucleotide and L is length of amplification unit in nucleotides.

Only newly synthesized strands can have new mutations. The fraction of strands having a correct sequence at the end of the first cycle, f, is given as

$$f = O + pN$$
$$= [1 + k \exp(-mL)]/(k + 1)$$

Therefore, the fraction of strands with a correct sequence after n cycles, $F(n)$, can be estimated by

$$F(n) = f^n = [1 + k \exp(-mL)]^n/(k + 1)^n$$

This estimate may not be appropriate if the reaction is initiated from a very small amount of DNA (e.g., less than 10^3 molecules), when the timing of occurrence of the first mutation can significantly alter the error rate. However, this situation is unusual since it is equivalent to less than 3 ng of human genomic DNA, or less than 0.01 pg of 10-kb plasmid DNA.

Table 1.1 shows the fractions of strands carrying correct sequences after 20 and 30 ampli-

TABLE 1.1. Fraction of fragments having correct sequences remaining after the PCR.[a]

	$m = 10^{-4}$		$m = 10^{-5}$	
kb	20 cycles	30 cycles	20 cycles	30 cycles
0.1	0.91	0.87	0.99	0.98
0.2	0.83	0.75	0.98	0.97
0.5	0.63	0.50	0.95	0.93
1.0	0.40	0.25	0.91	0.87
2.0	0.17	0.07	0.83	0.75
4.0	0.03	0.01	0.69	0.57

[a]Calculated from the equation in text, assuming that the efficiency of amplification (k) is 0.9. m is the error rate of the DNA polymerase per nucleotide.

fication cycles, as estimated by the previous equation. In this calculation, error rates of the polymerase are assumed to be 10^{-4} and 10^{-5} per nucleotide, respectively.

When the errors during PCR are distributed evenly throughout the fragment, no particular mutated sequence constitutes a major sub-population. In this case the predominant species at each nucleotide position in the product is that of the initial sequence, and direct sequencing of the product as a mixture is an appropriate method for determining the sequence in the initial DNA segments (Pääbo and Wilson, 1988). The situation is different when PCR products are used as cloning sub-strates. Each clone originates from a single molecule in the PCR product mixture, and therefore may represent errors occurring during the amplification process.

Although mutation sites are usually distributed throughout the amplified fragments (except in the primer regions), hot and cold spots of base substitutions exist that apparently depend on sequence contexts. The mechanism underlying this observation is not understood (Eckert and Kunkel, 1991).

Simple repeats, such as homopolymeric stretches and dinucleotide repeats, are particularly significant sites of PCR variation, which may be due to slippage of the polymerase. These phenomena appear common to all polymerases, and can be problematic, especially during genotype analysis of length polymorphisms of these repeats. CA repeats are used extensively as polymorphic DNA markers in human genome mapping, because they are abundant in the genome (Stallings et al., 1991), highly polymorphic in their number of repeats, and can be easily analyzed by PCR (Weber and May, 1989). When PCR products of fragments containing this repeat are separated by polyacrylamide gel electrophoresis, ladders of bands are usually observed, thus revealing the slippage. This is problematic when the objective is to distinguish between a homozygote and a heterozygote and the alleles differ by only a single repeat unit.

Sequence Manipulation

Primers with 5'-Tags

Addition of extraneous nucleotides at the 5'-end of a primer does not usually interfere with the process of primer–template annealing. Thus, miscellaneous sequences can be added to PCR primers for purposes including addition of restriction sites for subsequent cloning, as sequences for primers in secondary PCR, and as promoter sequences for *in vitro* transcription from PCR products by RNA polymerases (Higuchi, 1989). By using primers with terminal overlaps, two or more PCR products can also be assembled in any desired order into one contiguous stretch by secondary PCR (Higuchi et al., 1988). This "copy and paste" capability of PCR has revolutionized construction of chimeric DNA sequences because the joining sites are no longer dependent on the availability of the sites of restriction enzymes.

Degenerate Primer

The use of degenerate primers in PCR is a powerful method for isolating cDNA clones in which only limited information on the amino acid sequences of the coded proteins is available (Lee et al., 1988). Primers with nucleotide sequences deduced from reverse translation of the amino acid sequences are used to amplify the target region by the PCR of reverse-transcript of an mRNA mixture. Since unique primer sequences cannot be deduced because of degeneracy of genetic code, a mixture of oligonucleotides that is compatible with all possible codons is used. The PCR product usually consists of the target sequence and additional nonspecific products. After appropriate enrichment procedures, e.g., length selection by gel electrophoresis, the fragments are rescued by subcloning. The clone carrying the proper fragment, which also codes for the expected amino acid sequence, is selected as a probe for screening a cDNA library by conventional hybridization methods.

Inverse PCR, Vectorette PCR

The PCR, in its original form, requires prior knowledge of the primer sequences that bracket the target region to be amplified. This means that the amplification unit cannot be extended beyond the region of known sequences. However, there are now methods available to amplify unknown sequences adjacent to the region of a known sequence. One strategy is self-circularization. By this procedure, the known (self)-sequence is brought to the distal end of the adjacent unknown sequence. The sandwiched unknown region can then be amplified by PCR using a pair of primers that extends divergently from the known region, hence the term "inverse PCR" (Ochman et al., 1988; Triglia et al., 1988; Silver and Keerikatte, 1989). Another strategy is to attach a sequence tag, either by ligation of double-stranded oligonucleotides (Mueller and Wald, 1989) or tailing by terminal transferase (Frohman et al., 1988; Loh et al., 1989; Ohara et al., 1989) to a fragment with an unknown region adjacent to a known region. The unknown region is amplified by PCR between the known and the tag, making the reaction hemispecific. In some cases, the tag contains a region of nonhomology to avoid amplification between the two tags (vectorette PCR) (Arnold and Hodgson, 1991). These procedures have been used to clone 5'-ends of ϵDNA, chromosomal regions adjacent to insertion sites of retrovirus (Silver and Keerikatte, 1989), and for obtaining the ends of inserts of yeast artificial chromosomes (Ochman et al., 1989).

Primer Pairs That Amplify Everything

A mixture of DNA segments flanked by a pair of primer sequences will be amplified indiscriminately by PCR. If a selective pressure for a particular sequence subset is applied and PCR is repeated, the amplification product will be enriched with the subset. The selected sequence can be isolated by simply repeating this amplification–selection cycle. The products can then be characterized to determine which sequence the selective pressure is for.

The practicality of this strategy has been demonstrated in studies of recognition sequences of several DNA-binding nuclear proteins (Kinzler and Vogelstein, 1989; Blackwell and Weintraub, 1990; Bickmore et al., 1992). In these studies, DNA fragments with extensive divergence in the middle were used in cycles that included selection by gel retardation, followed by PCR amplification. These DNAs were either chemically synthesized or PCR amplified from terminal "catch" primer sequences ligated to fragments of total genome DNA. The effectiveness of this selection–amplification cycle for enrichment of particular sequences from mixture of random sequences is mathematically considered in more general terms (Irvine et al., 1991; also see Chapter 20 of this book).

Directed Mutagenesis

Using primers with mismatch, mutations that include base substitutions, insertions, and deletions can be introduced at the primer regions in the amplified products (Higuchi, 1989). With sufficiently long primers, multiple sites can be mutagenized in one amplification reaction (Clackson et al., 1991). The power of this directed mutagenesis by PCR is perhaps best highlighted in the construction of humanized murine monoclonal antibody for use as a cancer therapeutic agent (Carter et al., 1992), or construction of combinatorial antibody libraries for *in vitro* selection of antibodies (Huse et al., 1989).

Nondirected Mutagenesis

Errors produced by *Taq* DNA polymerase are base substitutions, while insertions/deletions are rare (Eckert and Kunkel, 1991). If PCR is performed for a sufficient number of cycles, the frequency of accumulated base substitutions becomes significant. Thus, PCR can be used to produce nondirected mutations, *in vitro*. Theoretically, this can be achieved simply by repeating PCR cycles and, when the amplification efficiency reaches a plateau, diluting and starting PCR again using the same set of primers. In practice, however, it is preferable to conduct PCR in conditions where nucleotide misincorporation is high, so that fewer cycles of the amplification reaction are required until accumulated mutations reach the desired level. Leung et al. (1989) studied conditions of PCR suitable for *in vitro* mutagenesis, showing that in the presence of Mn^{2+} ion and using an unbalanced nucleotide concentration, mutation frequencies as high as 2% can be reached after 25 cycles of PCR, without significant reduction in the efficiency of the amplification. One limitation of *in vitro* mutagenesis by PCR is that the induced mutations are not random. Previous reports have indicated that misincorporation of nucleotides by *Taq* DNA polymerase is sequence dependent, while the spectrum of error may differ depending on the conditions of the amplification reaction. Therefore, the library of mutated sequences produced by PCR may inadequately represent certain types of mutations.

Genome Structure Analysis

AP-PCR

A useful application of PCR in genomic studies is arbitrary primer PCR (AP-PCR) (Welsh and McClelland, 1990; also see Chapter 25 of this book). In this technique, many sites in genomic DNA are simultaneously amplified by using short primers that have arbitrary sequences, and performing the PCR under relaxed conditions. Amplification with a single primer is feasible, because the stringency of annealing is so reduced that the same primer can start chain elongation from multiple sites in the template DNA. In the second cycle of PCR, a subset of the elongation products in the first cycle can serve as templates of the following cycles because it has the second sites for primer annealing within the distance suitable for PCR amplification. Products are usually analyzed by denaturing polyacrylamide electrophoresis, and length polymorphisms in multiple sites can be detected by the presence or absence of bands at various positions of gel migration follows electrophoresis.

This method of detection of sequence differences effectively allows polymorphisms to be interpreted as a two-allele system (that is, presence or absence of a band per locus), and the method is suited for one general problem of mapping complex genomes (Welsh et al., 1991). Linkage maps of laboratory animals are usually constructed by analyzing segregation patterns of polymorphisms in the crosses of two strains, and a two-allele system is sufficient for these experiments. However, AP-PCR may be of limited use in linkage mapping of the human genome, in which pedigree analysis is the only available method. This is because multiallelic loci are much more informative than two allelic loci in pedigree analysis, and, so, the detection techniques that can identify multiple alleles of the same locus are more advantageous.

Alu-PCR

Alu repeats are a family of primate-specific repetitive sequences that appear about 500,000 times throughout the human genome. With the proper choice of primers complementary to the consensus sequence of this repeat, human sequences between *Alu*s can be specifically amplified from a background of DNAs of other species (Nelson et al., 1989; Ledbetter and Nelson, 1991). This method is frequently used for retrieval of human sequences from DNA of human–rodent hybrid cells, or from DNA of yeast cells that carry a yeast artificial chromosome (YAC) that contains an insert of human origin.

PCR-SSCP

Of the several PCR-based techniques for detecting mutations, PCR-SSCP analysis is perhaps the easiest to perform and one of the most sensitive (Orita et al., 1989; Hayashi, 1992). This technique has been widely used to detect mutations in genes responsible for various hereditary diseases, and somatic mutations of oncogenes or tumor-suppressor genes in cancer tissues, as well as polymorphisms.

In this analysis, the target sequence is amplified and labeled simultaneously by using primers or nucleotides that have been labeled with radioactivity. The amplified product is then heated to dissociate the strands and subjected to nondenaturing polyacrylamide gel electrophoresis. Mutations are detected as shifts in the mobility of the bands of separated single strands in the autoradiogram. Conformational change of the single-stranded DNA caused by mutation seems to be responsible for the mobility shift, hence the name "single-strand conformation polymorphism" (SSCP) analysis. PCR-SSCP enables detection of any type of mutation, including single base substitution, which occurs anywhere in target sequences up to several hundred nucleotides long.

Only a small amount of DNA is required for SSCP analysis if the product is labeled with radioactivity. An amplification reaction in 5 μl with limited concentrations of primers or nucleotides usually yields sufficient product for hundreds of electrophoretic runs. Convenient and economical PCR protocols for SSCP analysis have been reported (Mashiyama et al., 1990).

Figure 1.1 shows an example of PCR-SSCP analysis in which polymorphism within an *Alu* repetitive element was detected for the purpose of linkage mapping of human genome.

The ability of PCR-SSCP to detect mutations depends on how the mutation affects folding of the molecule, and how the folding affects electrophoretic mobility. No theory is currently available to predict these factors. Therefore, theoretical estimation of sensitivity of PCR-SSCP analysis is difficult. Empirical estimation of the sensitivity is also difficult, because the sensitivity obviously depends on the sequence context of the examined fragment, and available data are still too limited to enable prediction of sensitivity in all possible sequence contexts. However, based on the limited experience of our group and others, PCR-SSCP is able to detect more than 90% of all single base substitutions in 200-nucleotide fragments, and more than 80% in 400-nucleotide fragments (Gaidano et al., 1991; Hayashi, 1992).

PCR-SSCP is less sensitive for longer fragments. Therefore, long sequences should be divided into shorter segments before being analyzed by SSCP. This can be done either by separately amplifying the target sequence in overlapping subfragments, or by amplifying the entire fragments in one unit and then digesting them with suitable restriction enzymes. However, most exons in mammalian genomes are shorter than 300 nucleotides, and these can be directly analyzed by PCR-SSCP using intron primers without additional procedures.

Constant gel temperature during electrophoresis is important in obtaining reproducible results in SSCP analysis. Therefore, efficient release of heat using a thin gel (e.g., 0.3 mm) and vigorous air-cooling or cooling with a water-jacket is strongly recommended. Properties of the gel and the presence of additives in the solvent also affect the separation. A reduced concentration of cross-linker (N, N'-methylene bisacrylamide) relative to that of acrylamide (1:49 or 1:99) always improves separation. Addition of low concentrations of glycerol in gel is also generally beneficial (Orita et al., 1989).

Though optimal conditions for separation of mutations differ depending on the sequence context of the target, electrophoresis at 4 to 10°C in gel without glycerol usually results in a good separation. Addition of 5–10% glycerol to the gel and electrophoresis at 20–25°C will also give satisfactory results. It should be emphasized, however, that some mutations can be detected only under specific conditions (e.g., at 25°C without glycerol), although such mutations seem rare.

Although a growing amount of evidence suggests that PCR-SSCP is highly sensitive, false negative results cannot be excluded and some mutations may not be detected under the chosen conditions of electrophoresis. Therefore, the absence of mutation cannot be proven by this technique. This is especially important when applying PCR-SSCP for a clinical test. For example, suppose that a parent is a carrier of a detectable mutation of a gene for a hereditary disease. If a child shows a normal pattern in PCR-SSCP analysis of the gene, inheritance of the affected allele of the parent is excluded, but the child can still be a carrier of a new mutation.

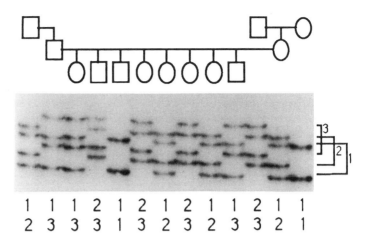

FIGURE 1.1. Polymorphism of an *Alu* repeat detected by PCR-SSCP. An anonymous *Alu* repetitive element was amplified using bracketing single copy sequences as primers and analyzed by SSCP (Iizuka et al., 1992). DNAs of a three generation family of CEPH were examined. Genotypes of the three alleles, 1 to 3, are indicated at the bottom.

Since fragments having different sequences are separated by SSCP analysis, a mutated allele can be isolated and reamplified for further analysis including sequence determination to define the mutation (Suzuki et al., 1991). Thus, mutations in cells that constitute only a small portion of the material examined can be detected and unambiguously characterized at the sequence level.

Development of nonradioactive PCR-SSCP analysis is important for its clinical or forensic applications. Several groups have reported detection of bands in SSCP gel by silver staining (Ainsworth et al., 1991). Small gels (5–6 cm long) were used in these studies because large gels are inconvenient in staining–destaining procedures. Several known mutations in genes responsible for hereditary diseases were detectable by this staining method, thus demonstrating its diagnostic value. However, reduced sensitivity is inevitable with smaller gels, and this method may not be suitable for detection of unidentified mutations.

Another nonradioactive PCR-SSCP method involves the use of fluorescein-labeled primers and detection of the bands in the gel by fluorescence (Makino et al., 1992). This method requires an automated DNA sequencer, and therefore may not be suitable for use in small laboratories. However, it does have the advantage that electrophoresis can be carried out under strictly controlled conditions, and data can be entered directly into a computer.

Denaturing Gradient Gel Electrophoresis

In denaturing gradient gel electrophoresis (DGGE), the double-stranded DNA is subjected to electrophoresis in gel that has an increasing concentration of denaturant along the length of the gel (Fischer and Lerman, 1980). The fragment melts while traveling through the gel. The melting proceeds in segments, called melting domains, because of the cooperative nature of the denaturation of the double-stranded DNA (Fischer and Lerman, 1983). When a domain melts, the fragment assumes a branched structure that causes significant retardation of movement by an unknown mechanism. Thus, the position of the fragment in the gel after a certain time of electrophoresis is determined by the history of melting of the fragment that is altered if the sequence is different.

The principle of separation in DGGE is such that sequence changes in the melting domain of highest stability cannot be detected by the technique, because the fragment no longer has a branched structure when the last domain melts. If, however, a stretch of sequence that serves as an extremely stable domain is attached to one side of the fragment, then mutations at any sites within certain types of sequence context can be detected by DGGE (Meyers et al., 1985). This extra sequence of extremely high stability can be conveniently attached to the target sequence of PCR by using one primer that has 35–40 nucleotides of an artificial GC-rich sequence (GC-clamp) extending at its 5'-end.

With the use of "GC-clamp," DGGE may be able to detect nearly all possible mutations in any given sequences (Sheffield et al., 1989). DGGE, however, requires special apparatus for electrophoresis because the gel must be maintained at a high temperature. Also, the need to synthesize longer primers can make the GC-clamp method costly.

RNase Mismatch and Related Techniques

In RNase mismatch cleavage and related techniques, the region of DNA to be examined is hybridized with a radioactively labeled RNA that has wild type or reference sequence. The resultant RNA–DNA hybrid is then treated with RNase. The RNA cannot properly base pair at the site of mutation, and is therefore cut by the enzyme. Analysis by gel electrophoresis of the digest and autoradiography reveals the position of the mismatch (Winter et al., 1985). However, certain mismatches in the DNA:RNA duplex are known to resist RNase digestion and cannot be detected by this technique. Chemical modification of unpaired nucleotide at the site of mutation in the heteroduplex and subsequent cleavage of the main chain by another chemical reaction have been developed as a related technique (Cotton et al., 1988). The principles underlying these methods are well understood, so that they may be modified to detect virtually all mutated sequences. Some possible disadvantages of these methods are that many biochemical steps are involved and therefore some skill is required.

Heteroduplex Gel Electrophoresis

Double-stranded DNA has a rod-like structure, the rigidity of which is maintained mainly by the stacking of paired bases along the chain. A mismatch somewhere in the chain disturbs this stack, and probably causes changes in the three-dimensional structure. A duplex carrying a mismatch, such as heteroduplex between wild type and mutated DNA fragments, and a perfectly base-paired duplex behave differently in polyacrylamide gel electrophoresis because of this structural difference (White et al., 1992). Many mutations in the p53 gene have been detected by this technique. The overall procedure is simple and suited for nonradioactive detection. However, the available data are too limited to assess its sensitivity.

Allele-Specific Oligonucleotide (ASO) Hybridization

In this technique, an oligonucleotide probe, usually radioactively labeled, is hybridized to test DNA under conditions that allow the probe to remain attached to a perfectly matched sequence, but to dissociate from a sequence with a mismatch (Wallace et al., 1981). If the fragment is short, the helix-destabilizing effect of a mismatch can be sufficiently large so that mismatched sequences can be distinguished from the perfectly matched under certain hybridizing/washing conditions. Various modifications of this method have reportedly been used with a large number of samples (e.g., Saiki et al., 1989). This method detects mutations in limited lengths of regions, approximately 20 nucleotides, and is therefore suitable for identification of known sequence differences in a fixed position in the genome, such as *RAS* mutations in cancer cells or HLA typing (van Mansfeld et al., 1992).

Allele-Specific PCR

All known DNA polymerases elongate the chains from base-paired ends, and mismatch at the 3'-end is unfavored for this elongation reaction. Allele-specific PCR uses this phenomenon to detect mutations by employing, as PCR primers, oligonucleotides that either do or do not match specific mutations at their 3'-ends (Wu et al., 1989). However, *Taq* DNA polymerase has been found to initiate chain elongation even from 3'-unpaired primers, at least under some conditions (Kwok et al., 1990). Selective amplification can be achieved in PCR using low concentrations of deoxynucleotides (as low as a few micromolar) and limiting the numbers of thermal cycles. Alleles of several polymorphic loci could be distinguished by these selective conditions in the second amplification of nested PCR starting from single sperm DNA (Li et al., 1990).

Restriction Fragment Length Polymorphism (RFLP)

By digesting products of PCR with appropriate restriction enzymes and analyzing by agarose gel electrophoresis, some mutations resided in the recognition sequences of the enzymes can be detected as RFLP in the ethidium bromide-stained gel. Mutations that can be detected by this method are limited, even though the numbers can be increased by using mismatched primers in PCR (Jiang et al., 1989). However, this method is widely used for the detection of various known mutations because obtained results are clear-cut, and radioactivity is not required.

Mutation-enriched PCR amplification is another important improvement in sensitive mutation detection using cleavage by restriction enzymes. In this method, the target sequence is first amplified using a mismatch primer that generates a restriction enzyme recognition site only in combination with the wild-type sequence. The PCR product is then digested by the restriction enzyme and reamplified using the same primers. The fragment is produced from the mutant sequence in the second PCR, but not from the wild-type sequence because it is digested. As a result, mutated sequences can be enriched even if they constitute a small fraction. A *RAS* mutation occurring in 1 per 103 cells can be detected by this method (Chen and Viola, 1991).

Acknowledgments. Some data presented derive from works using CEPH family DNA. This work was supported by a Grant-in-Aid for the Human Genome Project from the Ministry of Education, Science and Culture, and a grant from the Special Coordination Fund of the Science and Technology Agency, Japan.

References

Ainsworth PJ, Surh LC, Coulter-Mackie MB (1991): Diagnostic single strand conformational polymorphism, (SSCP): A simple non-radioisotopic method as applied to a Tay-Sachs B1 variant. *Nucl Acids Res* 19:405–406.

Arnold C, Hodgson IJ (1991): Vectorette PCR: A novel approach to genomic walking. *PCR Meth Appl* 1:39–42.

Bickmore WA, Oghene K, Little MH, Seawright A, van Heynigen V, Hastie ND (1992): Modulation of DNA binding specificity by alternative splicing of the Wilms Tumor wt1 gene transcript. *Science* 257:235–237.

Blackwell TK, Weintraub H (1990): Differences and similarities in DNA-binding preferences of MyoD and E2A protein complexes revealed by binding site selection. *Science* 250:1104–1110.

Carter P, Presta L, Gorman CM, Ridgway JBB, Henner D, Wong WLT, Rowland AM, Kotts C, Carver ME, Shepard HM (1992): Humanization of an anti-p185[HER2] antibody for human cancer therapy. *Proc Natl Acad Sci USA* 89:4285–4289.

Chen J, Viola MV (1991): A method to detect ras mutations in small subpopulations of cells. *Anal Biochem* 195:51–56.

Clackson T, Gussow D, Jones PT (1991): General applications of PCR to gene cloning and manipulation, In: *Polymerase Chain Reaction I: A Practical Approach.* McPherson MJ, Quirke P, Taylor GR, eds. Oxford: IRL Press.

Cotton RGH, Rodrigues NR, Campbell RD (1988): Reactivity of cytosine and thymine in single-base-pair mismatches with hydroxylamine and osmium tetroxide and its application to the study of mutations. *Proc Natl Acad Sci USA* 85:4397–4401.

Eckert KA, Kunkel TA (1991): The fidelity of DNA polymerase and the polymerases used in the PCR. In: *Polymerase Chain Reaction I: A Practical Approach.* McPherson MJ, Quirke P, Taylor GR, eds. Oxford: IRL Press.

Fischer SC, Lerman LS (1980): Separation of random fragments of DNA according to properties of their sequences. *Proc Natl Acad Sci USA* 77:4420–4424.

Fischer SC, Lerman LS (1983): DNA fragments differing by single base-pair substitutions are separated in denaturing gradient gels: Correspondence with melting theory. *Proc Natl Acad Sci USA* 80:1579–1583.

Frohman MA, Martin GR (1989): Cut, paste and save: New approaches to altering specific genes in mice. *Cell* 56:145–147.

Frohman MA, Dush MK, Martin GR (1988): Rapid production of full-length cDNAs from rare transcripts: Amplification using a single gene-specific oligonucleotide primers. *Proc Natl Acad Sci USA* 85:8998–9002.

Gaidano G, Ballerini P, Gong JZ, Inghirami G, Neri A, Newcomb EW, Magrath IT, Knowles DM, Dalla-Favera R (1991): p53 mutations in human lymphoid malignancies: Association with Burkitt lymphoma and chronic lymphocytic leukemia. *Proc Natl Acad Sci USA* 88:5413–5417.

Hayashi K (1990): Mutations induced during the polymerase chain reaction. *Technique* 1:216–217.

Hayashi K (1991): PCR-SSCP: A simple and sensitive method for detection of mutations in the genomic DNA. *PCR Meth Appl* 1:34–38.

Hayashi K (1992): PCR-SSCP: A method for detection of mutations. *Gen Anal Tech Appl* 9:73–79.

Higuchi R (1989): Using PCR to engineer DNA. In: *PCR Technology.* Erlich H ed. New York: Stockton Press.

Higuchi R, Krummel, Saiki R (1988): A general method of *in vitro* preparation and specific mutagenesis of DNA fragments: Study of protein and DNA interactions. *Nucl Acids Res* 16:7351–7367.

Huse WD, Sastry L, Iverson SA, Kang AS, Alting-Mies M, Burton DR, Benkovic SJ, Lerner RA (1989): Generation of a large combinatorial library of the immunoglobulin repertoire in phage lambda. *Science* 246:1275–1289.

Iizuka M, Mashiyama S, Oshimura M, Sekiya T, Hayashi K (1992): Cloning and polymerase chain reaction-single-strand conformation polymorphism analysis of anonimous *Alu* repeats on chromosome 11. *Genomics* 12:139–146.

Irvine D, Tuerk C, Gold L (1991): SELEXION. Systematic evolution of ligands by exponential enrichment with integrated optimization by nonlinear analysis. *J Mol Biol* 222:739–761.

Jiang W, Kahn SM, Guillem JG, Lu S-H, Weinstein IB (1989): Rapid detection of ras oncogenes in human tumors: Application to colon, esophageal and gastric cancer. *Oncogene* 4:923–928.

Kinzler KW, Vogelstein B (1989): Whole genome PCR: Application to the identification of sequences bound by gene regulatory proteins. *Nucl Acids Res* 17:3645–3652.

Krawczak M, Reiss J, Schmidke J (1989): Polymerase chain reaction: Replication error and reliability of gene diagnosis. *Nucl Acids Res* 17:2197–2201.

Kwok S, Kellogg DE, Spasic D, Goda L, Levenson C, Sninsky JJ (1990): Effects of primer-template mismatches on the polymerase chain reaction: Human immunodeficiency virus type 1 model studies. *Nucl Acids Res* 18:999–1005.

Ledbetter SA, Nelson DL (1991): Genome amplification using primers directed to interspersed repetitive sequences (IRS-PCR). In: *Polymerase Chain Reaction I: A Practical Approach.* McPherson MJ, Quirke P, Taylor GR, eds. Oxford: IRL Press.

Lee CC, Wu X, Gibbs RA, Cook RG, Muzny DM, Caskey T (1988): Generation of cDNA probes directed by amino acid sequence: cloning of urate oxydase. *Science* 239:1288–1291.

Leung DW, Chen E, Goeddel DV (1989): A method for random mutagenesis of a defined DNA segment using a modified polymerase chain reaction. *Technique* 1:11–15.

Li H, Cui X, Arnheim N (1990): Direct electrophoretic detection of the allelic state of single DNA molecules in human sperm by using the polymerase chain reaction. *Proc Natl Acad Sci USA* 87:4580–4584.

Loh EY, Elliot JF, Cwirla S, Lanier LL, Davis MM (1989): Polymerase chain reaction with single-sided specificity: Analysis of T-cell reception of chain. *Science* 243:217–220.

Makino R, Sekiya T, Hayashi K (1992): F-SSCP: Fluorescence-based polymerase chain reaction-single-stranded conformation polymorphism (PCR-SSCP) analysis. *PCR Meth Appl* 2:10–13.

Mashiyama S, Sekiya T, Hayashi K (1990): Screening of multiple DNA samples for detection of sequence changes. *Technique* 2:304–306.

Meyers R, Fischer SG, Lerman L, Maniatis T (1985): Nearly all single base substitutions in DNA fragments joined to a GC-clamp can be detected by denaturing gradient gel electrophoresis. *Nucl Acids Res* 13:3131–3146.

Mueller PR, Wold B (1989): In vivo footprinting of a muscle specific enhancer by ligation mediated PCR. *Science* 246:780–786.

Nelson DL, Ledbetter SA, Corbo L, Victoria MF, Ramirez-Solis R, Webster TD, Ledbetter DH, Caskey CT (1989): *Alu* polymerase chain reaction: A method for rapid isolation of human-specific sequences from complex DNA source. *Proc Natl Acad Sci USA* 86:6686–6690.

Ochman H, Ajioka JW, Garza D, Hartl DL (1989): Inverse polymerase chain reaction. In: *PCR Technology.* Erlich H, ed. New York: Stockton Press.

Ochman H, Gerber AS, Hartl DL (1988): Genetic application of an inverse polymerase chain reaction. *Genetics* 120:621–623.

Ohara O, Dorit RL, Gilbert W (1989): One-sided polymerase chain reaction: The amplification of cDNA. *Proc Natl Acad Sci USA* 86:5673–5677.

Orita M, Suzuki Y, Sekiya T, Hayashi K (1989): A rapid and sensitive detection of point mutations and genetic polymorphisms using polymerase chain reaction. *Genomics* 5:874–879.

Pääbo S, Wilson AC (1988): Polymerase chain reaction reveals cloning artifacts. *Nature* 334:387–388.

Saiki R, Gelfand DH, Stoffel S, Scharf SJ, Higuchi R, Horn GT, Mullis KB, Erlich HA (1988): Primer-directed enzymatic amplification of DNA with thermostable DNA polymerase. *Science* 239:487–491.

Saiki RK, Walsh PS, Levenson CH, Erlich HA (1989): Genetic analysis of amplified DNA with immobilized sequence-specific oligonucleotide probe. *Proc Natl Acad Sci USA* 86:6230–6234.

Sambrook J, Fritch EF, Maniatis T (1989): *Molecular Cloning: A Laboratory Manual*, 2nd ed. Cold Spring Harbor, NY: Cold Spring Harbor Laboratory Press.

Sheffield VC, Cox R, Lerman LR, Meyer RM (1989): Attachment of a 40-base-pair G+C rich sequence (GC-clamp) to genomic DNA fragments by the polymerase chain reaction results in improved detection of single-base changes. *Proc Natl Acad Sci USA* 86:232–236.

Silver J, Keerikatte V (1989): Novel use of polymerase chain reaction to amplify cellular DNA adjacent to an integrated provirus. *J Virol* 63:1924–1928.

Stallings RL, Ford AF, Nelson D, Torney DC, Hildebrand CE, Moyzis RK (1991): Evolution and distribution of (GT)n repetitive sequences in mammalian genomes. *Genomics* 10:807–815.

Suzuki Y, Sekiya T, Hayashi K (1991): Allele-specific polymerase chain reaction: A method for amplification and sequence determination of a single component among a mixture of sequence variants. *Anal Biochem* 192:82–84.

Triglia T, Peterson MG, Kemp DJ (1988): A procedure for *in vitro* amplification of DNA segments that lie outside the boundaries of known sequences. *Nucl Acids Res* 16:8186.

van Mansfeld ADM, Boss JL (1992): PCR-based approaches for detection of mutated ras genes. *PCR Meth Appl* 1:211–216.

Wallace RB, Johnson MJ, Hirose T, Miyake T, Kawashima EH, Itakura K (1981): The use of synthetic oligonucleotides as hybridization probes. II. Hybridization of oligonucleotides of mixed sequence to rabbit β-globin DNA. *Nucl Acids Res* 9:879–894.

Weber JL, May PE (1989): Abundant class of human DNA polymorphisms which can be typed using the polymerase chain reaction. *Am J Hum Genet* 44:388–396.

Welsh J, McClelland M (1990): Fingerprinting genomes using PCR with arbitrary primers. *Nucl Acids Res* 18:7213–7218.

Welsh J, Petersen C, McClelland M (1991): Polymorphisms generated by arbitrarily primed PCR in the mouse: Application to strain identification and genetic mapping. *Nucl Acids Res* 19:303–304.

White MB, Calvalho M, Derse D, O'Brien SJ, Dean M (1992): Detecting single base substitutions as heteroduplex polymorphisms. *Genomics* 12:301–306.

Winter E, Yamamoto F, Almoguera C, Perucho M (1985): A method to detect and characterize point mutations in transcribed genes: Amplification and overexpression of the mutant c-K-ras allele in human tumor cells. *Proc Natl Acad Sci USA* 82:7575–7579.

Wu DY, Ugozzoli L, Pal BK, Wallace RB (1989): Allele-specific enzymatic amplification of β-globin genomic DNA for diagnosis of sickle cell anemia. *Proc Natl Acad Sci USA* 86:2757–2760.

2

Cloning PCR Products

Michael A. Frohman

Introduction

It is often necessary to clone PCR products. In this chapter, the advantages and disadvantages of various strategies are discussed. It should be kept in mind, however, that PCR can be used to achieve many objectives—such as obtaining sequence information, preparing probes for hybridization analysis, and constructing new hybrid genes—without ever cloning the PCR products. In some instances, it is even advantageous not to clone the products, as described in other chapters.

There are three main scenarios in which PCR products are cloned:

1. When two gene-specific primers are used to amplify and clone a defined gene fragment or family of fragments.

2. When a gene-specific primer and a "universal" primer are used to amplify and clone a cDNA or gene fragment for which only one end has previously been determined.
3. When two universal primers are used to amplify and clone libraries of cDNAs or gene fragments.

For each of these scenarios, an additional decision has to be made—whether to employ a "blunt-ended" or an "overhanging-ended" (also known as "sticky-ended") cloning strategy (Figs. 2.1 and 2.2). In addition, two major variations exist for each strategy. Given the wide variation of experimental settings, there is no "best" way to clone PCR products. However, the points discussed below should provide a rational way to choose the most appropriate approach for an individual setting.

In the following sections, each of these topics will be discussed in order of decreasing generality. However, our discussion begins at the PCR step, which has to be carried out under optimal conditions to generate clones containing desirable products.

Portions of this chapter have been adapted and reprinted by permission of the publisher from "Rapid Amplification of Complementary DNA Ends for Generation of Full-Length Complementary DNAs: Thermal RACE," by Michael A. Frohman in *Methods in Enzymology*, Volume 218, pages 340–356. Copyright © 1993 by Academic Press, Inc.

The Polymerase Chain Reaction
K.B. Mullis, F. Ferré, R.A. Gibbs, editors
© 1994 Birkhäuser Boston

After PCR, the reaction mixture contains the product in several forms:

Strategy 1A

Before PCR: Kinase primers.

After PCR: Remove any extraneous terminal A's.
-      - Separate from residual primers, dNTPs, and primer-dimer products.
-      - Ligate to plasmid that has been linearized with a blunt-cutting restriction enzyme and
            dephosphorylated using CIP.

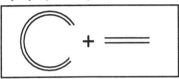

Strategy 1B

Before PCR: -

After PCR: Separate from residual primers and primer-dimer products.
-      - Ligate to plasmid linearized with a blunt-cutting restriction enzyme and extended by one nt
            using TTP to produce overhanging dT's complementary to the A's overhanging the PCR product.

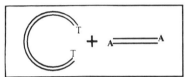

Advantages of blunt cloning

- Employs primers of minimal length and maximal specificity
- Does not risk cleavage of product at internal site (assuming sequence of product is not known)
- Requires relatively little post-PCR manipulation of product.

Disadvantages of blunt cloning

- Cloning is inefficient.
- Requires kinasing primers and preparing blunt-cut and phosphatased plasmid (Strategy 1A) or preparing /
        purchasing dT-extended blunt-cut plasmid (Strategy 1B).
- Is non-directional.
- Does not select against artifactual products generated through the use of a single primer at both ends of the
        DNA fragment.
- Often generates recombinant plasmids containing multiple inserts.

FIGURE 2.1. Blunt cloning.

Strategy 2A

Before PCR: Synthesize hybrid primers containing a) sequences specific to gene under study;
b) restriction endonuclease sites and
c) 3 additional nt, to enable restriction enzymes to cut the PCR product at its ends.

After PCR: Separate product from residual primers, dNTPs, Taq polymerase,
& primer-dimers.
- Digest with the restriction enzymes selected above.
- Ligate to plasmid linearized with the same restriction enzymes.

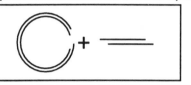

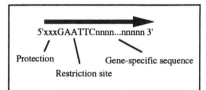

Strategy 2B

Before PCR: Synthesize hybrid primers containing a) sequences specific to gene under study;
b) partial restriction endonuclease sites.

After PCR: Separate product from residual primers, dNTPs, Taq polymerase, & primer-dimers.
- Add back selected dNTP's and T4 DNA Polymerase to remove 3' nts as depicted
and thus create 5' overhangs.
- Ligate to plasmid linearized with the corresponding restriction enzymes.

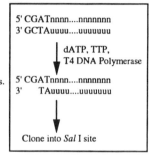

Advantages of cloning PCR products with overhanging ends

- Cloning is efficient.
- Does not require kinasing primers, phosphatased plasmid, or preparing / purchasing a T-extended blunt-cut plasmid.
- Is directional.
- Selects against artifactual products generated through the use of a single primer at both ends of the DNA fragment.
- Does not (usually) generate recombinant plasmids containing multiple inserts.

Disadvantages of cloning PCR products with overhanging ends

- Requires extra non-gene-specific nt to be added to primer, increasing cost and decreasing specificity. (Strategy 2A = 9 nt;
Strategy 2B = 4-5 nt)
- Requires more post-PCR manipulation of product.
- (Strategy 2A only) Risks cleavage of product at internal sites (assuming sequence of product is not known)

FIGURE 2.2. Overhanging ends.

Optimizing PCR Conditions Prior to Cloning

For some applications intended for cloned PCR products, such as expressing cDNAs to generate proteins, it is critically important to minimize the rate at which mutations occur during amplification. In other applications, such as using the cloned DNA as a probe in hybridization experiments, the presence of a few mutations is relatively unimportant and thus it is most convenient to use PCR conditions that maximize the likelihood of generating the desired product the first time a set of primers is used. Unfortunately, PCR conditions that result in a minimum of mutations are finicky and often the desired product cannot be generated until the PCR conditions have been optimized, whereas PCR conditions that reliably produce desired products result in a relatively high mutation rate ($\sim 1\%$ after 30 rounds). Thus, appropriate conditions must be chosen to generate the PCR products required prior to undertaking cloning steps.

PCR conditions that result in a minimum of mutations require the use of nucleotides (dNTPs) at low concentrations (Eckert and Kunkel, 1990). Using the conditions recommended for *Taq* polymerase by Perkin–Elmer–Cetus (0.2 mM) results in an error rate of $\sim 0.05\%$ after 30 rounds of amplification. However, the conditions recommended often have to be optimized, meaning that the pH of the buffer and the concentration of magnesium have to be adjusted until the desired product is observed. In addition, inclusion of dimethyl sulfoxide (DMSO) or formamide may be required. For those who do not wish to prepare their own reagents to carry out optimization experiments, such kits are commercially available (e.g., from Invitrogen).

PCR conditions that work much more frequently in the absence of optimization steps require the use of dNTPs at high concentrations (1.5 mM). One such set of conditions, described initially by New England Biolabs, is employed as follows: PCR is performed in the presence of 10% DMSO (Fluka), 1.5 mM dNTPs, and $1 \times$ PCR buffer that contains 67 mM Tris-HCl, pH 8.8, 6.7 mM MgCl$_2$, 170 μg/ml BSA, and 16.6 mM (NH$_4$)$_2$SO$_4$. The PCR buffer and the dNTPs can be prepared and stored as $10 \times$ solutions. It should be noted that the inclusion of DMSO to 10% decreases primer melting temperatures (and thus optimal annealing temperatures) by about 5–6°C.

General Cloning Strategies and Protocols

Background Information for Cloning

What Is Really in a PCR Tube

Following PCR, the reaction tube contains a complex mixture of (1) the desired product in several molecular forms, (2) a number of artifactual (undesired) amplification products including very short DNA fragments often referred to erroneously as "primer-dimers," but denoted here as "ampli-schmutz," and (3) residual reaction components, i.e., salts, dNTPs, primers, and *Taq* polymerase. The extent to which (2) and (3) negatively impact on cloning depends on the approach used; but in general, even for those situations in which cloning can be accomplished straight out of a PCR reaction mixture, better and more consistent results will be obtained after separating the desired product from contaminants. In some instances, failure will be virtually certain if separation is not carried out.

Definitions

After PCR, the desired reaction products are present in three forms, as depicted in Figure 2.1 and here. The top form is the one usually associated with PCR reactions. In each cycle, primers (boxes) anneal to the 3′-end of complementary single-stranded DNA and become extended to form a double-stranded product.

In theory, because the primers anneal precisely to the very 3′-end of their target DNA, and because the extension continues through the last nucleotide of the target DNA but no further, a "blunt" product should be created, meaning that there should be no single-

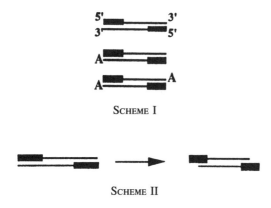

SCHEME I

SCHEME II

stranded extensions on either the 5'- or the 3'-ends. However, the real reaction is a little more complicated. To varying extents, *Taq* polymerase also appends an extra nucleotide, usually dA, to the 3'-ends of blunt double-stranded DNA (also known as "template-independent polymerization"). Therefore, some molecules have an extra dA appended to one of the two strands; some have extra dAs appended to both strands, as depicted in the second and third forms of Scheme I, respectively. In cloning such products using a "blunt-end" strategy, the goal is to ligate them "as is" to an appropriately prepared vector, by either removing or taking advantage of the extraneous dAs. Technically, products containing the extra dA are not "blunt," but since most of the considerations are similar, they will be discussed at the same time.

In contrast, when cloning PCR products using an "overhanging-end" strategy, the goals are to change the ends of the product so as to create single-stranded overhangs of several nucleotides (Scheme II), and then to ligate the product to coordinately prepared vector (Fig. 2.2). In the two most popular current strategies, restriction enzymes or T_4 DNA polymerase are used to cut the double-stranded DNA or "chew-back" 3'-ends, respectively.

Blunt Cloning

The extent to which *Taq* polymerase appends dAs to PCR products depends on the activity of the enzyme near the end of the run and the ratio of the *Taq* polymerase to the entire mass

of double-stranded DNA present in the reaction mixture. If enzyme activity is low, then most molecules will not have dAs appended. In addition, large amounts of ampli-schmutz, which can vastly outnumber the specific product on a molar basis, may competitively inhibit addition of dA to the desired product. In practice, some of both forms should be present in most PCR samples. However, it is advisable to manipulate either the PCR run or the product after PCR to maximize recovery of the desired form.

Cloning without Extraneous dAs (Strategy 1A)

The PCR Product

To remove the extraneous dAs, PCR products are incubated with the Klenow fragment of DNA polymerase in the presence of all four dNTPs. Klenow exhibits a strong $3' \rightarrow 5'$ single-stranded exonuclease activity and will remove the overhanging dAs. Note that it is necessary to have the dNTPs present, or else Klenow will continue its $3' \rightarrow 5'$ exonuclease activity on the double-stranded DNA. It is not necessary to remove *Taq* polymerase in order to "polish" the PCR product with Klenow, since Klenow exhibits much greater activity than *Taq* polymerase at room temperature.

The Vector

Under normal circumstances, only a few percent of plasmids recovered from simple blunt cloning experiments actually contain inserts. This is because the most frequent reaction is unimolecular in which the blunt-cut, linear plasmid recircularizes without insert. This can be countered by increasing insert concentration, at the risk of generating frequent multimers of insert, or by dephosphorylating the free 5'-ends of the plasmid DNA to render it incapable of religating without an exogenous energy source (e.g., a phosphate group on the 5'-end of some other fragment of DNA, such as the insert). This step is conceptually straightforward, but in practice it is found to be challenging to digest plasmid to completion, and perform extensive dephosphorylation

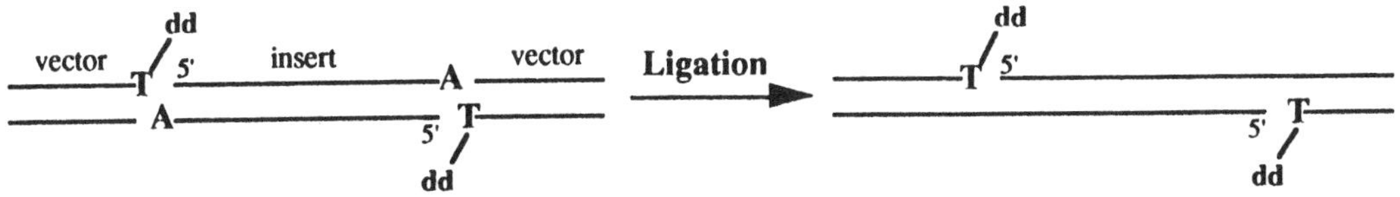

dd
vector   T⁄ 5'   insert   A   vector   **Ligation**   dd   T⁄ 5'

A   5' T⁄
          dd   5' T⁄
                           dd

SCHEME III

without additional DNA damage. If attempted, a large quantity of plasmid should be prepared, so that it can be properly tested and used for many experiments.

Back to the PCR Product

Unfortunately, PCR primers, from which the 5'-ends of the PCR products are derived, do not normally bear the 5'-phosphate group required to energize a ligation reaction. Therefore, to enable ligation of insert to the vector, it is necessary to kinase the PCR primers, either before or after the PCR reaction. In general, it is advisable to kinase the primers prior to PCR, since primer can therefore be prepared for multiple experiments and since the kinase reaction is more efficient in the absence of PCR reaction contaminants. Alternatively, the phosphate groups may be added during chemical synthesis.

Cloning Using Extraneous dAs (Strategy 1B)

The PCR Product

To maximize the percentage of products that contain appended dAs, it is advisable not to carry out more than 20 cycles of PCR, since after this point decreased enzyme activity or increased template concentration may decrease the frequency at which dAs are appended to newly synthesized 3'-ends. If difficulty recovering clones is encountered, dA-tails can be appended to the PCR products after the PCR run by separating the PCR products from the previous reaction components and contaminants (primers, dNTPs, *Taq* polymerase, and ampli-schmutz), and then incubating the products in fresh PCR reaction buffer containing fresh dNTPs and *Taq* polymerase for 15 min at 72°C.

The Vector

To carry out a successful ligation reaction using dA-tailed PCR products, the plasmid vector must be tailed with dT. Plasmid vector so prepared can be purchased commercially at high cost, or made easily in bulk. Among several approaches, the most popular is to incubate blunt-cut linear vector with terminal deoxynucleotidyltransferase (TdT) and dideoxy-TTP (ddTTP). TdT will add ddTTP onto the plasmid's free 3'-ends, and only one ddTTP will be added, since dideoxy nucleotides terminate such reactions. Since this vector cannot recircularize (due to the overlapping ddTs) nor religate (since the ddTs do not have free 3'-hydroxyl groups), it is not necessary to dephosphorylate it; moreover, since the vector can now energize a ligation reaction to the insert through its own 5'-phosphate groups, kinasing the PCR product's primers is also not required. On completion of the ligation reaction, the insert-containing plasmid will still have a nick in each DNA strand, where the ddT nucleotide abuts the 5'-end of the inserted PCR product (Scheme III). This does not create difficulties, however, because such nicks will be repaired efficiently by the bacteria after transformation.

General Comments on Blunt Cloning

The effects of short-length products (ampli-schmutz) on cloning experiments are not generally appreciated. Such PCR products can be present in vast molar excess as compared to the desired product, and therefore become the predominant species cloned and recovered from ligation reactions. If short PCR products are observed after the PCR run, it is imperative to separate them from the desired product prior to carrying out the ligation reaction. Either spin filtration (described below) or gel isolation is acceptable for this purpose.

In practice, there is rarely a good reason for planning to carry out blunt ligation on PCR products, given the disadvantages listed in Figure 2.1. The small cost saving and gain in sensitivity that is realized over the method described for Strategy 2B, or even 2A, does not compensate for the increased effort required to carry out blunt cloning. However, it is necessary to be able to carry out blunt cloning in two settings: when gene-construction constraints dictate it, or when it becomes desirable to clone a PCR product using primers that were not initially designed to be used for a cloning project, and thus that are not compatible with Strategy 2A or 2B.

Overhanging End Cloning (also Known as "Sticky-Ended," Forced, or Directional Cloning)

The best strategy, whenever possible, is to use unmodified primers that flank restriction enzyme sites already present in the target DNA (Scheme IV). This offers at least two advantages over the addition of artificial restriction site on the end of the primers.

First, unmodified primers are less expensive and more specific than ones encoding synthetic restriction sites. Second, it is unlikely that undesired amplification products, including ampli-schmutz, will encode both of the naturally occurring restriction sites present in the desired PCR product. Therefore, since the corresponding restriction enzymes will not digest the undesired amplification products and ampli-schmutz, only the desired PCR product will provide clonable DNA fragments to the ligation reaction.

The next best strategy, when it is possible, is to choose a region for the primer at which the substitution of a single nucleotide will result in a new restriction site (Scheme V).

The two rules governing the choice of sequence are (1) the mismatched nucleotide should be as far away from the 3′-end of the primer as possible and (2) the restriction site should be flanked by at least 3 bp on its 5′-end (see Strategy 2A for discussion of this "protection" region). DNA analysis computer programs that search for such almost correct sites are available in the public and commercial domains.

In contrast to blunt end cloning, it is unimportant in overhanging end cloning whether terminal dAs are added to the PCR product or not, since they are removed if present. In addition, since energy for the ligation is supplied by the vector's 5′-phosphates, it is not necessary to kinase the primers before PCR. Instead, the most crucial tactical element is to carry out the post-PCR manipulations [restriction enzyme digestion or T_4 DNA polymerase $3' \rightarrow 5'$ exonuclease digestion (also known as "chew-back")] in the absence of PCR reaction "contaminants" that will change the outcome of the strategy.

Cloning with Primers that Contain Built-In Restriction Endonuclease Sites (Strategy 2A)

The Primers

Primers are generally designed as shown depicted in Figure 2.2 (Strategy 2A). The 3′-end of the primer consists of 17–30 nucleotides of sequence specific to the gene under study; this is followed by six nucleotides corresponding to a restriction endonuclease site of choice; and finally, three more nucleotides are added to "protect" the restriction site.

What factors influence the choice of restriction enzyme?

1. Empirically, it has been found that many restriction enzymes will not cleave DNA if the recognition site is less than three nucleotides from the end of the DNA fragment. With three nucleotides of protection, most enzymes will function efficiently. However, there are some exceptions. Commercial catalogs (such as Stratagene) often contain

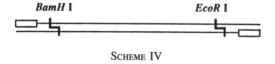

BamH I   *EcoR* I

SCHEME IV

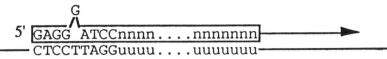

New *BamH* I site created

SCHEME V

such lists, and it is advisable to check them before synthesizing your primers.

2. If you do not know the sequence of your product (and you do not instead want to use Strategy 2B, which is what should be used in such circumstances), use restriction enzymes that recognize sequences found infrequently in the genome ("rare-cutters"). In mammalian DNA, enzymes sites containing "CG" (e.g., *Sal*I, *Xho*I, *Cla*I) are found relatively infrequently. Frequencies differ in DNA from other species.

3. Cost of the restriction enzyme.

4. Buffer compatibility for simultaneous digestion with the enzyme chosen for the other primer.

5. Whether the restriction enzyme can be heat inactivated after the digestion.

The PCR Product

If not removed, by-products and leftover ingredients from PCR will interfere with restriction enzyme cleavage of the intended product. Specifically, the principal villains are amplischmutz, and active *Taq* polymerase enzyme + dNTPs. Since, on a molar basis, amplischmutz can vastly outnumber the desired product, and since the restriction enzyme site may be intact in the ampli-schmutz molecules, large amounts of ampli-schmutz may competitively inhibit digestion of the specific product by tying up all of the enzyme. If significant ampli-schmutz is observed, the product should be separated prior to digestion. Even more importantly, if *Taq* polymerase and dNTPs are present during the digestion reaction, overhanging ends will be trimmed or filled back in as fast as they are created—resulting in unclonable blunt-ended fragments! Finally, salts, additives, and proteins from the PCR reaction

can also interfere with enzyme digestion, depending on the specific enzyme used.

Although short-cuts (e.g., heating the PCR tube to 100°C for 10 min and cooling to 37°C followed by immediate enzymatic digestion) will work in some instances, clonable material will be obtained *reliably* only if the contaminants described above are removed first. There are numerous easy and quick methods to purify the DNA and the cost and time required to do so are wisely invested.

Cloning with Primers that Contain Restriction Endonuclease Sites Activated by Limited 3′–5′-Exonuclease Digestion (Strategy 2B; also see Stoker, 1990)

The Primers

Primers are generally designed as depicted in Figure 2.2 (Strategy 2B). The 3′-end of the primer consists of 17–30 nucleotides of sequence specific to the gene under study; this is followed by four to five nucleotides corresponding to a partial restriction endonuclease site of limited choice.

What factors influence the choice of restriction enzyme site?

1. Nucleotide composition of the overhanging sequence. To carry out the limited exonuclease reaction, the appropriate dNTP(s) must be absent before T_4 DNA polymerase will begin to digest the 3′-strand, since T_4 DNA polymerase's synthesis speed exceeds its exonuclease speed. In addition, the appropriate nucleotide(s) should be present to stop the digestion from proceeding beyond the desired 5′ overhang. This is illustrated in Scheme VI and in Figure 2.2 (Strategy 2B). Thus, restriction enzymes that create 5′ overhangs containing all four nucleotides (e.g., *Bam*HI-GATC) cannot be used.

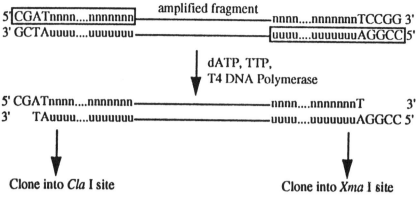

5' CGATnnnn....nnnnnnn ——————— nnnn....nnnnnnnnT   3'
3'   TAuuuu....uuuuuuu ——————— uuuu....uuuuuuuAGGCC 5'

Clone into *Cla* I site   Clone into *Xma* I site

SCHEME VI

Moreover, both primers must use the same sets of "missing" and "present" nucleotides, since the reaction cannot be carried out on each end at different times. A compatible set of restriction sites (boxed) are *Cla*I and *Xma*I, as shown here (note, the *Xma*I/*Sma*I site is not regenerated on ligation to the vector).

2. (Relevant to vector preparation only) Cost of restriction enzymes and buffer compatibility for simultaneous digestion with both enzymes chosen.

The PCR Product

As in Strategy 2A, by-products and leftover ingredients in the PCR tube will interfere with T₄ DNA polymerase exonuclease digestion of the intended product. Since ampli-schmutz can vastly outnumber the desired product on a molar basis, ampli-schmutz can competitively inhibit exonuclease digestion of the specific product. If ampli-schmutz is observed, the product should be separated from it prior to digestion. Even more importantly, if dNTPs are present during the reaction, T₄ DNA polymerase will not be able to chew back at all! Finally, salts, additives, and proteins from the PCR reaction can also interfere with T₄ DNA polymerase activity. Clonable material will be obtained *reliably* only if the contaminants described above are removed first, and there are numerous easy and quick methods to purify the DNA (discussed below).

Protocols

Listed below are some sample protocols. For additional details, refer to Sambrook et al. (1989), *Molecular Cloning: A Laboratory Manual*, or other sources, for basic molecular biology techniques.

Alternatives for Separation of PCR Products from Undesired Reactants

1. *Taq* polymerase.
   a. The PCR reaction can be heated at 100°C for 10 min to inactivate the *Taq* polymerase. The desired product will also be denatured, but it should reanneal quickly on cooling, if present in significant quantity (e.g., visible by ethidium bromide on a 1% agarose gel).

  b. The reaction mixture can be extracted with phenol/chloroform, then chloroform, and finally filtered by gravity centrifugation using a commercial spin filter such as Microcon-100 (Amicon Corp.). Filtration by itself is not sufficient to remove *Taq* polymerase without organic extraction.
  c. Gel isolation of the desired product (glass bead isolation kits are convenient for this step).
  d. Treatment with proteinase K may improve cloning by digesting *Taq* polymerase bound to the DNA, which may be resistant to other forms of removal (Crowe et al., 1991).

 2. Ampli-schmutz, primers, dNTPs, salts, additives to the PCR reaction.
  a. Spin filtration. Note: you may have to "wash" the product in the filter up to three times; assume a 95% reduction in concentration of contaminants for each wash cycle. In addition, check the molecular weight cutoff for DNA for any product you select! The effective size cutoff for DNA on spin filters is not the same as for proteins.
  b. Gel isolation.

Kinasing Primers

Mix:
  300 pmol primer (~2 μg of a 18-nucleotide primer)
  2 μl 10× Kinase buffer
  1 μl 10 mM ATP
  water to 10 μl
  2 U T$_4$ polynucleotide kinase

  Incubate 37°C for 60 min
  Incubate 65°C for 5 min to inactivate kinase
  Dilute to 20 μl with water
  Use 1 μl of kinased primer for a 50 μl PCR reaction

Vector Preparation for Strategy 1A

Cut 10 μg plasmid vector with a restriction enzyme that produces blunt ends (e.g., *Sma*I or *Eco*RV)
Extract with phenol/CHCl$_3$, CHCl$_3$, precipitate, and redissolve in 90 μl TE, pH 8.3

Add:
  10 μl of 10× CIP buffer
  0.25 units of calf intestinal phosphatase (CIP)
  incubate at 37°C for 30 min

Add:
  EGTA to 20 mM
  heat at 65°C for 10 min

Extract with phenol/CHCl$_3$, CHCl$_3$, dilute to 400 μl, precipitate, and redissolve in 100 μl TE
Adjust concentration to 40 ng/μl

Insert Preparation for Strategy 1A

Carry out PCR using kinased primers

After PCR, add 1 U Klenow and incubate at room temperature for 15 min; purify using organic extraction and spin filtration or gel isolation as described above

Blunt End Ligation for Strategy 1A

Mix on ice:

 40 ng blunt-cut, dephosphorylated vector

 An equal number of moles of purified PCR product amplified with kinased primers and polished with Klenow

 2 μl 5× Ligation buffer (including ATP)

 water to 9 μl

 1 μl T$_4$ DNA ligase (1–2 Weiss units)

Incubate at 12°C overnight, then transform using standard techniques

Vector Preparation for Strategy 1B

Cut 10 μg plasmid vector with a restriction enzyme that produces blunt ends (e.g., SmaI or EcoRV)

Extract with phenol/CHCl$_3$, CHCl$_3$, precipitate, and redissolve in 68 μl TE

Add:

 20 μl of 5× terminal transferase buffer

 1 μl of 1 mM dideoxy-TTP

 6 μl of 25 mM CoCl$_2$

 ~5 μl (125 U) terminal transferase

Incubate at 37°C for 15 min; then 65°C for 30 min

Extract with phenol/CHCl$_3$, CHCl$_3$, precipitate, and redissolve in 100 μl TE

Adjust concentration to 40 ng/μl

Insert Preparation for Strategy 1B

Carry out PCR using regular (nonkinased) primers, for no more than 20 cycles

After PCR, purify using organic extraction and spin filtration or gel isolation as described above

Blunt End Ligation for Strategy 1B

Mix on ice:

 40 ng blunt-cut, ddT-tailed vector

 An equal number of moles of purified PCR product

 2 μl 5× Ligation buffer (including ATP)

 water to 9 μl

 1 μl T$_4$ DNA ligase (1–2 Weiss units)

Incubate at 12°C overnight, then transform using standard techniques

Insert Preparation for Strategy 2A

Either extract PCR product with phenol/CHCl$_3$, then CHCl$_3$; filter through a Microcon-100 spin column; or gel isolate insert from a 1% agarose gel
Then, digest products using standards conditions and heat inactivate the restriction enzymes

Insert Preparation for Strategy 2B

Either extract PCR product with phenol/CHCl$_3$, then CHCl$_3$; filter three times through a microcon-100 spin column; or gel isolate insert from a 1% agarose gel
Then, on ice:

Add:
the selected dNTPs to a final concentration of 0.1 mM
1/10th volume 10× T$_4$ DNA polymerase buffer
1–2 U T$_4$ DNA polymerase

Incubate 12°C for 15 min; then 75°C for 10 min to heat inactivate the T$_4$ DNA polymerase

Overhanging End Ligation

Mix on ice:
20 ng vector digested with the chosen enzymes
An equal number of moles of PCR products prepared as described above in Strategy 2A or 2B
2 μl 5× Ligation buffer (including ATP)
water to 9 μl
1 μl T$_4$ DNA ligase (1 Weiss unit)

Incubate at 12°C overnight, then transform using standard techniques

---

Cloning cDNA Ends

A common result when attempting to isolate a DNA copy of a novel transcript is the recovery of a cDNA clone that contains only part of the sequence present in the original mRNA. The missing cDNA ends can be cloned by PCR using the rapid amplification of cDNA ends (RACE) procedure (Frohman et al., 1988), also known as Anchored PCR (Loh et al., 1989), or using one of the many variant protocols published subsequently. A commercial RACE kit is available from Bethesda Research Laboratories (Schuster et al., 1992) that is convenient but is not as powerful as more recent versions of RACE (Frohman and Martin, 1989; Frohman, 1993).

Scheme VII represents the circumstance in which RACE plays a role in cDNA cloning strategies. Depicted is a mRNA for which a cDNA representing only a small and internal portion of the transcript has been cloned. Such circumstances arise frequently, for example (1) when closely related family members are

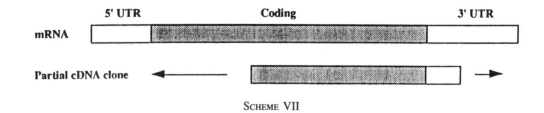

SCHEME VII

cloned using PCR and degenerate primers encoding sequences homologous to amino acids found in all known members of the family; and (2) when incomplete cDNAs are obtained after screening conventional or PCR libraries.

Overview

Why use PCR (RACE) to clone cDNA ends instead of screening additional libraries? RACE cloning offers several advantages over traditional library screens. First, it takes weeks to screen libraries, obtain individual cDNA clones, and analyze the clones to determine if the missing sequence has been obtained; using RACE, such information can be generated in 1–2 days. As a consequence, reverse transcription conditions can be modified until full length cDNAs are generated and observed, ensuring that the missing sequence will be obtained.

Second, generally only a single to a few cDNA clones are recovered from a library screen. Using RACE, larger numbers of independent clones can be generated, providing confirmation of nucleotide sequence and allowing the isolation of unusual transcripts that are alternately spliced or that begin at infrequently used promoters.

Principles

PCR is used to amplify partial cDNA copies of the region between a single point in an mRNA transcript and its 3'- or 5'-end. A short, internal stretch of sequence must already be known from the mRNA of interest. From this sequence, gene-specific primers are chosen that are oriented in the direction of the missing sequence. Extension of the partial cDNAs from the ends of the message back to the known region is achieved using primers that anneal to the natural (3'-end) or a synthetic (5'-end) poly(A) tail. By using RACE, enrichments in the range of 10^6- to 10^7-fold can be obtained for a specific cDNA end. As a consequence, relatively pure partial cDNA "ends" are generated that can be easily cloned or rapidly characterized using conventional techniques.

To generate 3'-end partial cDNA clones, mRNA is reverse transcribed using a "hybrid" primer (Q_T) that consists of 17 nucleotides of oligo(dT) followed by a unique 35 base oligonucleotide sequence (Q_I-Q_O; Fig. 2.3a and c). Amplification is then performed using a primer containing part of this sequence (Q_O) that now binds to each cDNA at its 3'-end, and using a primer derived from the gene of interest (GSP1). A second set of amplification cycles is then carried out using "nested" primers (Q_I and GSP2) to achieve greater specificity. To generate 5'-end partial cDNA clones, reverse transcription (primer extension) is carried out using a gene-specific primer (GSP-RT; Fig. 2.3b). Then, a poly(A) tail is appended using terminal deoxynucleotidyltransferase (TdT) and dATP to tail the first strand reaction products. Amplification is then achieved using the hybrid primer Q_T described above to form the second strand of cDNA, the Q_O primer, and a gene-specific primer upstream of and distinct from the one used for reverse transcription. Finally, a second set of PCR cycles is carried out using nested primers (Q_I and GSP2) to increase specificity.

Alternatively, the 5'-end can be tailed with Cs and then amplified using a hybrid primer with a tail containing a mixture of Gs and inosines (I) (Fig. 2.3d; see Schuster et al.,

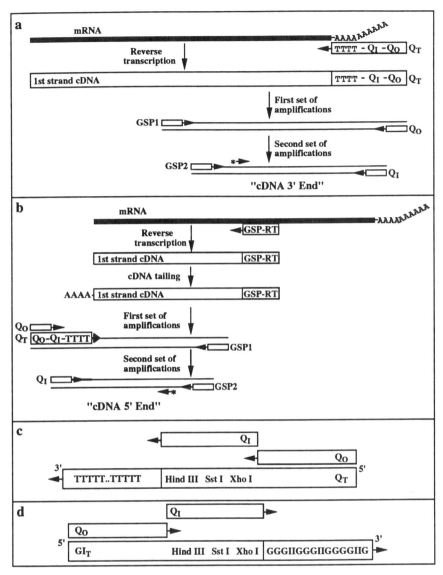

FIGURE 2.3. Schematic representation of thermal RACE. Explanations are given in the text. At each step, the diagram is simplified to illustrate only how the new product formed during the previous step is utilized. GSP1, gene-specific primer 1; GSP2, gene-specific primer 2; GSP-RT, gene-specific primer used for reverse transcription; *→, GSP-Hyb/Seq or gene-specific primer for use in hybridization and sequencing reactions. (a) Amplification of 3' partial cDNA ends. (b) Amplification of 5' partial cDNA ends. (c) Schematic representation of the primers used in thermal RACE. The 52 nucleotide Q_T primer (5' Q_O-Q_I-TTTT 3') contains a 17-nucleotide oligo(dT) sequence at the 3'-end followed by a 35-nucleotide sequence encoding HindIII, SstI, and XhoI recognition sites. The Q_I and Q_O primers overlap by 1 nucleotide; the Q_I primer contains all three of the recognition sites. (d) Schematic representation of an alternate primer for 5' thermal RACE, to be used in conjunction with C-tailed cDNAs.

Primers:

Q_T: 5'-CCAGTGAGCAGAGTGACGAGGACTCGAGCTCAAGCTTTTTTTTTTTTTTTTT-3'

Q_O: 5'-CCAGTGAGCAGAGTGACG-3'

Q_I: 5'-GAGGACTCGAGCTCAAGC-3'

GI_T: 5'-CCAGTGAGCAGAGTGACGAGGACTCGAGCTCAAGCGGGIIGGGIIGGGGIIG-3'

1992). Although this approach entails synthesizing a primer that can be used for 5′ RACE only [since a T-tailed primer must be used to anneal to the poly(A) tail of the 3′-end], there may be sufficient benefits from using a mixed G:I tail to justify the extra cost, since the G:I region should behave like a normal primer in PCR. In contrast, it is believed that homopolymers of either Ts or Gs present problems in PCR (Frohman, unpublished data; see Schuster et al., 1992).

Protocols

Materials

The materials required for this procedure can be purchased, along with the appropriate $5 \times$ or $10 \times$ enzyme reaction buffers, from most major suppliers. MMLV reverse transcriptase can be obtained from Bethesda Research Labs (BRL), heat-stable reverse transcriptase from Epicentre Technologies, RNasin and *Taq* polymerase from Promega Biotech (or Tfl polymerase from Epicentre Technologies), and TdT from either BRL or Boehringer Mannheim. Enzymes are used as directed by the suppliers, except for *Taq* polymerase: Instead of using the recommended reaction mixture, a $10 \times$ buffer consisting of 670 mM Tris-HCl, pH 9.0, 67 mM MgCl$_2$, 1700 μg/ml BSA, and 166 mM (NH$_4$)$_2$SO$_4$ is substituted (as discussed in the beginning of the chapter), and reaction conditions are altered as further described below. Oligonucleotide primer sequences are listed in the legend to Figure 2.3. Primers can be used "crude" except for Q$_T$ or GI$_T$, which should be purified to ensure that they are uniformly full length. dNTPs can be purchased as 100 mM solutions from PL-Biochemicals/Pharmacia or Boehringer Mannheim.

3′-End cDNA Amplification

Step 1. Reverse Transcription to Generate cDNA Templates

Procedure. Assemble reverse transcription components on ice: 4 μl of $5 \times$ reverse transcription buffer, 1.3 μl of dNTPs (stock concentration is 15 mM of each dNTP), 0.25μl (10 units) of RNasin, and 0.5 μl of Q$_T$ primer (100 ng/μl). Heat 1 μg of poly(A)$^+$ RNA or 5 μg of total RNA in 14 μl of water at 80°C for 3 min and cool rapidly on ice. Add to reverse transcription components. Add 1 μl (200 units) of MMLV reverse transcriptase, and incubate for 2 hr at 37°C. Dilute the reaction mixture to 1 ml with TE (100 mM Tris-HCl, pH 7.5/1 mM EDTA) and store at 4°C ("3′-end cDNA pool").

Comments. Poly(A)$^+$ RNA is preferentially used for reverse transcription to decrease background, but it is unnecessary to prepare it if only total RNA is available. An important factor in the generation of full length 3′-end partial cDNAs concerns the stringency of the reverse transcription reaction. Reverse transcription reactions were historically carried out at relatively low temperatures (37–42°C) using a vast excess of primer ($\sim$1/2 the mass of the mRNA, which represents an $\sim$30:1 molar ratio). Under these low stringency conditions, a stretch of A residues as short as 6–8 nucleotides will suffice as a binding site for an oligo(dT)-tailed primer. This may result in cDNA synthesis being initiated at sites upstream of the poly(A) tail, leading to truncation of the desired amplification product. One should be suspicious that this has occurred if a canonical polyadenylation signal sequence (Wickens and Stephenson, 1984) is not found near the 3'-end of the cDNAs generated. This can be minimized by controlling two parameters: primer concentration and reaction temperature. The primer concentration can be reduced dramatically without decreasing the amount of cDNA synthesized significantly (Coleclough, 1987) and will begin to bind preferentially to the longest A-rich stretches present [i.e., the poly(A) tail]. The quantity recommended above represents a good starting point; it can be reduced 5-fold further if significant truncation is observed.

Until recently, reaction temperatures could not be increased because reverse transcriptase became inactivated by elevated temperatures. However, heat stable reverse transcriptases are now available from several suppliers (Perkin–Elmer–Cetus, Amersham, Epicentre Technologies, and others). As in PCR reactions, the stringency of reverse transcription can thus be controlled by adjusting the temperature at which the primer is annealed to the mRNA. The optimal temperature depends on the specific reaction buffer and reverse transcriptase used and should be determined empirically, but it will usually be found to be in the range of 48–56°C for a primer terminated by a 17-nucleotide oligo(dT) tail.

Step 2. Amplification

Procedure. First round: Add an aliquot of the cDNA pool (1 μl) and primers (25 pmol each of GSP1 and Q_O) to 50 μl of PCR cocktail [1× *Taq* polymerase buffer (described above), each dNTP at 1.5 mM, and 10% DMSO] in a 0.5-ml microfuge tube and heat in a DNA thermal cycler for 5 min at 98°C to denature the first strand products. Cool to 75°C. Add 2.5 U *Taq* polymerase, overlay the mixture with 30 μl of mineral oil (Sigma 400-5; preheat it in the thermal cycler to 75°C), and incubate at the appropriate annealing temperature (52–60°C) for 2 min. Extend the cDNAs at 72°C for 40 min. Carry out 30 cycles of amplification using a step program (94°C, 1 min; 52–60°C, 1 min; 72°C, 3 min), followed by a 15 min final extension at 72°C. Cool to room temperature.

Second round: Dilute a portion of the amplification products from the first round 1:20 in TE. Amplify 1 μl of the diluted material with primers GSP2 and Q_I using the procedure described above, but eliminate the initial 2 min annealing step and the 72°C, 40 min extension step.

Comments. It is important to add the *Taq* polymerase *after* heating the mixture to a temperature above the T_m of the primers ("Hot Start" PCR). Addition of the enzyme prior to this point allows one "cycle" to take place at room temperature, promoting the synthesis of nonspecific background products dependent on low stringency interactions.

An annealing temperature close to the effective T_m of the primers should be used. The Q_I and Q_O primers work well at 60°C under the PCR conditions recommended here, although the actual optimal temperature may depend on the PCR machine used. Gene-specific primers of similar length and GC content should be chosen. Computer programs to assist in the selection of primers are widely available and should be used. An extension time of 1 min/kb expected product should be allowed during the amplification cycles. If the expected length of product is unknown, try 3–4 min initially.

Very little substrate is required for the PCR reaction: 1 μg of poly(A)$^+$ RNA typically contains $\sim 5 \times 10^7$ copies of *each* low abundance transcript. The PCR reaction described here works optimally when 10^3–10^5 templates (of the desired cDNA) are present in the starting mixture; thus as little as 0.002% of the reverse transcription mixture suffices for the PCR reaction! Addition of too much starting material to the amplification reaction will lead to production of large amounts of nonspecific product and should be avoided. The RACE technique is particularly sensitive to this problem, since every cDNA in the mixture, desired and undesired, contains a binding site for the Q_O and Q_I primers.

It was found empirically that allowing extra extension time during the first amplification round (when the second strand of cDNA is created) sometimes resulted in increased yields of the specific product relative to background amplification, and, in particular, increased the yields of long cDNAs versus short cDNAs when specific cDNA ends of multiple lengths were present (Frohman et al., 1988). Prior treatment of cDNA templates with RNA hydrolysis or a combination of RNase H and RNase A infrequently improves the efficiency of amplification of specific cDNAs.

5'-End cDNA Amplification

Step 1. Reverse Transcription to Generate cDNA Templates

Procedure. Assemble reverse transcription components on ice: 4 μl of 5 × reverse transcription buffer, 1.3 μl of dNTPs (stock concentration is 15 mM of each dNTP), 0.25 μl (10 units) of RNasin, and 0.5 μl of GSP-RT primer (100 ng/μl). Heat 1 μg of poly(A)$^+$ RNA or 5 μg of total RNA in 14 μl of water at 80°C for 3 min and cool rapidly on ice. Add to reverse transcription components. Add 1 μl (200 units) of MMLV reverse transcriptase, and incubate for 2 hr at 37°C. Dilute the reaction mixture to 1 ml with TE (10 mM Tris-HCl, pH 7.5/1 mM EDTA) and store at 4°C ("5'-end cDNA pool-1").

Comments. Many of the remarks made above in the section on reverse transcribing 3'-end partial cDNAs are also relevant here and should be noted. There is, however, one major difference. The efficiency of cDNA extension is now critically important, since each specific cDNA, no matter how short, is subsequently tailed and becomes a suitable template for amplification. Thus, the PCR products eventually generated directly reflect the quality of the reverse transcription reaction. Extension can be maximized by using clean, intact RNA, by selecting the primer for reverse transcription to be near the 5'-end of region of known sequence, and by using heat-stable reverse transcriptase at elevated temperatures or a combination of MMLV and heat-stable reverse transcriptase at multiple temperatures. Synthesis of cDNAs at elevated temperatures diminishes the amount of secondary structure encountered on GC-rich regions of the mRNA.

Step 2. Appending a Poly(A) Tail to First-Strand cDNA Products

Procedure. Remove excess primer using Microcon-100 spin filters (Amicon Corp.) or an equivalent product, following the manufacturer's instructions. Wash the material by spin filtration twice more using TE. The final volume recovered should not exceed 10 μl.

Add 4 μl 5× tailing buffer (125 mM Tris-HCl, pH 6.6, 1 M Kcacodylate, and 1250 μg/ml BSA), 1.2 μl 25 mM CoCl$_2$, 4 μl 1 mM dATP, and 10 U TdT. Incubate 5 min at 37°C and 5 min at 65°C. Dilute to 500 μl with TE ("5'-end cDNA pool-2").

Comments. To attach a known sequence to the 5'-end of the first strand cDNA, a homopolymeric tail is appended using TdT. We prefer appending poly(A) tails rather than poly(C) tails for several reasons. First, the 3'-end strategy is based on the naturally occurring poly(A) tail; thus the same adapter primers can be used for both ends, decreasing variability in the protocol and cost. Second, since A : T binding is weaker than G : C binding, longer stretches of A residues ($\sim 2\times$) are required before the oligo(dT)-tailed Q$_T$ primer will bind to an internal site and truncate the amplification product. Third, vertebrate coding sequences and 5' untranslated regions tend to be biased toward G/C residues; thus, use of a poly(A) tail further decreases the likelihood of inappropriate truncation. However, the amplification may work best if the products are tailed with C residues and amplified with a hybrid G : I tail, as described in Figure 2.3.

Unlike many other situations in which homopolymeric tails are appended, the actual length of the tail added here is unimportant, as long as it exceeds 17 nucleotides. This is because although the oligo(dT)-tailed primers subsequently bind all along the length of the appended poly(A) tail, only the innermost one becomes incorporated into the amplification product, and, consequently, the remainder of the poly(A) tail is lost. The conditions described in the procedure above result in the addition of 30–400 nucleotides.

Step 3. Amplification

Procedure. First round: Add an aliquot of the "5'-end cDNA pool-2" (1 μl) and primers [25 pmol each of GSP1 and Q$_O$ (shown in Fig. 2.3b), and 2 pmol of Q$_T$] to 50 μl of PCR cocktail [1× *Taq* polymerase buffer (described above), each dNTP at 1.5 mM, and 10% DMSO] in a 0.6-ml microfuge tube and heat in a DNA Thermal Cycler for 5 min at 97°C to denature the first strand products. Cool to 75°C. Add 2.5 U *Taq* polymerase, overlay the mixture with 30 μl of mineral oil (Sigma 400-5; preheat it in the thermal cycler to 75°C), and incubate at the appropriate annealing temperature (48–52°C) for 2 min. Extend the cDNAs at 72°C for 40 min. Carry out 30 cycles of amplification using a step program (94°C, 1 min; 52–60°C, 1 min; 72°C, 3 min), followed by a 15 min final extension at 72°C. Cool to room temperature.

Second round: Dilute a portion of the amplification products from the first round 1 : 20 in TE. Amplify 1 μl of the diluted material with primers GSP2 and Q$_I$ using the procedure described above, but eliminate the initial 2 min annealing step and the 72°C, 40 min extension step.

Comments. Many of the remarks made above in the section on amplifying 3'-end partial cDNAs are also relevant here and should be noted. There is, however, one major difference. The annealing temperature in the first step (48–52°C) is lower than that used in successive cycles (52–60°C). This is because cDNA synthesis during the first round depends on the interaction of the appended poly(A) tail and the oligo(dT)-tailed Q_T primer, whereas in all subsequent rounds, amplification can proceed using the Q_O primer which is composed of ~60% GC and which can anneal at a much higher temperature to its complementary target. This part of the cycle program should be adjusted if a hybrid G:I primer is used with a poly(C) tail.

Analysis of Amplification Products during Execution of the RACE Protocol

The production of specific partial cDNAs by the RACE protocol is assessed using Southern blot hybridization analysis. After the second set of amplification cycles, the first and second set reaction products are electrophoresed in a 1% agarose gel, stained with ethidium bromide (EtBr), denatured, and transferred to nylon membrane. After hybridization with a labeled oligomer or gene fragment derived from a region contained within the amplified fragment (e.g., GSP-Hyb/Seq in Fig. 2.3a and b), gene-specific partial cDNA ends should be detected easily. Yields of the desired product relative to nonspecific amplified cDNA in the first round products should vary from <1% of the amplified material to nearly 100%, depending largely on the stringency of the amplification reaction, the amplification efficiency of the specific cDNA end, and the relative abundance of the specific transcript within the mRNA source. In the second set of amplification cycles, ~100% of the cDNA detected by EtBr staining should represent specific product. If specific hybridization is not observed, then trouble shooting steps should be initiated.

Information gained from this analysis should be used to optimize the RACE procedure. If low yields of specific product are observed because nonspecific products are being amplified efficiently, then annealing temperatures can be raised gradually (~2°C at a time) and sequentially in each stage of the procedure until nonspecific products, and almost until specific products, are no longer observed. Optimizing the annealing temperature is also indicated if multiple species of specific products are observed which could indicate that truncation of specific products is occurring. If multiple species of specific products are observed after the reverse transcription and amplification reactions have been fully optimized, then the possibility should be entertained that alternate splicing or promoter use is occurring. If a nearly continuous smear of specific products is observed up to a specific size limit after 5'-end amplification, this suggests that polymerase pausing occurred during the reverse transcription step. To obtain nearly full length cDNA ends, the amplification mixture should be electrophoresed and the longest products recovered by gel isolation. An aliquot of this material can then be reamplified for a limited number of cycles.

Further Analysis and Use of RACE Products

Cloning. RACE products can be cloned like any other PCR products. To assist in this step, the Q_I primer encodes *Hind*III, *Sst*I, and *Xho*I restriction enzyme sites. Products can be efficiently cloned into vectors that have been double-cut with one of these enzymes and with a blunt-cutting enzyme such as *Sma*I. If clones are not obtained, determine whether the restriction enzyme chosen is cutting the amplified gene fragment a second time, at some internal location in the new and unknown sequence.

Sequencing. RACE products can be sequenced directly using a variety of protocols, including cycle sequencing, from the end at which the gene-specific primers are located. Note that the products cannot be sequenced without subcloning using the Q_I primer at the unknown end, since individual cDNAs contain different numbers of A residues in their poly(A) tails and, as a consequence, the sequencing ladder falls out of register after reading through the tail. 3'-end products can be sequenced from their unknown end using the following set of primers (TTTTTTTTT TTTTTTTTA, TTTTTTTTTTTTTTTTTG, TTTTTTTTTTTTTTTTTTC). The non-T nucleotide at the 3'-end of the primer forces the appropriate primer to bind to the inner end of the poly(A) tail (Thweatt et al., 1990). The other two primers do not participate in the sequencing reaction. Individual cDNA ends, once cloned into a plasmid vector, can be sequenced from either end using gene-specific or vector primers.

Hybridization Probes. RACE products are generally pure enough that they can be used as probes for RNA and DNA blot analyses. It should be kept in mind that small amounts of contaminating nonspecific cDNAs will always be present. It is also possible to include a T_7 RNA polymerase promoter in one or both primer sequences and to use the RACE products in *in vitro* transcription reactions to produce RNA probes (Frohman and Martin, 1989). Primers encoding the T_7 RNA poly-

merase promoter sequence do not appear to function as amplification primers as efficiently as the ones listed in the legend to Figure 2.3 (personal observation). Thus, the T_7 RNA polymerase promoter sequence should not be incorporated into RACE primers as a general rule.

Construction of Full Length cDNAs. It is possible to use the RACE protocol to create overlapping 5'- and 3'-cDNA ends that can later, through judicious choice of restriction enzyme sites, be joined together through subcloning to form a full length cDNA. It is also possible to use the sequence information gained from acquisition of the 5'- and 3'-cDNA ends to make new primers representing the extreme 5'- and 3'-ends of the cDNA, and to employ them to amplify a *de novo* copy of a full length cDNA directly from the "3'-end cDNA pool." Despite the added expense of making two more primers, there are several reasons why the second approach is preferred.

First, a relatively high error rate is associated with the PCR conditions for which efficient RACE amplification takes place, and numerous clones may have to be sequenced to identify one without mutations. In contrast, two specific primers from the extreme ends of the cDNA can be used under inefficient but low-error rate conditions (Eckert and Kunkel, 1990) for a minimum of cycles to amplify a new cDNA that is likely to be free of mutations. Second, convenient restriction sites are often not available, thus making the subcloning project difficult. Third, by using the second approach, the synthetic poly(A) tail can be removed from the 5'-end of the cDNA. Homopolymer tails appended to the 5'-end of cDNAs have in some cases been reported to inhibit translation. Finally, if alternate promoters, splicing, and polyadenylation signal sequences are being used and result in multiple 5'- and 3'-ends, it is possible that one might join two cDNA halves that are never actually found together *in vivo*. Employing primers from the extreme ends of the cDNA as described confirms that the resulting amplified cDNA represents an mRNA actually present in the starting population.

Trouble-Shooting and Controls

Problems with Reverse Transcription

1. *Damaged RNA.* Electrophorese RNA in 1% formaldehyde mini-gel and examine integrity of the 18 S and 28 S ribosomal bands. Discard the RNA preparation if ribosomal bands are not sharp.
2. *Contaminants.* Ensure that the RNA preparation is free of agents that inhibit reverse transcription, e.g., LiCl and SDS (see Sambrook et al., 1989) regarding the optimization of reverse transcription reactions).
3. *Bad Reagents.* To monitor reverse transcription of the RNA, add 20 μCi of [^{32}P]dCTP to the reaction, separate newly created cDNAs using gel electrophoresis, wrap the gel in saran wrap, and expose it to X-ray film. Accurate estimates of cDNA size can best be determined using alkaline agarose gels, but a simple 1% agarose mini-gel will suffice to confirm that reverse transcription took place and that cDNAs of reasonable length were generated. Note that adding [^{32}P]dCTP to the reverse transcription reaction results in the detection of cDNAs synthesized both through the specific priming of mRNA and through RNA self-priming. When a gene-specific primer is used to prime transcription (5'-end RACE) or when total RNA is used as a template, the majority of the labeled cDNA will actually have been generated from RNA self-priming. To monitor extension of the primer used for reverse transcription, label the primer using T_4 DNA kinase and [γ-^{32}P]ATP prior to reverse transcription. Much longer exposure times will be required to detect the labeled primer-extension products than when [^{32}P]dCTP is added to the reaction.

    To monitor reverse transcription of the gene of interest, one may attempt to amplify an internal fragment of the gene containing a region derived from two or more exons, if sufficient sequence information is available.

Problems with Tailing

1. *Bad Reagents.* Tail 100 ng of a DNA fragment of approximately 100–300 bp in length for 30 min. In addition, mock tail the same fragment (add everything but the TdT). Run both samples in a 1% agarose minigel. The mock-tailed fragment should run as a tight band. The tailed fragment should have increased in size by 20–200 bp and should appear to run as a diffuse band that trails off into higher molecular weight products. If this is not observed, replace reagents.
2. Mock tail 25% of the cDNA pool (add everything but the TdT). Dilute to the same final concentration as the tailed cDNA pool. This serves two purposes. First, while amplification products will be observed using both tailed and untailed cDNA templates, the actual pattern of bands observed should be different. In general, discrete bands are observed using untailed templates after the first set of cycles, and a broad smear of amplified cDNA accompanied by some individual bands is typically observed using tailed templates. If the two samples appear different, this confirms that tailing took place and that the oligo(dT)-tailed Q_T primer is annealing effectively to the tailed cDNA during PCR. Second, observing specific products in the tailed amplification mixture that are not present in the untailed amplification mixture indicates that these products are being synthesized off the end of an A-tailed cDNA template, rather than by annealing of the dT-tailed primer to an A-rich sequence in or near the gene of interest.

Problems with Amplification

1. *No Product.* If no products are observed for the first set of amplifications after 30 cycles, add fresh *Taq* polymerase and carry out an additional 15 rounds of amplification (extra enzyme is not necessary if the entire set of 45 cycles is carried out without interruption at cycle 30). Product is always observed after a total of 45 cycles if efficient amplification is taking place. If no product is observed, carry out a PCR reaction using control templates and primers to ensure the integrity of the reagents.

2. *Smeared Product from the Bottom of the Gel to the Loading Well.* Too many cycles, or too much starting material.

3. *Nonspecific Amplification, But No Specific Amplification.* Check sequence of cDNA and primers. If all are correct, examine primers (using computer program) for secondary structure and self-annealing problems. Consider ordering new primers. Determine whether too much template is being added, or if the choice of annealing temperatures could be improved.

   Alternatively, secondary structure in the template may be blocking amplification. Consider adding formamide (Sarker et al., 1990) or ^{7}aza-GTP (in a 1:3 ratio with dGTP) to the reaction to assist polymerization. ^{7}aza-GTP can also be added to the reverse transcription reaction.

4. *The Last Few bp of the 5'-End Sequence Do Not Match the Corresponding Genomic Sequence.* Be aware that reverse transcriptase can add on a few extra template-independent nucleotides.

5. *Inappropriate Templates.* To determine whether the amplification products observed are being generated from cDNA or whether they derive from residual genomic DNA or contaminating plasmids, pretreat an aliquot of the RNA with RNase A.

Conclusions for RACE

The RACE protocol offers several advantages over conventional library screening to obtain additional sequence for cDNAs already partially cloned. RACE is cheaper, much faster, requires very small amounts of primary material, and provides rapid feedback on the generation of the desired product. Information regarding alternate promoters, splicing, and polyadenylation signal sequences can be obtained and a judicious choice of primers (e.g., within an alternately spliced exon) can be used to amplify a subpopulation of cDNAs from a gene for which the transcription pattern is complex. Furthermore, differentially spiced or initiated transcripts can be separated by electrophoresis and cloned separately, and essentially unlimited numbers of independent clones

can be generated to examine rare events. Finally, for 5'-end amplification, the ability of reverse transcriptase to extend cDNAs all the way to the ends of the mRNAs is greatly increased since a primer extension library is created instead of a general purpose one.

A number of modifications of the RACE protocol have been developed. It has been suggested that ligation of oligonucleotides to first strand cDNA (Dumas et al., 1991) or linkers to double-stranded cDNA (Ko et al., 1990) provides an alternative to appending a poly(A) tail to cDNA ends produced in the 5' amplification procedure. The use of a 3'-end reverse transcription primer terminating in random nucleotides instead of oligo(dT) has also been suggested to be of use when the poly(A) tail is too far away from the region of sequence already known to be amplified in a single RACE step (Fritz et al., 1991). It is probable that these and future modifications will continue to increase the utility of the RACE protocol for cDNA cloning.

Amplifying and Cloning Libraries of Fragments

A number of approaches have been described to use PCR to amplify cDNA or genomic libraries, using a universal primer that binds to both ends of the DNA templates (Kalman et al., 1990; Ko et al., 1990), or using different primers to bind to each end (Kaiser, 1990). The experimental approaches differ significantly, and for that reason several references, but no specific protocols, are presented here.

The advantages of PCR-created libraries are that they can be prepared rapidly using little starting material. This is particularly important when it is not practical to attempt to collect sufficient poly(A)$^+$ RNA to create a standard library. As a result, very restricted tissue-specific or subtracted libraries can be prepared (Hla et al., 1990; Lebeau et al., 1991; Swaroop et al., 1991). In addition, PCR can be used to "normalize" or "equalize" cDNA libraries, meaning that the frequency of individual cDNA species (such as actin and rare messages) can be adjusted until they are all equal, making it easier to find novel messages in a nonsubtracted population (Ko, 1990; Patanjali et al., 1991).

The disadvantage of a PCR library is that of unequal representation: Different DNA templates amplify with different efficiencies; thus, after 30–40 rounds of amplification, DNA or cDNA fragments that were initially present in equal quantity may now differ by several orders of magnitude in their relative concentrations. A number of approaches have been described to minimize this problem. First, the amplification should be carried out for as few rounds as possible. Second, extension times should be increased up to as much as 7 min per cycle to allow all molecules sufficient time to become fully extended (Ko et al., 1990). Third, the amplification should be carried out under optimal conditions (e.g., using the high nucleotide, DMSO containing buffer described in the beginning of the chapter) to avoid selective enrichment for DNA fragments that amplify efficiently under suboptimal conditions. Fourth (optional), ^{7}aza-GTP should be added to the nucleotide mixture in a 1:3 ratio with dGTP to increase the efficiency of amplification of GC-rich sequences.

With all of these caveats in mind, PCR-generated libraries make possible a wide range of experiments that can be approached from no other direction, and are invaluable for many fields.

References

Chomczynski P, Sacchi N (1987): Single step method of RNA isolation by acid guanidinium thyocyanate-phenol-chloroform extraction. *Anal Biochem* 162:156.

Coleclough C (1987): Use of primer-restriction end adapters in cDNA cloning. *Methods Enzymol* 154:64.

Crowe JS, Cooper HJ, Smith MA, Sims MJ, Parker D, Gewert D (1991): Improved cloning efficiency of polymerase chain reaction (PCR) products after proteinase K digestion. *Nucl Acids Res* 19:184.

Dumas JB, Edwards M, Delort J, Mallet J (1991): Oligodeoxyribonucleotide ligation to single-stranded cDNAs: A new tool for cloning 5' ends

of mRNAs and for constructing cDNA libraries by *in vitro* amplification. *Nucl Acids Res* 19:5227.

Eckert KA, Kunkel TA (1990): High fidelity DNA synthesis by the *Thermus aquaticus* DNA polymerase. *Nucl Acids Res* 18:3739.

Fritz JD, Greaser ML, Wolff JA (1991): A novel 3' extension technique using random primers in RNA-PCR. *Nucl Acids Res* 19:3747.

Frohman MA (1993): Rapid amplification of cDNA for generation of full-length cDNA ends: Thermal RACE. *Methods in Enzymology* 218:340–356.

Frohman MA, Martin GR (1989): Rapid amplification of cDNA ends using nested primers. *Technique* 1:165.

Frohman MA, Dush MK, Martin GR (1988): Rapid production of full-length cDNAs from rare transcripts by amplification using a single gene-specific oligonucleotide primer. *Proc Natl Acad Sci USA* 85:8998.

Hla T, Maciag T (1990): Isolation of immediate-early differentiation mRNAs by enzymatic amplification of subtracted cDNA from human endothelial cells. *Biochem Biophys Res Commun* 167:637–643.

Kaiser K (1990): New directions in cDNA cloning: 2. Towards a library from a single cell. *Technique* 2:51–64.

Kalman M, Kalman ET, Cashel M (1990): Polymerase chain reaction (PCR) amplification with a single specific primer. *Biochem Biophys Res Commun* 167:504–506.

Ko MSH (1990): An 'equalized cDNA library' by the reassociation of short double-stranded cDNAs. *Nucl Acids Res* 18:5706+.

Ko MSH, Ko SBH, Takahashi N, Nishiguchi K, Abe K (1990): Unbiased amplification of a highly complex mixture of DNA fragments by 'lone linker'-tagged PCR. *Nucl Acids Res* 18:4293–4294.

Lebeau M-C, Alvarez-Bolado G, Wahli W, Catsicas S (1991): PCR driven DNA-DNA competitive hybridization: A new method for sensitive differential cloning. *Nucl Acids Res* 19:4778.

Loh EL, Elliott JF, Cwirla S, Lanier LL, Davis MM (1989): Polymerase chain reaction with single sided specificity: Analysis of T cell receptor delta chain. *Science* 243:217.

Patanjali SR, Parimoo S, Weissman SM (1991): Construction of a uniform-abundance (normalized) cDNA library. *Proc Natl Acad Sci USA* 88:1943–1947.

Sambrook J, Fritsch EF, Maniatis T (1989): *Molecular Cloning: A Laboratory Manual*, 2nd ed. Cold Spring Harbor, NY: Cold Spring Harbor Laboratory.

Sarker G, Kapelner S, Sommer SS (1990): Formamide can dramatically improve the specificity of PCR. *Nucl Acids Res* 18:7465.

Schuster DM, Buchman GW, Rastchian A (1992): A simple and efficient method for amplification of cDNA ends using 5' RACE. *Focus* 14:46–52.

Stoker AW (1990): Cloning of PCR products after defined cohesive termini are created with T4 DNA polymerase. *Nucl Acids Res* 18:4290.

Swaroop A, Xu J, Agarwal N, Weissman SM (1991): A simple and efficient cDNA library subtraction procedure: Isolation of human retina-specific cDNA clones. *Nucl Acids Res* 19:1954.

Thweatt RS, Goldstein S, Reis RJS (1990): A universal primer mixture for sequence determination at the 3' ends of cDNAs. *Anal Biochem* 190:314.

Welsh J, Liu J-P, Efstratiadis A (1990): Cloning of PCR-amplified total cDNA: Construction of a mouse oocyte cDNA library. *GATA* 7:5–17.

Wickens M, Stephenson P (1984): Role of the conserved AAUAAA sequence: Four AAUAAA point mutants prevent mRNA 3' end formation. *Science* 226:1045.

3

Optimization of Multiplex PCRs

Jeffrey S. Chamberlain and Joel R. Chamberlain

Introduction

The development of the polymerase chain reaction (PCR) has enabled rapid and efficient analysis of specific DNA sequences (Mullis and Faloona, 1987). Most PCR strategies are designed to amplify one or more target sequences with a single set of oligonucleotide primers. However, many experimental approaches require the analysis of a variety of DNA sequences, which necessitates that multiple PCRs be performed on the same or related DNA templates. Considerable savings of time and effort can be achieved by simultaneously amplifying multiple sequences in a single reaction, a process referred to as multiplex PCR (Chamberlain et al., 1988, 1989).

Theoretical considerations suggest that multiplex PCR should display nearly the same degree of specificity and efficiency as a single target reaction. The specificity of PCR amplification results from the proximity and relative orientation of sequences within a complex template that anneal with a pair of oligonucleotide primers (Mullis, 1992). The increased number of primer pairs used in a multiplex PCR increases the chance of obtaining spurious am-

plification products. However this problem generally can be overcome by replacement of any primer that generates an unwanted product. As a result, highly specific multiplex PCRs can be developed that enable different sequences to be amplified using mixtures of primer pairs.

Optimization of a PCR to produce large quantities of a single, specific amplification product often requires testing a variety of reaction conditions. Establishing conditions that enable amplification of multiple targets using mixtures of primers can require a proportionately greater effort. Multiplex PCRs require that primers lead to amplification of unique regions of DNA, both in individual pairs and in combinations of many primers, under a single set of reaction conditions. In addition, methods must be available for the analysis of each individual amplification product (amplicon) from within the mixture of all the products. While there is no clear theoretical limit to the number of sequences that can be amplified simultaneously, the constraints on establishing conditions for specific and interpretable reactions generally limit the useful number of target sequences. In many cases PCR primer pairs retain their target specificity when com-

The Polymerase Chain Reaction
K.B. Mullis, F. Ferré, R.A. Gibbs, editors
© 1994 Birkhäuser Boston

bined into a single reaction using the amplification conditions established for the individual pairs. Unfortunately, the development of an efficient multiplex PCR usually requires strategic planning and multiple attempts to optimize reaction conditions. This chapter describes a variety of parameters that we have found to affect the reliability and interpretability of multiplex PCRs. Many of these variables were identified while developing a reaction to amplify nine segments of the human dystrophin gene (Chamberlain et al., 1988, 1989). Several examples are described to illustrate these principles, and we provide a general strategy for developing future reactions.

matic DNA sequencer. The advantage of this approach is that four separate fluorescent dyes can be used to label PCR products. The software developed by Applied Biosystems can resolve fragments that overlap in size as long as separate dyes were used to label each product (Ziegle et al., 1992).

An additional spacing problem can result from the proximity of the amplificaton targets. Our experiences with multiplex PCR have been limited to coamplification of targets separated by at least several kilobases of DNA. Overlapping amplicons should result in amplification of nested products, rather than the intended products, and related problems could be encountered with closely spaced amplicons.

Basic Considerations

Establishing efficient multiplex amplifications is simplified by the availability, in advance, of sequence data flanking each of the PCR targets. While it is possible to add primer pairs to existing reactions as new sequence data become available, choosing all primer binding sites in advance provides greater flexibility in designing optimal primer combinations. The greater the available sequence data at each target region, the easier it is to design primer pairs that display similar annealing temperatures. Longer sequences also provide increased flexibility in designing resolvable target amplicons. We have generally resolved amplicons by size differences on agarose gels. Greater resolution is obtained with acrylamide gels, but these require more effort for analysis. Identifying suitable primer pair binding regions in a short DNA sequence sometimes can be difficult, particularly from regions rich in the bases A and T. While computer programs such as "PRIMER" (available from Eric S. Lander) can simplify this problem, one must be able to identify primer binding sites that generate amplification products that are resolvable by size from the other reaction products. Spacing problems can be overcome by using fluorescently labeled primers (Chamberlain et al., 1992a,b; Clemens et al., 1992), but this approach assumes one has access to an auto-

Primers

The key to successful PCRs of any type lies in the design of appropriate primers. Ideally, all the primers in a multiplex reaction should enable identical amplification efficiencies for each amplicon. While it is difficult to predict the efficiency that any given primer pair will display, oligonucleotides with nearly identical optimum annealing temperatures should work under fairly similar conditions if they anneal with single copy sequences.

Similar annealing temperatures can be achieved by designing primers that are the same length and display not only the same G/C base content but also a similar distribution of G and C bases within their length. We have achieved the best results using primers with a G/C base composition near 50% and with a fairly even distribution of G/C bases versus A/T bases. Primers that anneal with sequences displaying lower G/C contents can be compensated for by an increase in length. The 3'-end of a primer is more important in determining the annealing temperature than the 5'-end, and thus a primer rich in G/C content at the 3'-end often can be made shorter than those with a more even distribution of bases. Primers should not display significant homology either internally or to one another. We generally use primers 25 bases in length.

Primer concentration is a critical parameter for successful multiplex PCR. If all the primers in a reaction anneal with equal efficiencies they can generally be used at the same concentration. This concentration should be empirically determined for each type of reaction. Figure 3.1 displays the results obtained by using two different primer concentrations in a multiplex PCR. In this experiment 18 primers were combined to amplify nine exons of the human dystrophin gene. Reactions containing 0.5 μM of each primer produce similar ratios of all nine amplification products. However, increasing the concentration of each primer to 1 μM leads to the generation of several artifacts. An extra band at approximately 1.2 kb is produced, there is a considerable increase in primer artifacts, and the relative ratio of the amplified exons is altered.

Enzyme Concentration

Multiplex PCR can lead to a greater total concentration of amplification products than is obtained with a single target reaction. The efficiency of a typical PCR is limited in higher cycle numbers by the rate at which amplified fragments anneal with each other rather than the primers. In contrast, we have observed that multiplex reactions can produce such large amounts of product that amplification efficiency becomes limited by the kinetics of polymerase binding to templates. This can lead to distortions in the relative amplification efficiency of individual amplicons, presumably due to differences in the relative efficiency of primer/template annealing. Thus in later stages of amplification if enzyme concentration becomes rate limiting, the amplicons that most efficiently anneal with a primer will preferentially bind free enzyme and will be amplified to a greater degree than the other amplicons in a reaction.

To compensate for problems that may arise from amplifying microgram quantities of multiple fragments we alter the polymerase concentration and lengthen the polymerase exten-

sion times for PCR cycles. Both of these changes increase the probability that each primer/template hybrid can be extended by the polymerase. For the nine-plex dystrophin gene PCR we achieved the best results using 5 units of Taq polymerase per 50 μl reaction, with a 4 min extension time (Chamberlain et al., 1989). Each of these parameters is four to five times greater than is required to amplify any one of the nine amplicons in the reaction. Optimal enzyme consideration and extension time are also dependent on the total number of PCR cycles (see below).

Buffer Composition

Most PCRs are performed with a standard buffer composed of 1.5 mM Mg^{2+}, 50 mM Tris, and 50 mM KCl (Cetus buffer). However, many of the early PCR protocols used a buffer with greater Mg^{2+} concentrations (>5 mM) and 10% dimethyl sulfoxide (DMSO) (Kogan et al., 1987). The original DMSO buffer also called for the use of higher Mg^{2+} concentrations, presumably to counterbalance the elevated levels of dNTPs. The DMSO acts to lower the melting temperature of the primers, in a similar manner to that of formamide in hybridizations. For reasons that are unclear, we have always been able to generate more specific multiplex amplification reactions in the DMSO buffer than in the Cetus buffer, and we thus routinely prepare both buffers in our lab. At least three examples of multiplex PCR in the DMSO buffer have been reported (Chamberlain et al., 1988; Ballabio et al., 1990; Gibbs et al., 1990).

A number of publications describe the effect of various Mg^{2+} concentrations on the specificity of PCR primers (e.g., Saiki, 1989). Some labs routinely test each new primer pair under a variety of magnesium concentrations prior to routine use. In our experience such tests rarely lead to a significantly better PCR, and primers that do not work under standard conditions are best replaced. This is particularly true for multiplex PCRs, where all the primer pairs must work under identical reaction conditions. When considering the amount

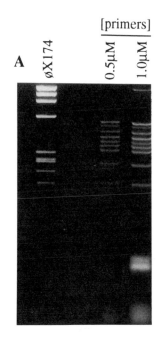

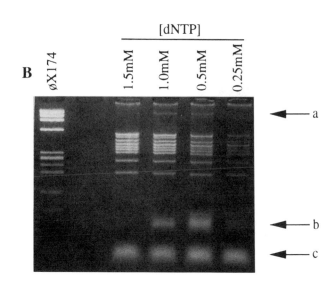

FIGURE 3.1. Effect of nucleotide and primer concentrations on multiplex PCR. A human genomic DNA sample was amplified using a mixture of 18 primers for nine exons of the dystrophin gene. Reactions contained 250 ng genomic DNA, and 5 units *Thermus aquaticus* (*Taq*) polymerase, in a buffer of 16 mM (NH$_4$)$_2$SO$_4$, 65 mM Tris-HCl, pH 8.3, 10 mM 2-mercaptoethanol, 0.1 mg/ml bovine serum albumin, 7 μM EDTA, and 10% dimethyl sulfoxide. Amplification conditions were 94°C for 5 min, followed by 23 cycles of 94°C for 30 sec, 53°C for 30 sec, and 65°C for 4 min. A final extension at 65°C for 5 min was used. Primer sequences and exon locations have been described elsewhere (Chamberlain et al., 1989). (**A**) Amplification with 0.5 or 1.0 μM of each primer [1.5 mM each deoxynucleotide triphosphate (dNTPs)]. (**B**) Reactions were performed as described in (**A**) except that primers were used at 0.5 μM each, and various concentrations of dNTPs were tested. Lower dNTP concentrations result in a loss of specificity (band a), an increase in primer artifacts (b), and a distortion in the relative yield of the amplicons. Primers migrate at position c. ϕX174, *Hae*III-digested ϕX174 DNA.

of Mg^{2+} to add to a reaction, it is important to keep in mind that a balance must be achieved between the total Mg^{2+} and dNTP concentrations. To optimize the buffer concentration of multiplex PCRs we performed a series of titrations of the enzyme and primer concentrations (described above), and then titrated the Mg^{2+} and dNTPs levels. Optimal results were obtained with 6.7 mM Mg^{2+}, and this level was used to determine the optimal dNTPs concentration.

Figure 3.1B illustrates the effect of four different levels of dNTPs on multiplex PCR. Optimal amplification was produced with 1.5 mM dNTPs, while lower levels resulted in a de-crease in the efficiency and specificity of amplification. Lower levels of dNTPs also led to inconsistent amplification results, and frequently the reactions produced only a subset of the targeted amplicons. Note that reduction of the dNTP concentrations can lead to a considerable increase in the formation of primer artifacts (Fig. 3.1B), a likely consequence of the excess free Mg^{2+} resulting from the lowered dNTP concentration. It is possible that lowered dNTP concentrations could be used in conjunction with alternate Mg^{2+} chelators such as EDTA, but this has not been attempted. If three of the dNTPs are maintained at a high level the fourth dNTP can be lowered

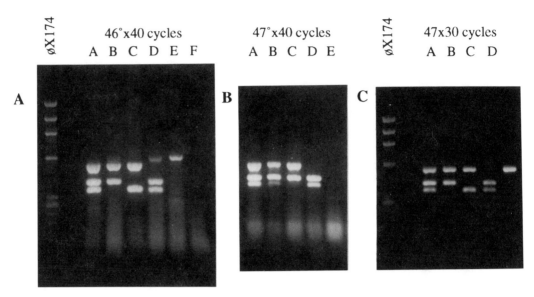

FIGURE 3.2. Effect of annealing temperature and cycle number on multiplex PCR. Three exons of the human dystrophin gene were coamplified essentially as described in the legend to Figure 3.1. (A) Amplification was performed with a 46°C annealing temperature for 40 cycles. A nonspecific amplification product is observed in lanes B, D, and E. A–E are separate template DNAs from DMD patients with various intragenic deletions. The sample in lane A is not deleted for these regions of the gene, that in lane E is deleted for the entire dystrophin locus. F is a control (no template). (B) Amplification with a 47°C annealing temperature for 40 cycles. The nonspecific band observed in (A) is lost. Lanes A and E are amplification products from the same samples as in lanes A and E from (A); the other lanes contain different samples. (C) Amplification at 47°C for 30 cycles. The reactions are specific and there is a lower background. The samples in lanes A–D correspond to those in (A); lane E contains a separate sample.

to approximately 0.1 mM without dramatically affecting the reaction, which facilitates adding radioactive tracers (not shown).

Cycle Parameters

The cycle conditions used for multiplex PCR will dramatically affect the reliability of the reactions. As with any PCR, the most important cycle parameter is the annealing temperature. Figure 3.2A illustrates the effect that even a slight change in annealing temperature can have on a multiplex reaction. In this example, primers for three exons of the dystrophin gene were amplified for 40 cycles at an annealing temperature of 46°C. Two undesirable consequences resulted from these cycle conditions. First, an extra band was amplified that did not arise from within the dystrophin gene (Fig. 3.2A). Second, large amounts of nonspecific amplification products were obtained that were of lower size than the targeted exons. Figure 3.2B displays the results of a similar experiment in which the annealing temperature was raised by a single degree. The extra band is no longer detected, and there has been a reduction in the amount of low-molecular-weight products. Subsequent experiments indicated that it was unnecessary to perform 40 cycles of PCR. Figure 3.2C displays the results of a similar reaction that was amplified for 30 cycles; fewer low-molecular-weight artifacts were obtained.

The experiments in Figure 3.2 illustrate two important principles. The annealing temperature should be kept as high as possible, and the fewest number of cycles as will permit easy detection of the products should be performed.

As more amplicons were added to the dystrophin multiplex reaction it was necessary to raise the annealing temperature to 53°C. At this temperature nine amplicons were analyzed without production of nonspecific products. A dramatic effect of cycle number on multiplex PCR is illustrated in Figure 3.3. In this experiment various numbers of PCR cycles were performed on a Duchenne muscular dystrophy (DMD) patient DNA sample that had been mixed with increasing amounts of normal control DNA. At low cycle number the deletion in the patient's DNA is evident, even with 10% normal DNA added to the reaction. At higher cycle numbers the ratio of amplified fragments is distorted, and the contaminating fragment approaches the level of some of the patient DNA fragment (Fig. 3.3). This is likely a consequence of the limited amounts of enzyme available for fragment extension at high cycle numbers, as well as the relative annealing efficiency of each of the PCR primers. These results demonstrate that coamplification of multiple DNA targets may not always proceed at an equal efficiency for each amplicon, and that excess cycles of PCR can lead to results that may not be easily intepreted.

Other Considerations

A potential source of problems with multiplex PCR is the relative degree of sequence similarity between amplicons in a reaction. It is important to avoid repetitive DNA sequences in the regions that anneal with primers. Although it is possible to amplify sequences using one unique primer and one primer in an ALU repeat (Economou et al., 1990), such reactions produce a large amount of nonspecific amplification and it is unlikely that they could be incorporated into an efficient multiplex PCR. Repetitive sequences can be avoided by screening the Genbank DNA sequence data base and through the use of primer analysis software such as "PRIMER." Repetitive DNA can be amplified as long as the primers anneal with unique regions of DNA flanking the repeat. Jeffreys et al. (1988) described a multiplex PCR that amplifies six different VNTR se-

quences. This VNTR reaction produces amplified fragments that can be resolved via incorporation of radioactive nucleotides and autoradiography, but resolution is lost at higher cycle numbers thus preventing visualization by staining with ethidium bromide.

Another example of multiplex amplification of repetitive DNA is the analysis of microsatellite repeat polymorphisms (such as $[dC-dA]_n$ repeats) for linkage studies. Several groups have amplified multiple $[dC-dA]_n$ repeats in a single reaction (Weber and May, 1989; Clemens et al., 1992; Ziegle et al., 1992). In our experiences multiplex amplification of $[dC-dA]_n$ repeats is more difficult than for sequences that do not contain repetitive DNA. Many duplex PCRs can be established with little difficulty, but in general the development of reactions to amplify three or more repeats can require considerable effort to optimize reaction conditions. Figure 3.4 displays the results of multiplex PCR of three $[dC-dA]_n$ repeats that map to chromosome 17q. Each of these repeats displays multiple alleles, and the amplicons can be resolved by size and visualized by autoradiography of acrylamide gels. Despite testing a variety of conditions these PCRs always display a few extra bands that are not detected when any of the three primer pairs are used individually. Nonetheless, these extra bands do not comigrate with the targeted amplicons and do not interfere with interpretation of the reaction. It is likely that $[dC-dA]_n$ repeats are difficult to amplify because of the high degree of sequence similarity in each of the amplicons, namely the alternating $[dC-dA]_n$ motif.

Another source of difficulty can arise when trying to amplify sequences that are members of a related gene family or for which one or more pseudogenes are present in the genome of interest. Reactions can be developed for such sequences, but it is important that the primers be designed to anneal with regions that are unique among the related sequences. Ballabio et al. (1990) developed a multiplex PCR that amplified three segments of the human steroid sulfatase (STS) gene. This gene has a Y-linked pseudogene, but the X-linked STS gene was specifically amplified using

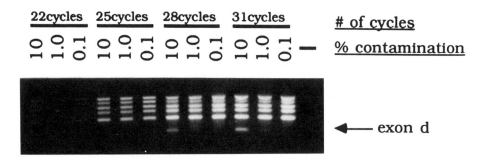

FIGURE 3.3. The effect of cycle number on multiplex PCR. Six exons of the human dystrophin gene were amplified essentially as described in Figure 3.1. The template DNA was deleted for exon d (Chamberlain et al., 1988). Various amounts of normal control (nondeleted) DNA were mixed into the template DNA and amplified for the indicated number of cycles. After 22 cycles a uniform ratio of amplified fragments is observed. By 31 cycles some exons have amplified to a greater degree than others. Reprinted from Chamberlain et al. (1988) with permission of Oxford University Press.

primers that had at least three unique bases at their 3'-end.

In addition to the parameters discussed in the preceding sections, two additional factors could potentially improve the specificity of multiplex PCR reactions that do not work well. Spermidine has been suggested as a potential ingredient to reduce nonspecific amplification in multiplex PCRs, however, we have generally not observed a significant improvement in the quality of reactions containing spermidine. A second factor that is as yet untested is gene 32 protein from *Escherichia coli*. This protein is a single-stranded DNA binding protein that is reported to improve the efficiency of some PCR reactions that produce a large amount of nonspecific amplification. Such a protein may improve the quality of multiplex PCRs as well, but this remains to be determined.

Development of Multiplex PCRs

The combined experiences from a number of labs that have reported successful multiplex PCRs suggest a strategy for the development of future reactions. Multiplex PCRs that amplify two to three sequences simultaneously can often be performed with little or no change in reaction conditions from those used to amplify single sequences. Difficulties generally arise as more primers are added to a reaction. In each case one must decide whether the effort required to develop optimal conditions will be justified in terms of the time that would be required for nonmultiplex amplification of their samples. Each system likely will have an inherent limit on the number of amplicons that can be multiplexed, but this needs to be experimentally determined.

Initially one should check their sequence data with a primer analysis software package to identify sets of primers that display nearly identical annealing temperatures and that will amplify fragments that can be resolved by size. All of the primers should be mixed together at several concentrations between 0.1 and 1 μM, and tested in Cetus PCR buffer as well as in the DMSO buffer using the annealing temperature predicted from the primer program. The buffer that works best can be further optimized by testing a variety of different concentrations of *Taq* polymerase between 1 and 5 units per 50 μl reaction. If nonspecific amplification is observed the annealing temperature should be raised as high as possible until loss of specific amplification is observed. Finally, the polymerase extension time can be extended from 30 sec to 4–5 min if some fragments amplify less well than others. If these conditions fail to produce specific multiplex amplification additional variables involving the primers can be tested. If some amplicons are produced at much greater efficiency than others, it may

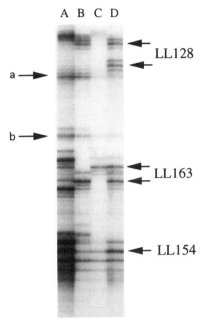

FIGURE 3.4. Three primer pairs for separate [dC-dA]$_n$ repeats isolated from human chromosome 17 were used for multiplex PCR of four unrelated human DNA samples (A–D). Each repeat displays a variety of alleles which can be scored for each locus and used for linkage analysis. The three repeats are LL128 (UM4), LL163 (UM3), and LL154 (UM5). Sample (A) is heterozygous for all three markers; (B) is heterozygous for LL128 and LL154, but homozygous for LL163; (C) is heterozygous for LL128 and homozygous for the other two markers; (D) is homozygous for LL154 and heterozygous for the other two markers. Multiplex PCR of these types of repeats can be difficult to optimize, and spurious amplification products are frequently observed (a and b). The allele sizes are indicated by arrows for sample (D).

sequentially add additional primer pairs to the reactions while optimizing the above mentioned variables for each additional pair. Those pairs that produce nonspecific amplification can then be replaced as needed. Occasionally it may be necessary to replace a primer pair that works well to accommodate the amplification product size of a replacement pair of primers. Both the dystrophin gene and the HPRT gene multiplex PCRs that amplify nine and eight separate sequences (Chamberlain et al., 1992b; Gibbs et al., 1990) were developed using this approach of mixing a variety of primers to find the best initial multiplex conditions, and then optimizing conditions as additional primer pairs were added to the reaction. The most important variable has always been with the primers themselves. The most important reaction parameters have been the annealing temperature, the amount of enzyme, and the polymerase extension time. With the proper combinations of primers and reaction conditions it is likely that many additional multiplex reactions can be developed for the analysis of a variety of different sequences.

Acknowledgments. We thank Drs. Richard Gibbs and C. Thomas Caskey for advice and discussions and for assistance with development of the dystrophin multiplex PCRs. We also thank Virginia Willour for assistance with the microsatellite repeat analysis. J.S.C. is a recipient of a Basil O'Conner Starter Scholar Research Award from The March of Dimes Birth Defects Foundation. Supported by Grants AR40864, HG00209, and DK42718 from the National Institutes of Health.

help to lower the concentration of primers for the amplicons that produce the greatest yields, while raising the concentration of those that produce low yields, within the limits of 0.1–1 μM. If nonspecific amplification products are observed alternate primer pairs should be designed.

An efficient approach to tracing those primer pairs that work poorly is to try combinations of primers representing a subset of the total. By starting with a reaction that uses the largest possible subset of primer pairs, one can

References

Ballabio A, Ranier JE, Chamberlain JS, Zollo M, Caskey CT (1990): Screening for steroid sulfatase (STS) gene deletions via multiplex DNA amplification. *Hum Genet* 84:571–573.

Chamberlain JS, Gibbs RA, Ranier JE, Nguyen PN, Caskey CT (1988): Deletion screening of the Duchenne muscular dystrophy locus via multiplex DNA amplification. *Nucl Acids Res* 16:11141–11156.

Chamberlain JS, Gibbs RA, Ranier JE, Caskey CT (1989): Multiplex PCR for the diagnosis of Duchenne muscular dystrophy. In: *PCR Protocols: A Guide to Methods and Applications*. Innis M, Gelfand D, Sninski J, White T, eds. Orlando: Academic Press, 272–281.

Chamberlain JS, Chamberlain JR, Fenwick RG, Ward PA, Dimnik LS et al. (1992a): Diagnosis of Duchenne and Becker muscular dystrophy by polymerase chain reaction: A multicenter study. *JAMA* 267:2609–2615.

Chamberlain JS, Gibbs RA, Ranier JE, Caskey CT (1992b): Detection of gene deletions using multiplex polymerase chain reactions. In: *Methods in Molecular Biology,* Vol. 9. Mathew C, ed. Clifton, NJ: *Humana Press*, 299–312.

Clemens PR, Fenwick RG, Chamberlain JS, Gibbs TA, de Andrade M et al. (1992): Carrier detection and prenatal diagnosis in Duchenne and Becker muscular dystrophy families, using dinucleotide repeat polymorphisms. *Am J Hum Genet* 49:951–960.

Economou EP, Bergen AW, Warren AC, Antonarakis SE (1990): The polydeoxyadenylate tract of Alu repetitive elements is polymorphic in the human genome. *Proc Natl Acad Sci USA* 87:2951–2954.

Gibbs RA, Nguyen PN, Edwards AO, Civitello A, Caskey CT (1990): Multiplex DNA deletion detection and exon sequencing of the hypoxanthine phosphoribosyltransferase gene in Lesch-Nyhan families. *Genomics* 7:235–244.

Jeffreys AJ, Wilson V, Neumann R, Keyte J (1988): Amplification of human minisatellites by the polymerase chain reaction: towards DNA fingerprinting of single cells. *Nucl Acids Res* 16:10953–10971.

Kogan SC, Doherty M, Gitschier J (1987): An improved method for prenatal diagnosis of genetic diseases by analysis of amplified DNA sequences. Application to hemophilia A. *N Engl J Med* 317:985–990.

Mullis KB (1992): The polymerase chain reaction in an anemic mode: How to avoid cold oligodeoxyribonuclear fusion. *PCR Meth Applic* 1: 1–4.

Mullis KB, Faloona FA (1987): Specific synthesis of DNA in vitro via a polymerase-catalyzed chain reaction. *Methods Enzymol* 155:335–350.

Saiki RK (1989): The design and optimization of the PCR. In: *PCR Technology: Principles and Applications for DNA Amplification*. Erlich HA, ed. New York: Stockton Press, 7–16.

Weber JL, May PE (1989): Abundant class of human DNA polymorphisms which can be typed using the polymerase chain reaction. *Am J Hum Gent* 44:388–396.

Ziegle JS, Su Y, Corcoran P, Nie L, Mayrand E et al. (1992): Application of automated DNA sizing technology for geneotyping microsatellite loci. *Genomics* 14:1026–1031.

4

Preparation of Nucleic Acids for Archival Material

Darryl Shibata

The PCR, with its ability to amplify short fragments of nucleic acids, has greatly extended the types of specimens available for molecular genetic analysis. Specimens can be categorized into essentially three different classes based on the length of time since collection and analysis—fresh, archival, and ancient.

The methods used to prepare nucleic acids for PCR analysis have an additional important criteria that can differ from those of other molecular techniques. The enhanced sensitivity provided by amplification demands rigorous attention to possible cross-contamination between different specimens, PCR products, plasmids, or standards. This is especially important if the target of interest is expected in very low numbers or the DNA from the specimen is severely degraded, since greater amplification efforts are generally required. Therefore, PCR on nucleic acids isolated without careful attention to possible contamination should be attempted with great caution. Ideally, only nucleic acids prepared specifically for PCR should be analyzed. The specimens should be prepared and stored at a site physically separated from areas in which PCR products are manipulated. The DNA should also be prepared such that multiple replicates of independent isolations can be tested for verification. This may entail dividing a single specimen at the time of collection or obtaining multiple independent specimens. In addition, because neither high-molecular-weight nor highly purified nucleic acids are needed for PCR, fast and simple procedures that minimize the chances of specimen contamination are possible.

Estimation of the amount of DNA added to a PCR reaction can be difficult. If the specimen is degraded or present in extremely low amounts, absorbance or fluorometric methods may be misleading. "Unmeasurable" amounts of DNA can be easily detected by PCR and "large" amounts of DNA can produce no signal if it is extensively degraded. If sufficient amounts of DNA are present, the quantity and quality can be estimated after electrophoresis with an ethidium bromide stained 0.7% agarose gel. In many cases, the desired information is the number of target sequences. This can be estimated by using the PCR itself as a sensitive DNA detector. Quantitative PCR or serial dilutions of specimens followed by PCR of various targets allows the estimation of the relative abundance of intact targets both between and within a specimen.

The Polymerase Chain Reaction
K.B. Mullis, F. Ferré, R.A. Gibbs, editors
© 1994 Birkhäuser Boston

Fresh Specimens

DNA and RNA can be prepared from fresh or frozen specimens using traditional standard extraction techniques. However, the relatively large number of steps, large amounts of tissues, and reagents used for these procedures make contamination, especially between specimens, a problem. Therefore, rapid and relatively simple alternative procedures have been developed by many investigators to prepare DNA suitable for PCR analysis.

The ability of PCR to amplify nucleic acids from relatively crude extracts has fostered many types of rapid isolation procedure. These techniques utilize crude lysis (heat, osmotic, freeze–thaw, detergents, enzymatic, etc.) and balance the inherent high sensitivity of PCR with the relative abundance of expected targets. For most PCR protocols, at least 100 and often fewer targets are easily detected. Therefore instead of purifying nucleic acids from possible inhibitors, it is often possible to effectively remove inhibitors by dilution and analyzing small amounts of crude extracts. Alternatively, positive capture of desired cells or organisms prior to lysis, usually by immunological criteria (Jansen et al., 1990), can reduce background and enhance sensitivity.

Perhaps the simplest method of DNA preparation is to boil intact cells (Saiki et al., 1986). This process simultaneously denatures and "purifies" the DNA sufficiently to allow PCR, and illustrates how resilient the reaction can be to extraneous materials. However, if too many cells ($>50,000$) are boiled, inhibition of the PCR (like any enzymatic reaction) can occur. For many specimens, this inhibition can be avoided by adding lesser amounts of the specimen to the PCR. Notable inhibitors of the *Taq* DNA polymerase include red blood cell components and SDS (Gelfand and White, 1990). Other possible inhibitors of the PCR present in added specimens include high salt, chelating agents, too much DNA, and other unknown agents.

Since it is not always possible to predict the presence of potential inhibitors or extensive template degradation, it is prudent to test each DNA sample with primers that can amplify a genomic sequence (of a length similar to the target) to verify that the specimen contains DNA and it is suitable for PCR. A specimen negative by a single pair of target primers may either lack the target or may not be suitable for PCR (false negative). The sensitivity of PCR on crude extracts is often less than on purified nucleic acids secondary to inhibition and the smaller amounts of added templates. This reduced sensitivity, however, is usually sufficient for most applications.

Rapid Methods of DNA Isolation

In general crude extracts from specimens with relatively defined compositions (blood, CSF, buccal smears, colony plaques, etc.) are a more reliable source of PCR templates compared to heterogeneous specimens (urine, cervical swabs, feces, etc.). Nonbloody body fluids with low numbers of cells can be analyzed directly. For instance, cerebral spinal fluid (CSF) is generally obtained in small amounts, contains low numbers of nucleated cells, and can be boiled for 7 min before being added directly to a PCR reaction. Up to 50 μl of CSF can be added to a 100 μl reaction. Similarly, urine can be boiled and then added directly. The variable cellular, inorganic, and organic composition of urine, however, can result in marked inhibition of the PCR. Some of this inhibition has been attributed to high concentrations of urea (Khan et al., 1991). The large numbers of pathogens (such as cytomegalovirus) typically present in positive urine specimens allow the direct assay of small urine volumes (5 μl), which limits the inhibition problems (Demmler et al., 1988).

With the limitations to the boiling of isolated intact cells, a number of other rapid methods have been developed. One general solution is the utilization of PCR buffer (50 mM KCl, 20 mM Tris-Cl, 2.5 mM MgCl$_2$, pH 8.3) without gelatin containing 1% Laureth 12 or 0.5% Tween 20 ["K buffer" (Kawasaki, 1990)] with

100 μg/ml added fresh proteinase K. Cellular material, relatively free of red blood cells (visibly nonbloody), can be incubated at 55°C in this buffer for 1 hr, and then boiled for 5 min to inactivate the proteinase K. Approximately 10 μl, representing up to 100,000 cells equivalents, can be added to a 50–100 μl PCR reaction. Examples of specimens that work well with this procedure are buccal scraps (obtained with a toothpick), Ficoll–Hypaque fractionated mononuclear cells, tissue culture pellets, and small fragments of fresh tissues (such as cryostat single slices of frozen tissues). Extraneous material (Ficoll–Hypaque, OTC, tissue culture media, etc.) should be eliminated prior to the incubation by washing the cells in normal saline or phosphate-buffered saline.

The marked inhibition of the PCR by red blood cells requires steps for their removal or neutralization. A simple method to assay bloody specimens utilizes a styrene divinylbenzene copolymer resin, Chelex 100 (Bio-Rad Laboratories), which chelates divalent ions (Singer-Sam and Tanguary, 1989). A 5% (w/v) Chelex suspension is prepared in sterile distilled water. Whole blood (1–10 μl) is added to 1 ml of distilled water for 15 min at room temperature. The solution is centrifuged (2 min, 12,000 g) and all but 20–50 μl is discarded. Approximately 200 μl of the 5% Chelex suspension is added (with a large bore (1-ml) pipette tip or dropper) and then incubated at 55°C for 30 min. The specimen is then boiled for 7 min and briefly centrifuged. Approximately 5–20 μl is used for a 100 μl PCR reaction (Cetus, 1990).

Archival Specimens

Vast collections of archival specimens have been stored since and before the turn of the century in nonfresh/frozen states. These specimens include museum collections of various species, hospital files of patient specimens, forensic evidence, and generally any cellular specimen of interest. The advantage of utilizing archival specimens is that they provide a unique "window" or molecular "snapshot" of past events.

The majority of human archival specimens are formalin-fixed, paraffin-embedded tissues. Undoubtedly, the majority of individuals (North American industrialized) will have some of their tissues stored in this manner sometime during or after their lifetimes. These fixed tissues are carefully labeled and filed, and can be linked to specific patients and pathology. Since most of these tissues are stored for years, broad retrospective studies of both common and rare diseases are practical. An example is the amplification of HIV provirus from the fixed autopsy tissues of a sailor who died in England in 1959 (Corbitt et al., 1990).

A typical single thin 5- to 10-μm slice (identical in thickness to a section on a microscope slide) usually provides sufficient DNA for 10–50 PCR assays and scores or more of such slices can be obtained from the average block. Therefore, independent replicate sections can be taken to validate a result and ample tissue is available for later studies. In addition, a section can be stained and examined microscopically to estimate the number and types of cells analyzed (Fig. 4.1).

Fresh tissues are placed in 10% buffered neutralized formalin (BNF), dehydrated with xylene (or another suitable agent), and then infiltrated with liquid paraffin. The result is a tissue "sealed" in wax. The formaldehyde molecules rapidly form Schiff bases with the nitrogen atoms in the purine and pyrimidine rings that are readily reversible in aqueous solutions (Goelz et al., 1985; Dubeau et al., 1986; Impraim et al., 1987). Longer fixation times allow the slower progressive accumulation of stable products of the reaction of formaldehyde with the purine and pyrimidine rings (Feldman, 1973). Experimentally, prolonged fixation of the tissue in 10% BNF results in a decreased ability to amplify longer target sequences (Greer et al., 1991). The optimal time of fixation is identical to the period routinely used clinically—3–48 hr. Tissues fixed for longer than 1 week are significantly poorer PCR substrates. Therefore, tissues stored "wet" in formalin solutions are significantly poorer PCR substrates than their paraffin-embedded counterparts. Ironically, some modern fixatives apparently irreversibly dam-

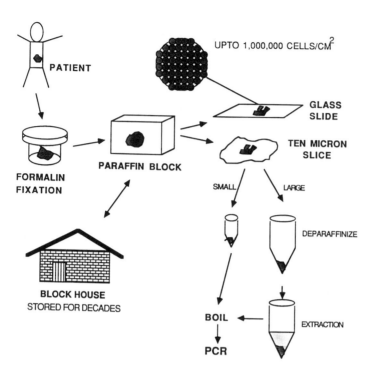

FIGURE 4.1. Processing of fixed tissues.

age DNA even with short fixation times and amplification is generally impossible. Fixatives and their effects on the PCR are listed in Table 4.1. It is noteworthy that fixation continues, usually in BNF ("soak file"), in most automated tissue processors until the unit is actually cycled.

Paraffin blocks greater than 5 years old sometime yield poorer results (Greer et al., 1991) although most older sets of blocks are excellent PCR substrates. Blocks greater than 40 years old have been successfully analyzed (Shibata, 1988b). Fixation conditions are the greater source of DNA degradation compared to the overall age of the block. Unbuffered formalin solutions were commonly used before the 1960s and the acidic conditions present during this type of tissue fixation may have contributed to the greater DNA degradation evident in older blocks.

In general, the efficiency of amplification is less with DNA extracted from fixed tissues compared to conventional high-molecular-weight DNA extracted from fresh tissues, and typically 40 to 50 cycles are necessary. In addi-

tion, higher backgrounds and artifact bands are much more commonly present in the PCR products. Because of these drawbacks, a hybridization step is often useful to increase sensitivity and specificity.

Target size is a critical factor in successfully applying the PCR to DNA extracted from fixed tissues. Since fixation times, type of fixative, age of the block, and type of tissue are factors that may be unknown or are typically not controlled by the investigator, the DNA extracted will be of variable quality. Therefore, a small target is desirable in order to amplify even the most degraded specimens. A target size less than 200 bases can usually be detected from most fixed tissues and, if possible, primers that amplify a shorter segment (less than 100 bases) are desirable. Targets greater than 1000 bases can be amplified from optimally fixed tissues, but, in general, lower degrees of success will be experienced with the longer targets. A genomic primer set to a target of similar length to the desired target should be utilized as an amplification control.

TABLE 4.1. Variables that effect PCR of fixed tissues.

Variable	Optimal	Adequate	Poor
Fixation time	3–24 hr	1–3 days	>7 days
Age of block[a]	Less than 5 years		
Fixative[b]	10% BNF	Carnoy's	Bouin's
	Alcohol	Clarke's	Zenker's
	Acetone	Methacarn	"B5"
	Omnifix	Zamboni's	Decalcifying agents
		Alcoholic-formalin	
		Paraformaldehyde	
Target size	<200 bases	<500 bases	>1000 bases
Type of tissue	Most		Brain[c]

[a]This effect has not been formally determined and is a general impression. However, blocks greater than 40 years old have been successfully analyzed.

[b]See Greer et al. (1991), Rogers et al. (1990), and Ben-Ezra et al. (1991).

[c]Many autopsy brains are fixed for many weeks in 20% formalin in order to allow complete fixation and kill slow viruses. These autopsy brains are generally poor PCR substrates.

Processing of Formalin-Fixed, Paraffin-Embedded Tissues

The microtome area should be clean, isolated from PCR products, and organized. Tubes should be labeled beforehand. The paraffin blocks do not require special precautions as the outer layers will be discarded in the process of producing a flat surface ("facing" the block).

A 5- to 10-μm slice or slices are carefully placed in a sterile 1.5-ml microfuge tube (or a sterile 0.5-ml PCR tube for small sections). One section can be stained to verify the identity of the tissue. A guide to the number of slices is provided in Table 4.2. Of note, this procedure is extremely difficult with gloves and we have found that gloves are not necessary. We use our fingers to place the sections in the tubes, although many other investigators use forceps cleaned by various methods (acid, flame, chemwipes) between specimens. The blade and microtome areas (and our fingers) in

contact with the tissues are cleaned with chemwipes between specimens. To check technique, control blocks can be alternatively cut and then assayed for cross-contamination. For instance, blocks from two unrelated individuals can be alternatively cut and then tested for cross-contamination by PCR of a polymorphic locus. It is important that the sections not be "floated" on a water bath prior to placement in the microfuge tube as water will interfere with the subsequent deparaffinization.

At times it is desirable to select only certain portions of the tissue for analysis. The entire tissue block may be deparaffinized, cut into appropriate sections, and then reembedded separately by a histotechnician. Alternatively, the paraffin block may be scored with a sterile scalpel into the desired quadrants. On sectioning, the desired portions are placed into separate tubes. The skill of the operator determines the precision of the dissection. It is important to verify with stained sections that the desired separations are achieved.

The sections are deparaffinized by adding xylene (or alternatively octane (Wright and Manos, 1990) or histoclear). The section will turn clear and be difficult to see. This is essentially instantaneous with xylene. The tissue is pelleted in a microfuge for 1 min, and the xylene is carefully decanted. The xylene is removed by two washes (as above) with 95–100% ethanol. The tissue will turn white in the

TABLE 4.2. Amounts of tissue for PCR.

Area of section (mm²)	Number of slices	Processing
<1	1–3	"Direct"
1–4	1–3	"Direct or extraction"
>4	1	"Extraction"

ethanol. The section is desiccated under a vacuum until dry.

For small sections (Table 4.2), 20–50 μl of water is added and then the closed microfuge tube is placed in a boiling water bath for 7 min (Shibata et al., 1988a). The tube is cooled on ice and a 50–100 μl final volume PCR is performed on the entire section.

For larger sections (Table 4.2), the amount of DNA or inhibiting factors present is generally too much to be directly assayed by the *Taq* DNA polymerase, although this inhibition was not a major problem using the heat labile Klenow fragment of the *Escherichia coli* DNA polymerase. A DNA extraction solution (100 mM Tris-HCl, 2 mM EDTA, pH 8.0) sufficient to cover the tissue (typically 50–100 μl) is added along with 1–2 μl of proteinase K (20 mg/ml) (Shibata et al., 1989). The desiccated pellet must be disrupted with the pipette tip for rehydration and exposure to the extraction solution. The tissue is incubated at 37°C overnight or at 50°C for 3–4 hr. The tube is boiled for 7 min to inactivate the proteinase K, vortexed for 10–20 sec, and then the residual tissue fragments are pelleted in a microfuge for 1 min. These tubes may be stored (with the residual tissue) at −20 to 4°C for several months to years. Another similar procedure which includes detergents has been described by Wright and Manos (1990).

Additional purification with phenol/chloroform extraction is usually unnecessary and a possible source of contamination. The major cause of failure is the addition of too much of the DNA containing extraction solution to the PCR. The extraction of DNA from formalin-fixed, paraffin-embedded tissues is usually a robust procedure. With optimally fixed tissues, the majority of the DNA can be extracted and amplified. As there are approximately 1,000,000 cells/cm^2 in a single 10-μm-thick slice (assuming the cells are 10 μm in diameter and packed "back to back"), large amounts of DNA can be extracted. This cell density is commonly present in tumors and lymph nodes, with lesser numbers of cells in other tissues. The cell density can be estimated by counting the cells under the microscope. Usually 1–10% of the extraction solution is added to the

PCR. If this amount is unsuccessful, a 10-fold dilution is recommended.

A second major source of failure is the fixative used (see Table 4.1). Unfortunately, little can be done to repair this template damage, although amplification of extremely short targets (less than 100 base pairs) may be possible. In general, a single copy genomic sequence can be easily amplified from greater than 90% of all formalin fixed, paraffin-embedded tissues.

Microscope Slides

DNA can also be extracted from fixed paraffin tissues or cellular smears (such as "PAP" smears) stored on glass slides (Jackson et al., 1989a). The tissue may be stained or unstained. A coverslip may be removed by soaking the entire slide in xylene. This removal may take several days. The tissues are scrapped off the glass slide with a sterile scalpel blade into a 0.5- or 1.5-ml microfuge tube and then processed as above. The tissues in unstained slides are usually infiltrated with paraffin and they must be deparaffinized. This step is unnecessary with stained slides as they have already been deparaffinized. The usual amounts of hematoxylin and eosin dyes do not inhibit the PCR, but can produce a fluorescent smear at about 200–500 base pairs in an agarose gel that may obscure faint PCR product bands.

Unfortunately, the analysis of stained slides usually destroys the only record of the specimen, and a replicate sample for verification of the PCR is therefore not possible. The task of scrapping tissues off slides is difficult and creates numerous small tissue fragments that can be lost or play a role in cross-contamination. For these reasons, it is desirable to use the paraffin block as the DNA source.

RNA in Fixed Tissues

RNA can also be extracted from formalin-fixed, paraffin-embedded tissues (Rupp and Locker, 1988) or glass slide smears (Hanson et al., 1990), and amplified by reverse PCR (Jackson et al., 1989b, 1990; Weizsacker et al., 1991). The RNA isolation is technically more difficult, probably secondary to the ubiquitous presence of RNases, and most studies of fixed tissues have used DNA as the PCR target.

Ancient Specimens

Ancient specimens are the rare and extremely old tissue remnants that have been preserved, usually in haphazard manners. Their rarity precludes specific comments and the reader is referred to Chapter 22 of this volume and an excellent article by Paabo (1989) for specific details. Generally primers that amplify extremely short (less than 100 bp) targets are employed and the PCR products are sequenced to verify the origin of the DNA.

References

Ben-Ezra J, Johnson DA, Rossi J, Cook N, Wu A (1991): Effect of fixation on the amplification of nucleic acids from paraffin-embedded material by the polymerase chain reaction. *J Histochem Cytochem* 39:351–354.

Cetus Corporation (1990): *Amplitype User Guide, Version 2*, 3-14-15.

Corbitt G, Bailey AS, Williams G (1990): HIV infection in Manchester, 1959. *Lancet* 336:51.

Demmler GJ, Buffone GJ, Schimbor CM, May RA (1988): Detection of cytomegalovirus in urine from newborns using polymerase chain reaction DNA amplification. *J Infect Dis* 158:1177–1184.

Dubeau L, Chandler LA, Gralow JR, Nichols PW, Jones PA (1986): Southern blot analysis of DNA extracted from formalin-fixed pathology specimens. *Cancer Res* 46:2964–2969.

Feldman MY (1973): Reactions of nucleic acids and nucleoproteins with formaldehyde. *Progr Nucl Acid Res Mol Biol* 13:1–49.

Gelfand DH, White TJ (1990): Thermostable DNA polymerases. In: *PCR Protocols: Guide to Methods and Applications*. Innis MA, Gelfand DH, Sninsky JJ, White TJ, eds. San Diego: Academic Press, 129–141.

Goelz SE, Hamilton SR, Volgelstein B (1985): Purification of DNA form formaldehyde-fixed and paraffin-embedded human tissues. *Biochem Biophys Res Commun* 130:118–126.

Greer CE, Peterson SL, Kiviat NB, Manos MM (1991): PCR amplification from paraffin-embedded tissues: Effects of fixative and fixation time. *Am J Clin Pathol* 95:117–124.

Hanson CA, Holbrook EA, Sheldon S, Schnitzer B, Roth MS (1990): Detection of Philadelphia chromosome-positive cells from glass slide smears using the polymerase chain reaction. *Am J Pathol* 137:1–6.

Impraim CC, Saiki RK, Erlich HA, Teplitz RL (1987): Analysis of DNA extracted from formalin-fixed, paraffin-embedded tissues by enzymatic amplification and hybridization with sequence-specific oligonucleotides. *Biochem Biophys Res Commun* 142:710–716.

Jackson DP, Bell S, Payne J, Lewis FA, Sutton J, Taylor GR, Quirke P (1989a): Extraction and amplification of DNA from archival haematoxylin and eosin sections and cervical cytology Papnicalaou smears. *Nucl Acid Res* 17:10134.

Jackson DP, Quirke P, Lewis F, Boylston AW, Sloan JM, Robertson D, Taylor GR (1989b): Detection of measles virus RNA in paraffin-embedded tissue. *Lancet* 1:1391.

Jackson DP, Lewis FA, Taylor GR, Boylston AW, Quirke P (1990): Tissue extraction of DNA and RNA and analysis by the polymerase chain reaction. *J Clin Pathol* 43:499–504.

Jansen RW, Siegl G, Lemon SM (1990): Molecular epidemiology of human hepatitis A virus defined by an antigen-capture polymerase chain reaction method. *Proc Natl Acad Sci USA* 87:2867–2871.

Kawasaki ES (1990): Sample preparation from blood, cells, and other fluids. In: *PCR Protocols: A Guide to Methods and Applications*. Innis MA, Gelfand DH, Sninsky JJ, White TJ, eds. San Diego: Academic Press, 146–152.

Khan G, Kangro HO, Coates PJ, Heath RB (1991): Inhibitory effects of urine on the polymerase chain reaction for cytomegalovirus DNA. *J Clin Pathol* 44:360–365.

Paabo S (1989): Ancient DNA: Extraction, characterization, molecular cloning and enzymatic amplification. *Proc Natl Acad Sci USA* 86:1939–1943.

Rogers BB, Alpert LC, Hine EAS, Buffone GJ (1990): Analysis of DNA in fresh and fixed tissue by the polymerase chain reaction. *Am J Pathol* 136:541–548.

Rupp GM, Locker J (1988): Purification and analysis of RNA from paraffin-embedded tissues. *Biotechniques* 6:56–60.

Saiki RK, Bugawan TL, Horn GT, Mullis KB, Erlich HA (1986): Analysis of enzymatically amplified b-globin and HLA-DQa DNA with allele-specific oligonucleotide probes. *Nature (London)* 324:163–166.

Shibata D, Arnheim N, Martin WJ (1988a): Detection of human papilloma virus in paraffin-embedded tissue using the polymerase chain reaction. *J Exp Med* 167:225–230.

Shibata D, Martin WJ, Arnheim N (1988b): Analysis of DNA sequences in forty-year-old paraffin-embedded tissue sections: A bridge between molecular biology and classical histology. *Cancer Res* 48:4564–4566.

Shibata D, Brynes RK, Nathwani BN, Kwok S, Sninsky JJ, Arnheim N (1989): Human immunodeficiency viral DNA is ready found in lymph node biopsies from seropositive individuals: Analysis of fixed tissues using the polymerase chain reaction. *Am J Pathol* 135:697–702.

Singer-Sam J, Tanguay R (1989): Use of Chelex to improve the PCR signal from small number of cells. Amplifications, A Forum for PCR Users, September, Issue 3.

Weizsacker FV, Labeit S, Koch HK, Oehlert W, Gerok W, Blum HE (1991): A simple and rapid method for the detection of RNA in formalin-fixed, paraffin-embedded tissues by PCR amplification. *Biochem Biophys Res Commun* 174:176–180.

Wright DK, Manos MM (1990): Sample preparation from paraffin-embedded tissues. In: *PCR Protocols: A Guide to Methods and Applications.* Innis MA, Gelfand DH, Sninsky JJ, White TJ, eds. San Diego: Academic Press, 153–158.

5

PCR Amplification of Viral DNA and Viral Host Cell mRNAs *in Situ*

Janet Embretson, Katherine Staskus, Ernest Retzel, Ashley T. Haase, and Peter Bitterman

Introduction

The hallmark and power of *in situ* hybridization methodology are its ability to determine the levels of gene expression in an individual cell in a population or determine which cells in a population have acquired new genes by infection or other processes. In this way one can gain insight into how levels of gene expression can vary within a population with the same complement of genes, how different genes within a cell are coordinately regulated, and how newly introduced genes are regulated and interact with genes in the host cell. In contrast to other techniques that measure the average number of molecules per cell in the population, *in situ* analyses measure the number of molecules in a particular cell in a particular spatial and temporal context. With double-labeling techniques, one can also appreciate, for example, the relative abundancy of specific nucleic acid and protein in the same cell.

One of the limitations, however, of *in situ* hybridization is detection and quantitation of very low levels of nucleic acid targets where the signal is insufficient to distinguish it clearly from background noise. The advent of poly-merase chain reaction (PCR) technology to amplify targets provided an opportunity to develop new technologies to examine this end of the spectrum of gene expression or infection. In this chapter we describe conditions and primers for PCR *in situ*.

Amplification of DNA *in Situ:* Viral Experimental Systems

Because of our interest in chronic and latent viral infections, we have focused much of our efforts on developing PCR *in situ* techniques in experimental systems. In these systems it is important to know if a cell harbors a viral genome and, if so, to what extent that viral genome is being expressed, since one mechanism for persistence of viruses is restricted gene expression in which there is insufficient expression for detection and destruction of the infected cell by host defenses. Lentiviruses such as visna and human immunodeficiency virus (HIV), the causative agent of AIDS, fulfill these criteria as they may persist inside cells in a state where the viral genome, like all retroviruses, is stably associated with the

The Polymerase Chain Reaction
K.B. Mullis, F. Ferré, R.A. Gibbs, editors
© 1994 Birkhauser Boston

genome of the host cell but can remain in a transcriptionally inactive state. Manifest disease occurs after a long incubation period during which the viral genome is activated in some infected cells and virus is produced (Fauci, 1988; Levy, 1988; Harper et al., 1986; Haase et al., 1990; Staskus et al., 1991). The consequent dissemination of infection leads to cumulative damage to individual organ systems. In these alternative states of gene expression, the number of copies of viral nucleic acid ranges from a single to a few copies of viral DNA per cell and several hundred copies to more than a thousand copies of viral RNA. These levels of RNA occur occasionally in cells in an animal and routinely in productive infection of infected tissue cultures.

Lentivirus infections thus offer an experimental system that is at once amenable to method development, in productively infected cells, and a testing ground for PCR *in situ* approaches to examine virus–host cell relationships that are inaccessible to conventional *in situ* hybridization techniques. This is particularly important for HIV infections where we want (1) to know whether there are other reservoirs in addition to the macrophage, (2) to estimate the true extent of infection or "viral burden" in the course of disease and response to treatment, and (3) to understand the mechanisms of persistence and destruction of the host immune system through insights into patterns of viral gene expression in identified cell types.

Visna

We initially used visna virus infection of tissue culture cells to establish conditions for amplifying and retaining lentiviral DNA in fixed cells for several reasons. First, in tissue culture, in contrast to the slow infection this lentivirus causes in sheep, viral replication is not restricted. Large quantities of virus are produced in a few days and viral DNA increases from a single copy per cell in the early hours of infection to a few hundred copies 72 hr later. With this large founder population we could anticipate quicker assessment of the critical parameters for success in PCR amplification of

viral DNA. Once we had established optimal conditions we could then determine, based on previously established copy numbers per cell at designated times after infection, the amplification achieved and the sensitivity of the method. With confidence in our ability to detect a single copy of the viral genome we could then return to the animal model where gene expression is restricted and where we suspected that there was a reservoir of latently infected cells with a single copy of viral DNA with very little or no viral RNAs being expressed.

In these experiments we harvested cells infected with 3 plaque-forming units (PFU)/cell of visna virus at three time points when the cells had about 1, 20, or 200 copies of viral DNA per cell (Haase et al., 1990). We trypsinized the cultures or their uninfected counterparts, fixed the cell suspension in 4% paraformaldehyde for 2 min, and then in 70% ethanol for at least 1 hr, or longer for storage. Prior to amplification we collected the cells by centrifugation, washed the pellet with phosphate-buffered saline (PBS), and resuspended them in a PCR reaction mixture with 0.1–1 μM primers described below. After an initial denaturation for 10 min at 94°C we added *Thermus aquatiqus* (*Taq*) DNA polymerase, denatured the DNA for 2 min at 94°C, annealed primers for 2 min at 42°C, and extended for 15 min at 72°C. We repeated this cycle 25 times, added fresh *Taq* polymerase and cycled the reaction 25 times more before collecting and washing the cells in PBS and depositing them by cytocentrifugation onto glass slides. We subsequently treated the cells with ribonucleases, cross-linked DNA by fixation in paraformaldehyde, and denatured the DNA with formamide prior to hybridization to ^{125}I-labeled probes specific for the amplified region of the visna genome, regions of the genome that should not have been amplified, or heterologous viral DNA.

We chose primers for PCR *in situ* positioned at 200–300 nt intervals on the plus and minus strands of a 1.2 kbp region of the *gag* gene of visna virus (Fig. 5.1). Because the amplified segments overlap, the individual fragments can form larger fragments through base pairing at

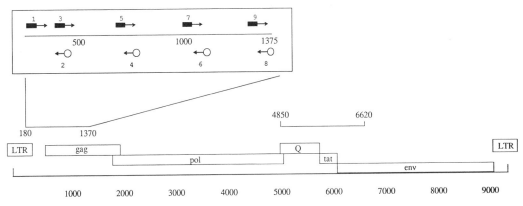

FIGURE 5.1. Positions of the multiple primer set (MPS) relative to the visna virus genome. Primers spanned a total of 1.2 kbp in the *gag* gene, separated by 200–300 nt. Reprinted from Haase et al., *Proc Natl Acad Sci USA* 87:4971–4975, 1990, with permission.

their cohesive termini and this, we reasoned, would increase retention of the product. At the same time, amplification should be relatively efficient as the individual DNA products would not exceed a few hundred bases until the last cycles where presumably overlapping DNA fragments are extended to form long covalently linked products.

This strategy proved successful and we found that we could amplify and retain visna DNA in single cells that hybridized only to a probe specific for the amplified region. In comparisons of the multiple primer set (MPS), which yielded a 1.2 kb product from four ca. 300-bp fragments, with individual primer pairs that would yield amplified DNA of 600, 900, or 1200 bp, we found that we obtained the best yield of retained product with the MPS, which was nonetheless orders of magnitude less than amplification of DNA in solution (300-fold increase in DNA in cells in 50 cycles compared to a million-fold in solution in 25 cycles). This presumably reflects inefficiency in amplifying DNA in cells fixed under our conditions and the loss of shorter amplified products from cells. In support of this interpretation are three observations: (1) amplification with individual primer pairs that generated DNA products of less than 900 bp appeared to be less efficient than larger products; (2) the product detected by *in situ* hybridization was distributed in a ring-like pattern around the

perimeter of the cell, as though the product had diffused and bound at the surface (Fig. 5.2); and (3) the background binding of probe to the slides with visna virus-infected cells was much higher than uninfected cells, reflecting leakage of visna-related product from the infected cells.

The 300-fold increase in visna DNA in cells with the PCR amplification *in situ* under the conditions described was also the maximal yield. Other conditions for fixation, pretreatments to increase diffusion of enzymes and reactants into the cell, and manipulation of PCR variables proved to be even less efficient. Because, however, we needed only about a 10-fold increase in target sequences to detect a single copy of the genome, we turned from the studies of PCR *in situ* in suspended cells to the development of methods applicable to tissue sections so that we could investigate latent infections in animals.

For this application we modified the procedure as follows (Fig. 5.3): we cut sections of formalin-fixed and paraffin-embedded tissues, adhered these to slides, and after removing the paraffin with xylene and ethanol, we denatured the DNA in cells by heating to 65°C in 95% formamide for 15 min. Following rapid cooling to 4°C, we dehydrated and added the PCR reaction mixture and *Taq* polymerase to the sections. We spread the mixture over the section by covering it with a coverslip, placed the

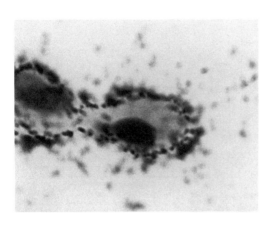

FIGURE 5.2. Pattern of hybridization to small PCR product generated during amplification, *in situ*. A single primer pair which gives rise to a 600 bp fragment in the PCR was used for amplification *in situ* of visna virus DNA in productively infected sheep cells, fixed in solution 20 hr postinfection. As seen in this cell, subsequent *in situ* hybridization with radiolabeled probe specific for this fragment results in the deposition of silver grains in the autoradiograph in a ring-like pattern at the periphery of the cell. This is consistent with the ability of smaller molecules to diffuse easily into or out of cells during the amplification. Magnification: 400×. Reprinted with modification from Haase et al., *Proc Natl Acad Sci USA* 87:4971–4975, 1990, with permission.

slides in a plastic bag, and covered the slides with mineral oil to prevent evaporation. We put the heat-sealed bags into a Bios Thermal Cycler oven and amplified for 25 cycles. A slide to which a thermal sensor had been attached by the manufacturer was similarly sealed in an oil-filled bag and placed in a rack adjacent to sample slides in a Bios Oven Thermal Cycler. After 25 cycles (92°C denaturation for 2 min, 42°C annealing for 2 min, 72°C extension for 15 min), we removed the slides from the bags, placed them in $CHCl_3$ (twice, 5 min each) to remove residual oil. We removed the slides from the $CHCl_3$ and, as soon as the $CHCl_3$ volatilized, we removed the coverslips with the tip of a scalpel and forceps. We quickly added fresh PCR mixture, *Taq* polymerase, and coverslip and placed the slides back in the oil-filled plastic bags for an additional 25 cycles.

We again removed oil in $CHCl_3$ and washed the sections twice in PBS (5 min each) and dehydrated in graded alcohols. After pretreatments with ribonucleases, postfixation in paraformaldehyde, and denaturation in formamide, sections were hybridized for 12–16 hr to a gel-purified fragment of cloned visna virus DNA corresponding to the amplified segment, labeled with ^{125}I-labeled dCTP by nick translation to specific activities of 5–10×10^8 dpm/ μg (1–3×10^6 dpm per section), or to an HIV-specific probe labeled similarly to comparable specific activities.

We thus far have achieved even less amplification of target DNA in cells in tissue sections but the roughly 30-fold amplification proved sufficient to show that visna virus can establish latent infections in sheep where cells contain probably a single copy of the viral genome and fewer than 10 copies of viral RNA (Staskus et al., 1990) (Fig. 5.4). These cells were 10 times as frequent as those with even modest levels of viral RNA (50–100 copies per cell) compared to productive infections (1000–8000 copies per cell) establishing for the first time the existence of a reservoir of infected cells.

HIV

While work is progressing on PCR *in situ* analysis of the pathogenesis of animal lentiviral infections, we have concurrently been engaged in similar efforts to develop comparable methods for studies of HIV infections. These have the promise of telling us more about the progression of infection to disease and the mechanisms that induce the immunodeficient state than has been learned thus far from less sensitive single cell techniques or population analysis of extracted nucleic acids.

In adapting PCR *in situ* techniques developed with the visna virus system to HIV, we began with a $CD4^+$ cell line, H9, and its chronically HIV-infected counterpart, IIIB (IIIB). We fixed these cells in paraformaldehyde and delipidated them in 70% ethanol as described for visna and used individual primer pairs 500–1200 bp apart, or an HIV-specific MPS spanning 1500 bp, for PCR *in situ*. We again achieved the greatest amplification with

FIGURE 5.3. *In situ* PCR applied to tissue sections. Diagrammatic representation of the primary steps of the method.

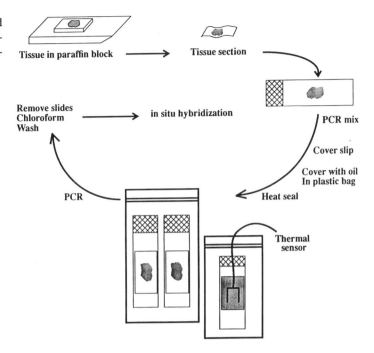

the MPS and found that smaller amplified products (500 bp) diffused and bound to the cell surface or glass. We also discovered in these initial experiments a new problem not present in the visna system: if infected and uninfected cells were mixed prior to amplification, nearly all the cells scored as infected; if we mixed the cells after amplification, we scored the appropriate ratio of infected to uninfected cells. We suspect that smaller products made in earlier cycles with this MPS leak from infected cells, diffuse into the uninfected cells, and then are amplified and retained. This interpretation is supported by analysis of the DNA in these supernatants and cell pellets where we have documented PCR products of the correct size in both. Our attempts to correct the problem of leakage of the PCR product by varying conditions of fixation were unsuccessful and we turned to amplification on slides with the expectation that diffusion and leakage would be less likely to confound the analysis.

For these experiments we have begun to define optimal conditions for PCR *in situ* by drying H9 or IIIB cells on slides, fixing them for varying periods of time, and then dehydrating them in graded ethanols. After pretreatment and denaturing we then amplify with the MPS, or individual primer sets, for 25 cycles in the Bios Thermal Cycler oven as described for visna virus-infected tissues. In this analysis we compared paraformaldehyde (1%, 4%) with glutaraldehyde (1%) and ethanol (95%) and found that fixing in 1% paraformaldehyde for 20 min followed by pretreatment of the cells with proteinase K (5–30 μg/ml, 55°C, 1 hr) prior to denaturation generated the greatest yield of detectable product and the lowest background.

Because the efficiency of amplification even with these conditions was lower than expected, we wondered whether there were something peculiar to HIV DNA in fixed cells inhibiting amplification. We therefore compared amplification of HIV DNA in IIIB cells, present on average at least one copy of provirus per cell, with a single copy gene, β-globin. We sampled equivalent numbers of fixed cells on slides and amplified DNA, released into solution by digestion with proteinase K, with either HIV or β-globin-specific primers. We consistently obtained at best 10-fold less amplification of HIV in infected cells, possibly reflecting copurification of an inhibitor or some preferential effect

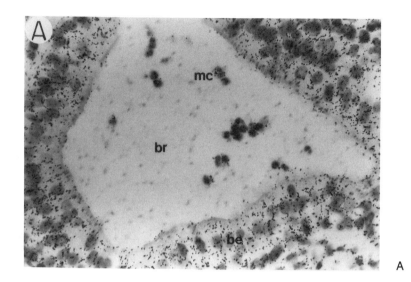

A

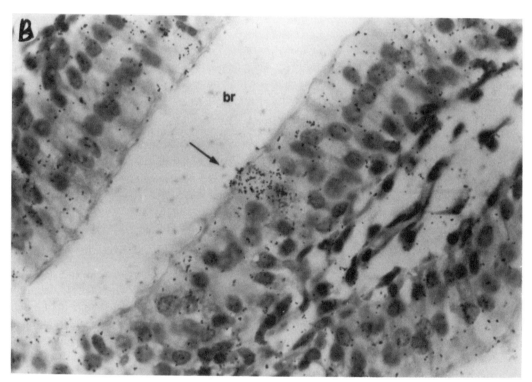

B

FIGURE 5.4. *In situ* PCR performed on tissue sections taken from the lung of a lamb experimentally infected with visna virus reveals a previously undescribed reservoir of latently infected cells. Amplification of viral genomic sequences within cells in tissue sections taken from infected regions of the lung, followed by *in situ* hybridization, demonstrates that nearly every cell of the bronchiolar epithelium contains viral DNA (**A**). In contrast, *in situ* hybridization for viral RNA shows that few of these infected cells (**B**, arrow) are transcriptionally active for viral sequences. Magnification: 240× (mc = mononuclear cells; br = bronchioles; be = bronchiolar epithelium). Reprinted with modification from Staskus et al., *Microbial Path* 11:67–76, 1991, with permission of Academic Press.

FIGURE 5.5. (**A**) A lymph node section was incubated with a PCR mixture without HIV-specific MPS primers and cycled as described in the text. After pretreatments, sections were hybridized with a ^{125}I-labeled HIV probe. (**B**) Subjacent section to that in **A** was incubated with a PCR mixture with HIV-specific (MPS) primers, cycled, pretreated and hybridized as in **A**.

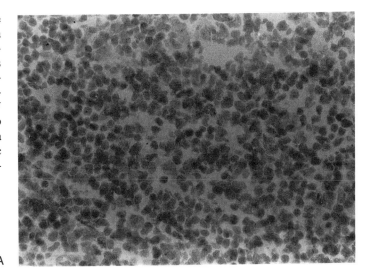

A

B

of fixation in HIV DNA. Whatever the explanation, it may limit our ability currently to detect HIV DNA in tissue specimens and we have qualified accordingly one conclusion drawn from preliminary work we now describe.

Even though there is considerable room for improvement in PCR *in situ* to detect HIV DNA we achieved some amplification and for this reason embarked on a pilot study of lymph node specimens from HIV-infected individuals. Sections from frozen samples fixed either in buffered formalin or paraformaldehyde were cut and adhered (with Elmer's glue) to glass slides coated with Denhardt's medium. We used conventional *in situ* hybridization techniques to detect viral RNA in cells and PCR *in situ* amplification and hybridization to look for HIV DNA in cells in the sections. We also manually removed sections from slides and digested them with proteinase K and amplified DNA in solution for 25 cycles with either HIV MPS or β-globin primers. We reamplified the HIV DNA with a nested set of primers for 25 more cycles and analyzed the DNA products from both amplifications by gel electrophoresis and Southern blotting.

There was excellent concordance between detection of DNA by either method (*in situ* or solution PCR) and some specimens positive for viral DNA lacked detectable RNA, in accord with the latent infection model of persistence of lentiviruses supported by our experience with visna virus. However, only a few cells in the sections had HIV DNA even by a PCR *in situ* method (Fig. 5.5). We do not know as yet if this reflects the limits of current methodology or the true situation, but the results clearly point to the need for further work in the HIV system.

Recently (Embretson et al., 1993), we have succeeded in amplifying HIV DNA in tissue sections. Unlike our early studies, these tissues contained large numbers of infected cells. We were able to determine the number of latently infected cells in two different cell populations in the tissue and have worked out conditions to double label sections with both antibody via immunocytochemistry and labeled HIV probes for viral DNA.

Others (Bagasra et al., 1992; Nuovo et al., 1991a,b) have documented amplification of both HIV and other viral DNAs. These methods involve different amplification parameters including different thermocycling profiles, different primers, and the use of a single primer pair instead of a MPS, detection using a nonradiolabeled probe and different fixation conditions. All of these variations have been empirically defined and optimized for each system.

Amplification of RNA *in Situ:* Growth Factors and Lung Disease

In the course of studies of the role PDGF plays in the development of intraalveolar fibrosis following acute lung injury, we wanted to establish the temporal and spatial relationships of cells in the lung containing PDGF mRNA to the tissue lesions observed. Conventional *in situ* hybridization methods proved insuffi-

ciently sensitive to reproducibly detect PDGF mRNA in many cells that contained PDGF protein. By adapting PCR *in situ* methods, developed in the viral systems, to amplification of mRNAs in single cells in tissue section, in preliminary analyses we showed that the increased expressions of mRNA and protein were congruent. These studies provide evidence that PDGF expression is important for development of fibrosis following lung injury and more generally provide a new approach to analyzing the spatial patterns of mRNAs in cells in tissue sections when the mRNAs are of low abundance or are undetectable because of fixation or other uncontrolled aspects of specimen acquisition and preservation.

For PCR *in situ* for RNA, a solution containing reverse transcriptase was applied to deparaffinized tissue sections. After incubation (2 cycles of 37°C, 1 hr), a solution containing primers and *Taq* polymerase was added to the slides, and the slides were placed in a Bios Thermal Cycler (Bitterman et al., 1993). The primers were a multiple overlapping primer set which spanned 1000 bp. Postamplification, slides were pretreated and hybridized to an end-labeled PDGF oligonucleotide for probe. Signal was present over cells in regions that were also positive for PDGF protein by immunocytochemistry in a pattern consistent with the known anatomic evolution of intraalveolar fibrosis, in which buds of granulation tissue grow into the airspace (Fig. 5.6). Prior to amplification, only occasional intraalveolar buds contained cells with signal. Following amplification, every bud had cells with a positive *in situ* signal. Moreover, the signal intensity was much greater than in nonamplified cells, and was specific for PDGF probe. Thus, there was close correlation between cells expressing PDGF message and protein at the advancing edge of intraalveolar fibrosis after injury to the lung.

Conclusions and Summary

By joining the technologies of *in situ* hybridization with PCR amplification it should now be possible to detect in individual cells single

FIGURE 5.6. (**A**) Human lung section hybridized with a ^{35}S-labeled PDGF probe. (**B**) Human lung section that was first incubated with reverse transcriptase, then with *Taq* in the presence of PDGF-specific primers. Sections were pretreated then incubated with a ^{35}S-labeled PDGF probe.

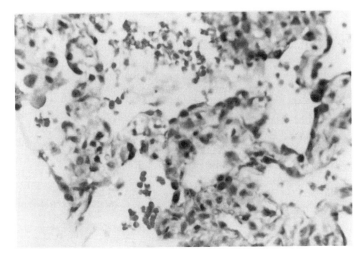

A

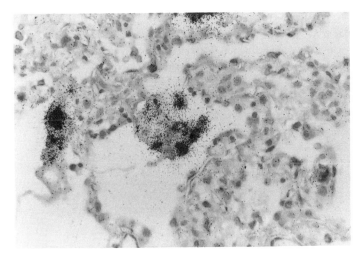

B

copies of viral genomes or low levels of transcripts. There are still many problems that reflect differences inherent in any experimental system, differences in the fixation and condition of the tissues, and no doubt other confounding variables that will be discovered. In this chapter we have presented some approaches to overcoming some of the difficulties such as leakage of amplified product and have emphasized the need to substantiate the PCR *in situ* results by additional methods such as immunocytochemistry and conventional *in situ* hybridization. We conclude on the encouraging note that PCR *in situ* has already deepened our insight into lentiviral latency and pathogenic mechanisms of lung disease, justifying our hope that these early analyses presage a future in which we can look to single cells for the answers to many interesting questions. These include the coordination of expression of low abundancy transcripts, splice junction usage, and more about the role of viruses and oncogenes in tissue injury and cancer.

References

Bagasra O, Hauptman SP, Lischner HW, Sachs M, Pomerantz RJ (1992): Detection of human immunodeficiency virus type 1 provirus in mononuclear cells by in situ polymerase chain reaction. *N Engl J Med* 326:1385–1391.

Bitterman P, Haase A, Embretson J, Peterson M, Harman K, Jessurum J (1993): Combination of the polymerase chain reaction with in situ hybridization to define the spatial pattern of mRNA in tissue. Manuscript submitted.

Embretson J, Zupanocic M, Beneke J, Till M, Wolinsky S, Ribas JL, Burke A, Haase AT (1993): Analysis of human immunodeficiency virus infected tissues by amplification and in situ hybridization reveals latent and permissive infections at single cell resolution. *Proc Natl Acad Sci USA* 90:357–361.

Fauci AS (1988): The human immunodeficiency virus: Infectivity and mechanisms of pathogenesis. *Science* 239:617–622.

Haase AT, Retzel EF, Staskus KA (1990): Amplification and detection of lentiviral DNA inside cells. *Proc Natl Acad Sci USA* 87:4971–4975.

Harper ME, Marselle LM, Gallo RC, Wong-Staal F (1986): Detection of lymphocytes expressing human T-lymphotropic virus III in lymph nodes and peripheral blood from infected individuals by in situ hybridization. *Proc Natl Acad Sci USA* 83:722–776.

Levy JA (1988): Mysteries of HIV: Challenges for therapy and prevention. *Nature (London)* 333:519–522.

Nuovo GJ, Gallery F, MacConnell P, Becker J, Bloch W (1991a): An improved technique for the in situ detection of DNA after polymerase chain reaction amplification. *Am J Pathol* 139:1239–1244.

Nuovo GJ, MacConnell P, Forde A, DeIvenne P (1991b): Detection of human papilloma virus DNA in formalin-fixed tissues by in situ hybridization after amplification by polymerase chain reaction. *Am J Pathol* 139:847–854.

Staskus KA, Couch L, Bitterman P, Retzel EF, Zupancic M, List JF, Haase AT (1991): In situ amplification of visna virus DNA in tissue sections reveals a reservoir of latently infected cells. *Microbial Path* 11:67–76.

PART ONE
Methodology

SECTION II
Quantitation

6

Quantitative PCR: An Overview

F. Ferré, A. Marchese, P. Pezzoli, S. Griffin, E. Buxton, and V. Boyer

Introduction

John Maddox recently wrote (Maddox, 1992) that "molecular biology seems well on the way to becoming a largely qualitative science. . . . It would be a worthwhile precaution against the quantitative days that lie ahead that people should make sure that published data are capable of quantitative interpretation by those who have the zeal for that." Well, with the current outburst of publications on quantitative PCR (Q-PCR) methods and their applications, it looks like the "quantitative days" are already on us and here to stay. Quantitation of nucleic acids by PCR has been used in an array of situations in both basic and clinical research (for review see, Bej et al., 1991; Volkenandt et al., 1992; Ferré, 1992; Clementi et al., 1993). To name a few, Q-PCR methods have been developed to study gene expression (for review see Chapter 24), to assess the progress of a therapeutic (for review see Chapters 27–30), to estimate the amount of the HIV-1 virus load (Ferré, 1992; Clementi et al., 1993), to diagnose genetic deletions (Abbs and Bobrow, 1992), to determine the carrier frequency of a recessive disease in a population (Syvanen et al., 1992), or to quantitate plant's biotrophs (Simon et al., 1992).

With its impressive sensitivity and specificity set aside, PCR technology does not seem to be poised to conduct quantitative analyses. The amplification process, which is exponential and thus potentially difficult to control, is the natural suspect for anyone dubious about the quantitative ability of PCR and rightfully so. Therefore, why is PCR so widely used to quantitate nucleic acids? We will address this issue in the first part of this chapter. Since there cannot be quantitation without a fair assessment of the amount of starting material, it being cell lysate or extracted nucleic acids, we have devoted a full section to this topic. In the course of this chapter, we will also present some of the numerous PCR approaches that have been developed to perform relative quantitation. Lastly, we will entertain the concept of absolute quantitation using PCR.

Quantitation of the Fewest

Despite the numerous obstacles that PCR faces as a quantitative tool, the fact that it can reproducibly detect 10 or fewer specific nucleic acid

The Polymerase Chain Reaction
K.B. Mullis, F. Ferré, R.A. Gibbs, editors
© 1994 Birkhäuser Boston

molecules in a background of hundreds of millions, makes the challenges worthwhile. Prior to PCR, quantitation of specific nucleic acid sequences from eukaryotic cells was mainly obtained using blotting procedures such as Southern, Northern, and slot blots. With these techniques, the lower limits of detection/quantitation are in the range of 10^5 to 10^7 target molecules (Sambrook et al., 1989). These batch procedures are laborious and require considerable amounts of nucleic acids (10–20 μg/lane) to yield credible quantitative results. Furthermore, meticulous care is required at all stages of the procedure to generate blots of sufficiently good quality for reliable dosage analysis. Recently, Feddersen and Van Ness, using a modified Southern blot assay, have shown that the limit of detection of their assay is in the range of 5×10^4 copies of target DNA (Feddersen and Van Ness, 1989).

At the RNA level, the RNase protection assay has been shown to be at least 10-fold more sensitive than the Northern blot with a limit of detection in the range of 5×10^5–10^6 target molecules (Melton et al., 1984). Farrell has recently reported an S1 nuclease procedure capable of detecting 1 pg of specific mRNA (representing 2×10^{-7} of the poly(A)$^+$ component) in 100 μg of total RNA (Farrell, 1993). This represents 10^6 target copies if one assumes an average RNA size of 2 kb. Thus, using the above batch procedures, a minimum of 5×10^4 target molecules is required for detection with a limit of quantitation probably substantially higher.

The sensitivity for detection of DNA/RNA targets can be dramatically increased by using the *in situ* hybridization technique. This method, which quantitates the amount of positive cells instead of the absolute amount of nucleic acid, possesses a limit of detection of 10 to 100 molecules per cell. However, the *in situ* hybridization method is technically difficult and does not lend itself to the processing of a large number of samples. Furthermore, even if single copy detection has been reported (Spadoro et al., 1990), this method has not been routinely used for the detection and quantitation of very low levels of nucleic acid targets such as single copy proviral integrated DNA or

low-copy-number mRNA transcripts (1–10 copies per cell).

To detect and quantitate small amounts of nucleic acid targets, an amplification step is required. Recently, methods have been developed in which the signal rather than the target, as in PCR, is amplified. Kramer and co-workers used replicatable hybridization probes (Lomell et al., 1989; Lizardi and Kramer, 1991), which consist of RNA engineered to be amplified with the QB replicase. With this technique, it was found, quantitating HIV-1 mRNA as targets, that the limit of quantitation is about 10^4 mRNA molecules. Urdea and co-workers also developed an assay to quantitate small amounts of HIV-1 mRNA (Kern et al., 1992). In this procedure, an HIV-1 RNA-probe complex is captured onto a microtiter well surface, followed by hybridization of branched DNA (bDNA) molecules, which mediate signal amplification. The lower limit of quantitation of this method is about 2×10^4 HIV-1 mRNA molecules per ml of plasma. Thus, these methods are still a couple of orders of magnitude less sensitive than PCR.

In addition to PCR, methods for target amplification, such as the transcription-based amplification system (TAS) (Kwoh et al., 1989; Davis et al., 1990) or its most recent version termed the self-sustained sequence replication (3SR) reaction (Guatelli et al., 1989; Fahy et al., 1991) have been developed. In these technologies, the production of RNA copies of the target sequence provides the principal means of amplification. As PCR, TAS is extremely sensitive, i.e., one target molecule detectable in a background of 10^6 human genomes. However, quantitation with TAS offers less precision and reproducibility than PCR (Davis et al., 1990).

Q-PCR methods were not made equal. The choice of a quantitative method should be linked to the quantitative needs. Monitoring the relative 20-fold transient increase in the expression of progesterone receptor mRNA after the preovulatory luteinizing hormone surge (Park and Mayo, 1991) does not require the same quantitative power as monitoring the effect of therapy on viral burden in HIV-1-infected individuals for which increases (or decreases) of 2- to 3-fold in the amount of integrated virus might matter and should then be detected. At another level, one may have to decide if an accurate assessment of the absolute amount of a given target is necessary or if a relative evaluation will suffice.

For the selection of a suitable PCR method, choices have to be made at many levels. For example, one will have to decide which procedures for nucleic acids preparation should be used, which standards should be selected, or which methods for detection and quantitation of the amplicons should be implemented. Decisions taken at these levels will ultimately impact not only the sensitivity, precision, reproducibility, and accuracy of the assay but also its practicality.

Nucleic Acid Preparation in Quantitative Settings

Darryl Shibata (Chapter 4) extensively describes numerous methods of nucleic acid preparation suitable for PCR, and we would encourage its reading concomitantly with this chapter. We will nonetheless elaborate on some of the implications pertinent to quantitation that are associated with the choice of a particular method. The need for optimization of the amplification per se as well as the value of the different methods for detection and quantitation are discussed elsewhere (Ferré, 1992) and are not reviewed in this chapter.

Preparation of DNA

Two major methods for the preparation of DNA have been implemented. One involves the lysis of cells with a so-called lysis buffer that contains mild detergents (Laureth 12 and Tween 20) and freshly added proteinase K, followed by a boiling step for 5–60 min (Aoki et al., 1990; Ferré et al., 1992a; Kellogg et al., 1990; Lee et al., 1990; Oka et al., 1990; Ou et al., 1990; Schnittman et al., 1990). The other

utilizes the classical phenol/chloroform DNA extraction (Dickover et al., 1990; Genesca et al., 1990; Katz et al., 1990; Landgraf et al., 1991; Simmonds et al., 1990; Sugiyama et al., 1991). The cell lysis procedure has the advantage of simplicity but does not permit a direct estimation of the starting amount of DNA. It is possible to estimate the amount of DNA by counting the number of starting cells (Ferré et al., 1992a; Schnittman et al., 1989; Simmonds et al., 1990) but this is not applicable to source of materials like small pieces of tissue. A more sophisticated way to evaluate the amount of starting material when utilizing this cell lysis procedure is to quantitate retrospectively the amount of total DNA by PCR (Aoki et al., 1990; Kellogg et al., 1990; Lee et al., 1990; Michael et al., 1992; Oka et al., 1990; Ferré et al., 1992a). This estimation of total DNA can then be used to normalize the calculated number of specific DNA copies. This normalization process should add to the quantitative power of assays in which the control DNA is coamplified because any fluctuation in the amplification efficiency should be reflected on both amplicons. Thus, a loss of efficiency in the amplification of the studied amplicon may be compensated through the normalization process using the coamplified single copy genomic DNA target (Ferré et al., 1993).

Preparation of RNA

We have just mentioned that crude lysate could be directly used for DNA quantitation by PCR. However, even if RNA PCR can also be performed on crude extract (Kawasaki, 1990; Ferré and Garduno, 1989; Wilkinson, 1988), the somewhat low levels of sensitivity and reproducibility achieved in those conditions are not adequate in quantitative settings. The most important consideration in the preparation of RNA is to rapidly and efficiently inhibit the endogenous ribonucleases (Chirgwin et al., 1979; Sambrook et al., 1989; Farrell, 1993) that are present in virtually all living cells. All Q-PCR RNA procedures described until now utilize RNA extraction methodologies, which still represent the best way to eliminate ribonucleases. Indeed, contrary to DNases, RNases are heat-resistant enzymes that are not destroyed by boiling (Sambrook et al., 1989; Farrell, 1993). In most procedures of RNA preparation commonly implemented in Q-PCR analyses, a very strong denaturant of ribonucleases, guanidinium thiocyanate, in combination with a reducing agent such as 2-mercaptoethanol, serves as the basic ingredients.

In quantitative settings, it is often instrumental to estimate the amount of total extracted RNA. Quantitation by spectrophotometry with measurement of A_{260}/A_{280} ratios to control purity has been the method of choice even if it has been regarded as being somewhat too imprecise (Murphy et al., 1990; Masters et al., 1992). When dealing with very small quantities of starting material, it is generally recommended to add carrier molecules (tRNA or glycogen) for the precipitation step. This implies that the carrier of choice in Q-PCR becomes glycogen since this polysaccharide does not absorb at A_{260}/A_{280}.

The classical cesium chloride cushion preparation (Chirgwin et al., 1979) has been implemented with some modifications to make it suitable for very small amounts of starting material (Brenner et al., 1989). As expected, very high quality RNA can be obtained with this method but it has the drawback of being cumbersome, which renders it almost useless when dealing with more than a few samples. The most widely used methodology consists of a clever single-step procedure in which RNA is isolated by acid guanidinium thiocyanate–phenol–chloroform (AGPC) extraction (Chomczynski and Sacchi, 1987). The AGPC procedure allows the simultaneous processing of a large number of samples. In addition, this method permits recovery of total RNA from very small quantities of tissue or cells (less than 3 mg of tissue or 10^6 cells). Direct extraction from whole blood is not recommended since inhibitors of PCR such as porphyrins and hematin are still present in the purified RNA (Higuchi, 1989). Still, this method can be implemented after addition of a cationic surfactant solution (Catrimox-14) to whole blood resulting in lysis of the cells and in the precipitation of RNA and DNA complexed with the surfactant (Macfarlane and Dahle, 1993). We and others (Yamaguchi et al., 1992), using the AGPC methods, have observed, however, that the A_{260}/A_{280} ratios are quite variable and span a wide range from 1.4 to 1.99. These variations in the purity of RNA obtained by the AGPC method might prevent precise mRNA quantitation by affecting the efficiency of RT/PCR reactions (Ferré et al., 1992b, 1994; Yamaguchi et al., 1992). To address this issue, we have modified the AGPC procedure by including a glass bead binding step after RNA extraction in guanidinium (Ferré et al., 1992b, 1994). This procedure takes advantage of the property of RNA to bind to glass beads in high salt solutions. Reproducible A_{260}/A_{280} ratios in the 1.8–1.9 range can be obtained this way. However, because glass beads do absorb at 260, very careful elution of the RNA from the bead is strongly recommended.

Glass bead methods have also been particularly useful in isolating RNA from virus particles such as HIV or hepatitis from plasma or serum (Yamada et al., 1990; McCaustland et al., 1991; Boom et al., 1990; Koopmans et al., 1991). However, the amount of RNA recovered from these sources being minuscule, quantitation of extracted RNA by spectrophotometry is not feasible. This lack of quantitation of the starting material might significantly curtail the precision of the subsequent quantitation of a given target by PCR. To alleviate this limitation, a known quantity of a specific RNA such as ribosomal RNA is added to a guanidinium lysate of plasma or serum. The amount recovered after extraction can be monitored by spectrophotometry and the efficiency of extraction calculated (F. Ferré, P. Pezzoli, and E. Buxton, unpublished data).

Recently, automated RNA extraction technologies became available and the need for a fast, reliable, efficient, user friendly RNA extractors that would perform at least a dozen extraction at a time on very limited amounts of material, such as 10^6 blood cells, has been recognized.

Relative versus Absolute Quantitation

In this section, we will first review PCR methods capable of relative quantitation. Next, we will discuss the feasibility of absolute quantitation using PCR. Because the accurate quantitation of HIV-1 targets is seropositive individuals can be regarded as a key step in our quest for the understanding of HIV-1 pathogenesis, we will use this example to illustrate how difficult a task absolute quantitation by PCR still is.

Relative Quantitation

In relative quantitation settings, the goal is to evaluate differences in nucleic acid content among samples. Comparing relative amounts of nucleic acid molecules instead of determining their absolute number (absolute quantitation) is often sufficient for a number of applications. Examples of the usefulness of this approach abound in the literature. In some methodologies, the distinction between relative and absolute quantitation is not highlighted. For example, the copy number of a target can be reported but the focus and conclusions are on relative assessment of the amount of nucleic acids. Thus, for the sake of clarity, in methodologies that we labeled relative quantitation, either the quantitative interpretation was obtained without reference to exact copy numbers or if exact copy numbers were reported then it was made clear that those were relative values.

DNA Quantitation

At the DNA level, relative quantitation as defined above is rarely implemented. This is due mainly to the fact that rather accurate controls are easily available. Thus, even if only relative quantitation is required, it is somewhat tempting to report absolute values. Nevertheless, examples of relative DNA quantitation can be found in the literature. Abbs and Bobrow have used multiplex PCR for the diagnosis of deletion and duplication carriers in the dystrophin gene (Abbs and Bobrow, 1992; see Chapter 3

for multiplex PCR). The method, verified in blind trials, can differentiate between the 2:1 dosage ratio (control locus:deleted locus) observed in carriers and the 1:1 ratio in normals as well as the 2:3 ratio in a female duplication carrier. Using relative quantitation, estimation of the frequency of a 7436 bp deletion in mitochondrial DNA in the heart of humans of various ages has been performed. The frequency of the deletion has been shown to increase exponentially with age (Sugiyama et al., 1991). PCR has been used also in drug susceptibility testing to determine relative amounts of virus DNA in cultures maintained in different drug concentrations following *in vitro* infection (Eron et al., 1992). Relative assessment of the amount of HIV-1 DNA in PBMCs has also been implemented (1) in research settings to study the life cycle of the virus (Zack et al., 1990), and (2) in clinical settings to compare HIV-1 DNA load in patients in different disease stages (Pang et al., 1990; Genesca et al., 1990; Ou et al., 1990).

RNA Quantitation

Contrary to DNA, relative quantitation of mRNA has been widely implemented. This type of PCR format has been used to analyze temporal and differential expression of mRNA (Rappolee et al., 1988; Arrigo et al., 1989, 1990; Choi et al., 1989; Chelly et al., 1988, 1990a,b; Singer-Sam et al., 1990b; Makino et al., 1990; Murphy et al., 1990; Park and Mayo, 1991; Golay et al., 1991; Birnbaum and Van Ness, 1992; Mohler and Butler, 1991; Abe et al., 1992; Wood et al., 1992; Horikoshi et al., 1992; Hall and Finn, 1992), to study alternative splicing (Neve et al., 1990; Mochizuki et al., 1992), to evaluate the amount of allele-specific transcripts differing by a single nucleotide (Singer-Sam et al., 1992), or to anatomize the reverse transcription process of HIV-1 in quiescent cells (Zack et al., 1990, 1992).

The fact that relative quantitation has been so widely performed is linked to the difficulty in generating accurate RNA controls. Several groups have even reported relative quantitation of target RNA without referring to standards

(Choi et al., 1989; Arrigo et al., 1989; Makino et al., 1990; Singer-Sam et al., 1990b; Hall and Finn, 1992; Boyer et al., 1993). The biggest advantage of these PCR assays is the simplicity of their implementations. However, because of the lack of standards, their quantitative frame is rather loose and thus it is difficult to ascertain their quantitative power. Still, estimation of the quantitative ability of these assays can be obtained by (1) ensuring robustness in crucial steps such as total RNA preparation and quantitation, reverse-transcription, and amplification, and (2) testing samples with known differences in their RNA target contents and reevaluating these relative differences periodically. Hall and Finn have reported that this type of PCR format suits quite well the analysis of gene expression within a multigene family. The quantitative ability of their assay could discriminate less than 3-fold differences in mRNA target levels (Hall and Finn, 1992). Generally, however, the limited precision and reproducibility of such PCR assays must be acknowledged to avoid misinterpretation of results.

A number of groups have relied on standards to estimate relative difference in RNA targets. In the majority of these quantitative methods the relative levels of mRNAs are determined by (1) coamplifying the target RNA with an internal control, and (2) comparing the ratio target RNA : control RNA in which the internal control is either an endogenous (Singer-Sam et al., 1992; Golay et al., 1991; Park and Mayo, 1991; Neve et al., 1990; Wood et al., 1992; Birnbaum and Van Ness, 1992; Abe et al., 1992; Noonan et al., 1990) or an exogenous mRNA (Chelly et al., 1990; Chapter 8, this volume; Rappolee et al., 1988; Wood et al., 1992; Ferré et al., 1992b, 1994).

The rationale for having a control RNA co-reverse transcribed and coamplified with the target is to compensate for the poor reproducibility of RT-PCR. Specifically, it has been reported that the efficiency for the cDNA synthesis step is variable ranging from 5 to 90% (Noonan et al., 1990; Henrard et al., 1992; Simmonds et al., 1990). It has also been reported that the yield of amplification of a cDNA fragment can vary as much as 6-fold among duplicates (Gilliland et al., 1990).

The advantage of using an endogenous RNA as an internal control over an exogenous RNA is that it provides a control on the yield of amplifiable targets from the pool of successfully isolated total RNA. RNA from highly expressed genes such as β_2-microglobulin or ribosomal RNA has been used as internal standards (Horikoshi et al., 1992; Noonan et al., 1990; Park and Mayo, 1991). RNA species connected through function or structure to the actual target have also been used. For example, for the estimation of relative level of the different T-cell receptor Vβ chain mRNA, the Cα chain mRNA can be coamplified to normalize the expression of the Vβ chains (Birnbaum and Van Ness, 1992; Abe et al., 1992). The Cα mRNA is better suited to play the role of an internal control than the β_2-microglobulin or ribosomal RNA because its level of expression is closer to that of the target's.

Indeed, one of the major drawbacks in using endogenous RNA such as β_2-microglobulin or ribosomal RNA in coamplification settings has been their very high level of expression. It has been reported that simultaneous amplification of highly expressed control and target genes results in lower levels of target amplicons due to competition, which varies from sample to sample (Horikoshi et al., 1992; Murphy et al., 1990). Even the Cα control is far from being ideal since its level of expression, too high for Vβ chains expressed at very low levels, leads, through competition with the Vβ target, to an underestimation of the amounts of those Vβ transcripts (Hall and Finn, 1992; Boyer and Ferré, unpublished data; Chapter 9, this volume). It has been suggested that a housekeeping gene should be a better denominator for estimating gene expression per cell. The ideal endogenous internal standard should be one whose expression does not vary significantly during the cell cycle. In addition, its expression should be very close to the expression of the target RNA and should be amplified with equivalent efficiency, so that their linear regions of amplification would coincide. Such an ideal situation can be found when estimating the relative expression of mRNAs through alternative splicing (Neve et al., 1990; Mochizuki et al., 1992) or when measuring the relative abundance of allele-specific transcripts differing by a single nucleotide (Singer-Sam et al., 1992). Needless to say, however, that for most applications finding the ideal endogenous internal control is a real challenge.

Relative quantitation has also been performed in a coamplification format using an exogenous source of mRNA as a control (Chelly et al., 1988, 1990; Wood et al., 1992; Fonknechten et al., 1992; Ferré et al., 1992b, 1994). The advantage of this approach over the endogenous internal control lies in the fact that the amount of standard RNA added to the reaction can be adjusted to the target's level and that it should represent a more consistent source of standard because contrary to endogenous RNA, it is not subject to temporal variation in expression.

We have utilized a synthetic standard RNA (HIR) in a coamplification format to quantitate HIV-1 *gag* RNA in PBMCs for use in the monitoring of patients under therapy (Ferré et al., 1992b, 1994). In this assay, 10^3 copies of HIR are coamplified with the HIV-1 target. After amplification with a ^{32}P-labeled primer, both amplicons are detected and quantitated from the gel using the AMBIS radioanalytic imaging system (Fig. 6.1A). Note that both amplicons are coamplified with similar efficiencies (Fig. 6.1B). The amount of HIV-1 target is directly obtained from a simple equation: [(cpm target − cpm background)/(cpm HIR − cpm background)] × 1000. At high target:HIR ratio (> 10), competition between both amplicons can negatively affect the amount of control amplicon. Still, in the measurable linear part of the amplification, i.e., when enough labeled amplicons are generated to yield adequate cpm, the efficiency of both reactions remains equivalent. This suggests that the aforementioned competition occurs in the early cycles or at the reverse transcription level. Despite such competition, however, the precision of the assay in this range of target concentration, as compared to the precision evaluated at the optimal target:HIR ratio of 1, does not seem to be significantly affected as long as enough cpm for the HIR amplicon are gener-

ated. At low target:HIR ratio ($0.01 < R < 0.1$), the quantitation is significantly dependent on the background level and the assay starts to lose proportionality (Fig. 6.2). Thus, the linear range of the assay spans at least 2 logs from 100 to 10,000 HIV-1 RNA copy equivalents (Fig. 6.2). These copy numbers should be interpreted as relative values. Evaluating the precision of this assay, we have shown that a 2.2-fold difference in the amount of HIV-1 RNA targets represents a significant change (Ferré et al., 1992b, 1994).

A number of reports challenge the common view that an internal control is mandatory for maximum precision and/or reproducibility in relative quantitation settings (Horikoshi et al., 1992; Murphy et al., 1990; Hall and Finn, 1992). Murphy et al. (1990) prefer an endogenous control amplified in a different reaction vessel. They, and others (Masters et al., 1992), argued that the major source of error in any target RNA quantitation lies in the measurement in terms of quantity as well as integrity of the RNA material itself. Thus, an endogenous external control takes care of this variable by allowing normalization of the amount of amplified target to the amount of total RNA. Furthermore, a number of investigators (Noonan et al., 1990; Murphy et al., 1990; Horikoshi et al., 1992) also disputed the gain in precision/reproducibility brought by a coamplified control since, as stated previously, this very control can interfere with the amplification of the target. Yet, from our own experience with the HIV-1 RNA assay previously mentioned, we can attest that a coamplification format can yield more precision. As exemplified in Figure 6.3, the variance in cpm from the HIV-1 target is equivalent with or without coamplification. However, after normalization with the coamplified HIR control there is a significant gain in precision compared to normalization without coamplification. The mean RNA copy number without coamplification is 621 ± 265 (CV = 43%) compared to 565 ± 107 (CV = 19%) with coamplification. Similar results were obtained with 7 independent experiments (data not shown).

To summarize, a number of different PCR formats have been implemented to perform rel-

A   B

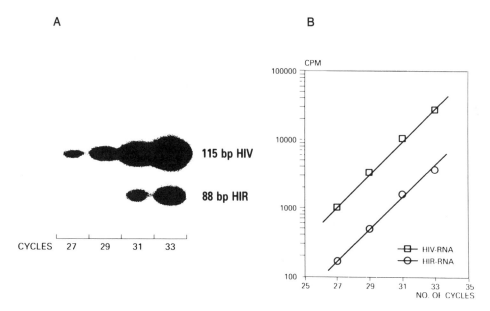

FIGURE 6.1. (**A**) AMBIS scan of a kinetic analysis of HIV-1/HIR coamplification. (**B**) Plot of the coamplification's kinetic.

ative quantitation. It is difficult from the literature to compare the quantitative power of these different assays specifically in terms of precision and reproducibility. Indeed, as reported previously (Ferré, 1992), almost everyone has different criteria on what is an appropriate assessment of the limits of a quantitative assay. It

is clear, however, that regardless of the PCR format, to perform precise and reliable determination of relative differences between samples, one has to analyze them in the same PCR assay. Indeed, with most Q-PCR methodologies, the between-assay variability spans a rather large range from 2- to 10-fold (Oka

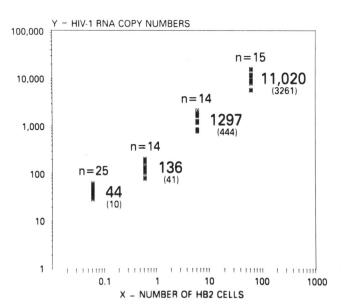

FIGURE 6.2. Quantitation of HIV-1 RNA copies in HB2 cells (chronically infected with HIV-1). n, number of replicates; 11,020, 1297, 136, 44 = mean HIV-1 copy numbers; (3261), (444), (41), (10) = standard deviations.

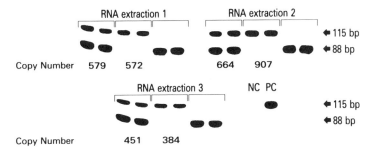

FIGURE 6.3. Assessment of the precision of the HIV-1 RNA PCR assay. Three HIV-1 RNA extractions were performed (HIR controls were from the same source), each PCR was essayed in duplicates as follows: coamplification HIV-1/HIR (left duplicate), HIV-1 RNA amplification alone (middle duplicate), HIR amplification alone (right duplicate). The copy number without coamplification (middle copy number) was obtained by dividing the cpm from the duplicated HIV-1 target bands by the mean of the cpm from the 3 duplicated HIR control bands. PC, HIV-1 DNA positive control; NC, negative control.

et al., 1990; Ferré et al., 1992a, 1993; Holodniy et al., 1991a,b; Feldman et al., 1991; Davis et al., 1990). It has recently been reported that relative Q-PCR can discriminate as little as 2-fold difference in gene expression (Horikoshi et al., 1992; Ferré et al., 1992b, 1994). Such levels of precision should be adequate for most applications. External and internal controls can add robustness to the quantitation. However, additions of controls such as an exogenous internal standard bring new variables into the system and thus their overall benefit, specifically in terms of precision, should be thoroughly investigated.

Absolute Quantitation

The aim of absolute quantitation is the determination of the exact number of molecules of target in a given sample. This type of information can be extremely valuable for a number of applications. For example, in research settings, estimation of the exact copy number of a given mRNA per cell can be instrumental in evaluating its physiological role (see Montarras et al., Chapter 24). The need for accurate evaluations, instead of estimates, of HIV-1 viral load in the different lymphoid tissues is of the utmost importance in understanding the pathology of HIV infections and represents another good example of the tremendous potential of absolute PCR quantitation. The same is true for the assessment of therapy effectiveness

in cancer treatments (see Chapters 27 and 28). Relative quantitation can help to judge efficacy but ultimately absolute quantitation is needed to evaluate the clinical status of a patient, i.e., is the patient entering molecular remission, still in remission, or resuming relapse?

But first, is PCR really capable of absolute quantitation? To answer this question we will first analyze the many quantitative approaches in which the amount of target has been reported in absolute numerical terms. As previously mentioned, most of the quantitative DNA methods, as well as more and more of the RNA work, fall into that category.

Absolute DNA Quantitation

The accuracy of any quantitation is intimately linked to the exactness of the standards. Not only does the standard need to be accurate in numbers, it also needs to be very close in composition to what is being tested. Accurate standards are fairly easy to obtain for DNA quantitation. A cell line containing only one (or two) copy(ies) of a given target should be a good source of standards (Oka et al., 1990; Lee et al., 1990; Kellog et al., 1990; Aoki et al., 1990; Ferré et al., 1992a; Billadeau et al., 1991, 1992; Ou et al., 1990). We will discuss absolute quantitation of HIV-1 DNA targets as a case example.

To quantitate HIV-1 proviruses in PBMCs, dilutions of cells harboring only one provirus into seronegative PBMCs have been used. These types of standards present some advantages compared to other sources of standards such as plasmid HIV DNA diluted in PBMCs. For example, cells and thus targets can be counted accurately prior to dilutions down to 5×10^5 cells (targets)/ml using a simple hemocytometer, but 20 μg/ml of plasmid is needed to have an adequate reading on the spectrophotometer. This represents, for a 5-kb plasmid, 4×10^{12} targets. Thus, to quantitate by PCR from 10^4 targets down, a starting 50-fold dilution for the cell standard will be needed compared to 4×10^8-fold dilution for the plasmid. Needless to say that through this process, labeling the final dilution of plasmid DNA with a real number of molecules becomes hazardous. It has been mentioned that the broad differences, reported throughout the literature (up to 100-fold), in the amount of HIV-1 DNA in PBMCs in similar patient populations might in part reflect possible flaws in the estimation of HIV standards (Genesca et al., 1990).

To increase the precision and accuracy of HIV-1 DNA quantitation, a gene control such as the globin locus can be coamplified. We have utilized this type of approach to monitor the amount of HIV-1 DNA in the PBMCs of asymptomatic HIV-1 seropositive individuals under immunotherapeutic treatment for 1 year. An example of this Q-PCR format is shown in Figure 6.4. A drop in the HIV-1 band intensity occurs at bleed 36 in this otherwise stable individual for HIV-1 copy numbers. Normalization of this bleed value with globin brings it in the range of the other bleed values, i.e., 70, 76, and 92 HIV-1 copy numbers for bleed 32, 36, and 40 weeks, respectively (instead of 63, 19, and 120 copies obtained without globin adjustment). To further evaluate the impact of the globin control on the precision of the assay, five duplicates from the same cell lysate from six different bleeds have been analyzed in two separate PCR reactions. The copy number values reported in Table 6.1 corresponds to the mean of these five duplicates. Since the amount of HIV-1 and globin DNA should be equivalent in all duplicates, the calculated mean fold difference between the highest value

and the four others gauges the whithin-assay variability. It is apparent from Table 6.1 that, in the first PCR assay, the HIV-1 DNA values obtained without globin adjustment are less precise as compared to the adjusted ones. Furthermore, the precision of the globin-adjusted assay is more consistent. From these examples, it can be concluded that normalization of HIV-1 copy numbers with the globin control affects positively the precision of the assay.

Since the equivalent of 4×10^5 cells is added to the reaction vessel, the amount of globin targets (8×10^5) is at least two orders of magnitude higher than the amount of HIV-1 targets (0–10^4). If the same number of cycles is performed for both amplicons (typically 30), the globin target is overamplified, which implies that it is no longer in the linear range and competition with the HIV-1 target may occur (Lee et al., 1990; F. Ferré, A. Marchese, unpublished data). Thus, to coamplify both targets and still stay in their linear range of amplification, 30 cycles are used for HIV-1 and only 15 for globin. This can be achieved by adding the globin primers after 15 cycles of HIV-1 amplification. Alternatively, globin primers with lower T_m than HIV-1 primers can be used (G. Cimino, personal communication). In this format, the first 15 cycles are run at high stringency permitting only HIV-1 amplification and for the last 15 cycles, the stringency is reduced to allow coamplification of globin. Using the HLA locus as a control, Kellogs et al. reported another way to eliminate interference in coamplification settings. It consists of reducing the amount of HLA primers (down to 1 pmol each) such that the efficiency of the HLA amplifications is attenuated sufficiently to allow simultaneous quantitation of both targets (Kellogs et al., 1990). However, experimenting with the same approach, we have found that by lowering the amount of primers to 1 pmol, the reproducibility of the globin amplification is seriously affected (F. Ferré, A. Marchese, unpublished data).

A number of observations made us believe that our HIV-1 quantitation method in which the globin gene is coamplified for fewer cycles is reasonably accurate. First, it has been shown by Southern technology (Roques and Dor-

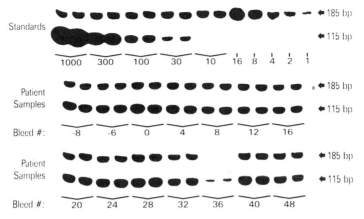

FIGURE 6.4. HIV-1 and globin targets were coamplified; (upper panel, left side) Autoradiograms of duplicated serial dilutions of 85-14-F2 cells from 1000 to 10 cells (or HIV-1 copies) in 4×10^5 PBMCs (HIV-1 standard); (upper panel, right side) autoradiograms of serial dilutions of blood bank PBMCs from 16×10^5 to 10^5 cells (globin standard); HIV-1 amplicon = 115 bp, globin amplicon = 185 bp. Fifteen consecutive bleed samples (-8, -6, 0, 4 . . . 48 weeks) of a given HIV-1-infected individuals were analyzed in the same PCR assay (middle/lower panels). The HIV-1 and globin copy numbers were extrapolated from the respective standards, then the HIV-1 values can be expressed per 4×10^5 PBMCs after normalization using the globin internal control.

mont, 1991; S.Z. Salahuddin, personal communication) that the 85-14-F2 cell line used to produce the HIV-1 standard contains a unique copy of a truncated HIV virus per cell. Since 10^6 85-14-F2 cells can be counted accurately, their dilution down to 1000 cell equivalent per 4×10^5 blood bank PBMCs should also be accurate.

Second, by analyzing the kinetics of coamplification of the 10^3 HIV-1 standard and the globin control (8×10^5 copies), we can demonstrate that if the amount of globin targets is

accurate then the amount of HIV-1 targets is also accurate. Indeed, from the standard curves shown in Figure 6.5, one can observe that 8×10^5 globin targets (4×10^5 PBMCs) yield 7500 cpm after 15 cycles and both amplicons accumulate with a similar efficiency of amplification of 93% (the specific activities of both HIV-1 and globin ^{32}P-labeled primers have also been shown to be equivalent). Thus, the number of additional cycles (n) necessary for the HIV-1 amplification to recover its original handicap of 800-fold compared to globin is

TABLE 6.1. Impact of the globin control on the assay's precision.

PCR assay number	Sample number	Without globin adjustment		With globin adjustment	
		Mean DNA copy number	Mean fold difference (SD)	Mean DNA copy number	Mean fold difference (SD)
1	1	359	1.5 (0.3)	637	1.2 (0.1)
	2	111	2.2 (0.9)	314	1.4 (0.3)
	3	44	1.8 (0.4)	79	1.3 (0.3)
2	4	18	1.1 (0.1)	38	1.3 (0.2)
	5	468	1.2 (0.2)	692	1.3 (0.3)
	6	99	1.4 (0.2)	153	1.3 (0.1)
	Mean		1.5 (0.4)		1.3 (0.1)
	Range		1.1–2.2		1.2–1.4

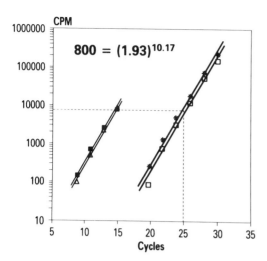

$$800 = (1.93)^{10.17}$$

FIGURE 6.5. Kinetic analyses of the globin (■, △) and HIV-1 (*, □) coamplifications for the 1000 copy standard from two PCR assays; cpm values versus cycle numbers were plotted for both amplicons.

given by the equation $800 = (1.93)^n$ or $n = \log 800/\log 1.93 = 10.17$. It follows that 25 cycles $(15 + 10)$ of HIV-1 amplification should yield an amount of cpm equivalent to the globin amplification; as shown in Figure 6.5, this is effectively the case. Therefore since 4×10^5 PBMCs can be obtained rather accurately, we conclude that the 1000 HIV-1 copies are also reasonably accurate.

Third, we have previously reported that the 10 copy level from the HIV-1 standard is effectively in the range of 10 copies (Ferré et al., 1992a). This was achieved through the amplification of 10-fold dilutions of the 10 copy standards in 10 duplicates and by showing that the number of HIV-1 positive and negative samples obeyed the laws of Poisson distribution.

Lastly, 30 of 33 HIV-1-infected individuals (91%) showed similar viral load (less than a 2-fold difference) when utilizing a second set of HIV-1 primers M667/M668 (Arrigo et al., 1989) (data not shown). The other 3 patients showed a 10-fold increase or more in the amount of HIV-1 DNA targets when using the M667/M668 primer set. This might be explained by mismatches between the SK38/

SK39 primer set and the HIV-1 strains in these 3 patients. These data indicate, however, that the estimation of the HIV-1 DNA load is independent of the choice of primers for the majority of infected individuals and therefore if the HIV-1 standard is accurate then the extrapolated copy number for a given patient sample should also be accurate.

The principle of limiting dilution can also be called on to achieve absolute DNA quantitation. It is based on the use of a qualitative all-or-none end point and on the premise that one or more targets in the reaction mixture give rise to a positive end point. This quantitative format was first proposed to obtain relative quantitation (Zhang et al., 1991; Brillanti et al., 1991; Steuler et al., 1992). Accurate quantitation can be achieved by performing multiple replicates at serial dilutions of the material to be assayed (Simmonds et al., 1990; Lee et al., 1990; Sykes et al., 1992). At the limit of dilution, where some end points are positive and some are negative, the number of targets present can be calculated from the proportion of negative end points by using Poisson statistics. Unlike the previously mentioned standard PCR procedures that quantitate PCR products, this method quantitates the total number of initial DNA targets present in a sample. In this type of quantitative format, it is mandatory that PCR be optimized so that reliable detection of one or a few DNA targets occurs. Therefore, as long as the one copy level still gives a positive signal, the quantitation is not dependent on the amplification efficiency. This represents a major advantage of this PCR format. However, for many applications this means that a relatively high number of cycles (usually over 40) and/or two-stage PCR is performed, thus increasing the risk of false-positive through carryover. On a different level, because many PCR reactions per sample are required, this approach is time consuming, costly, and of limited application when analyzing a large number of samples.

A recent approach, PCR in situ hybridization, described in detail in Chapter 5, combines the power of in situ hybridization and PCR. As in in situ hybridization per se, this method has been designed to accurately quantitate the amount of positive cells rather than the total amount of initial targets present in the sample. One of the main advantages of this technology resides in the fact that the results of amplification and thus quantitation can be directly associated with a specific cell type (Haase et al., 1990; Spann et al., 1991; Nuovo, 1992; Nuovo et al., 1991a, 1992a,b; Bagasra et al., 1992, 1993a,b; Embretson et al., 1993; Patterson et al., 1993). This methodology can be implemented, for example, to better identify the cell types that carry significant amounts of HIV-1 *in vivo* (Bagasra et al., 1993a). Because the exact number of positive HIV-1-infected cells as estimated using this method is significantly higher than the number obtained through extrapolation using conventional Q-PCR, it has been suggested that the *in situ* PCR format is more sensitive (Bagasra et al., 1992). Our current reading of the literature is that the jury is still out on this issue.

Finally, we shall mention that competitive PCR procedures have been used for the accurate quantitation of DNA targets (Simon et al., 1992; Lundeberg et al., 1991). This technique, extensively utilized with RNA targets, will be described in some detail in the RNA section.

In summary, it seems that despite the numerous restrictions and pitfalls previously described, fairly accurate assessment of the amount of DNA targets is achievable by PCR.

Absolute Quantitation of RNA

At the RNA level more obstacles lie in the way. As previously mentioned, the first hurdle to overcome for accurate quantitation of RNA targets is finding the right source of standards. Some investigators have used internal DNA standards in a competitive PCR format for the quantitation of RNA targets (Gilliland et al., 1990; Uberla et al., 1991; Li et al., 1991). As discussed previously, DNA standards are usually not considered optimum because they cannot be utilized to control the reverse-transcription step that is relatively inefficient and represents one of the most important sources of variability. Furthermore, because the yield of the reverse transcription reaction is not calcu-

lated (but usually in the range of 5–90%), the mRNA amounts inferred by cDNA measurements (i.e., considering 100% of reverse transcription efficiency) are undervalued (Silani et al., 1991). Thus, for accurate quantitation of RNA, a RNA standard is preferable.

Contrary to the situation encountered in PCR DNA settings, however, there is no cell line that can be utilized as a reliable provider of standard mRNA simply because the amount of most mRNA species fluctuates significantly throughout the cell cycle. The amount of a specific RNA can be estimated by Northern analysis or nuclease protection assay but both methods are limited in accuracy.

Recently, a growing number of investigators have turned to recombinant RNA templates as the ultimate RNA standard for absolute quantitation. *In vitro* transcribed specific RNA (cRNA) similar to the RNA target can be purified, quantitated by spectrophotometry, and diluted to generate standard curves. Such external controls have been utilized, for example, to estimate the amount of HIV-1 RNA in PBMCs and plasma (Michael et al., 1992; Seshamma et al., 1992; Winters et al., 1992; Holodniy et al., 1991a,b) or to monitor gene expression (Hoof et al., 1991; Ballagi-Pordany et al., 1991). Since these cRNAs should have secondary structures equivalent to the target, such controls seem suitable to monitor the reverse-transcription step and the amplification efficiency. Michael et al. also used actin primers and actin RNA control to evaluate the amount of starting RNA (Michael et al., 1992). What is left out of these methods is the monitoring of the tube-to-tube variability that, as described previously, is needed to increase precision.

Similar to the approach reported by Gilliland et al. (1990), Becker-Andre and Hahlbrock developed a quantitative assay based on the competition between the target and an internal cRNA standard that differs by a single base compared to the target mRNA. Since both target and control are virtually identical, the efficiency of their amplification should be equivalent, leading to a fair competition and therefore to an accurate measurement (Becker-Andre and Hahlbrock, 1989; Lin et al., 1991; Furtado et al., 1990, 1993). Although, elegant in its concept, this method has not been widely applied plausibly due to a number of limitations. To differentiate both amplicons, the point mutation introduced in the cRNA control is engineered to reveal a new restriction site. The need for restriction analysis of the amplified sequences represents the first limitation since this added step is not always 100% efficient. Furthermore, it has been reported that heteroduplexes, containing target and control strands, are generated during the amplification and thus affect the reliable calculation of transcript concentration (Gilliland et al., 1990; Becker-Andre and Hahlbrock, 1989). However, to eliminate the complication generated by the heteroduplex formation, the use of a sequencing gel that separates single-stranded molecules has been implemented (Porcher et al., 1992).

Today, it seems that the cRNA standard of choice, first developed by Alice Wang and her colleagues, utilizes the same primer sequences as the target mRNA but yields a PCR product of different size (Wang et al., 1989). Such a cRNA standard can be coamplified with the target and both amplicons separated by gel electrophoresis. This approach has become so popular that a need for efficient ways in creating those cRNA controls has emerged (Simon et al., 1992; Vanden Heuvel et al., 1993). Two quantitative formats have been developed around this type of cRNA standard.

The first one, pioneered by Wang and co-workers, capitalizes on the fact that throughout the coamplification process, the efficiency of the reactions stays equivalent for both amplicons (Wang et al., 1989). Thus, in the exponential phase of the amplification, the amount of target mRNA can be quantitated by extrapolating against the standard curve. These authors have shown that for up to 5×10^5 copies of IL-1α mRNA, the amplification is exponential between 14 and 22 cycles with an efficiency of 88% for both amplicons. Variations of this method have been implemented to determine the levels of production of a number of growth factors or cellular genes such as the LDL receptor (Powell and Kroon, 1992; Baldwin and Zhang, 1992; Kanangat et al., 1992; Feldman et al., 1991).

Interestingly, it has been reported that just after a plateau is reached (around 30 cycles), the accumulation of both control and target amplicons still occurs at the same rate, which indicates that the plateau effect results from a general slowdown of the PCR machinery (Powell and Kroon, 1992; Ferré et al., 1992b, 1994). This also implies that quantitation should still be feasible shortly after the plateau. From a practical standpoint, running serial dilutions of cDNA or performing kinetic analysis of the amplification for each sample can rapidly become cumbersome for a number of applications. Once the equivalency of the amplification efficiency for both target and control has been established, only one time-point per sample should be sufficient for quantitative analysis (Powell and Kroon, 1992; Ferré et al., 1992b, 1994).

The second quantitative format is based on the previously mentioned competitive approach. The target RNA is coamplified with serial dilutions of the synthetic cRNA control and both amplicons are separated by gel electrophoresis (for review, Clementi et al., 1993). A minimum of four to five competitor dilutions within the expected range of the target RNA needs to be performed (Stieger et al., 1991; Simon et al., 1992; Scadden et al., 1992; Li et al., 1991; Kaneko et al., 1992; Lin et al., 1991; Piatak et al., 1993a,b). The PCR products can be quantitated by a variety of different techniques. The densitometric evaluation of ethidium bromide-stained gels represents the simplest way. Contrary to the approach developed by Wang et al. (1989), this method does not require the quantitation be done in the exponential phase of both amplicons, which represents a major advantage. Indeed, in principle, a ratio of 1 obtained from the amplified products reflects the initial concentration of both template species, regardless of the total amounts produced by the amplification reaction. Thus, as for the limited dilution approach, the sensitivity of this method can be boosted by increasing the number of cycles. In fact, in most procedures at least 40 cycles are run. The major drawback of this procedure, however, resides in the fact that it requires on average six amplification reactions per sample, thus it is expensive and cumbersome.

To conclude this review of RNA PCR methods presumably capable of absolute quantitation, we should mention the advent of a potentially very promising mean of absolute RNA quantitation, namely the *in situ* RT-PCR methodology (Nuovo, 1992; Patterson et al., 1993). But the crucial question remains unanswered: how accurate is the quantitation of any transcript using the aforementioned methodologies? As previously specified, we will utilize material extracted from the HIV-1 literature in our efforts to address this point. The concern over accuracy comes from at least two different angles.

The first one pertains to the fact that a significant difference in HIV-1 RNA copy numbers in similar patient populations has been published. For example, the group of Thomas Merigan has reported a mean HIV-1 copy number of 2700 ± 875 in patients eligible for dideoxynucleoside therapy (CDC II and III) (Holodniy et al., 1991) compared to a mean of 78,000 copies/ml of plasma for patients in CDC stage II and III (asymptomatic), 352,000 in CDC IVC2 (ARC) or 2,448,000 in CDC IVC1 (AIDS) as recently published by Piatak and co-workers (Piatak et al., 1993a). Both teams utilized a cRNA control that was quantitated on a spectrophotometer to obtain correct copy numbers. The first group used this cRNA as an internal control to generate a standard curve whereas the other team developed a competitive format. Interestingly, Aoki-Sei and co-workers have published that the geometric mean of HIV-1 RNA targets in asymptomatic patients is 958 copies (Aoki-Sei et al., 1992) whereas Bagnarelli et al., utilizing a competitive assay, found values closer to the range reported by Piatak and co-workers (mean 27,800 copies/ml in CDC II and III) (Bagnarelli et al., 1992). Thus, different methods give significantly different results. It is also possible that different methods of RNA extraction as well as slightly different cRNA per se could lead to these different estimations. Indeed, changes in the secondary structure of the cRNA could modify the processivity of the reverse transcriptase and therefore could bias

the absolute quantitation (Sperison et al., 1992). It has been reported that the competitor cRNA is often amplified more efficiently than the target RNA (Horikoshi et al., 1992; Volkenandt et al., 1992). Thus, the point where the amplification products are of equal intensity on the gel may not actually represent equal concentrations of the competing RNA segments. Then, should it be concluded that absolute RNA quantitation by PCR is not achievable? This leads us to the second point.

Most of the current methods that describe absolute quantitation of nucleic acid targets do not establish the validity of the reported numbers by comparing them to numbers obtained using other means of nucleic acids quantitation. This is of crucial importance for RNA quantitation since, as previously mentioned, the exactness of RNA standards is rather difficult to demonstrate and thus should be assessed using a number of different methods. Lets illustrate this point through a couple of examples. The easiest case scenario is found when high copy numbers of target RNA are reported ($> 10^7$ copies per μg of total RNA or ml of plasma). Indeed, such high numbers of targets should also be quantifiable by Northern blot or RNase protection analysis. In the case that only a few copies are present, the above analysis will require that the starting material be concentrated, which is usually possible using a few abundant sources of targets. For example, it has been reported that 10 HIV-1 infectious doses represent about 750 RNA molecules (Piatak et al., 1993b). By pelleting the equivalent of 10,000 HIV-1 infectious doses, one should reach the limit of sensitivity of RNase protection assay; with 100,000 infectious doses, the sample should be quantifiable by Northern blot. Finally, as sophisticated and sensitive quantitative assays such as the branched DNA (bDNA) signal amplification becomes more available, they will certainly be useful in challenging the accuracy of PCR methods. It seems logical that those types of evaluations be performed before reporting any accurate measurement of RNA by Q-PCR. They will not guarantee the accuracy of the PCR measurement but should help in the process of legitimizing it and thus should boost the credibility of the PCR data. For example, Wang et al. have reported that the amount of IL-1α mRNA in LPS-induced macrophages as estimated by Q-PCR correlated with the results of Northern blot analysis (Wang et al., 1989).

Conclusion

In the last few years, the quantitative side of PCR grew from being a lab curiosity to representing a key technology for the understanding of a complex biological entity such as the pathology of AIDS (Temin and Bolognesi, 1993). We have reviewed in this chapter the tremendous amount of work, accruing almost exponentially, that accompanied the development and maturation of Q-PCR methodologies. We have previously mentioned that, as is often the case with exponential growth, certain aspects of Q-PCR methods have been overlooked. For example, if it is true that Q-PCR methodologies have reached the maturation stage, it is also very clear that, contrary to wishful thinking recently expressed by Clementi and colleagues (Clementi et al., 1993), more methods need to be validated to boost the credibility of Q-PCR assays (Ferré, 1992). This viewpoint has recently been strengthened through our interaction with governmental regulatory agencies. Indeed, they expressed some distrust in Q-PCR methods, which is rooted, in essence, in the lack of validated methodologies in the published literature.

On the upside, though, it is now well recognized that Q-PCR is capable of relative quantitation with great precision, i.e., low within-assay variability. One challenge of the future will be the development of even more robust assays in which the between-assay variability will be reduced. For example, this might be partly achieved by improving reproducibility at the thermo-cycler level (see Chapter 14). Indeed, it has been suggested that the thermo-cycler itself represents an important source of variability (Hoof et al., 1991). We have shown that, despite the presence of an internal control in HIV-1 RNA quantitation, the use of different thermo-cyclers increases significantly the between-assay variability (F. Ferré, P. Pezzoli,

and E. Buxton, unpublished data). For the quantitation of RNA, diminishing the variability associated with the reverse-transcription step should also be a tangible goal. Enzymes such as the *Thermus thermophilus* DNA polymerase (Thl pol) represent reasonable candidates (Myers and Gelfand, 1991). Indeed, the ability of Thl pol to perform both reverse-transcription and DNA amplification might prove useful in tightening the reproducibility of RNA quantitation. Finally, by automating most of the PCR procedures from nucleic acid extraction to the final quantitation of the amplified product, the daunting specter of irreproducibility might become a thing of the past (DiCesare et al., 1993).

We have devoted a great deal of this chapter to tackling the problem of absolute quantitation using PCR. We have stressed that PCR methods are not genuinely gifted for accuracy and therefore other means of nucleic acid quantitation have to be implemented at some level to validate the PCR findings. Interestingly, recent developments such as quantitative analyses using *in situ* PCR of DNA targets, which fueled the controversy over the accuracy of standard PCR assays, represent powerful tools for absolute quantitation. One drawback of such methodology is that it is still quite cumbersome and thus, for it to be more widely usable, it will be necessary to facilitate the technology perhaps through increased automation.

Will we, one day, be able to quantitate the exact amount of RNA targets inside a given cell using technology such as *in situ* PCR? A positive answer to this question will without doubt fulfill John Maddox's dream.

References

Abbs S, Bobrow M (1992): Analysis of quantitative PCR for the diagnosis of deletion and duplication carriers in the dystrophin gene. *F Med Genet* 29:191–196.

Abe J, Kotzin BL, Jujo K, Melish ME, Glode MP, Kohsaka T, Leung DYM (1992): Selective expansion of T cells expressing T-cell receptor variable regions Vβ2 and Vβ8 in Kawasaki disease. *Proc Natl Acad Sci USA* 89:4066–4070.

Aoki S, Yarchoan R, Thomas RV, Pluda JM, Marczyk K, Broder S, Mitsuya H (1990): Quantitative analysis of HIV-1 proviral DNA in peripheral blood mononuclear cells from patients with AIDS and ARC: Decrease of proviral DNA content following treatment 2',3'-dideoxyinosine (ddI). *AIDS Res Human Retrovirus* 6:1331-1339.

Aoki-Sei S, Yarchoan R, Kageyama S, Hoekzema DT, Pluda JM, Wyvill KM, Broder S, Mitsuya H (1992): Plasma HIV-1 viremia in HIV-1 infected individuals assessed by polymerase chain reaction. *AIDS Res Human Retrovirus* 7:1263-1270.

Arrigo SJ, Weitsman S, Rosenblatt JD, Chen ISY (1989): Analysis of rev gene function on human immunodeficiency virus type 1 replication in lymphoid cells by using a quantitative polymerase chain reaction method. *J Virol* 63:4875-4881.

Arrigo SJ, Weitsman S, Zack JA, Chen ISY (1990): Characterization and expression of novel singly spliced RNA species of human immunodeficiency virus type 1. *J Virol* 64:4585-4588.

Bagasra O, Hauptman SP, Lischner HW, Sachs M, Pomerantz RJ (1992): Detection of human immunodeficiency virus type 1 provirus in mononuclear cells by in situ polymerase chain reaction. *N Engl J Med* 326:1385-1391.

Bagasra O, Pomerantz RJ (1993a): Human immunodeficiency virus type I provirus is demonstrated in peripheral blood monocytes in vivo: A study utilizing an in situ polymerase chain reaction. *AIDS Res Human Retrovirus* 9:69-76.

Bagasra O, Seshamma T, Pomerantz RJ (1993b): Polymerase chain reaction in situ: Intracellular amplification and detection of HIV-1 proviral DNA and other specific genes. *J Immunol Methods* 158:131-145.

Bagnarelli P, Menzo S, Valenza A, Manzin A, Giacca M, Ancarani F, Scalise G, Varaldo PE, Clementi M (1992): Molecular profile of human immunodeficiency virus type 1 infection in symptomless patients and in patients with AIDS. *J Virol* 66:7328-7335.

Baldwin GS, Zhang Q-X (1992): Measurement of gastrin and transforming growth factor α messenger RNA levels in colonic carcinoma cell lines by quantitative polymerase chain reaction. *Cancer Res* 52:2261-2267.

Ballagi-Pordany A, Ballagii-Pordany A, Funa K (1991): Quantitative determination of mRNA phenotypes by the polymerase chain reaction. *Anal Biochem* 196:89-94.

Becker-Andre M, Hahlbrock K (1989): Absolute mRNA quantification using the polymerase chain reaction (PCR). A novel approach by a PCR aided transcript titration assay (PATTY). *Nucl Acids Res* 17:9437-9446.

Bej AK, Mahbubani MH, Atlas RM (1991): Amplification of nucleic acids by polymerase chain reaction (PCR) and other methods and their applications. *Crit Rev Biochem Mol Biol* 26:301-334.

Billadeau D, Blackstadt M, Greipp P, Kyle RA, Oken MM, Kay N, Van Ness B (1991): Analysis of B-lymphoid malignancies using allele-specific polymerase chain reaction: A technique for sequential quantitation of residual disease. *Blood* 78:3021-3029.

Billadeau D, Quam L, Thomas W, Kay N, Greipp P, Kyle R, Oken MM, Van Ness B (1992): Detection and quantitation of malignant cells in the peripheral blood of multiple myeloma patients. *Blood* 80:1818-1824.

Birnbaum G, Van Ness B (1992): Quantitation of T-cell receptor Vβ chain expression on lymphocytes from blood, brain, and spinal fluid in patients with multiple sclerosis and other neurological diseases. *Ann Neurol* 32:24-230.

Boom R, Sol CJ, Salimans MM, Jansen CL, Wertheim van Dillen PM, van der Noordaa J (1990): Rapid and simple method for purification of nucleic acids. *J Clin Microbiol* 28:495-503.

Boyer V, Smith LR, Ferré F, Pezzoli P, Trauger RJ, Jensen FC, Carlo DJ (1993): T cell receptor Vβ repertoire in HIV-infected individuals: Lack of evidence for selective Vβ deletion. *Clin Exp Immunol* 92:437-441.

Brenner CA, Tam AW, Nelson PA, Engleman EG, Suzuki N, Fry KE, Larrick JW (1989): Message amplification phenotyping (MAPPing): A technique to simultaneously measure multiple mRNAs from small numbers of cells. *BioTechniques* 7:1096-1103.

Brillanti S, Garson JA, Tuke PW, Ring C, Briggs M, Masci C, Miglioli M, Barbara L, Tedder RS (1991): Effect of α-interferon therapy on hepatitis C viraemia in community acquired chronic non-A, non-B hepatitis: A quantitative polymerase chain reaction study. *J Med Virol* 34:136-141.

Chelly J, Kaplan JC, Maire P, Gautron S, Kahn A (1988): Transcription of the dystrophin gene in human muscle and non-muscle tissues. *Nature (London)* 333:858-860.

Chelly J, Hamard G, Koulakoff A, Kaplan J-C, Kahn A, Berwald-Netter Y (1990a): Dystrophin gene transcribed from different promoters in neuronal and glial cells. *Nature (London)* 344:64-65.

Chelly J, Montarras D, Pinset C, Berwald-Netter Y, Kaplan JC, Kahn A (1990b): Quantitative estimation of minor mRNAs by cDNA-polymerase chain reaction: application to dystrophin mRNA in cultured myogenic and brain cells. *Eur J Biochem* 187:691–698.

Chirgwin J, Przybyla A, MacDonald R, Rutter W (1979): Isolation of biologically active ribonucleic acid from sources enriched in ribonuclease. *Biochemistry* 18:5294–5299.

Choi Y, Kotzin B, Herron L, Callahan J, Marrack P, Kappler J (1989): Interaction of *Staphylococcus aureus* toxin "superantigens" with human T cells. *Proc Natl Acad Sci USA* 86:8941–8945.

Chomcynski P, Sacchi N (1987): Single-step method of RNA isolation by acid guanidinium Thiocyanate-phenol-chloroform extraction. *Anal Biochem* 162:156–159.

Clementi M, Menzo S, Bagnarelli P, Manzin A, Valenza A, Varaldo PE (1993): Quantitative PCR and RT-PCR in virology. *PCR Methods Applic* 2:191–196.

Davis GR, Blumeyer K, DiMichele LJ, Whitfield KM, Chappelle H, Riggs N, Ghosh SS, Kao PM, Fahy E, Kwoh DY, Guatelli JC, Spector SA, Richman DD, Gingeras TR (1990): Detection of HIV-1 in AIDS patients using amplification-mediated hybridization analyses: Reproducibility and quantitative limitations. *J Infect Dis* 162:13–20.

DiCesare J, Grossman B, Katz E, Picozza E, Ragusa R, Woudenberg T (1993): A high-sensitivity electrochemiluminescence-based detection system for automated PCR product quantitation. *BioTechniques* 15:152–157.

Dickover RE, Donovan RM, Goldstein E, Dandekar S, Bush CE, Carlson JR (1990): Quantitation of human immunodeficiency virus DNA by using the polymerase chain reaction. *J Clin Microb* 28:2130–2133.

Embretson J, Zupancic M, Beneke J, Till M, Wolinsky S, Ribas JL, Burke A, Haase AT (1993): Analysis of human immunodeficiency virus-infected tissues by amplification and *in situ* hybridization reveals latent and permissive infections at single-cell resolution. *Proc Natl Acad Sci USA* 90:357–361.

Eron JJ, Gorczyca P, Kaplan JC, D'Aquila RT (1992): Susceptibility testing by polymerase chain reaction DNA quantitation: A method to measure drug resistance of human immunodeficiency virus type 1 isolates. *Proc Natl Acad Sci USA* 89:3241–3245.

Fahy E, Kwoh DY, Gingeras TR (1991): Self-sustained sequence replication (3SR): An isothermal transcription-based amplification system alternative to PCR. *PCR Methods Applic* 1:25–33.

Farrell RE (1993): *RNA Methodologies: A Laboratory Guide for Isolation and Characterization.* San Diego: Academic Press, 13:220.

Feddersen RM, Van Ness BG (1989): Single copy gene detection requiring minimal cell numbers. *BioTechniques* 7:44–49.

Feldman AM, Ray PE, Silan CM, Mercer JA, Minobe W, Bristow MR (1991): Selective gene expression in failing human heart: Quantification of steady-state levels of messenger RNA in endomyocardial biopsies using the polymerase chain reaction. *Circulation* 83:1866–1872.

Ferré F (1992): Quantitative or semi-quantitative PCR: Reality versus myth. *PCR Methods Applic* 2:1–9.

Ferré F, Garduno F (1989): Preparation of crude cell extract suitable for amplification of RNA by the polymerase chain reaction. *Nucl Acids Res* 17:2141.

Ferré F, Marchese A, Duffy PC, Lewis DE, Wallace MR, Beecham HJ, Burnett KG, Jensen FC, Carlo DJ (1992a): Quantitation of HIV viral burden by PCR in HIV seropositive Navy personnel representing Walter Reed staging 1 to 6. *AIDS Res Human Retrovirus* 8:269–275.

Ferré F, Pezzoli P, Jensen FC, Carlo DJ (1992b): Development and validation of quantitative PCR assay to precisely assess the amount of HIV-1 RNA in blood cells from patients undergoing a one year immunotherapeutic treatment. *VIII Int Conf AIDS, Amsterdam* (Abstract PoA2134).

Ferré F, Marchese AL, Griffin SL, Daigle AE, Richieri SP, Jensen FC, Carlo DJ (1993): Development and validation of a quantitative PCR assay to assess with precision the amount of HIV-1 DNA in blood cells from patients undergoing a one-year immunotherapeutic treatment. *AIDS*, in press.

Ferré F, Pezzoli P, Buxton E, Marchese A (1994): Quantitation of RNA targets using the polymerase chain reaction. In: *Molecular Methods for Virus Detection*, Wiedbrauk DL, Farkas DH, eds. San Diego: Academic Press, in press.

Fonknechten N, Chelly J, Lepercq J, Kahn A, Kaplan J-C, Kitzis A, Chomel J-C (1992): CFTR illegitimate transcription in lymphoid cells: Quantification and applications to the investigation of pathological transcripts. *Hum Genet* 88:508–512.

Furtado MR, Balachandran R, Gupta P, Wolinsky SM (1990): Analysis of alternatively spliced human immunodeficiency virus type-1 mRNA species, one of which encodes a novel tat-env fusion protein. *Virology* 185:258–270.

Furtado MR, Murphey R, Wolinsky S (1993): Quantification of human immunodeficiency virus type 1 tat mRNA as a marker for assessing the efficacy of antiretroviral therapy. *J Infect Dis* 167:213–216.

Genesca J, Wang RY, Alter HJ, Shih JW (1990): Clinical correlation and genetic polymorphism of the human immunodeficiency virus proviral DNA obtained after polymerase chain reaction amplification. *J Infect Dis* 162:1025–1030.

Gilliland G, Perrin S, Bunn HF (1990): Competitive PCR for quantitation of mRNA. In: *PCR Protocols*. Innis MA, Gelfand DH, Sninsky JJ, White TJ, eds. New York: Academic Press, 60–69.

Golay J, Passerini F, Introna M (1991): A simple and rapid method to analyze specific mRNAs from few cells in a semi-quantitative way using the polymerase chain reaction. *PCR Methods Applic* 1:144–145.

Guatelli JC, Gingeras TR, Richman DD (1989): Nucleic acid amplification in vitro: Detection of sequences with low copy numbers and application to diagnosis of human immunodeficiency virus type 1 infection. *Clin Microbiol Rev* 2:217–226.

Haase AT, Retzel EF, Staskus KA (1990): Amplification and detection of lentiviral DNA inside cells. *Proc Natl Acad Sci USA* 87:4971–4975.

Hall BL, Finn OJ (1992): PCR-based analysis of the T-cell receptor Vβ multigene family: Experimental parameters affecting its validity. *BioTechniques* 13:248–257.

Henrard DR, Mehaffey WF, Allain JP (1992): A sensitive viral capture assay for detection of plasma viremia in HIV infected individuals. *AIDS Res Human Retrovirus* 8:47–52.

Higuchi R (1989): Simple and rapid preparation of samples for PCR. In: *PCR Technology: Principles and Applications for DNA Amplification*. Erlich HA, eds. New York: Stockton Press, 31–38.

Holodniy M, Katzenstein DA, Sengupta S, Wang AM, Casipit C, Schwartz DH, Konrad M, Groves E, Merigan TC (1991a): Detection and quantification of human immunodeficiency virus RNA in patient serum by use of the polymerase chain reaction. *J Infect Dis* 163:862–866.

Holodniy M, Katzenstein DA, Israelski DM, Merigan TC (1991b): Reduction in plasma human immunodeficiency virus ribonucleic acid after dideoxynucleoside therapy as determined by the polymerase chain reaction. *J Clin Invest* 88:1755–1759.

Hoof T, Riordan JR, Tummler B (1991): Quantitation of mRNA by the kinetic polymerase chain reaction assay: A tool for monitoring P-glycoprotein gene expression. *Anal Biochem* 196:161–169.

Horikoshi T, Danenberg KD, Stadbauer THW, Volkenandt M, Shea LCC, Aigner K, Gustavsson B, Leichman L, Frosing R, Ray M, Gibson NW, Spears CP, Danenberg PV (1992): Quantitation of thymidylate synthase, dihydrofolate reductase, and DT-diaphorase gene expression in human tumors using the polymerase chain reaction. *Cancer Res* 52:108–116.

Kanangat S, Solomon A, Rouse BT (1992): Use of quantitative polymerase chain reaction to quantitate cytokine messenger RNA molecules. *Mol Immunol* 29:1229–1236.

Kaneko S, Murakami S, Unoura M, Kobayashi K (1992): Quantitation of hepatitis C virus RNA by competitive polymerase chain reaction. *J Med Virol* 37:278–282.

Katz JP, Bodin ET, Coen DM (1990): Quantitative polymerase chain reaction analysis of herpes simplex virus DNA in ganglia of mice infected with replication-incompetent mutants. *J Virol* 64:4288–4295.

Kawasaki ES (1990): Sample preparation from blood, cells, and other fluids. In: *PCR Protocols*. Innis MA, Gelfand DH, Sninsky JJ, White TJ, eds. New York: Academic Press, 146–152.

Kellogg DE, Sninsky JJ, Kwok S (1990): Quantitation of HIV-1 proviral DNA relative to cellular DNA by the polymerase chain reaction. *Anal Biochem* 189:202–208.

Kern DG, Sheridan PJ, Stempien MS, Yeghiazarian Y, Todd JA, Neuwald PD, Pachl CA, Urdea MS, Lindquist C, El-Beik T, Feinberg M (1992): Quantitation of HIV-1 RNA in plasma using branched DNA technology. Presented at 15th AIDS Clinical Trial Group Meeting, Washington, D.C.

Koopmans M, Snijder EJ, Horzineck MC (1991): cDNA probes for the diagnosis of bovine totovirus (Breda virus) infection. *J Clin Microbiol* 29:493–497.

Kwoh DY, Davis GR, Whitfield KM, Chappelle HL, DiMichele LJ, Gingeras TR (1989): Transcription-based amplification system and detection of amplified human immunodeficiency virus type 1 with a bead-based sandwich hybridization format. *Proc Natl Acad Sci USA* 86:1173–1177.

Landgraf A, Reckmann B, Pingoud A (1991): Quantitative analysis of polymerase chain reaction (PCR) products using primers labeled with biotin and a fluorescent dye. *Anal Biochem* 193:231–235.

Lee T, Sunzeri FJ, Tobler LH, Williams BG, Busch MP (1990): Quantitative assessment of HIV-1 DNA load by coamplification of HIV-1 gag and HLA-DQ-α genes. *AIDS* 5:683–691.

Li B, Sehajpal PK, Khanna A, Vlassara H, Cerami A, Stenzel KH, Suthanthiran M (1991): Differential regulation of transforming growth factor B and interleukin 2 genes in human T cells: Demonstration by usage of novel competitor DNA constructs in the quantitative polymerase chain reaction. *J Exp Med* 174:1259–1262.

Lin JH-C, Grandchamp B, Abraham NG (1991): Quantitation of human erythroid-specific porphobilinogen deaminase mRNA by the polymerase chain reaction. *Exp Hematol* 19:817–822.

Lizardi PM, Kramer FR (1991): Exponential amplification of nucleic acids: New diagnostics using DNA polymerases and RNA replicases. *Tibtech* 9:53–58.

Lomell H, Tyagi S, Pritchard CG, Lizardi PM, Kramer FR (1989): Quantitative assays based on the use of replicatable hybridization probes. *Clin Chem* 35:1826–1831.

Lundeberg J, Wahlberg J, Uhlen M (1991): Rapid colorimetric quantification of PCR-amplified DNA. *BioTechniques* 10:68–75.

Macfarlane DE, Dahle CE (1993): Isolating RNA from whole blood—the dawn of RNA-based diagnosis? *Nature (London)* 362:186–188.

Maddox J (1992): Is molecular biology yet a science? *Nature (London)* 355:201.

Makino R, Sekiya T, Hayashi K (1990): Evaluation of quantitative detection of mRNA by the reverse transcription-polymerase chain reaction. *Technique* 2:295–301.

Masters DB, Griggs CT, Berde CB (1992): High sensitivity quantification of RNA from gels and autoradiograms with affordable optical scanning. *BioTechniques* 13:902–911.

McCaustland KA, Hi S, Purdy MA, Bradley DW (1991): Application of two RNA extraction methods prior to amplification of hepatitis E virus nucleic acid by the polymerase chain reaction. *J Virol Methods* 35:331–342.

Melton PA, Drieg PA, Rebagliati MR, Maniatis J, Zinn K, Green MR (1984): Efficiant in vitro syn-

thesis of biologically active RNA and RNA hybridization probes from plasmids containing bacteriophage SP6 promoter. *Nucl Acids Res* 12:7035.

Michael NL, Vahey M, Burke DS, Redfield RR (1992): Viral DNA and mRNA expression correlate with the stage of human immunodeficiency virus (HIV) type 1 infection in humans: evidence for viral replication in all stages of HIV disease. *J Virol* 66:310–316,

Mochizuki H, Nishi T, Bruner JM, Lee PSY, Levin VA, Saya H (1992): Alternative splicing of neurofibromatosis type 1 gene transcript in malignant brain tumors: PCR analysis of frozen-section mRNA. *Mol Carcinogen* 6:83–87.

Mohler KM, Butler LD (1991): Quantitation of cytokine mRNA levels utilizing the reverse transcriptase-polymerase chain reaction following primary antigen-specific sensitization *in vivo*—I. Verification of linearity, reproducibility and specificity. *Mol Immunol* 28:437–447.

Murphy LD, Herzog CE, Rudick JB, Fojo AT, Bates SE (1990): Use of the polymerase chain reaction in the quantitation of mdr-1 gene expression. *Biochemistry* 29:10351–10356.

Myers TW, Gelfand DH (1991): Reverse transcription and DNA amplification by a *Thermus thermophilus* DNA polymerase. *Biochemistry* 30:7661–7666.

Neve RL, Rogers J, Higgins GA (1990): The Alzheimer amyloid precursor-related transcript lacking the β/A4 sequence is specifically increased in Alzheimer's disease brain. *Neuron* 5:329–338.

Noonan KE, Beck C, Holzmayer TA, Chin JE, Wunder JS, Andrulis IL, Gazdar AF, William CL, Griffith B, Von Hoff DD, Roninson IB (1990): Quantitative analysis of MDR1 (multidrug resistance) gene expression in human tumors by polymerase chain reaction. *Proc Natl Acad Sci USA* 87:7160–7164.

Nuovo GJ (1992): *PCR in Situ Hybridization: Protocols and Applications.* New York: Raven Press.

Nuovo GJ, Gallery F, MacConnell P, Becker J, Bloch W (1991a): An improved technique for the detection of DNA by in situ hybridization after PCR-amplification. *Am J Pathol* 139:1239–1244.

Nuovo GJ, MacConnell P, Forde A, Delvenne P (1991b): Detection of human papillomavirus DNA in formalin fixed tissues by in situ hybridization after amplification by PCR. *Am J Pathol* 139:847–854.

Nuovo GJ, Becker J, MacConnell P, Margiotta M, Comite S, Hochman H (1992a): Histological distribution of PCR-amplified HPV 6 and 11 DNA in penile lesions. *Am J Surg Pathol* 16:269–275.

Nuovo GJ, Margiotta M, MacConnell P, Becker J (1992b): Rapid in situ detection of PCR-amplified HIV-1 DNA. *Diagn Mol Pathol* 1:98–102.

Oka S, Urayama K, Hirabayashi Y, Ohnishi K, Goto H, Mitamura K, Kimura S, Shimada K (1990): Quantitative analysis of human immunodeficiency virus type-1 DNA in asymptomatic carriers using the polymerase chain reaction. *Biochem Biophys Res Commun* 167:1–8.

Ou C-Y, McDonough SH, Cabanas D, Ryder TB, Harper M, Moore J, Schochetman G (1990): Rapid and quantitative detection of enzymatically amplified HIV-1 DNA using chemiluminescent oligonucleotide probes. *AIDS Res Human Retrovirus* 6:1323–1329.

Pang S, Koyanagi Y, Miles S, Wiley C, Vinters HV, Chen ISY (1990): High levels of unintegrated HIV-1 DNA in brain tissue of AIDS dementia patients. *Nature (London)* 343:85–89.

Park O-K, Mayo KE (1991): Transient expression of progesterone receptor messenger RNA in ovarian granulosa cells after the preovulatory luteinizing hormone surge. *Mol Endocrinol* 5:967–978.

Patterson BK, Till M, Otto P, Goolsby C, Furtado MR, McBride LJ, Wolinsky SM (1993): Detection of HIV-1 DNA and messenger RNA in individual cells by PCR-driven in situ hybridization and flow cytometry. *Science* 260:976–979.

Piatak M Jr, Saag MS, Yang LC, Clark SJ, Kappes JC, Luk K-C, Hahn BH, Shaw GM, Lifson JD (1993a): High levels of HIV-1 in plasma during all stages of infection determined by competitive PCR. *Science* 259:1749–1754.

Piatak M Jr, Luk K, Williams B, Lifson JD (1993b): Quantitative competitive polymerase chain reaction for accurate quantitation of HIV DNA and RNA species. *BioTechniques* 14:70–80.

Porcher C, Malinge M-C, Picat C, Grandchamp B (1992): A simplified method for determination of specific DNA or RNA copy number using quantitative PCR and an automatic DNA sequencer. *BioTechniques* 13:106–113.

Powell EE, Kroon PA (1992): Measurement of mRNA by quantitative PCR with nonradioactive label. *J Lipid Res* 33:609–614.

Rappolee DA, Mark D, Banda MJ, Werb Z (1988): Wound macrophages express TGF-α and other growth factors in vivo: Analysis by mRNA phenotyping. *Science* 241:708–712.

Roques P, Dormont D (1991): *Quantitative PCR and Viral Burden of HIV-1 Infected Individuals: Analysis of Mother/Newborn Pairs.* Andrieu J-M, ed. Paris: John Libbey Eurotext, 177–185.

Sambrook J, Fritsch EF, Maniatis T (1989): *Molecular Cloning: A Laboratory Manual.* Cold Spring Harbor, NY: Cold Spring Harbor Lab., 7.01–7.87.

Scadden DT, Wang Z, Groopman JE (1992): Quantitation of plasma human immunodeficiency virus type 1 RNA by competitive polymerase chain reaction. *J Infect Dis* 165:1119–1123.

Schnittman S, Psallidopoulos MC, Lane HC, Thompson L, Baseler M, Massari F, Fox CH, Salzman NP, Fauci AS (1989): The reservoir for HIV-1 in human peripheral blood is a T cell that maintains expression of CD4. *Science* 245:305–308.

Schnittman SM, Lane HC, Greenhouse J, Justement JS, Baseler M, Fauci AS (1990): Preferential infection of CDR⁺ memory T cells by human immunodeficiency virus type 1: Evidence for a role in the selective T-cell functional defects observed in infected individuals. *Proc Natl Acad Sci USA* 87:6058–6062.

Seshamma T, Bagasra O, Trono D, Baltimore D, Pomerantz RJ (1992): Blocked early-stage latency in the peripheral blood cells of certain individuals infected with human immunodeficiency virus type 1. *Proc Natl Acad Sci USA* 89:10663–10667.

Silani V, Pizzuti A, Falini A, Borsani G, Rugarli EI, Melo CA, Sidoli A, Villani F, Baralle F, Scarlato G (1991): β-Nerve growth factor (β-NGF) mRNA expression in the Parkinsonian adrenal gland. *Exp Neurol* 113:166–170.

Simmonds P, Balfe P, Peutherer JF, Ludlam CA, Bishop JO, Leigh Brown AJ (1990): Human immunodeficiency virus infected individuals contain provirus in small numbers of peripheral mononuclear cells and at low copy numbers. *J Virol* 64:864–872.

Simon L, Levesque RC, Lalonde M (1992): Rapid quantitation by PCR of endomycorrhizal fungi colonizing roots. *PCR Methods Applic* 2:76–80.

Singer-Sam J, LeBon JM, Tanguay RL, Riggs AD (1990a): A quantitative Hpall-PCR assay to measure methylation of DNA from a small number of cells. *Nucl Acids Res* 18:687.

Singer-Sam J, Robinson MO, Bellve AR, Simon MI, Riggs AD (1990b): Measurement by quantitative PCR of changes in HPRT, PGK-1, PGK-2, APRT, MTase, and Zfy gene transcripts during mouse spermatogenesis. *Nucl Acids Res* 18:1255–1259.

Singer-Sam J, LeBon JM, Dai A, Riggs AD (1992): A sensitive, quantitative assay for measurement of allele-specific transcripts differing by a single nucleotide. *PCR Methods Applic* 1:160–163.

Spadoro JP, Payne H, Lee Y, Rosenstraus MJ (1990): Single copies of HIV proviral DNA detected by fluorescent *in situ* hybridization. *BioTechniques* 9:186–195.

Spann W, Pachmann K, Zabnienska H, Pielmeier A, Emmerich B (1991): In situ amplification of single copy gene segments in individual cells by the polymerase chain reaction. *Infection* 19:242–244.

Sperison P, Wang SM, Reichenbach P, Nabholz M (1992): A PCR-based assay for reporter gene expression. *PCR Methods Applic* 1:164–170.

Steuler H, Munzinger S, Wildemann B, Storch-Hagenlocher B (1992): Quantitation of HIV-1 proviral DNA in cells from cerebrospinal fluid. *J Acquired Immun Defic Syndromes* 5:405–408.

Stieger M, Demolliere C, Ahlborn-Laake L, Mous J (1991): Competitive polymerase chain reaction assay for quantitation of HIV-1 DNA and RNA. *J Virol Methods* 34:149–160.

Sugiyama S, Hattori K, Hayakawa M, Ozawa T (1991): Quantitative analysis of age-associated accumulation of mitochondrial DNA with deletion in human hearts. *Biochem Biophys Res Commun* 180:894–899.

Sykes PJ, Neoh SH, Brisco MJ, Hughes E, Condon J, Morley AA (1992): Quantitation of targets for PCR by use of limiting dilution. *BioTechniques* 13:444–449.

Syvanen A-C, Ikonen E, Manninen T, Bengtstrom M, Soderlund H, Aula P, Peltonen L (1992): Convenient and quantitative determination of the frequency of a mutant allele using solid-phase minisequencing: Application to aspartylglucosaminuria in Finland. *Genomics* 12:590–595.

Temin HM, Bolognesi DP (1993): Where has HIV been hiding? *Nature (London)* 362:292–293.

Uberla K, Platzer C, Diamanstein T, Blankenstein T (1991): Generation of competitor DNA fragments for quantitative PCR. *PCR Methods Applic* 1:136–139.

Vanden Heuvel JP, Tyson FL, Bell DA (1993): Construction of recombinant RNA templates for use as internal standards in quantitative RT-PCR. *BioTechniques* 14:395–398.

Volkenandt M, Dicker AP, Banerjee D, Fanin R, Schweitzer B, Horikoshi T, Danenberg K, Danenberg P, Bertino JR (1992): Quantitation of gene copy number and mRNA using the polymerase chain reaction. *Proc Soc Exp Biol Med* 200:1–6.

Wang M, Doyle MV, Mark DF (1989): Quantitation of mRNA by the polymerase chain reaction. *Proc Natl Acad Sci USA* 86:9717–9721.

Wilkinson M (1988): RNA isolation: A mini-prep method. *Nucl Acids Res* 16:10933.

Winters MA, Holodniy M, Katzenstein DA, Merigan TC (1992): Quantitative RNA and DNA gene amplification can rapidly monitor HIV infection and antiviral activity in cell culture. *PCR Methods Applic* 1:257–262.

Wood JN, Lillycrop KA, Dent CL, Ninkina NN, Beech MM, Willoughby JJ, Winter J, Latchman DS (1992): Regulation of expression of the neuronal POU protein Oct-2 by nerve growth factor. *J Biol Chem* 267:17787–17791.

Yamada O, Matsumoto T, Nakashima M, Hagari S, Kamahora T, Ueyama H, Kishi Y, Uemura H, Kurimura T (1990): A new method for extracting DNA or RNA for polymerase chain reaction. *J Virol Methods* 27:203–209.

Yamaguchi M, Dieffenbach CW, Connolly R, Cruess DF, Baur W, Sharefkin JB (1992): Effect of different laboratory techniques for guanidiniumphenolchloroform RNA extraction on A_{260}/A_{280} and on accuracy of mRNA quantitation by reverse transcriptase-PCR. *PCR Methods Applic* 4:286–290.

Zack JA, Arrigo SJ, Weitsman SR, Go AL, Haislip A, Chen ISY (1990): HIV-1 entry into quiescent primary lymphocytes: Molecular analysis reveals a labile, latent viral structure. *Cell* 61:213–222.

Zack JA, Haislip AM, Krogstad P, Chen I (1992): Incompletely reverse-transcribed human immunodeficiency virus type 1 genomes in quiescent cells can function as intermediates in the retroviral life cycle. *J Virol* 66:1717–1725.

Zhang LQ, Simmonds P, Ludlam CA, Leigh Brown AJ (1991): Detection, quantification and sequencing of HIV-1 from plasma of seropositive individuals and from factor VIII concentrates. *AIDS* 5:675–681.

7

Quantification of DNAs by the Polymerase Chain Reaction Using an Internal Control

Donald M. Coen

Introduction

Polymerase chain reaction (PCR) technology provides the most sensitive methods for detecting nucleic acids. These methods have proven exceedingly useful in detection of infectious agents in experimental and clinical settings (Kwok et al., 1987) and in analyses of unusual and precious small samples of tissue, such as those from extinct animals (Pääbo, 1989). They also have considerable potential for forensic applications (von Beroldingen et al., 1989). Most initial efforts to utilize the sensitivity of PCR were geared to issues of detection. For example, Saiki et al. (1988) showed that they could detect single target sequences (a β-globin gene) in 10^5 to 10^6 cells. Similarly, procedures for amplification of DNA from single cells exist (Li et al., 1988). However, these procedures were not designed to quantify amounts of target sequence in different samples.

The methodology presented below to quantify DNAs was developed to measure the amount of herpes simplex virus (HSV) DNA in the ganglia of mice infected with various HSV mutants. Initial efforts used slot-blot hybridization, but failed to detect viral sequences reliably below 0.01 to 0.1 copy of HSV DNA per mouse cell equivalent (Leib et al., 1989). For this reason, a number of parameters in standard PCR protocols were varied to keep the replication machinery in excess to the number of templates. Using this approach, it has been possible to quantify HSV DNA over a 10^4-fold range, from a few molecules per 100 ng ganglion DNA from mice infected with mutants with serious growth impairments to tens of thousands of molecules in ganglion DNA from mice infected with wild-type virus (Katz et al., 1990). In addition, this approach helps assess the presence of contaminating sequences, the bane of this kind of procedure. The methodology should be pertinent to numerous other applications where small amounts of nucleic acid needed to be detected and quantitated, including diagnostics and forensics. In fact, similar assays have been developed to quantify nucleic acids and can be found elsewhere in this book.

Portions of this work were adapted with permission of the publisher from "Quantitation of rare DNAs by polymerase chain reaction. In: *Current Protocols in Molecular Biology.* F. M. Ausubel et al., eds. © 1990 Greene Publishing Associates and Wiley-Interscience.

The Polymerase Chain Reaction
K.B. Mullis, F. Ferré, R.A. Gibbs, editors
© 1994 Birkhauser Boston

The protocol outlined below has been adapted from one detailed in *Current Protocols in Molecular Biology* (Coen, 1990). The essential steps entail (1) preparing the DNA of interest and determining its concentration, (2) mixing a known amount of this DNA with two PCR primer pairs, one pair specific for the DNA of interest such as viral DNA and the other pair specific for an internal control, such as a single copy gene of a host organism, (3) amplifying the DNA between the primers by PCR, and (4) electrophoresing the PCR products on a gel, transferring them to a filter, and probing with oligonucleotides specific for each PCR product. The amounts of the amplified products from the DNA of interest can then be quantified by comparison to the internal control relative to a series of standard dilutions. For simplicity, the protocol is written in terms of quantifying viral DNA molecules relative to host cellular sequences; however, it can be adapted readily for other applications.

Protocol

Reagents and Solutions

$10 \times$ Amplification buffer:
> 500 mM KCl; 100 mM Tris-HCl, pH 8.4; and a concentration of MgCl$_2$ that is optimal for the primer-pairs and templates (Coen, 1990). Autoclave and then add gelatin to 1 mg/ml. Store at $-20°$C.

Proteinase digestion buffer:
> 20 mM Tris-HCl, pH 7.4 (prepared from autoclaved stock)
> 20 mM EDTA, pH 8 (prepared from autoclaved stock)
> 0.5% sodium dodecyl sulfate (SDS)
> Store at room temperature

Reaction mix cocktail (per amplification reaction):
> 10 μl $10 \times$ amplification buffer (recipe above)
> 10 μl 2 mM mix of dATP, dCTP, dGTP, and dTTP
> 1 μl each of 50 pmol/μl oligonucleotide primer for amplification (4 μl total)

Precautions to Avoid Contamination

Use sterile, distilled water to prepare all reagents. Do *not* use diethylpyrocarbonate to treat reagents. To avoid contamination with unwanted nucleic acids, prepare reagents and solutions solely for use in this protocol. Wear disposable gloves and change them frequently. Take care not to contaminate cells or tissue samples with unwanted DNA sequences. It is best to process samples in the order of increasing likelihood of their containing the sequences of interest. Perform all manipulations away from where products of the amplification reactions (PCR) or large amounts of plasmid DNA containing the sequence of interest are handled. Always include several negative control samples that contain no viral sequences. For further discussion of precautions, see Coen (1990).

Procedures

1. Place cells or tissue sample in a screw-cap microcentrifuge tube. Add ~100 μl proteinase digestion buffer per ~2×10^6 cells and 20 mg/ml proteinase K to 100 μg/ml. Incubate sample overnight at 50°C.

2. Mix sample gently up and down with a 200-μl microcapillary pipet to shear the DNA slightly, allowing more efficient extraction, but not too much to permit easier quantitation in step 10. Add 100 μl buffered phenol to digestion mixture, mix gently, add 100 μl of 24 : 1 chloroform/isoamyl alcohol, and mix gently.

3. Microcentrifuge 5 min and transfer aqueous phase (which contains DNA) to a new microcentrifuge tube.

4. Back-extract organic phase with proteinase digestion buffer ($\sim 1/2$ original volume).

5. Microcentrifuge 5 min and add aqueous phase from step 3.

6. Extract pooled aqueous phases twice with an equal volume of 24 : 1 chloroform/isoamyl alcohol, centrifuging 5 min each time to separate the phases.

7. Add 10 M ammonium acetate to 2.5 M in the final aqueous phase and mix gently. Add 2.5 vol cold ethanol and mix gently. Place on crushed dry ice 30 min. Microcentrifuge 15 min at 4°C to pellet DNA, and pour off supernatant.

8. Wash DNA pellet with 1 ml of 70% ethanol by inverting the tube several times. Microcentrifuge 15 min, pour off supernatant, and dry pellet under vacuum.

9. Resuspend pellet in TE buffer (100 μl for a sample prepared from 2×10^6 cells should yield optimally 100 μg/ml or less if losses occur). Store DNA at 4°C.

10. Estimate DNA concentration either by running an aliquot on an agarose gel alongside known amounts of standard DNA or by ethidium bromide dot quantitation.

11. Prepare one tube containing 110 ng, one tube containing 90 ng, and several tubes each containing 100 ng DNA from uninfected cells or tissue. Use these tubes to make a set of 10-fold serial dilutions of the sequence of interest as follows: Add a known amount (e.g., 20,000 molecules) of DNA containing the sequence of interest to the tube containing 110 ng DNA and mix. Add one-tenth of this material to a new tube containing 100 ng of DNA and mix. Repeat several more times until a tube contains ≤ 10 molecules of the sequence of interest. Then add one-tenth of the material from that tube to the tube containing 90 ng of DNA. The final total volume in each tube should be ≤ 71 μl.

12. For each amplification reaction, prepare a scew-cap microcentrifuge tube containing 24 μl reaction mix cocktail and enough sterile distilled water for a final column of 100 μl (after addition of DNA and *Taq* DNA polymerase, steps 13 and 15). Mix and overlay each reaction with two drops (~ 100 μl) mineral oil, to completely cover the surface of the reaction mixture.

13. Open only those tubes that will contain equivalent samples (e.g., duplicate samples or samples from animals infected with the same virus inocula). Add 100 ng sample DNA to each appropriate tube and close the tubes. Microcentrifuge briefly to mix.

14. Heat-denature the samples 1 min at 94°C, either in a water bath or in an automated cycler.

15. Open tubes (containing equivalent samples) and add 5 μl of 0.8 U/μl *Taq* DNA polymerase to each tube. Close tubes and repeat steps 13 to 15 with the next set of equivalent samples.

16. Microcentrifuge tubes briefly. Cycle tubes one time for 2 min at 55°C (reannealing) and 3 min at 72°C (extension).

17. Cycle tubes 29 times for 1 min at 94°C, 2 min at 55°C, and 3 min at 72°C. Extend for an additional 7 min at 72°C. Store completed reactions at 4°C.

18. Electrophorese product aliquots (one-tenth of the reaction should be sufficient) on an appropriate agarose or polyacrylamide gel. Include lanes with DNA molecular weight markets that will be visible both on ethidium bromide staining and by autoradiography.

19. Stain and photograph the gel.

20. Transfer gel to nylon filter and UV crosslink DNA to filter.

21. Prehybridize the filter and hybridize with end-labeled oligonucleotide specific for the sequence of interest. Analyze by autoradiography.

22. For more quantitative analysis, strip the filter of the previous probe by boiling in water 15 min (if necessary) and hybridize with a probe specific for the host single-copy sequence. Quantify the signals by densitometric scanning (following the densitometer manufacturer's instructions) and compute a standard curve from the dilution series, normalizing to the host signals. Determine the number of molecules in the experimental samples by interpolation from the standard curve.

Expected Results

Results are obtained at different stages of the protocol. The DNA preparation should yield relatively intact and pure DNA, but due to the precautions described (e.g., step 2), yields may not be as high as ordinarily obtained. After the PCR products are electrophoresed on a gel, ethidium bromide staining should reveal an easily visible band corresponding to the internal control product in every product lane. A visible band corresponding to the experimental product of interest should appear in the lane containing the 1-copy-per-cell-equivalent reconstruction and in any lanes that contain similar amounts of the sequence of interest. Because the sequences of interest are relatively nonabundant, a variety of nonspecific products may be seen as well.

After hybridization to the sequence of interest and autoradiography, the expected results are labeled bands of the appropriate size in the reconstructed dilution series, no bands that size in the negative controls, and bands with varying intensities in the experimental samples (Fig. 7.1). Depending on the probe and the stringency of the hybridization and wash conditions, nonspecific sticking of the probe to the abundant internal control product may be seen. It is also common to see minor specific PCR products of slightly greater or lower mobility than the major specific product, especially at a high copy number.

If each reaction is amplified with similar efficiency (which can be assessed by the intensity of the internal control PCR product in the ethidium bromide-

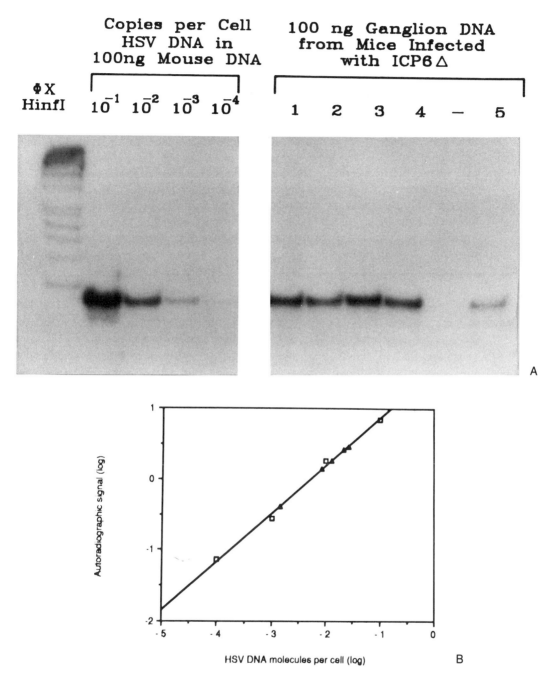

FIGURE 7.1. Quantitative PCR analysis of HSV DNA in trigeminal ganglia from mice infected with a ribonucleotide reductase mutant, ICP6Δ. (A) The indicated mixtures of HSV DNA and uninfected mouse DNA and the samples of trigeminal ganglion DNA from mice infected with ICP6Δ were analyzed as described in the protocol. (B) Densitometric analysis of quantitative PCR. The autoradiographs shown in A were scanned on an LKB laser scanner and integrals of the signals were computed. The logs of the computed signals were plotted relative to the logs of the amounts of HSV DNA present in the mixtures with the mouse DNA, as indicated by the open squares. The signals from the ganglia are shown as closed triangles. The internal control signals were indistinguishable in all samples. Taken from Katz et al. (1990) with permission of the ASM. Note that in other instances where there is greater variation in internal control signals among samples, normalizing to those signals permits a more linear standard curve.

stained gel), the dilution series should give monotonically decreasing signals of one predominant band with increasing dilution. It should be possible to detect a signal from dilutions containing only one or a few molecules. Note that the signal under 10^{-4} copies per cell in Figure 7.1A corresponds theoretically to 2 molecules. A reasonable estimate for the number of molecules of the sequence of interest in each sample can be obtained by comparison with the dilution series, assuming that each reaction amplified with similar efficiency. The dilution series will ideally give a linear relationship between the log of the autoradiographic signal and the log of the amount of DNA (Fig. 7.1). However, it may not necessarily be completely linear, and it is unlikely to have a slope of 1. At the high end (>1 copy per cell equivalent), it may plateau. This can be ascertained by determining whether increasing or decreasing amounts of input DNA correspondingly increases or reduces formation of both the viral and internal control products. If this is a problem, it may be necessary to reduce the number of amplification cycles.

Discussion

All parameters that are critical in PCR are also critical here. Several additional points, particular to this protocol, bear emphasis.

DNA

The amount of added DNA is critical for achieving a quantitative assay. Too much DNA will saturate the replication machinery, in terms of not only specific products generated, but also nonspecific products. In the protocol presented above, 100 ng of DNA is used per 100 μl reaction. This concentration of DNA may not be optimal in every instance, so it is advisable to test a dilution series of the sequence of interest mixed with the endogenous sequences at various amounts of total sample DNA to see how much sample DNA will allow a monotonically increasing signal with increasing amounts of the sequence of interest. In addition, impurities in DNA preparations can interfere with PCR; additional organic extractions and/or ethanol precipitations in the presence of ammonium acetate may help.

Internal Control

A set of primers to yield an internal control sequence is critical for two major reasons.

First, if no signal from the sequence of interest is obtained in a given sample, the internal control will verify whether this is a true or a false negative. It is not uncommon for amplifications to fail, especially since some experimental samples contain contaminants that interfere with PCR. Second, the internal control allows for quantification, since it normalizes for several factors including variation in the amount of sample DNA, efficiency and amplification, and the amount loaded on the gel. The internal control PCR product should be different enough in size to be resolved easily from the PCR product of interest, but close enough in size so there is no concern about differences in transfer efficiency due to size differences. It should also be clearly distinguished in size from any short artifactual PCR products.

In the protocol described here, the internal control product is derived from endogenous cellular sequences. For some applications, this would not be appropriate or practical. An alternative is to spike one's samples with a known amount of a foreign sequence and to include primers specific for this DNA in the amplification reaction. This would control for the efficiency of the reaction and certain other factors, but not for variation in the amount of sample DNA.

DNA Polymerase

The amount of *Taq* DNA polymerase added per reaction is critical in achieving a quantitative assay (unpublished results). The protocol outlined above uses more polymerase than many typical protocols to ensure that the replication machinery is in excess of the number of templates.

Contamination

It is critical in any procedure that can detect only a few molecules to be absolutely scrupulous in avoiding contamination. Certain basic precautions are outlined above; more details can be found elsewhere (Coen, 1990; other chapters in this book). The quantitative protocol described here can be helpful in assessing contamination because unlike nonquantitative assays, it can give one an estimate of the level of contamination. Even if negative controls yield positive signals, if they are much lower than those in experimental samples, it provides at least tentative assurance that the experimental signals are real.

Transfer and Crosslinking

It is very important that the PCR products be transferred and retained completely to ensure a quantitative assay in the protocol above. An alternative approach to transfer and hybridization is to use PCR primers, prelabeled to high-specific activity with polynucleotide kinase. The products can then be quantified by direct autoradiography of the gel (Arrigo et al., 1989). Potential disadvantages of this approach are that it adds steps where contamination can be introduced and detects more nonspecific products.

Quantitative Aspects of the Technique

In discussing the quantitative aspects of this protocol, two separate questions arise. The first question is "How sensitive is it?" It is basically as sensitive as can be. The procedure can readily detect single molecules of a sequence of interest (e.g., viral DNA) within 100 ng of mammalian genomic DNA (ca. 10^4 cell equivalents) or other nonspecific DNA. The amount of nonspecific DNA can be increased substantially without diminishing the sensitivity of the method (unpublished results). The second question is "How quantitative is it?" or, more operationally, "What fold-differences can one detect?" This question is not as easy to answer and depends on performing multiple measurements. In our hands, we can very readily distinguish 10-fold differences and probably 3-fold differences between DNA concentrations. This resolution diminishes with decreasing amounts of target DNA because, when there are only a few molecules, stochaistic effects come into play. For example, if there are on average 3 molecules of HSV DNA per 100 ng of mouse ganglionic DNA, then just by chance, one is likely to detect 0 molecules in one assay and as many as 10 in another. Variability of course can also arise from experimental manipulation and from normal biological variation. Regardless, the technique gives values in agreement with blot-hybridization methods and permits reasonably firm conclusions to be drawn (Katz et al., 1990).

References

Arrigo SJ, Weitsman S, Rosenblatt JD, Chen ISY (1989): Analysis of *rev* gene function on human immunodeficiency virus type 1 replication in lymphoid cells by using a quantitative polymerase chain reaction. *J Virol* 63:4875–4881.

Coen D (1990): Quantitation of rare DNAs by polymerase chain reaction. In: *Current Protocols in Molecular Biology*. Ausubel FM, Brent R, Kingston RE, Moore DD, Smith JA, Seidman JG, Struhl K, eds. New York: Greene Publishing Associates and Wiley-Interscience.

Katz JP, Bodin ET, Coen DM (1990): Quantitative polymerase chain reaction analysis of herpes simplex virus DNA in ganglia of mice infected with replication-incompetent mutants. *J Virol* 64:4288–4295.

Kwok S, Mack DH, Mullis KB, Poiesz B, Ehrlich G, Blair D, Friedman-Kien A, Sninsky JJ (1987): Identification of human immunodeficiency virus sequences by using in vitro enzymatic amplification and oligomer cleavage detection. *J Virol* 61:1690–1694.

Leib DA, Coen DM, Bogard CL, Hicks KA, Yager DR, Knipe DM, Tyler KL, Schaffer PA (1989): Immediate-early regulatory gene mutants define different stages in the establishment and reactivation of herpes simplex virus latency. *J Virol* 63:759–768.

Li H, Gyllensten UB, Cui X, Saiki RK, Erlich HA, Arnheim N (1988): Amplification and analysis of DNA sequences in single human sperm and diploid cells. *Nature (London)* 335:414–417.

Pääbo S (1989): Ancient DNA: Extraction, characterization, molecular cloning and enzymatic amplification. *Proc Natl Acad Sci USA* 86:1939–1943.

Saiki RK, Gelfand DH, Stoffel S, Scharf SJ, Higuchi R, Horn GT, Mullis KB, Erlich HA (1988): Primer-directed enzymatic amplification of DNA with a thermostable DNA polymerase. *Science* 239:487–488.

von Beroldingen CH, Blake ET, Higuchi R, Sensabaugh GF, Erlich HA (1989): Applications of PCR to the analysis of biological evidence. In: *PCR Technology: Principles and Applications for DNA Amplification.* Erlich HA, ed. New York: Stockton Press.

8

RT-PCR and mRNA Quantitation

Jamel Chelly and Axel Kahn

Introduction and Theoretical Considerations

Quantitative analysis of RNA is an important aspect of gene expression studies and central to the understanding of the mechanisms that regulate gene activity. Northern gels, dot or slot blots, are currently used for analyzing RNA levels, however, Northern analysis requires large quantities of RNA and is not very sensitive for quantitative use in detecting low abundance mRNA. S1 nuclease assays, RNase A protection, and *in situ* hybridization methods are more sensitive and quantitative, however, these methods are time consuming, can be technically difficult, and are not useful for a simultaneous processing of a large number of samples. Although these methods are more sensitive than Northern analysis, for many practical purposes, i.e., analyzing low copy number of transcripts or small amount of cells, the very low levels of mRNA limit their widespread use.

The adaptation of the polymerase chain reaction (Saiki et al., 1985) to amplify specific mRNA sequences after a first step of reverse transcription has permitted not only the detection of low abundance mRNAs whatever their initial amount, but also the development of a number of quantitative procedures for the analysis of steady-state RNA levels (Chelly et al., 1988, 1990a; Rappolee et al., 1989; Becker-Andre and Hahlbrock, 1989; Wang et al., 1989; Singer-Sam et al., 1990; Gilliland et al., 1990; Robinson and Simon, 1991). In addition, this method is so sensitive that it allowed us to demonstrate a basal level of transcription of any highly tissue-specific genes in any non-specific cells (Chelly et al., 1990b; Sarkar and Sommer, 1989). The extreme sensitivity of this amplification raises the possibility that RNA might be detected below levels where it has a physiological significance, therefore attention must be given to quantitation.

Theoretically, the amplification of a cDNA fragment is exponential with a doubling of each copy at each cycle of amplification. In fact, the efficiency is less than 100% and the extent of amplification (Y) is given by the formula $Y = A(1 + R)^n$ where A is the initial amount of cDNA obtained after the reverse transcription step, R is the efficiency of amplification at each cycle, and n is the number of cycles. To apply this theoretical formula for quantitative analysis of the initial amount of

The Polymerase Chain Reaction
K.B. Mullis, F. Ferré, R.A. Gibbs, editors
© 1994 Birkhauser Boston

template, it has been necessary to check experimentally the exponential nature of the PCR amplification. This has been verified with reasonable accuracy by measuring the extent of incorporation of 5′ ^{32}P-labeled primer into the amplified product. Figure 8.1 shows that the exponential increase of the extent (Y) with a constant efficiency (R) occurs only for a limited number of cycles, after which the amplification rate ceases to be exponential and reaches a plateau.

The initial amount of template that is roughly proportional to the initial amount of the specific mRNA under investigation depends essentially on the yield of the reverse transcription step, whereas, the efficiency (R) depends on several variables including the nature of primers and amplified sequences, components concentrations, and PCR temperatures. Because the amplification is initially an exponential process, small differences in any of the factors that influence the reaction efficiency will dramatically affect the level of specific PCR products. In addition, even when these parameters are controlled precisely, there is sometimes unexpected sample-to-sample and day-to-day variations. These constraints and the large number of reactions analyzed to specify the kinetics of amplification and to measure the extent (Y) of PCR amplification limit direct and accurate quantitation of initial amount of mRNA. Relative quantitation (or comparison of levels of a target mRNA in different samples) is easier but requires that certain principles are strictly observed: (1) comparison of specific cDNA-PCR products in different samples must be performed at the exponential phase of the amplification process, (2) when the abundance of different cDNA-PCR products is compared, they must be amplified by an identical efficiency, (3) and to overcome nonspecific variations inherent to each sample, we chose to standardize results by comparison with an internal standard mRNA, which is coreverse transcribed and coamplified with the transcript under investigation.

In the PCR amplification process the number of cycles after which the total product (Y) increase ceases to be exponential and reaches a plateau, depends on the efficiency of amplification R, and the abundance of the starting material (specific mRNA and cDNA). For a given amplified fragment the more abundant the starting material, the shorter is the range of exponential amplification (Fig. 8.2). When the plateau is reached, it is usual to obtain the same amount of amplified fragments regardless of the abundance of initial transcript in the original sample (for example see MyoD transcript in permissive myoblasts and myotubes samples in Fig. 8.2A and dilutions 1/10 and 1/100 of cardiac actin and mlc1a transcripts after 15 and 30 cycles in Fig. 8.2B, respectively). In general, previous analysis of the kinetics amplification of the investigated fragment allowed us to establish the limits of the exponential phase of amplification. In our experience, cDNA-PCR amplification of a fragment (100–200 bp) derived from a minor mRNA ceases to be exponential after approximately 15–20 cycles. For abundant transcripts, the plateau is reached after 8–12 cycles.

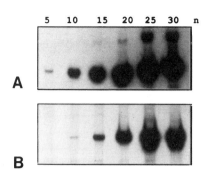

FIGURE 8.1. Kinetics of the amplification of 108-bp fragment of the H-type aldolase A mRNA. The samples were a cloned cDNA insert in single-strand M13 phage (A) and total lymphoblast RNA (B). One of the primers was labeled by kination before amplification. The amplified fragments were electrophoresed in polyacrylamide gels; the gels were then dried and exposed to autoradiographic films for 30 min. n, number of cycles. (C) The logarithm of the radioactivity incorporated into the amplified fragments was plotted versus the number of cycles n. The efficiency of amplification, R, of the fragment remained constant whatever the stating material. Reproduced from Chelly et al. (1990a), *Eur J Biochem* 187:691–698 by copyright permission of Springer-Verlag.

FIGURE 8.2. RT-PCR analysis of MyoD1, cardiac actin MLC1a in permissive and inducible myoblasts. (A) MyoD1 and cardiac actin were coamplified from 2 μg of total RNA from proliferating myoblasts (mb), myotubes (MT), and nonmuscle cells. MLC1a was coamplified together with the L-type pyruvate kinase transcript used as a standard. After 15 cycles the plateau is reached and the same level of the amplified MyoD1 fragment was observed in permissive myoblasts and myotubes. The plateau is also reached in (B) where fractions 1/10, 1/100, and 1/1000 of total RNA from permissive myotubes corresponding to 200, 20, and 2 ng were used to compare levels of cardiac actin and MLC1a transcripts in myotubes and myoblasts (ind, inducible cells; indq, quiescent inducible cells; per, permissive cells; T$_4$, aza-myoblasts; Sol8, myoblasts from the soleus muscle of adult C3H mice). Figure kindly provided by D. Montarras and C. Pinset (Institut Pasteur).

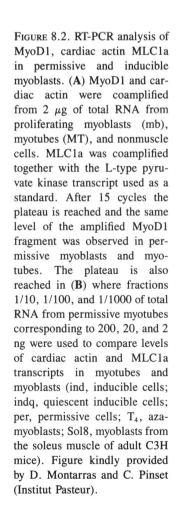

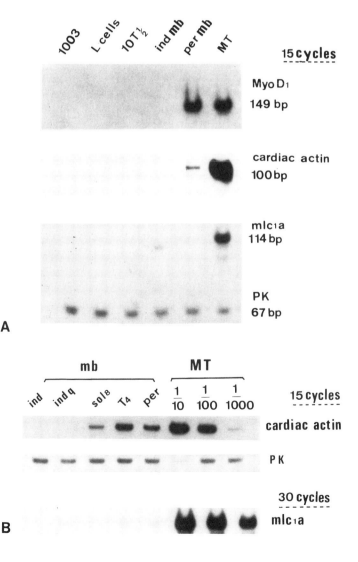

Protocol

Experimental Conditions and Reagents

RNA Purification

Total cellular and tissues RNA were prepared by a method that uses guanidinium thiocyanate to disrupt cells and homogenization of samples. The resulting homogenate is then layered and centrifuged on a cushion of a dense solution of CsCl according to Chirgwin or by similar methods (Chirgwin et al., 1979; Sambrook et al., 1989). Extraction of RNA from blood cells requires a preparation of mononuclear cells by any standard method. Pellets of cells [mononuclear cells, cells growing in monolayers or in suspension and harvested as described in Sambrook et al. (1989)] are processed as indicated above. Homogenization in guanidinium thiocyanate solution of the tissues was carried out using polytron or potters glass. Using this method RNAs can be extracted from very small quantities of starting material, such as skin or muscle biopsies of less than 10 mg. To extract RNA from very small numbers of cells (obtained by cell sorter), we used a modification of methods described by Strohman et al. (1977), MacDonald et al. (1987), and Sambrook et al. (1989). Cells are homogenized in guanidine-HCl buffer (Sambrook et al., 1989) and the nucleic acids are precipitated with 0.6 volume of ethanol (95%) and recovered by centrifugation at 5000 g. The pellet is resuspended in 100 to 200 μl of TE-sodium lauryl sarcosinate solution. (Tris 10 mM, EDTA, 1 mM, sodium lauryl sarcosinate, 0.5%) and RNAs are recovered by a second precipitation using dextran 40 as carrier (10 μg/ml), 1/10 volume of Na-acetate (3 M, pH 5.2), and 2.5 volumes of ethanol (100%). The pellet is then washed, dried, and resuspended in RNase free sterile water.

The yield of total RNA from different types of mammalian cells and tissues varies greatly—3–15 μg of RNA per 10^6 cells—depending on their sizes and states of differentiation and tissue structure; the muscle tissue is the most difficult to homogenize. The concentration of total RNA extracted from small samples was estimated only by agarose gel electrophoresis and ethidium bromide staining. The purification of poly(A)$^+$ RNA is not required since one can amplify specific mRNA sequences from the equivalent of 0.01 mg (or less) of total RNA. In addition, scarce mRNA and species of large size are most easily lost on an oligo(dT) column, and so alter the true proportions of such species in total RNA samples.

mRNA Used as Internal Standard

We add to the total RNA samples under investigation exactly the same amount of a standard transcript. In the present protocol the internal standard is the exogenous rat L-type pyruvate kinase mRNA (which is a liver-specific mRNA). A large amount of liver RNA was prepared from adult rats that were fasted for 3 days, and then fed with a high carbohydrate diet for 16 hr. In these conditions, the accumulation of the L-type pyruvate kinase mRNA is maximal (Cognet et al., 1987). Therefore, we can add a minimal amount (10–100 ng) of total RNA as a source of internal standard mRNA. From this large preparation, several aliquot are stored at $-70°C$ and used according to the details described below. This strategy requires only the use of the same quantity of total RNA, consequently, the same amount of standard transcript is added to each sample under investigation. We systematically checked that oligonucleotides used to amplify the internal standard do not amplify the pyruvate kinase transcript from mouse (or human) tissues RNA and that oligonucleotides used to amplify the investigated transcripts do not amplify the similar rat transcripts. Sequence of the primers used to amplify the internal standard transcript could be found in Chelly et al. (1990a).

Choice of Primers

We usually use nonpurified 20- to 24-mers with noncomplementary 3'-ends and 50–60% G + C content. Primers are chosen in different exons, so that the amplified products are readily distinguished from contaminating genomic DNA that may be present in the total RNA preparations. Generally, we choose primers that amplify the target mRNA without background and give the cleanest results. Amplification of fragments between 100 and 200 bp is usually selected to facilitate their amplification and their polyacrylamide blotting.

cDNA-PCR Amplification

Reverse transcription might be primed by using a specific antisense primer for the gene of interest, oligo(dT), or random hexanucleotide primers. In our hand and in almost cases, the latter approach is most consistent and results in the highest amplification of target sequence. This method also allows amplification of any desired target transcript from the same sample.

Analysis of the cDNA-PCR Products

Southern blot is used to estimate levels of specific amplified products and, because of their high resolution, we regularly use nondenaturing polyacrylamide gels to separate PCR products. Hybridization of filters (after southern blot) with an internal labeled primer allows unambiguous identification of the specific band over background amplification products.

Rational Selection of Controls

Because of the likelihood of contamination problems and because this method permits amplification from only one template molecule, extreme care must be taken to avoid false positive or overestimation of analyzed transcripts. In addition to some technical precautions, such as aliquotting reagents and especially oligonucleotides, use of special pipettes for oligonucleotides, rational selection of controls must be systematically run with each set of quantitative assays: (1) use a sample of total RNA that contains a high level of the investigated mRNA (this sample should facilitate the evaluation of results), (2) use well-characterized negative controls: either total RNA prepared from cells that do not express the investigated gene (cells exhibiting a genomic deletion of the gene of interest could be used as a source of negative control), or total RNA containing a similar transcript (such as RNA from a different species) that is not amplifiable by the selected oligonucleotides (in some of our quantitative studies, total RNA used as a source of internal standard was used as a negative control), and (3) use a sample in which the reverse transcriptase step was omitted to detect either eventual contamination by previously amplified cDNA, or amplification from DNA if primers are localized in the same exon. Also, it is recommended that a sample containing only the exogenous RNA, source of standard transcript, with primers corresponding to the investigated transcript and a sample of RNA containing the investigated transcript with primers corresponding to the standard transcript be used. Include reagent controls with each amplification. The reagent control should contain all the necessary components for PCR but without the addition of any template.

Reagents

$10 \times$ PCR buffer: 670 mM Tris-HCl (pH 8.3), 166 mM ammonium sulfate, 10 mM 2-mercaptoethanol, 45 mM MgCl$_2$ (for each fragment, we select the MgCl$_2$ concentration that gives an optimal efficiency of amplification, see Fig. 8.3); other buffers could be used

Random hexamer oligonucleotides, 100 pmol/μl and dNTP, 25 mM of each nucleoside triphosphate are from Pharmacia

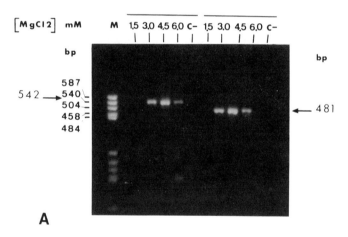

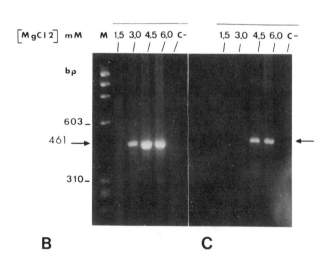

FIGURE 8.3. Effect of magnesium concentration on the efficiency of amplification and comparison of random hexamers and oligonucleotide-specific extension in the RT-PCR. Ethidium bromide-stained 2.5% nusieve gel electrophoresis of RT-PCR products corresponding to the amplification of different fragments of the α-hexosaminidase A transcript. (**A**) Effect of magnesium concentration. (**B**) RT-PCR using random hexamers extension. (**C**) RT-PCR using specific oligonucleotide extension. c−, negative control. In each line 1 μg of fibroblast RNA was used. Figure kindly provided by S. Akli (Institut Cochin de Génétique Moléculaire).

Reverse transcriptase: Moloney murine leukemia virus (MoMuLV) from Bethesda Research Laboratories (BRL) at 200 units/μl

RNasin: RNase inhibitor from Promega corporation at 40 units/μl

Taq polymerase, 5 units/μl from Perkin-Elmer Cetus

DMSO and light white mineral oil are from Sigma

Microfuge tubes and thermal cycler: we have regularly used Perkin-Elmer Cetus materials

Protocols

To improve the accuracy of the relative quantitation method, we always use master mixes for reverse transcription and polymerase chain reaction steps.

Reverse Transcription

In addition to all the components (except the mRNA source under investigation), the master mix contains the source of the transcript used as an internal standard (in our protocol, the L-type pyruvate kinase mRNA amplified from total rat liver RNA). When nine samples (including negative controls) are to be analyzed for comparison of a given mRNA, prepare reverse transcription mixture containing necessary components for 10 reactions: $10\times$ PCR buffer: 4 μl $\times$ 10 (40 μl); hexanucleotide primers 100 pmol/μl: 1 μl $\times$ 10 (10 μl) [5 pmol of specific antisense primer or 20 pmol of oligo(dT) could be used instead of hexanucleotide primers]; dNTP solution 25 mM of each: 2 μl $\times$ 10 (20 μl); source of internal standard (L-type pyruvate kinase), rat liver total RNA 200 ng/μl: 1 μl $\times$ 10 (10 μl); water to a final volume of 40 μl: 27 μl $\times$ 10 (RNA samples and enzymes will be added after). Add 33 μl of this mix to 2 μg of each total RNA under investigation (RNA suspended in water, 1 μg/μl). Heat the mixed RNA samples for 5 min at 65°C; spin down and quench on ice. Add 5 μl of the above mix in which reverse transcriptase (2 μl $\times$ 10) and RNasin (1 μl $\times$ 10) were diluted. Incubate at 42°C for 45–60 min (less than 2 μg of total RNA could be used, in this case components should be proportionally diminished).

PCR Amplification

For each PCR amplification, we use only 10 μl of reverse transcription product; the rest could be used (1) to confirm results, (2) to analyze another fragment of the same transcript, and (3) or to analyze other transcripts.

Prepare the following master mix (for 10 samples): $10\times$ PCR buffer: 4 μl $\times$ 10 (40 μl); primers: each upstream and downstream primer corresponding to the analyzed and the internal transcript is diluted at 50 pmol/μl: 1 μl $\times$ 4 $\times$ 10 (40 μl); DMSO (10%, final concentration): 5 μl $\times$ 10 (50 μl); water to a final volume of 40 μl: 27 μl $\times$ 10 (*Taq* polymerase enzyme will be added). It is not necessary to add dNTP. To 10 μl of each reverse transcription product (as a source of cDNA) add 35 μl of PCR master mix. To prevent evaporation of liquid during thermal cycling, layer one drop of mineral oil on top of PCR solution. Heat the mixed cDNA samples for 10 min at 85°C in the thermal cycler to inactivate the reverse transcriptase, at this temperature and to prevent a nonspecific elongation during the first few cycles, add to each sample (through mineral oil) 5 μl of PCR master mix in which *Taq* polymerase was diluted at 0.5 U/μl and start the coamplification by denaturation.

A thermal cycle profile that we usually use for amplification is (1) denaturing for 30 sec at 94°C, (2) annealing primers for 30 sec at 55°C, extending the primers for 30 sec at 72°C. After 15 cycles (and in the exponential phase of the amplification), stop the thermal cycler in the course of an extension and remove (through mineral oil) from each vial 25 μl of the reaction volume. Subject the remaining 25 μl of reaction volume to 15 additional cycles of amplification.

Analysis of the cDNA-PCR Amplified Products

An aliquot (10 μl) of each PCR product obtained after 15 and 30 cycles is electrophoresed in 8% (w/v) polyacrylamide gel in TBE buffer (use gel: 1.5 mm of thickness, 7.6% monoacrylamide, 0.4% bisacrylamide to separate fragments smaller than 200 bp of length and 7.8% monoacrylamide, 0.2% bisacrylamide to separate fragments larger than 200 bp). Stain the gel with ethidium bromide and photograph. PCR analysis performed after 30 cycles of amplification is used to assess the quality of cDNA-PCR coamplification and to detect contaminations. The amplified products obtained after 15 (or 20) cycles are used to perform the relative quantification. Generally, in the exponential phase of amplification, amplified specific fragments are not detectable by ethidium bromide staining. After alkaline denaturation for 30 min by 0.2 N NaOH/ 0.6 N NaCl solution and washing for 30 min (to minimize alterations of gel sizes) with a 7% (v/v) formaldehyde solution (to facilitate DNA blotting), transfer cDNA-PCR products onto nylon membrane (Hybond N) by overnight Southern blotting according to the procedure detailed by Wahl et al. (1987) and then fix the filter by UV light. Prehybridize (for 1 hr at 60°C) the filter in a Seal-a-Meal bag containing hybridization solution [different hybridization liquids could be used; usually we use the following solution: 30% formamide, 5% dextran sulfate, 0.75 M NaCl, 50 mg/ml heparin, 1% SDS, 50 mg/ml salmon DNA, 10 mg/ml poly(A)]. Hybridize overnight at 37–40°C with 5 × 10^6 cpm/ ml of ^{32}P-end-labeled internal oligonucleotides (or with specific probes labeled by random priming, in this case, use more stringent hybridization conditions). Wash in 2× SSC, 0.1% SDS at room temperature for 15 minutes, twice, and then at 37–40°C for 30 min. Filter is hybridized with internal oligoprobes corresponding to the cDNA fragment under investigation and the one used as internal standard successively (we can also hybridize with both probes together). Also, appropriate nusieve gels could be used to separate cDNA-PCR products.

Quantification by Densitometry

Filter was applied to X-omat Kodak X-ray film with an intensifying screen for different periods of time at −80°C. Levels obtained after 15 cycles of amplification of cDNA fragments were determined by densitometry. All the results were expressed as ratios of the intensity of the band of the investigated transcript to the intensity of the band used as a standard.

Discussion and Helpful Suggestions

In this chapter we describe a procedure for determining modification of mRNA levels in physiological or pathological conditions. In this method we used coreverse transcription and coamplification of the investigated transcript together with an exogenous mRNA used as a standard.

The use of the same buffer for both the reverse transcription reaction and the PCR has simplified the protocol without affecting the efficiency of amplification. To optimize the efficiency of cDNA-PCR amplification and to decrease the number of cycles, other buffers could be used. The first-strand cDNA has synthesized either, using a specific primer or a random hexamer extension. In general, we have found that the procedure using the random hexamer to accomplish the first step does not affect the specificity and gives the highest amount of final amplified products. We have not strictly tested the effect of the primer usage [specific, hexamers or oligo(dT) extension], but some preliminary results suggest that the efficiency of the reverse transcriptase step is in most cases significantly improved by the random hexamers extension (Fig. 8.3B and C). As reverse transcriptase, we have used only the MMLV enzyme from BRL. We did not try enzymes from other sources. For PCR amplification, we have often used the *Taq* polymerase from Perkin-Elmer Cetus. The equivalent enzyme from Boehringer Mannheim Biochemicals has been tested and gave the same results. Parameters such as magnesium concentration, concentration of dNTP, primer oligonucleotides, and enzymes have been tested (for example, see Fig. 8.3) to optimize efficiency of the cDNA-PCR procedure such that specific final products are detectable when the number of PCR cycles that gives exponential amplification is reduced.

To perform relative quantitation of specific transcripts, the prerequisite is to remain in the exponential phase of the amplification process, where the amount of amplified products is proportional to the abundance of starting material.

By judicious selection of a standard transcript that is amplified in the same conditions as the investigated transcript to evaluate nonspecific "tube to tube" variability of amounts of specific PCR products obtained in the exponential phase, we showed that we can reliably compare levels of a given mRNA analyzed in different samples. This method is simple, easy to set up, adaptable to any issue, and rapid: kinetics of accumulation of up to five mRNAs (obtained during *in vitro* differentiation or development), containing about 10 samples each, have been investigated during the same day. Also, by careful selection of primer oligonucleotides added in the master mix to avoid nonspecific amplification, using three couples of primers in addition to the internal standard primers, this method allows coamplification and relative quantitation of more than three different transcripts (Figs. 8.2A and Fig. 8.4). When accurate relative quantitation is required, the conditions have to be very strictly controlled and the amount of the PCR product corresponding to the standard transcript must be similar in all analyzed samples. Such a result could require an adaptation of the range of concentrations of both templates and primers. If the amount of the internal standard is the same in all samples, 2-fold differences in mRNA concentrations could be taken in account. Conversely, if a nonunderstandable high variability of the levels of the amplified standard transcript is observed, it is preferable to do the experiment again. In some cases this variability could be explained by a large disequilibrium between the initial amounts of the investigated and the standard transcripts. Such a situation always leads to an underestimation of the initial ratio of the investigated transcript (for example, see the coamplification of the cardiac actin: dilution 1/10, and the internal standard transcripts in Fig. 8.2B).

Because of the high sensitivity of the cDNA-PCR method, this protocol could be used to detect different levels of very low abundance transcripts. In addition to the prerequisites described above, such an application would require a large reduction of the RNA added as a source of standard transcript. Although this approach is powerful for determining the rela-

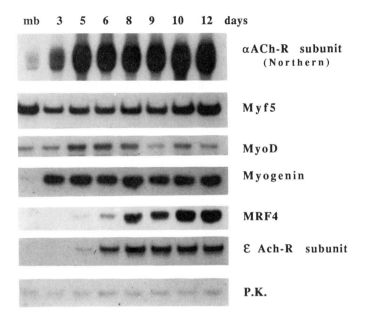

FIGURE 8.4. RT-PCR quantitative analysis of several transcripts during a time course of differentiation of Sol8 myoblasts. After reverse transcription using 2 μg of total RNA and random hexamers extension, Myf5, MyoD, and MRF4 were coamplified together in one tube and myogenin and ε-acetylcholine receptor subunit (ε Ach-R subunit) were coamplified in another one. L-PK transcript used as internal standard was amplified with each set of transcripts. The acetylcholine receptor α-subunit (αAch-R subunit) was assayed by Northern blot. Reproduced from Montarras et al. (1991), *New Biol* 3:592–600 by copyright permission of W.B. Saunders Company.

tive levels of a specific mRNA in different samples, in some cases it is difficult to determine whether the message levels detected are of physiological importance. For example, by comparing the level of dystrophin mRNA fragment (localized in the 5' of dystrophin transcript) obtained from brain total RNA (after 15 cycles) to that obtained from lymphoblasts RNA (after 30 cycles), and supposing that the amplification yield remains constant, we estimate that the amount of dystrophin transcript is about 20,000 times less abundant in the latter sample than in the former one. Such a very low level (much less than 1 copy per cell) corresponds to what we have already described as illegitimate transcription (Chelly et al., 1990b; Sarkar and Sommer, 1989; see also Chapter 24, this volume). On the other hand, the detection after 15 cycles in lymphoblasts of a significant level of dystrophin mRNA fragment localized in the 3'-end of dystrophin transcript

(Fig. 8.5) allowed us to characterize a new transcriptional unit that is produced by the distal part of the dystrophin gene and widely expressed (Hugnot et al., 1992).

In our protocol the specificity of the cDNA-PCR products is guaranteed by specific hybridization; we always try to avoid nonspecific amplification and to reduce the level of background bands. Adaptation of reaction components, annealing temperature, length of times required for primer annealing, extension and denaturation, and the adding of the *Taq* polymerase enzyme at high temperature could help to obtain clean results.

Although this approach is useful for comparing the levels of specific mRNA in different samples, it is not recommended for comparing the level of different mRNAs. Nevertheless, similar yields in amplifying fragments from two different mRNA species are a mandatory condition for comparative quantitation of these

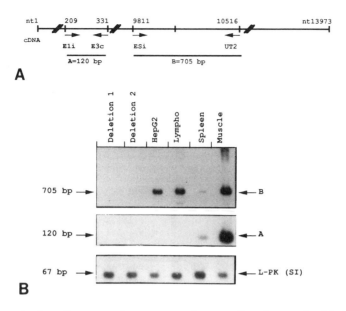

FIGURE 8.5. Characterization of nonmuscular transcript produced by the distal part of the dystrophin gene. (A) Position of the different oligonucleotide primers and their relation to the target cDNA region of human dystrophin gene and size of amplified fragments. (B) Autoradiographs of Southern blot of PCR products corresponding to the coamplification (15 cycles) of fragment A (located in the 5'-region of dystrophin cDNA), fragment B (located in the region encoding the cystein-rich domain), and L-PK transcript used as internal standard. Total RNA was extracted from skeletal muscle (muscle), spleen, control lymphoblasts (lympho), Hep G2 hepatoma cell lines (Hep G2), lymphoblasts from a patient with a deletion that removes the whole dystrophin gene (deletion 2), and lymphoblasts from a patient with a deletion of the distal part of the dystophin gene (deletion 1).

mRNAs. For example, we used this method to quantitate the relative amount of dystrophin mRNAs specifically transcribed from muscle and brain promoters in total RNA extracted from cultures of mouse brain neuronal and astroglial cells. In this case the primers were a common, forward primer, located in exon 2, and two specific reverse primers, located in the first muscle and brain exon, respectively (Chelly et al., 1990c and see Fig. 24.5 in Chapter 24, this volume). Sizes and sequences of the amplified fragments were so similar that one can assume an amplification of these fragments with equivalent yields.

This procedure cannot be used to determine the absolute value (proportion of mRNA toward total RNA) of a given mRNA in a given sample. Strategies using either a separate standard curve composed of serially diluted *in vitro* transcribed RNA run alongside the experimental samples (Robinson and Simon, 1991), or coamplification of the analyzed mRNA with (1) a competitive template or a synthetic cRNA as an internal standard that uses the same primers as those of the mRNA under investigation (Gilliland et al., 1990; Wang et al., 1989), or (2) an unrelated ubiquitously expressed mRNA used as an internal standard (Chelly et al., 1988) could be applied to deduce the amount of target mRNA present in the starting material. These methods use extrapolation against the standard curves that are established for each quantitative assay. However, because a significant variability of the efficiency of the reaction between experiments was observed, one can expect a significant variability of the results obtained by these methods. In our experience, day-to-day variability of efficiency of reverse transcriptase or PCR steps does not modify the evaluation of the results (comparison of the PCR products into the exponential phase) because this variability affects all investigated samples, so that the results expressed as a ratio of the amount of amplified investigated fragment to the amount of amplified standard fragment remain constant.

It is crucial to use controls for detecting contaminations that could lead to an overestimation of scarce transcripts. Multiple controls must always be run with each set of experiments. In our studies of the dystrophin gene expression, in addition to the amplification of a sample that contains all the necessary components for PCR but without template, an RNA sample corresponding to a patient with a 4-megabase deletion encompassing the whole dystrophin gene was regularly used as negative control. Otherwise, it is advantageous to avoid the use of PCR primers located in the same exon because such choice will require additional steps and controls (DNase treatment of the RNA, PCR amplification of a sample for which the reverse transcriptase was omitted, etc.) to obtain meaningful PCR results.

In summary, a quantitative PCR procedure using an exogenous mRNA as a standard is very useful for determining the accumulation of specific messengers. It has been applied to investigate modification of gene expression at levels that were under the limit of detectability by other techniques and to compare levels of an mRNA in different cells or tissues at different stages of physiological or pathological conditions. This strategy has also been used to coamplify multiple transcripts and to analyze concurrently the kinetics of expression of several genes.

Acknowledgments. We thank E. Clarke for critical reading of this manuscript.

References

Becker-André M, Hahlbrock K (1989): Absolute mRNA quantification using the polymerase chain reaction (PCR). A novel approach by a PCR aided transcript titration assay (PATTY). *Nucl Acids Res* 17:9437–9446.

Chelly J, Kaplan J-C, Maire P, Gautron S, Kahn A (1988): Transcription of the dystrophin gene in human muscle and non-muscle tissues. *Nature (London)* 333:858–860.

Chelly J, Montarras D, Pinset C, Berwald-Netter Y, Kaplan J-C, Kahn A (1990a): Quantitative estimation of minor mRNAs by cDNA-polymerase chain reaction. Application to dystrophin mRNA in cultures myogenic and brain cells. *Eur J Biochem* 187:691–698.

Chelly J, Concordet J, Kaplan J-C, Kahn A (1990b): Illegitimate transcription: Transcription of any gene in any cell type. *Proc Natl Acad Sci USA* 86:2617–2621.

Chelly J, Hamard G, Koulakoff A, Kaplan J-C, Kahn A, Berwald-Netter Y (1990c): Dystrophin gene transcribed from different promoters in neuronal and glial cells. *Nature (London)* 334:64–65.

Chirgwin J, Przybyla A, MacDonald R, Rutter W (1979): Isolation of biologically active ribonucleic acid from sources enriched in ribonuclease. *Biochemistry* 18:5294–5299.

Cognet M, Lone Y, Vaulont S, Kahn A, Marie J (1987): Structure of the rat L-type pyruvate kinase gene. *J Mol Biol* 196:11–25.

Gilliland G, Perrin S, Blanchard K, Bunn FF (1990): Analysis of cytokine mRNA and DNA: Detection and quantitation by competitive polymerase chain reaction. *Proc Natl Acad Sci USA* 87:2725–2729.

Hugnot J, Gilgenkrantz H, Vincent N, Chaffey P, Morris G, Monaco A, Koulakoff A, Berwald-Netter Y, Kaplan J, Kahn A, Chelly J (1992): Distal transcript of the dystrophin gene initiated from an alternative first exon and encoding a 75-kDa protein widely distributed in nonmuscle tissues. *Proc Natl Acad Sci USA* 89:7506–7510.

MacDonald R, Swift G, Przybyla A, Chirgwin J (1987): Isolation of RNA using guanidinium salts. *Methods Enzymol* 152:219–226.

Montarras D, Chelly J, Bober E, Arnold H, Ott M, Gros F, Pinset C (1991): Developmental patterns in the expression of Myf5, MyoD, myogenin, and MRF4 during myogenesis. *New Biol* 3:592–600.

Rappolee D, Wang A, Mark D, Werb Z (1989): Novel method for studying mRNA phenotypes in single or small numbers of cells. *J Cell Biochem* 39:1–11.

Robinson M, Simon M (1991): Determining transcript number using the polymerase chain reaction: PGK-2, mP2, and PGK-2 transgene mRNA levels during spermatogenesis. *Nucl Acids Res* 19:1557–1562.

Saiki R, Scharf S, Faloona F, Mullis K, Horn G, Erlich H, Arnheim N (1985): Enzymatic amplification of beta-globin genomic sequences and restriction site analysis for diagnosis of sickle cell anemia. *Science* 230:1350–1354.

Sambrook J, Fritsch E, Maniatis T (1989): *Molecular Cloning: A Laboratory Manual*. New York: Cold Spring Harbor Laboratory Press.

Sarkar G, Sommer S (1989): Access to a messenger sequence or its protein product is not limited by tissue or species specificity. *Science* 244:331–334.

Singer-Sam J, Robinson M, Bellvé A, Simon M, Riggs A (1990): Measurement by quantitative PCR of changes in HPRT, PGK-1, PGK-2, APRT, MTase, and Zfy gene transcripts during mouse spermatogenesis. *Nucl Acids Res* 18:1255–1259.

Strohman R, Moss P, Micou-Estwood J, Spector D, Przybyla A, Paterson B (1977): Messenger RNA for myosin polypeptides: Isolation from single myogenic cell cultures. *Cell* 10:265–272.

Wahl G, Meinkoth J, Limmel A (1987): *Methods Enzymol* 152. Orlando, FL: Academic Press, 572–581.

Wang A, Doyle M, Mark D (1989): Quantitation of mRNA by the polymerase chain reaction. Proc Natl Acad Sci USA 86:9717–9721.

9

Analysis of Human T-Cell Repertoires by PCR

Dominic G. Spinella and James M. Robertson

T cells recognize antigen by virtue of a hetero-dimeric T-cell receptor (TCR) molecule, each chain of which is encoded by several distinct germline gene segments. These variable (V), diversity (D), joining (J), and constant (C) region gene segments rearrange during T-cell ontogeny to give rise to enormous clonal diversity of receptor molecules, each with its own antigen specificity (for a review, see Wilson et al., 1988). A growing number of studies have demonstrated correlations between the expression of particular V_α or V_β genes, and human T-cell responses to specific antigen/MHC combinations (e.g., Moss et al., 1991; Boitel et al., 1992), superantigens (e.g., Choi et al., 1989; Kappler et al., 1989), or with autoimmune disease susceptibility (e.g., Palliard et al., 1991; Oksenberg et al., 1989). Because the receptor repertoire in a diverse population of T cells is heterogeneous, any marked skewing of this repertoire in a given population (reflected in significant elevation in the expression of individual receptors) is generally interpreted as evidence for antigen-driven expansion of one or more clones of cells that have come to predominate that population. This chapter will explore the use of the PCR for this kind of analysis.

Structure of the T-cell Receptor Genes

Antigen-specific T cells are divided into two categories based on their use of the so-called α/β receptor or γ/δ receptor. This chapter will focus on α/β receptors that are found in the vast majority of peripheral T cells and mediate standard MHC-restricted antigen recognition. Each of the polypeptide chains is encoded by a series of distinct gene segments that rearranges during development of an individual cell in a clonally distinct fashion. The germline organization of these genes is shown in Figure 9.1.

In the case of the α-chain, there are approximately 50 V-region genes, each with its own promoter elements, that are organized into families of several members based on their sequence homologies. Several kilobases 3' to the $V\alpha$ elements are a similar number of J_α elements, followed by a single $C\alpha$-region segment. During T-cell ontogeny, a DNA rearrangement occurs bringing one of these V gene segments next to a J-region segment. The locus then becomes transcriptionally active to produce an mRNA in which the intervening

The Polymerase Chain Reaction
K.B. Mullis, F. Ferré, R.A. Gibbs, editors
© 1994 Birkhäuser Boston

A

Rearrangement of Human T-Cell Receptor α Gene Locus

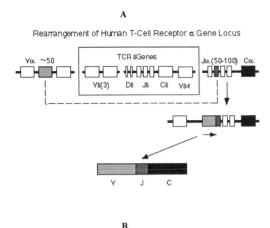

B

Rearrangement of Human T-Cell Receptor β Gene Locus

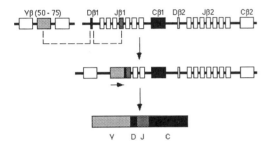

FIGURE 9.1. Germline organization and T-cell rearrangement of T-cell receptor α (**A**) and β (**B**) genes. The top line schematizes the locus in its germline (non-T-cell state), the center line depicts the DNA organization after specific rearrangement in an individual T cell, and the bottom line represents the mRNA transcribed from the rearranged locus.

material between the J_α and C_α regions is spliced away as a typical intron.

The β locus is organized similarly with the 50–60 V_β segments located 5' to two clusters of J_β elements and two C_β region genes. TCR β-chains also employ diversity (D) gene segments and transcriptional activation of this locus requires two rearrangements: An initial D_β–J_β rearrangement followed soon thereafter by a V_β to D_β–J_β rearrangement. The essentially random rearrangements between V and J segments and associations of independent α- and β-chains give rise to a great deal of "combinatorial" diversity in the expressed TCR repertoire. This diversity is further increased by

the fact that individual rearrangements are imprecise and often delete nucleotides from the 3'-end of the V segments, and the 5'-ends of the J elements (as well as from both ends of the D_β segments). Moreover, random nucleotides (N-regions) are inserted at the junctions of the rearranged gene segments. As a consequence of this diversity-generating mechanism, the nucleotide sequence through these junctions serves as a marker of clonality: It is very unlikely that independent rearrangements in separate T cells would bear the same sequence through this region.

PCR Analysis of the T-Cell Repertoire

Analysis of TCR gene expression in polyclonal populations of T cells is now becoming increasingly important to a variety of experimental and clinical programs. Such analysis has been greatly facilitated by the advent of PCR technology, which allows the specific amplification and quantitation of cDNAs derived from TCR transcripts. Typically, RNA is isolated from T-cell populations exposed to antigen or superantigen, or obtained from autoimmune lesions, and reverse transcribed. Individual TCR genes are then amplified in a series of independent PCR reactions using an antisense primer complementary to the C region and a panel of sense primers each specific for a single V gene or gene family.

Individual PCR products can be further analyzed by cloning them into plasmid vectors. Independent colonies can be prepared and plasmids subjected to sequence analysis with particular emphasis on the V–D–J junctions. Repeated isolation of a single junctional sequence implies that the PCR product was obtained by amplification of an identical starting template, i.e., a monoclonal population of cells.

The PCR products are resolved by gel electrophoresis and the relative quantities of each are measured. Typically, this is accomplished by radiolabeling the C-region primer prior to PCR amplification and excising the specific band for scintillation counting, or by preparing an autoradiogram of the gel and quantifying band intensity by densitometry. Variations on this standard theme abound and differ with respect to the method of quantitation, the coamplification of standard reporter genes (to control for differences in total template concentration among independent reactions), and the exact sequence of the oligonucleotide primers. In all cases the basic task is to use this PCR data concerning relative abundance of TCR transcripts to estimate the frequency in the starting population of the cells that produced them.

There are, however, a number of often-ignored factors that dramatically affect the accuracy of this estimate:

1. Differences in priming efficiency of upstream V-region-specific primers that could lead to differential amplification of TCR transcripts with distinct V regions regardless of their initial frequency in the starting population.
2. Limitations in the "dynamic range" of the PCR that become important when differences in starting concentrations of transcripts are such that abundant TCR transcripts are not exponentially amplified in later cycles, while rarer transcripts are. Such a phenomenon would tend to obscure or underestimate real differences in TCR gene expression.
3. Variations in amplification efficiency introduced by coamplification of reporter genes used as internal standards ("multiplexing").
4. Accuracy and sensitivity of the method used to quantify the PCR product.
5. Sampling artifacts that result from the use of small numbers of cells derived from limited samples (such as obtained from biopsy specimens). Of course, these variables influence not only TCR gene analysis, but any experiment in which PCR is used to measure relative levels of gene expression.

In this chapter we will explore some of these variables and their theoretical and practical effect on lymphocyte receptor analysis with particular emphasis on the widely studied TCR β-chain. We will attempt to develop a rational approach to the use of PCR for this purpose and to test the validity of our conclusions on populations of cells in which the frequency of cells bearing particular receptors is measured independently using flow cytometry and available monoclonal antibody probes.

Detection of PCR Products

A major factor to be considered in choosing a method to detect and quantify the PCR product is sensitivity. In contrast to "qualitative" PCR analyses, in which the mere presence of a product is the desired outcome, quantitative PCR experiments must pay rigorous attention to the stoichiometric variables of the reaction (Wang et al., 1989). Although the number of cycles in a PCR can, in principle, be increased until product is detectable, in practice amplification is truly exponential only in the early cycles. As the number of cycles increases beyond a certain number (the exact number depends a great deal on the starting concentration of the template), the fraction of available templates that becomes replicated decreases. This of course gives rise to the well-known "plateau effect" in PCR reactions. It is perhaps less widely appreciated that by the time most amplifications have generated sufficient product to visualize on an ethidium bromide gel, the PCR is already past the point of exponential amplification and into the "plateau" phase. This problem is compounded when comparing two templates whose starting concentration differs substantially because the more abundant template will enter the "plateau" phase before the less abundant one. Hence, the fewer cycles required to amplify the templates to detectable levels, the more accurate will be the quantitation.

Most investigators have relied on the use of radioactive primers to increase the sensitivity of the assay beyond that which can be achieved by simple electrophoresis in ethidium bromide-containing gels. The C region primer can be labeled using $[\gamma\text{-}^{32}P]ATP$ (or $[\gamma\text{-}^{33}P]ATP$) and T_4 polynucleotide kinase. The PCR product is then electrophoresed through agarose or acrylamide to separate the PCR product from the labeled primers, and the bands are quantified by autoradiography or scintillation counting. A variation of this theme employs unlabeled primers, and quantifies products by blotting the reactions and performing hybridizations with radioactive probes. This has the advantage of providing an additional level of specificity because of the use of nested probes. However, the variables introduced by blotting and hybridization as well as the increase in the time and tedium of the assay offset this potential advantage.

Aside from the hazards of isotope use, a potential drawback to using radioactivity is that primers or probes cannot be stored for any length of time due to their decay. Moreover, variations in the specific activity of the radioactive primers and in the labeling efficiency in different experiments increase interassay variability. Our laboratories now employ fluorescently tagged primers that generate PCR products that can be quantitated in real time using an automated DNA sequencer. The sensitivity of fluorescent product detection is comparable to that of ^{33}P detection by autoradiography (after overnight exposure) and somewhat less than ^{32}P detection. Nevertheless, product is detected with sufficient sensitivity to ensure that amplification is still "exponential" over the detection range. In our experience, most TCR V_β products derived from RNA isolated from 10,000 cells or more can be detected by this method after 22–25 cycles of amplification, and the amplification is still exponential in this range.

The data described in this chapter have been generated using the fluorescence detection system of the ABI 373A DNA Sequencer with the Genescan software package. Figure 9.2A is a photograph of the gel file that is assembled by the software following electrophoresis of TCR V_β PCR products. The software also assembles "electrophoretograms" in which the fluorescent peak heights and areas corresponding to any band are quantified (Fig. 9.2B).

A major advantage of this approach is that primers can be synthesized directly with the fluorescent tag (6-carboxyfluorescein) using a DNA synthesizer and commercially available fluorescent amidite. This ensures that all primers (and therefore all PCR product generated from them) are labeled. Because the label does not decay, the primers can be produced in quantity and stored indefinitely. However, regardless of the detection method chosen by a particular laboratory, it is important to perform a series of pilot experiments to verify that amplification is truly exponential over the range of cycles employed in the analyses.

Primer Selection

As in virtually all PCR-based experimentation, the selection of primers is of the utmost importance in ensuring the quality of the results. Typical PCR primers are 70–90% efficient and do not fully double the amount of product in each cycle of the PCR. When comparing the levels of two templates in a PCR using different primers to amplify them, small differences in primer efficiency can give rise to large differences in product yield. For example, a primer pair with an efficiency of 90% will yield nearly nine times more product than a pair with an efficiency of 70% after only 20 cycles. At 30 cycles (which is more typical of amplifications required to detect TCR transcripts from limited numbers of cells) the difference rises to more than 28fold.

Most of the published work on PCR analysis of T-cell repertoires is directed toward the TCR β-chain and employs the primers series originally described by Choi et al. (1989). These primers consist of a series of 20 V_β-region-specific oligonucleotides, each intended to amplify most members of the V_β 1–20 gene families. Each of these primers is paired with a single labeled antisense primer that is specific for the constant region of the TCR β-chain gene. Such an approach necessarily entails a compromise in choosing optimal amplification conditions. Because the same C-region primer is paired with different V-region primers, the amplification efficiency of each individual PCR reaction in the panel can vary widely.

This is particularly true because there are rather severe sequence constraints in the V-region primers that render them specific for

A

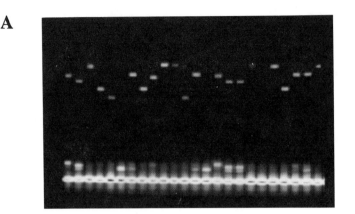

B

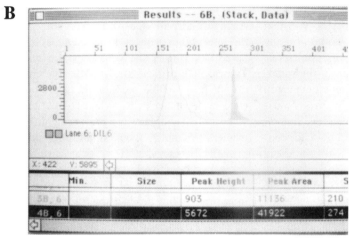

FIGURE 9.2. (**A**) Photograph (reproduced in black and white) of the computer screen displaying a "gene scan" run of normal peripheral blood T cells subjected to TCR V_β-specific PCR. The fluorescent PCR products corresponding to V_β families 1–24 were electrophoresed on an ABI 373A DNA sequencer with 6-cm plates. The displayed image is generated by the software after a 90-min run through 6% nondenaturing polyacrylamide. (**B**) Copy of the "electrophoretogram" in which the fluorescent peak heights and areas of the $V_\beta 1$ PCR product are displayed.

individual TCR V-gene families. In principle, one could design 20 individual sets of primers in which both the sense and antisense oligos are directed toward the V-gene segments. This would potentially provide more uniformity in primer efficiency as well as increasing the specificity of the amplifications. However, the need to radiolabel one of the primers makes this approach very cumbersome: one would need to perform 20 independent kinase reactions every time the assay is to be set up. Moreover, variations in specific activity of each radiolabeled primer would detract from the accuracy of the PCR-based quantitation. The use of fluorescent primers ameliorates this problem to a large extent.

A number of authors have attempted to design primer sets that improve upon the Choi series with respect to uniform efficiency of amplification (e.g., Genevee et al., 1992; Hall

and Finn, 1992). Nevertheless, all of these primer sets employ the same strategy—a common, C-region-specific antisense primer paired with different V-region primers, and therefore retain the theoretical drawbacks.

Our approach to the problem has been to employ a standard reference template in the PCR that consists of cloned TCR genes corresponding to each of the 24 known TCR V_β families. In order to produce this template, we began by cloning the 24 PCR products (obtained with our primers by amplification from T-cell derived cDNA) into plasmid vectors. For each plasmid, we then ligated an 86 bp XhoII fragment obtained from pUC 19 into a unique Bgl II site located in the C_β region 5' to the antisense priming site. The presence of this restriction fragment allows discrimination between the endogenous and reference templates after PCR amplification because products de-

FIGURE 9.3. Fluorescent peak areas of individual V_β PCR products produced by 20 cycles of amplification of a standard template in which all targets were present at equal concentration. Differences in peak area reflect relative priming efficiency of the V_β sense primers when paired with the common C_β antisense primer as described in the text.

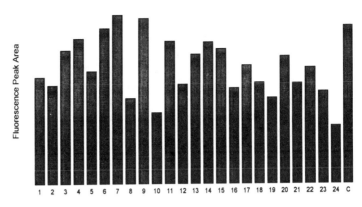

rived from the reference template are 86 bp larger. Finally, we prepared milligram quantities of each plasmid by CsCl banding. The standard template is prepared by mixing precise and equivalent molar quantities of each plasmid, and linearizing the DNA using a restriction enzyme that does not cut any of the PCR product inserts (typically Not I).

Figure 9.3 depicts the results of a typical assay in which the standard reference template has been diluted and then amplified for 22 cycles. Note that despite the uniformity in target concentration, there are wide variations in the amount of product generated after PCR amplification—reflecting the variability in the amplification efficiency of our primer series. It should be pointed out that this particular primer panel was selected in part for its relative uniformity of amplification efficiency. The more commonly used series described initially by Choi et al. (1989) is even more variable.

The use of a reference template in the PCR controls for these primer efficiency differences regardless of the number of cycles required to achieve product detection. In practice, one measures the quantities of each of the reference products and assigns a value of unity to the highest one (usually C_β). All other reference products are assigned values of less than one based upon their quantity relative to the highest. One then measures the quantity of product amplified from the endogenous template and divides by the value assigned to the analogous reference product. In this way, variations in priming efficiency are compensated for and any differences in the relative quantities of the PCR products reflect real differences in starting template concentration. The importance of this correction value to the accuracy of the analysis can hardly be overstated—particularly when analyzing material derived from small samples requiring many cycles of amplification.

Multiplexing

Most proponents of quantitative PCR analyses recommend the coamplification of reporter genes in every amplification. The reporter gene can be some constitutively expressed gene such as actin (which may not be as uniformly expressed as many would believe) or glyceraldehyde phosphate dehydrogenase. Choi et al. (1989) coamplified the TCR α-chain in each reaction, although there is no particular reason to choose another TCR gene as the standard reporter. The rationale behind this approach is that differences in concentrations of total RNA or cDNA in the various reactions or from one experiment to another are reflected in differences in amplification of the reporter gene.

Our alternative approach is to "spike" each reaction with synthetic targets that have the same priming sites as the gene of interests but are of different enough size to enable their resolution on gel electrophoresis. This has the advantage of ensuring that amplification efficiency of both the target and the reporter is the same, but does not control for differences in starting template concentration. For this purpose in TCR repertoire analysis, we perform a 25th amplification in which the C_β gene is amplified along with the synthetic reference template as described.

While the multiplex amplification of reporter targets may be of value in many quantitative PCR applications, we believe that its problems outweigh its benefits when used for TCR repertoire analysis. The use of endogenous templates as reporters requires that their amplification be completely independent of the amplification of the target. Unfortunately, this is not always true. It is certainly not true in the case of the TCR C_α gene coamplification because in at least some amplifications, as the V_β template increases, the levels of C_α product produced in the multiplex reaction decreases—sometimes dramatically (data not shown). In addition, multiplexing two independent PCR reactions in the same vessel increases the probability of nonspecific amplifications. Finally, multiplex amplification necessarily decreases assay sensitivity as both target amplicons must compete for the same pool of limited reagents in the reaction (particularly *Taq* polymerase).

The use of multiplex reporter amplification in TCR repertoire analysis is intended to control for two sources of error: pipetting error in which unequal quantities of template are added to each of the reactions, and cell quantitation errors in which variable amounts of target are compared from one experiment to the next. The former problem can be adequately controlled by the use of master mixes and simple care taken in pipetting. The latter problem can be addressed by amplification of an appropriate target in a separate reaction. If one is attempting to measure the V_β repertoire, the PCR master mix can simply be divided into one more aliquot in which a C_β-specific amplification is performed. If primer efficiencies are compensated for in advance, then the ratio of any V_β product to the C_β quantity ought to provide a useful estimate of the total proportion of T cells in the starting population that

employ the V gene of interest. When using the standard reference template described here it is important to recognize that each of the 24 plasmids that comprise the reference standard contains a C_β region. Therefore, the concentration of C_β target in the reference template is 24 times the concentration of any individual V gene target (this is approximately true of the endogenous template as well—all TCR genes contain a C region regardless of the V gene with which they are paired). In order to compensate for this, the cDNA and reference template that is added in the 25th (C_β) reaction is diluted 1:24 prior to amplification. The quantity of endogenous C_β product (but not the reference product) is then multiplied by 24 after the efficiency correction is made.

Activation State of the Cells

The major goal of the quantitative analysis of TCR transcripts in polyclonal T-cell populations is to draw inferences concerning the clonal diversity of the starting population. Thus, if transcripts bearing the $V_\beta 1$ segment comprise 5% of the TCR β-chain RNA, we would like to infer that $V_\beta 1$-bearing T cells comprise 5% of the original starting population. However, this is true only if the amount of TCR β-chain mRNA is equivalent in every cell in the population. We suspected that this was unlikely, and that the levels of TCR message varied with the activation state of the cell (i.e., its exposure to cognate antigen). To test this, we sorted two populations of T cells by flow cytometry using fluorescent antibodies to the interleukin-2 (IL-2) receptor (CD25). The IL-2 receptor is transiently expressed by T cells after antigenic stimulation, and provides a useful marker of activation. We obtained 10,000 cells that were strongly positive for this marker and 10,000 negative cells by FACS sorting as shown in Figure 9.4A.

We then amplified the C_β gene from cDNA derived from both populations. As seen in Figure 9.4B, the activated (CD25$^+$) pool yielded nearly five times more PCR product than the negative pool. To estimate cell frequencies us-

FIGURE 9.4. (A) A dot-plot representation of data produced by flow cytometric analysis of normal peripheral blood lymphocytes generated by double staining with fluorescein-labeled anti-CD3 (to discriminate T cells) and phycoerythrin-labeled anti-CD25 (to detect the IL-2 receptor). CD3-positive cells were sorted into IL-2R + (region R2) and negative (region R3) populations. RNA from 10,000 cells from each population was isolated, reverse transcribed, and subjected to quantitative PCR for 18 cycles using primers specific for the constant region of the TCR β-chain. (B) Graphs of the fluorescent peak areas of both PCR products clearly demonstrating that the IL-2R + cells produce a good deal more TCR mRNA than do the negative cells.

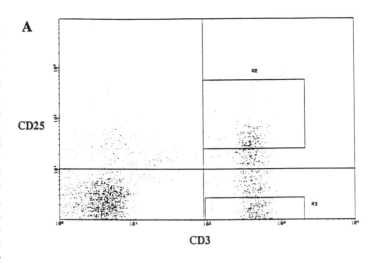

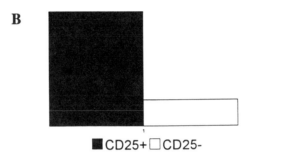

■CD25+□CD25-

ing the PCR then, it would appear to be important that some effort be made to analyze cells of equivalent activation state.

Sampling Artifacts

Assuming a sufficiently sensitive PCR assay, one could perform a T-cell repertoire analysis from RNA derived from a single cell. Presumably, such an analysis would show a single V gene product. If one cloned the PCR product and sequenced the junctional regions of several independent clones, one should find a single rearrangement. It would be folly, of course, to infer that the starting population from which the cell was derived was therefore monoclonal. While this argument is obvious and even trivial for single cells, considerations of cell sample size are important to the accuracy of the repertoire diversity estimates.

To demonstrate this, we performed a repertoire analysis for the TCR β-chain using RNA

derived from 50,000, 5,000, and 500 cells, respectively, from the same starting pool of peripheral blood T cells. We performed the study in duplicate using two separate RNA extractions from separate but equivalently sized sample of cells. If the repertoire analysis is accurate, the results between the replicates ought to be the same. Sampling artifacts should manifest themselves as marked variations in the expression of individual PCR products from one replicate to the next.

Figure 9.5 depicts the results of this experiment. When 50,000 cells are used, interassay variability is quite low, but that variability increases as the cell sample size decreases. Moreover, the variation is highest for those V genes that are the least abundant—again underscoring the importance of sample size. In a PCR such as this in which the cDNA is divided into 25 aliquots, each PCR reaction using cDNA derived from 500 cells should contain approximately 20 cell equivalents

50,000 Cells

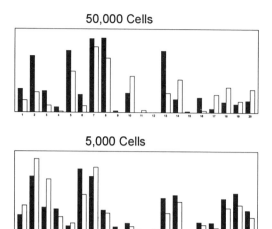

5,000 Cells

500 Cells

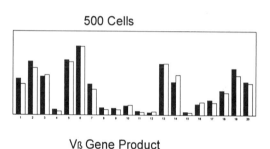

Vß Gene Product

FIGURE 9.5. Reproducibility of TCR repertoire analysis of RNA derived from 50,000, 5000, and 500 cells, respectively. The experiment was run in duplicate using aliquots of cells from the same starting pool. Dark and light bars represent peak fluorescent area of the replicates as described in the text.

Validation of the PCR Assay

To test our assay procedures and primer set, we decided to make use of available monoclonal antibodies directed against the V-gene products of several TCR β genes. Using flow cytometry, we measured the proportion of the total T cells bearing receptors of $V_\beta 2$, $V_\beta 3$, and $V_\beta 17$ families. We then isolated RNA from the same cell population and performed a standard repertoire analysis from 10,000 cells. In our analysis, we convert the RNA to cDNA and perform 25 independent PCR reactions on separate aliquots—corresponding to each of the 24 V_β families and a C_β control amplification. The products are quantified and the primer efficiencies are factored into the analysis. Performed correctly, the ratio of any given V_β gene product to the C_β gene product should reflect the frequency of cells in the starting population that employ that particular receptor.

Figure 9.6 depicts the results of our analysis with each V_β gene product expressed as a percent of the C_β product. The numbers over the $V_\beta 2$, $V_\beta 3$, and $V_\beta 17$ bars reflect the percentage estimates obtained by flow cytometry using the appropriate monoclonal antibodies. Our PCR estimates, for these three genes at any rate, are within 1% of the "true value" obtained by FACS.

of template. Statistical considerations alone would predict that random sampling error ought to be a significant component of between-sample variance in this sort of analysis.

One way around the problem is to use this interassay variability as a measure of the sampling error. Although this requires that precious sample be further diluted, equivalent results in two or more independent analyses increases confidence that unusual results are not due to sampling artifacts.

Conclusions

TCR repertoire analysis can be a powerful tool in the study of immune responses. An appreciation of the variables involved in quantitative PCR in general and in this specific application is essential to obtain accurate results. In the case of the TCR β-chain that is currently under wide study using a variety of PCR approaches, we have provided in Table 9.1 our list of V_β gene primers.

FIGURE 9.6. TCR repertoire analysis of normal, IL-2 receptor-negative peripheral blood T cells. Bars represent the proportion of the C_β product produced by each V_β-specific amplification. Numbers over bars from $V_\beta 2$, $V_\beta 3$, and $V_\beta 17$ are percentages of the total T-cell pool expressing these receptors as determined by flow cytometry with monoclonal antibodies to these gene products.

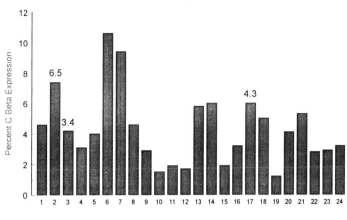

TABLE 9.1. TCR β family-specific oligonucleotide primers and their amplification efficiencies when paired with the $C_\beta a$ antisense primers.[a]

Family	Sequence
C_β RT	GCGGCTGCTCAGGCAGT
$C_\beta a$	CAGGCAGTATCTGGAGTCATTGA
$C_\beta s$	GTGTTCCCACCCGAGGTCGC
$V_\beta 1$	AAGAGAGAGCAAAAGGAAACATTCTT
$V_\beta 2$	TCAGGCCACAACTATGTTTTGGT
$V_\beta 3$	GTCTCTAGAGAGAAGAAGGAGC
$V_\beta 4$	ACAGAGCCTGACACTGATCGC
$V_\beta 5$	CTGATCAAAACGAGAGGACAGCA
$V_\beta 6$	CTCAGGTGTGATCCAATTTC
$V_\beta 7$	GGAATGACAAATAAGAAGTCTTTG
$V_\beta 8$	TTTACTTTAACAACAACGTTCCGA
$V_\beta 9$	GAACAAAATCTGGGCCATGATACT
$V_\beta 10$	GGATTGTGTTCCTATAAAAGCACA
$V_\beta 11$	GTTCTCAAACCATGGGCCATGA
$V_\beta 12$	CACCAGACTGAGAACCACC
$V_\beta 13$	TGTGCCCAGGATATGAACCAT
$V_\beta 14$	CAGAACCCAAGATACCTCATCAC
$V_\beta 15$	CTGGAATGTTCTCAGACTAAGGGT
$V_\beta 16$	AAAGAGTCTAAACAGGATGAGTCC
$V_\beta 17$	GAACAGAATTTGAACCACGATGCC
$V_\beta 18$	GCAGCCCAATGAAAGGACACAG
$V_\beta 19$	CAAAGATGGATTGTACCCCCGAA
$V_\beta 20$	TGTGGAGGGAACATCAAACCCC
$V_\beta 21$	GATTCACAGTTGCCTAAGGA
$V_\beta 22$	AAAGAGGGAAACAGCCACTCTG
$V_\beta 23$	CTGTGTCCCCATCTCTAATCAC
$V_\beta 24$	GTGACCCTGAGTTGTTCTCAGA

[a]The $C_\beta s$ sense primer is used together with $C_\beta a$ to amplify the C_β region in a separate PCR reaction. The C_β RT primer is used to reverse transcribe from total RNA prior to PCR amplification.

References

Boitel B, Ermonval M, Panina-Bordignon P, Mariuzza RA, Lanzavecchia A, Acuto O (1992): Preferential Vβ gene usage and lack of junctional sequence conservation among human T-cell receptors specific for a tetanus toxin-derived peptide: Evidence for a dominant role of a germline-encoded V region in antigen/major histocompatibility complex recognition. *J Exp Med* 175:765–777.

Choi Y, Kotzin B, Herron L, Callahan J, Marrack P, Kappler J (1989): Interaction of *Staphylococcus aureus* toxin "superantigens" with human T-cells. *Proc Natl Acad Sci USA* 86:8941–8945.

Hall BL, Finn OJ (1992): PCR-based analysis of the T-cell receptor Vβ multigene family: Experimental parameters affecting its validity. *BioTechniques* 13:248–257.

Genevee C, Diu A, Nierat J, Caignard A, Dietrich P-Y, Ferradini L, Roman-Roman S, Triebel F, Hercend T (1992): An experimentally validated panel of subfamily-specific oligonucleotide primers (Vα1-w29/Vβ1-w24) for the study of human T-cell receptor variable V gene segment usage by polymerase chain reaction. *Eur J Immunol* 22:1261–1269.

Kappler J, Kotzin B, Herron L, Gelfand EW, Bigler RD, Boylston A, Carrel S, Posnett DN, Choi Y, Marrack P (1989): Vβ-specific stimulation of human T-cells by staphylococcal toxins. *Science* 244:811–813.

Moss PAH, Moots RJ, Rosenberg WMC, Rowland-Jones SJ, Bodmer HC, McMichael AJ, Bell JI (1991): Extensive conservation of α and β chains of human T-cell antigen receptor recognition

HLA-A2 and influenza A matrix peptide. *Proc Natl Acad Sci USA* 88:8987–8990.

Oksenberg JR, Stuart S, Begovich AB, Bell RB, Erlich HA, Steinman L, Bernard CCA (1990): Limited heterogeneity of rearranged T-cell receptor Vα transcripts in brains of multiple sclerosis patients. *Nature (London)* 345:344–346.

Palliard X, West SG, Lafferty JA, Clements JR, Kappler JW, Marrack P, Kotzin BL (1991): Evidence for the effects of a superantigen in rheumatoid arthritis. *Science* 253:325–329.

Wang AM, Doyle MV, Mark DF (1989): Quantitation of mRNA by the polymerase chain reaction. *Proc Natl Acad Sci USA* 86:9717–9721.

Wilson RK, Lai E, Concannon P, Barth RK, Hood LE (1988): Structure, organization, and polymorphism of the human and murine T-cell α and β gene families. *Immunol Rev* 101:149–172.

PART ONE
Methodology

SECTION III
Nonisotopic Detection

10

Ultrasensitive Nonradioactive Detection of PCR Reactions: An Overview

Richard H. Tullis

Introduction

Nonradioactive detection in one of its many forms has been the touchstone of modern nucleic acid diagnostics. Typically, these detection systems involve the determination of a chemical compound through the use of reactions that alter the characteristic light absorption or emission of a reporter molecule. Classical techniques that fall in this category include photometry, fluorescence, and chemiluminescence, although one could argue that radioactivity might also be included since it is most often detected as a color change on X-ray film or as visible light in a liquid scintillation counter.

In DNA diagnostics, one of the principal goals has been to replace radioactive detection with equally sensitive nonradioactive techniques. Based on the experience garnered in immunodiagnostics, the paradigms are clear. The principal limitations to the direct application of immunochemical techniques have been (1) the need to develop reliable chemical techniques for labeling nucleic acids with reporter molecules such as enzymes, (2) the requirement for the survival of the reporter group in the relatively harsh conditions often encountered in hybridization reactions, and (3) the realization that nucleic acid hybridization targets most often are many orders of magnitude less abundant than immunochemical targets.

Development of reliable chemical labeling techniques for DNA probes has proceeded rapidly over the past 10 years to the point where virtually any desired reporter molecule can be attached. Similarly, methods for performing hybridization reactions under conditions that preserve reporter groups are now well known. However, it was not until the advent of PCR that the target limitation problem was clearly solved.

In this article, I intend to review the application of nonradioactive techniques to the detection of DNA and RNA hybridization reactions as they relate to PCR. It should be clear that the basic techniques for detecting the product of any hybridization reaction are applicable to the special case of PCR.

The Polymerase Chain Reaction
K.B. Mullis, F. Ferré, R.A. Gibbs, editors
© 1994 Birkhauser Boston

Detection of DNA Hybrids and PCR Reaction Products

Autoradiography is still the most sensitive DNA detection method (cf. Szabo and Ward, 1983). Autoradiographic detection limits using DNA hybridization probes for viruses and small DNA plasmids average 1–5 pg of target DNA using an overnight exposure (Brandsma and Miller, 1980; Kafatos et al., 1979). This is of course also true for PCR reaction products. Unfortunately, radiolabels pose significant health hazards. In addition, radiolabeled nucleic acids are relatively unstable. Thus simple, sensitive, and rapid nonradioactive detection methods for DNA and DNA hybrids have been sought. Table 10.1 compares the reported sensitivities of various nonradioactive methods in a dot blot format.

In general, nonradioactive detection systems fall into two classes, direct and indirect, based on the detectability of the label. In indirect systems the primary label (e.g., biotin) is detected through interaction with a secondary system that contains a detectable reporter group. In contrast, direct systems attach the reporter group (e.g., fluorescein) directly to the primer or probe. The major difference between these two approaches is found in the number of manipulations required to visualize the product.

Indirect Detection Methods

In the early stages, the most sensitive nonradioactive detection methods were indirect tech-niques based on the use of biotin-labeled DNA probes that were detected with avidin–enzyme conjugates. Other potential labeling groups, such as sugars detectable with lectin conjugates, were recognized but not well explored (Ward, 1982). As a recognition label biotin had several advantages. Biotin is quite stable and has an exceptionally high affinity for avidin ($K_d = 10^{-15}$). Methods were quickly developed for incorporating biotin into both cloned probes (Brigatti et al., 1983) and synthetic DNA and RNA (cf. Ruth, 1984; Ruth and Bryan, 1984; Coutlee et al., 1989). In the earliest studies, biotin–DNA hybrids were detected with enzyme–avidin complexes and fluorescent antibodies both for nick-translated probes (Langer et al., 1981; Langer-Safer et al., 1982; Ward, 1982; Brigatti et al., 1983) and synthetic oligonucleotide probes (Bryan and Arnold, 1984; Ruth and Bryan, 1984; Ruth, 1984).

Indirect DNA hybrid detection methods have classically been based either on the development of a precipitable dye or the detection of a fluorescent antibody. Several enzymatic systems have been applied to the detection of biotinylated compounds (Hsu et al., 1981, 1982; Sternberger et al., 1970; Gardner, 1983; Leary et al., 1983; Bryan and Arnold, 1984). The most sensitive indirect enzymatic detection methods are still based on chemically crosslinked, biotinylated alkaline phosphatase bound to avidin (Leary et al., 1983). This complex can detect single copy genes in Southern blots of human genomic DNA (Leary et al., 1983; Brigatti et al., 1983).

TABLE 10.1. Comparison of sensitivity for nonradioactive detection in dot blot format.

System	Via	Molecular sensitivity	Reference
A-poly-BAP	Color	1.8×10^6	Leary et al. (1983)
Avidin–G6PDH	CL	3.6×10^5	Balaguer et al. (1989)
			Tullis and Arnold (unpublished results)
APase oligomers	Color	ca. 1×10^8	Molecular Biosystems
Digoxigenin	Chemilumin.	9×10^4	Lanzillo (1990)
		2.6×10^8	Seibl et al. (1990)
^{32}P-labeled probes			
Oligomer	Film	1.8×10^7	Molecular Biosystems
Cloned	Film	ca. 1.0×10^5	Berninger et al. (1982)
Fluorescence quenching		9.6×10^4	Morrison et al. (1989)

More recently, a variety of indirect label systems have been used to advantage. These systems are of two types—immunochemically detectable labels and sequence-dependent labels. Examples of immunochemically reactive labels are digoxigenin and DNA:RNA hybrids while sequence-dependent labels include the lac operator and the GCN4 binding sequence. Examples of indirect detection systems are given in Table 10.2. In many cases, the application is strictly one of detection (cf. Inouye and Hondo, 1990; Hendy and Cauchi, 1990; Lanzillo, 1990). In most cases the hybridization event is detected via a color reaction based on alkaline phosphatase (cf. Gregerson et al., 1989) or horseradish peroxidase (cf. Keller et al., 1990; Saiki et al., 1989). In the case of the later enzyme, secondary signal amplification can be achieved using Au/Ag secondary staining (Teo and Griffin, 1990).

Other than biotin, the most widely used indirect label appears to be digoxigenin. This system, developed and marketed by Boehringer-Mannheim, typically employs hybridization probes labeled with digoxigenin, a plant alkaloid not normally present in clinical samples. Indirect detection is accomplished using an antidigoxin antibody conjugated to an enzyme reporter such as alkaline phosphatase. This system is remarkably sensitive, particularly when combined with chemiluminescent detection via stable dioxetanes.

Chemiluminescent detection, which may be employed either with direct or indirect labels, has recently gained popularity due to its high level of sensitivity. Chemiluminescent substrates are available for reactions employing either HRP or alkaline phosphatase. However, alkaline phosphatase labels are more commonly employed due to the ready availability of stable chemiluminescent substrates based on modified dioxetanes (Lanzillo, 1991; Syvanen et al., 1990; Zhang et al., 1991; Dissanayake et al., 1991). Alternatively, bioluminescent reaction systems can be employed to advantage, usually when coupled to other redox enzyme systems. For example, Balaguer et al. (1989) reported the use of a glucose-6-phosphate dehydrogenase (G6PDH)/luciferase couple to detect the formation of hybrids. This system can be quite sensitive. In some formats one can detect 10^{-21} mol of G6PDH and 10^{-19} mol of hybridized target (R.H. Tullis and L.J. Arnold, unpublished results).

Indirect labels may also be used to immobilize hybridization or amplification products to solid surfaces. One of the more common uses of biotin labeling is to trap PCR reaction products into avidin-coated beads or multiwell plates (cf. Saiki et al., 1988). This method takes advantage of the extremely high binding affinity of biotin for avidin. Similarly, immobilized probes can be used to bind PCR products to solid surfaces in order to simplify analysis of PCR products (cf. Saiki et al., 1989).

Among the more interesting methods for hybrid immobilizations is that employed by Mantero et al. (1991), who used a biotinylated RNA probe for immobilization and a monoclonal anti-DNA:RNA hybrid antibody for detection. Secondary detection was accomplished via an HRP-labeled antimouse antibody in a color development assay. Similarly, Coutlee and co-workers (1989) used an anti-biotin antibody to immobilize the biotinylated RNA hybrid, followed by detection with an anti-DNA:RNA hybrid antibody covalently coupled to β-galactosidase to visualize the PCR reaction products.

Kemp and co-workers (1990) also describe an unusual method of immobilizing amplicons. In their method, nested primers containing both a specific DNA binding site and biotin were used to amplify the target sequence. The amplified sequence was bound to the support surface via an immobilized DNA binding protein (GST-GCN4) that selectively bound the amplicons. Detection was then accomplished using an avidin–HRP conjugate and an ELISA reader.

One problem common to all assays employing peroxidase or alkaline phosphatase is that these enzymes may be confused with the native enzymes present in biological samples. Alkaline phosphatase and peroxidase are present in many mammalian tissues and fluids. In addition, other chemical entities such as hematin and Fe are known to have peroxidase activity. In the most sensitive assays, the background caused by these compounds must be reduced

TABLE 10.2. Indirect detection of PCR products.

Reporter group label	Detection method	References
Detection via hybridization probes		
Digoxigenin probe	Chemiluminescence	Lanzillo (1991)
		Kelly et al. (1990)
Biotin-labeled DNA probe	SAv-Apase via color	Said et al. (1990)
		Hendy and Cauchi (1990)
		Gregersen et al. (1989)
	SAv-HRP or SAv-βgal	Inouye and Hondo (1990)
		Ballagi-Pordany et al. (1990)
		Keller et al. (1989)
		Eliaou et al. (1989)
	G6PDH-Av conjugate	Balaguer et al. (1989)
	Detection via luciferase	
Biotin-labeled RNA probe	Anti-DNA:RNA hybrid	Coutlee et al. (1989)
	Antibody β-gal labeled	
	Fluorescence detection	
Unlabeled probe	Anti-DNA antibody	Mantero et al. (1991)
	Detection using HRP labeled antimouse—	
	color development	
Detection via label incorporation or secondary characteristics		
Digoxigenin incorporation	Chemiluminescence	Syvanen et al. (1990)
Biotin-labeled primers	Chemiluminescence	Zhang et al. (1991)
		Dissanayake et al. (1991)
	SAv-HRP color development	Keller et al. (1991)
		Kemp et al. (1989, 1990)
		Bugawan et al. (1990)
		Saiki et al. (1989)
	Bio-dUTP incorporation	Bej et al. (1990)
		Day et al. (1990)
Lac operator sequence primer	Lac-repressor/β-gal fusion	Lundeberg et al. (1991)
	Protein–fluorescence	Wahlberg et al. (1990a,b)
QB replicase primer	QB replicase	Pritchard and Stefano (1990)

by special pretreatments. Alternatively, one may look for enzymatic labels that are not normally present in the samples of interest. Among the current enzyme labels with turnover numbers in the range of 10^4 to 10^5 per second, β-galactosidase is one of the better candidates with low background in mammalian systems.

The main problem with indirect detection systems is that they require the addition of ancillary detection reagents. Excess detection reagent must then be removed by extended washing and binding steps, which are both cumbersome and time consuming. In addition, enzymatic detector complexes (e.g., alkaline phosphatase coupled to streptavidin) may bind nonspecifically both to DNA and to the support matrix, producing a background that can be eliminated only by extensive matrix blocking and washing. Direct detection systems that avoid some of these problems are therefore advantageous.

Direct Detection Systems

There are now three generally recognized direct techniques for the sensitive, nonisotopic detection of nucleic acids and their hybrids: (1) direct enzymatic detection, which requires the construction of enzyme DNA conjugates, (2) fluorescent detection, which depends on the ability to synthesize fluorescent DNA, and

(3) chemiluminescent detection via direct attachment of chemiluminescent labels to synthetic oligonucleotides. Clearly, these methods are interrelated in the sense that an enzyme can be used to generate both fluorescent and chemiluminescent products. Examples of these various direct methods are given in Table 10.3.

In 1983, Heller and Schneider reported the first synthetic DNA probe—enzyme conjugate. These authors attached equine cytochrome c microperoxidase to a simple oligonucleotide probe. This work was subsequently advanced when Renz and Kurz (1984) reported the construction and use of a direct detection system based on a DNA–alkaline phosphatase conjugate. The complex was made by coupling the enzyme (e.g., alkaline phosphatase) to a short polyethyleneimine core using benzoquinone. The unreacted amines on the complex were then used to couple it to the base arylamines in various long DNA probes via glutaraldehyde. These conjugates, which contained protein and DNA in a weight ratio of about 30 to 1, were shown to be capable of hybridizing to specific DNA target sequences in Southern blots with a detection limit of 1–5 pg of specific target DNA.

In 1985, Jablonski and co-workers published the first account detailing the synthesis and use of alkaline phosphatase-labeled synthetic oligonucleotide probes. Perhaps most surprisingly, these conjugated oligonucleotides proved capable of detecting less than 10 pg of plasmid target DNA bound to nitrocellulose filters using a precipitate formazan dye assay.

Direct detection schemes for defining PCR reaction products have most commonly employed HRP as the label (cf. Ehrlich et al., 1991; Bugawan et al., 1990). Beyond the remarkable stability of HRP to drying and its resistance to denaturation under the conditions used for hybrid formation, HRP is relatively inexpensive.

Fluorescence detection of DNA hybrids is currently under investigation by several research groups. Direct fluorescence detection of DNA hybrids has several advantages over enzymatic techniques.

1. Fluorescent molecules can be subjected to the rigorous conditions that are used in DNA synthesis and in performing hybridization reactions without substantial losses in detectability.
2. Fluorescence is mediated by relatively stable fluorophores that can undergo a large number of fluorescent transitions in very short time periods (i.e., more than 10^7 emissions per second under ideal conditions). Thus they are detectable with high sensitivity.
3. Fluorescent oligonucleotides are applicable in situations such as DNA sequencing that are difficult to perform with direct enzymatic labels.

Fluorescent labels provide for exceptionally sensitive detection. Under special laboratory conditions the laser-activated fluorescence of single molecules has been observed (Hirschfeld, 1976). In most laboratory conditions, however, fluorescence detection is limited by fluorescence quenching, photobleaching, background fluorescence from other materials in the sample, and scattered light. Some of these problems may be avoided through the use of fluorophores with highly discrete emission peaks and long fluorescent lifetimes (e.g., lanthanide chelates) in combination with time or phase resolved fluorescence detection systems. Scattered light and background fluorescence can be substantially reduced by limiting the sample to small volume elements (i.e., using microfluorometry) and by using fluorophores that emit toward the red end of the visible light spectrum.

Fluorescent labeling of oligonucleotides has generally been accomplished through the incorporation of strongly nucleophilic reaction centers into the structure of the molecule. For example, Ruth and co-workers (Ruth, 1983; Ruth and Bryan, 1984) successfully incorporated 5-allylamine deoxyuridine into synthetic DNA. The amine function was subsequently derivatized with FITC or Texas Red (sulfonyl chloride) to yield a stable fluorescent derivative. Hood and co-workers (Smith et al., 1985) using a slightly different strategy incorporated

TABLE 10.3. Direct detection of PCR products via hybridization probes.

Reporter group label	Detection method	References
Detection via hybridization probes		
Acridine esters	HPA chemiluminescence	Dhingra et al. (1991)
		Ou et al. (1990)
HRP-labeled DNA	Color development	Ehrlich et al. (1991)
		Scharf et al. (1991)
		Bugawan and Ehrlich (1991)
		Bugawan et al. (1990)
Rare earth metals	Eu^{3+}—time resolved fluorescence	Dahlen et al. (1991)
Fluorescence quenching	FITC probe donor	Morrison et al. (1989)
	Pyrene acceptor	
Detection via primer incorporation or secondary characteristics		
Fluorescent primers	Color complementation	Embury et al. (1990)
		Chehab and Kan (1990)
		Chehab and Kan (1989)
	Capillary electrophoresis fluorescence detection	Brownlee et al. (1990)
IEHPLC separation	Spectrophotometric	Katz et al. (1990)
Direct detection via sequencing		
Fluorescent primers	Fluorescent sequencing	Sullivan et al. (1991)
Unlabeled primers	Incorporate to amplicon sequence via fluorescent primers	McBride et al. (1989)
Biotin labeled primers	Immobilize on SAv then sequence	Syvanen et al. (1989)

5'-deoxy-5'-aminothymidine as the 5'-terminal nucleotide of a synthetic DNA sequencing primer. The reactive amine was subsequently derivatized with four different fluorescent labels and used in primer-directed sequencing reactions.

Fluorescent labeling of oligonucleotides has also been accomplished by the incorporation of a reactive sulfur atom at the 5'-terminus of synthetic DNAs. Connolly and Rider (1985) attached sulfhydryl terminated linker arms via a phosphodiester linkage to the 5'-hydroxyl of chemically synthesized oligonucleotides. At pH 8, these thiols react readily with iodoacetates and maleimides and have thus been used to form fluorescent derivatives with such fluorophores as 1,5-I-AEDANS [N-iodoacetyl-N'-(5-sulpho-1-naphthyl) ethylene diamine] and ANM [N-(1-anilinonaphthyl-4) maleimide].

Chu and Orgel (1985) recently described a nonisotopic DNA-labeling reaction based on the incorporation of a 5'-phosphoramidate. Such a technique was not unanticipated since

Letsinger and Schott (1981) previously succeeded in labeling an oligonucleotide via an internal phosphoramidate linker. In one of the earliest labeling techniques described for synthetic oligomers, a fluorescent or luminescent label was attached through a periodate oxidized 5'-terminal ribonucleotide (linked 5' to 5' to the product oligomer (Heller and Morrison, 1985). An analogous strategy has been employed by Bauman and co-workers to attach fluorescent labels to the 3'-ends of RNA (Bauman et al., 1983). In our view, the best approach favors the incorporation of primary amines due to the relative ease of derivatization.

Direct fluorescent labels have been employed usefully in PCR. Brownlee et al. (1990) used fluorescent PCR primers to detect amplicons separated by capillary electrophoresis. Morrison et al. (1989) used a fluorescence quenching assay employing fluorescein as the donor and pyrene as the nonfluorescent acceptor. Dahlen et al. (1991) employed time-resolved fluorescence techniques to detect rare earth metal-labeled probes. Rare earth metals have the advantage of relatively long fluorescence lifetimes allowing background fluorescence to decay prior to measurement.

One of the most interesting uses of fluorescent labels is the color complementation assay system of Chehab and Kan (1989, 1990). In this scheme, two different fluorophores are used to label the two primers. The combined fluorescence of the pair is chosen in such a fashion that the colors complement one another to form a unique visible color. Thus a wide variety of PCR reaction products can be differentiated solely on the basis of the visible color of the product.

Fluorescent enzyme substrates may also be used to advantage in some instances. β-galactosidase and alkaline phosphatase are perhaps the most useful of the enzyme labels due to the ready availability of fluorescent substrates most often based upon 4-methyl umbelliferone. One interesting use of this type of detection has been reported using primers incorporating the lac operator (Lundeberg et al., 1990, 1991; Wahlberg et al., 1990a,b). In this instance, the presence of the lac sequence is detected using a lac operator : β-galactosidase fusion protein and a fluorescent substrate.

Direct Chemiluminescent Detection of DNA

While indirect chemiluminescent techniques can be used to detect DNA hybrids, the most successful methods appear to be ones that rely on a direct enzymatic or chemiluminescent label. In 1983, Heller and Schneider described the use of a microperoxidase-labeled oligonucleotide for chemiluminescent detection of DNA hybrids through an energy transfer mechanism. However, it is not until 1987 that a truly successful chemiluminescent system was presented (Arnold et al., 1987). The principal impediment to labeling oligonucleotides with chemiluminescent reporter groups is that most such labels are unstable making synthesis difficult. Arnold and co-workers (1987) succeeded in postsynthetically attaching an acridine ester

to a modified base in the oligonucleotide. The acridine ester was found to be unstable when exposed to mildly basic conditions unless the probe containing it was hybridized to a suitable target. Thus excess probe could be readily stripped of label prior to analysis without the need for extensive washing. Dhingra et al. (1991) and Ou et al. (1990) used this system to advantage.

Summary

Nonradioactive detection systems employing colorimetry have been widely employed to detect PCR reaction products. These protocols typically involve the use of both indirect recognition labels (for immobilization) and direct reporter labels (for detection). Indirect recognition labels used include biotin and digoxigenin as well as structural features of the product that can be recognized immunochemically or through the use of DNA binding proteins. Reporter labels are used indirectly in the form of conjugates or fusion proteins as well as through direct attachment to probes or primers. Direct reporter labels include enzymes (e.g., alkaline phosphatase), fluorophores, and chemiluminescent molecules (e.g., acridinium esters and isoluminol derivatives). The most useful configurations are adapted to a modified ELISA format in which the recognition label is used to immobilize the PCR product for subsequent detection. It remains to be seen which of these alternative formats will prove most useful in clinical assays.

References

Arnold LJ, Hammond PW, Wiese WA, Nelson NC (1989): Assay formats involving acridinium ester labeled DNA probes. *Clin Chem* 35:1588–1594.

Balaguer P, Terouanne B, Eliaou JF, Humbert M, Boussioux AM, Nicolas JC (1989): Use of glucose-6-phosphate dehydrogenase as a new label for nucleic acid hybridization reactions. *Anal Biochem* 180(1):50–54.

Balaguer P, Terouanne B, Boussioux AM, Nicolas JC (1989): Use of bioluminescence in nucleic acid hybridization reactions. *J Biolumin Chemilumin* 4(1):302–309.

Ballagi-Pordany A, Klingeborn B, Flensburg J, Belak S (1990): Equine herpesvirus type 1: Detection of viral DNA sequences in aborted fetuses with the polymerase chain reaction. *Vet Microbiol* 22(4):373–381.

Bauman JG, Wiegant J, van Duijn P (1983): The development, using poly (Hg-U) in a model system, of a new method to visualize hybridization in fluorescence microscopy. *J Histochem Cytochem* 31:571–578.

Bej AK, Mahbubani MH, Miller R, DiCesare JL, Haff L, Atlas RM (1990): Multiplex PCR amplification and immobilized capture probes for detection of bacterial pathogens and indicators in water. *Mol Cell Probes* 4(5):353–365.

Berninger M, Hammer M, Hoyer B, Gerin JL (1982): An assay for the detection of the DNA genome of hepatitis B virus in serum. *J Med Virol* 9:57–68.

Brandsma J, Miller G (1980): Nucleic acid spot hybridization: Rapid quantitative screening of lymphoid cell lines for Epstein-Barr virus. *Proc Natl Acad Sci USA* 77:6851–6855.

Brigati DJ, Myerson D, Leary JL, Spalholz B, Travis SZ, Fong CKY, Hsiung GD, Ward DC (1983): Detection of viral genomes in cultured cells and paraffin embeded tissue sections using biotin labeled hybridization probes. *Virology* 126:32–50.

Brownlee RG, Sunzeri FJ, Busch MP (1990): Application of capillary DNA chromatography to detect AIDS virus (HIV-1) DNA in blood. *J Chromatogr* 533:87–96.

Bryan RN, Arnold LJ Jr (1984): Detection of HBV-DNA with modified synthetic oligonucleotides containing radioactive and non-radioactive reporter groups. *DNA* 3:124.

Bugawan TL, Erlich HA (1991): Rapid typing of HLA-DQB1 DNA polymorphism using non-radioactive oligonucleotide probes and amplified DNA. *Immunogenetics* 33(3):163–170.

Bugawan TL, Begovich AB, Erlich HA (1990): Rapid HLA-DPB typing using enzymatically amplified DNA and nonradioactive sequence-specific oligonucleotide probes. *Immunogenetics* 32(4):231–241.

Chehab FF, Kan YW (1989): Detection of specific DNA sequences by fluorescence amplification: A color complementation assay. *Proc Natl Acad Sci USA* 86(23):9178–9182.

Chehab FF, Kan YW (1990): Detection of sickle cell anaemia mutation by colour DNA amplification. *Lancet* 335(8680):15–17.

Chu BCF, Orgel LE (1985): Detection of specific DNA sequences with short biotin-labeled probes. *DNA* 4:327–331.

Connolly BA, Rider P (1985): Chemical synthesis of oligonucleotides containing a free sulphydryl group and subsequent attachment of thiol specific probes. *Nucl Acids Res* 13:4485–4502.

Coutlee F, Bobo L, Mayur K, Yolken RH, Viscidi RP (1989): Immunodetection of DNA with biotinylated RNA probes: A study of reactivity of a monoclonal antibody to DNA-RNA hybrids. *Anal Biochem* 181(1):96–105.

Dahlen P, Iitia A, Mukkala VM, Hurskainen P, Kwiatkowski M (1991): The use of europium (Eu3 +) labelled primers in PCR amplification of specific target DNA. *Mol Cell Probes* 5(2):143–149.

Day PJ, Bevan IS, Gurney SJ, Young LS, Walker MR (1990): Synthesis in vitro and application of biotinylated DNA probes for human papilloma virus type 16 by utilizing the polymerase chain reaction. *Biochem J* 267(1):119–123.

Dhingra K, Talpaz M, Riggs MG, Eastman PS, Zipf T, Ku S, Kurzrock R (1991): Hybridization protection assay: A rapid, sensitive, and specific method for detection of Philadelphia chromosome-positive leukemias. *Blood* 77(2):238–242.

Dissanayake S, Min X, Piessens WF (1991): Detection of amplified *Wuchereria bancrofti* DNA in mosquitoes with a nonradioactive probe. *Mol Biochem Parasitol* 45(1):49–56.

Eliaou JF, Humbert M, Balaguer P, Gebuhrer L, Amsellem S, Betuel H, Nicolas JC, Clot J (1989): A method of HLA class II typing using nonradioactive labelled olignucleotides. *Tissue Antigens* 33(4):475–485.

Embury SH, Kropp GL, Stanton TS, Warren TC, Cornett PA, Chehab FF (1990): Detection of the hemoglobin E mutation using the color complementation assay: Application to complex genotyping. *Blood* 76(3):619–623.

Erlich H, Bugawan T, Begovich AB, Scharf S, Griffith R, Saiki R, Higuchi R, Walsh PS (1991): HLA-DR, DQ and DP typing using PCR amplification and immobilized probes. *Eur J Immunogen* 18(1–2):33–55.

Gardner L (1983): Non-radioactive DNA labeling: Detection of specific DNA and RNA sequences on nitrocellulose and in situ hybridizations. *BioTechniques* 1:38–41.

Gregersen N, Winter V, Petersen KB, Koch J, Klvraa S, Rudiger N, Heinsvig EM, Bolund L (1989): Detection of point mutations in amplified single copy genes by biotin-labelled oligonucleotides: Diagnosis of variants of alpha-1-antitrypsin. *Clin Chim Acta* 182(2):151–164.

Heller MJ, Morrison LE (1985): Chemiluminescent and fluorescent probes for DNA hybridization systems. In: *Rapid Detection and Identification of Infectious Agents*, Kingsbury DT, Falkow S, eds. New York: Academic Press, 245–256.

Heller MJ, Schneider BL (1983): Chemiluminescent labeling of nucleic acids using azidophenyl glyoxal. *Fed Proc* 42:1954 (abst. 1149).

Hendy JG, Cauchi MN (1990): Direct detection of beta thalassemic mutations: Use of biotin labeled allele specific probes. *Am J Hematol* 34(2):151–153.

Hirschfeld T (1976): Optical microscope observation of single small molecules. *Appl Optics* 15:2965–2966.

Hsu SM, Raine L (1982): Versatility of biotin-labeled lectins and avidin-biotin-peroxidase complex for localization of carbohydrate in tissue sections. *J Histochem Cytochem* 30:157–161.

Hsu SM, Raine L, Fanger H (1981): The use of avidin-biotin-peroxidase complex (ABC) in immunoperoxidase techniques. A comparison between ABC and unlabeled antibody PAP procedures. *J Histochem Cytochem* 29:577.

Inouye S, Hondo R (1990): Microplate hybridization of amplified viral DNA segment. *J Clin Microbiol* 28(6):1469–1472.

Jablonski E, Moomaw E, Tullis RH, Ruth JL (1986): Preparation of oligodeoxynucleotide-alkaline phosphatase conjugates and their use as hybridization probes. *Nucl Acids Res* 14:6115–6128.

Kafatos FC, Jones CW, Efstradiadis A (1979): Determination of nucleic acid sequence homologies and relative concentrations by a dot hybridization procedure. *Nucl Acids Res* 7:1541.

Katz ED, Haff LA, Eksteen R (1990): Rapid separation, quantitation and purification of products of polymerase chain reaction by liquid chromatography. *J Chromatogr* 512:433–444.

Keller GH, Huang DP, Manak MM (1989): A sensitive nonisotopic hybridization assay for HIV-1 DNA. *Anal Biochem* 177(1):27–32.

Keller GH, Huang DP, Shih JW, Manak MM (1990): Detection of hepatitis B virus DNA in serum by polymerase chain reaction amplification and microtiter sandwich hybridization. *J Clin Microbiol* 28(6):1411–1416.

Keller GH, Huang DP, Manak MM (1991): Detection of human immunodeficiency virus type 1 DNA by polymerase chain reaction amplification and capture hybridization in microtiter wells. *J Clin Microbiol* 29(3):638–641.

Kelly DJ, Marana DP, Stover CK, Oaks EV, Carl M (1990): Detection of *Rickettsia tsutsugamushi* by gene amplification using polymerase chain reaction techniques. *Ann NY Acad Sci* 590:564–571.

Kemp DJ, Smith DB, Foote SJ, Samaras N, Peterson MG (1989): Colorimetric detection of specific DNA segments amplified by polymerase chain reactions. *Proc Natl Acad Sci USA* 86(7):2423–2427.

Kemp DJ, Churchill MJ, Smith DB, Biggs BA, Foote SJ, Peterson MG, Samaras N, Deacon NJ, Doherty R (1990): Simplified colorimetric analysis of polymerase chain reactions: Detection of HIV sequences in AIDS patients. *Gene* 94(2):223–228.

Langer PR, Waldrop AA, Ward DC (1981): Enzymatic synthesis of biotin-labeled polynucleotides: Novel nucleic acid affinity probes. *Proc Natl Acad Sci USA* 78:6633–6637.

Langer-Safer PR, Levine M, Ward DC (1982): Immunological method for mapping genes on *Drosophila* chromosomes. *Proc Natl Acad Sci USA* 79:4381–4385.

Lanzillo JJ (1990): Preparation of digoxigenin-labeled probes by the polymerase chain reaction. *Biotechniques* 8(6):620, 622.

Leary JJ, Brigati DJ, Ward DC (1983): Rapid and sensitive colorimetric method for visualizing biotin-labeled DNA probes hybridized to DNA or RNA immobilized on nitrocellulose: Bio-blots. *Proc Natl Acad Sci USA* 80:4045–4049.

Letsinger RL, Schott ME (1981): Selectivity in binding a phenanthridinium-dinucleotide derivative to homopolynucleotides. *J Amer Chem Soc* 103:7394.

Lundeberg J, Wahlberg J, Holmberg M, Pettersson U, Uhlen M (1990): Rapid colorimetric detection of in vitro amplified DNA sequences. *DNA Cell Biol* 9(4):287–292.

Lundeberg J, Wahlberg J, Uhlen M (1991): Rapid colorimetric quantification of PCR-amplified DNA. *Biotechniques* 10(1):68–75.

Mantero G, Zonaro A, Albertini A, Bertolo P, Primi D (1991): DNA enzyme immunoassay: General method for detecting products of polymerase chain reaction. *Clin Chem* 37(3):422–429.

McBride LJ, Koepf SM, Gibbs RA, Salser W, Mayrand PE, Hunkapiller MW, Kronick MN (1989): Automated DNA sequencing methods involving polymerase chain reaction. *Clin Chem* 35(11): 2196–2201.

Morrison LE, Halder TC, Stols LM (1989): Solution-phase detection of polynucleotides using interacting fluorescent labels and competitive hybridization. *Anal Biochem* 183(2):231–244.

Ou CY, McDonough SH, Cabanas D, Ryder TB, Harper M, Moore J, Schochetman G (1990): Rapid and quantitative detection of enzymatically amplified HIV-1 DNA using chemiluminescent oligonucleotide probes. *AIDS Res Hum Retrovirus* 6(11):1323–1329.

Pritchard CG, Stefano JE (1990): Amplified detection of viral nucleic acid at subattomole levels using Q beta replicase. *Ann Biol Clin (Paris)* 48(7):492–497.

Renz M, Kurz C (1984): A colorimetric method for DNA hybridization. *Nucl Acids Res* 12:3435–3444.

Rimstad E, Hornes E, Olsvik O, Hyllseth B (1990): Identification of a double-stranded RNA virus by using polymerase chain reaction and magnetic separation of the synthesized DNA segments. *J Clin Microbiol* 28(10):2275–2278.

Ruth JL (1984): Chemical synthesis of non-radioactively-labeled DNA hybridization probes. *DNA* 3:123.

Ruth JL, Bryan RN (1984): Chemical synthesis of modified oligonucleotides and their utility as non-radioactive hybridization probes. *Fed Proc* 43:2048 (abst. 3666).

Said JW, Sassoon AF, Shintaku IP, Corcoran P, Nichols SW (1990): Polymerase chain reaction for bcl-2 in diagnostic lymph node biopsies. *Mod Pathol* 3(6):659–663.

Saiki RK, Chang CA, Levenson CH, Warren TC, Boehm CD, Kazazian HH Jr, Erlich HA (1988): Diagnosis of sickle cell anemia and beta-thalassemia with enzymatically amplified DNA and nonradioactive allele-specific oligonucleotide probes. *N Engl J Med* 319(9):537–541.

Saiki RK, Walsh PS, Levenson CH, Erlich HA (1989): Genetic analysis of amplified DNA with immobilized sequence-specific oligonucleotide probes. *Proc Natl Acad Sci USA* 86(16):6230–6234.

Scharf SJ, Griffith RL, Erlich HA (1991): Rapid typing of DNA sequence polymorphism at the HLA-DRB1 locus using the polymerase chain reaction and nonradioactive oligonucleotide probes. *Hum Immunol* 30(3):190–201.

Seibl R, Holtke HJ, Ruger R, Meindl A, Zachau HG, Rasshofer R, Roggendorf M, Wolf H, Arnold N, Wienberg J et al (1990): Non-radioactive labeling and detection of nucleic acids. III. Applications of the digoxigenin system. *Biol Chem Hoppe Seyler* 371(10):939–951.

Smith LM, Fung S, Hunkapiller MW, Hunkapiller TJ, Hood LE (1985): The synthesis of oligonucleotides containing an aliphatic amino group at the 5′ terminus: Synthesis of fluorescent DNA primers for use in DNA sequence analysis. *Nucl Acids Res* 13:2399–2412.

Soderlund H (1990): DNA hybridization: Comparison of liquid and solid phase formats. *Ann Biol Clin (Paris)* 48(7):489–491.

Sternberger LA, Hardy PH, Cuculis JJ, Meyer HG (1970): The unlabeled antibody-enzyme method of immunohistochemistry. Preparation and properties of soluble antigen-antibody complex (horseradish peroxidase-antihorseradish peroxidase) and its use in identification of spirochetes. *J Histochem Cytochem* 18:315–333.

Sullivan KM, Hopgood R, Lang B, Gill P (1991): Automated amplification and sequencing of human mitochondrial DNA. *Electrophoresis* 12(1): 17–21.

Szabo P, Ward DC (1983): What's new with hybridization *in situ*. *Tech Biol Sci*, 425–427.

Syvanen AC, Aalto-Setala K, Kontula K, Soderlund H (1989): Direct sequencing of affinity-captured amplified human DNA application to the detection of apolipoprotein E polymorphism. *FEBS Lett* 258(1):71–74.

Syvanen AC, Aalto-Setala K, Harju L, Kontula K, Soderlund H (1990): A primer-guided nucleotide incorporation assay in the genotyping of apolipoprotein E. *Genomics* 8(4):684–692.

Teo CG, Griffin BE (1990): Visualization of single copies of the Epstein-Barr virus genome by in situ hybridization. *Anal Biochem* 186(1):78–85.

Wahlberg J, Lundeberg J, Hultman T, Holmberg M, Uhlen M (1990a): Rapid detection and sequencing of specific in vitro amplified DNA sequences using solid phase methods. *Mol Cell Probes* 4(4):285–297.

Wahlberg J, Lundeberg J, Hultman T, Uhlen M (1990b): General colorimetric method for DNA diagnostics allowing direct solid-phase genomic sequencing of the positive samples. *Proc Natl Acad Sci USA* 87(17):6569–6573.

Ward DC (1982): Modified nucleosides and methods of preparing and using same. European Patent Office Application Number 82311804.9.

Zhang Y, Coyne MY, Will SG, Levenson CH, Kawasaki ES (1991): Single-base mutational analysis of cancer and genetic diseases using membrane bound modified oligonucleotides. *Nucl Acids Res* 19(14):3929–3933.

11

Fluorescent Detection Methods for PCR Analysis

Michael J. Heller

Introduction

The polymerase chain reaction (PCR) has provided numerous scientists in biotechnology and biomedical research a powerful technique that has pushed many efforts a quantum leap forward. The ability of PCR to amplify small amounts of target nucleic acids has not only solved the main problem in DNA probe technology, but also has revolutionized molecular biology, and accelerated applications of other important technologies, such as DNA sequencing. However, the development of PCR technology still requires a considerable effort directed at the detection of PCR products. These efforts are required to improve the speed, reliability, quantitation, and sensitivity of PCR analysis. Improved detection methods are important for the secondary verification or corroboration of PCR products, and for the automation of the PCR process.

The detection and analysis of PCR products can be accomplished by a number of techniques. The most widely used method for PCR analysis is to simply run the PCR products on an agarose sizing gel, stain the gel with ethidium bromide, then observe and photograph the gel on a fluorescence transilluminator (Mullis et al., 1986; Mullis and Faloona, 1987; Saika et al., 1988). Comparison of the double-stranded PCR product bands to bands of known size on a DNA ladder allows one to verify that a given target DNA sequence is present in the sample. More sensitive and selective analysis and detection procedures involve the use of both isotopic and nonisotopic labeled PCR primers and DNA probes. Nonisotopic detection involves both direct or indirect techniques that produce color, chemiluminescence, or fluorescent responses. This chapter will cover the area of fluorescent detection and analysis of PCR products. The advantages and disadvantages of this methodology will be reviewed, and its potential for future applications discussed.

Fluorescent Analysis

Fluorescent methods of analysis have proven very useful in biomedical research and in clinical diagnostics (Taylor et al., 1986). Fluorescent analysis is frequently used in immunodiagnostics and other important areas of clinical diagnostics. Fluorescent detection was

The Polymerase Chain Reaction
K.B. Mullis, F. Ferré, R.A. Gibbs, editors
© 1994 Birkhäuser Boston

used very early in the DNA probe diagnostics area (Heller and Morrison, 1985). In the case of DNA sequencing technology, high sensitivity fluorescent detection is an active research area (Luckey et al., 1990; Smith, 1990; Wilson et al., 1990); and several commercially available automated DNA sequencing instruments are based on fluorescent detection methodology (Connell et al., 1987; Prober et al., 1987).

Fluorescent analysis offers many advantages over other detection methodologies. Fluorescent labels, when attached directly to a probe molecule, allow for almost instantaneous detection. Fluorescence analysis is very sensitive, especially when special optoelectronic detection equipment is used (photomultiplier tubes, microchannel plate detectors, intensified CCD detectors, etc.). Detection of less than 100 molecules is often possible in flow cytometers or with specialized epifluorescent microscopes. In very special cases single molecules have been detected (Nguyen et al., 1987).

One of the disadvantages of fluorescent analysis is that certain fluorophores are susceptible to quenching from the excitation light itself or from environmental effects. Fluorescent analysis is frequently limited by the background or autofluorescence from the sample itself. While sensitive detection equipment is available, it is rather expensive and thus out of reach for many researchers.

Preparation of Fluorescent Probes, Primers, and PCR Products

Much of the underlying technology for the functionalization and labeling of DNA (includes RNA, oligonucleotides, etc.) was a result of the large effort to develop DNA probe diagnostics (Keller and Manak, 1989; Symons, 1989). Some of this effort preceded the advent of PCR by approximately 5 years. During this time, technology was developed for the labeling of both large DNA fragments (which are usually produced by cloning procedures)

and small DNA fragments or oligonucleotides (which are produced by automated synthetic procedures). Detection procedures involving nonisotopic labels can be indirect or direct. Indirect or secondary detection is achieved by the incorporation of a primary affinity label (biotin, digoxigenin) into the DNA (RNA) probe sequence. The affinity labeled probe is then hybridized to the target DNA. Detection of the hybridized labeled DNA probe/target DNA is carried out using a secondary label. This is the complement of the affinity group (avidin for biotin, or the specific antibody for digoxigenin) to which a reporter group has been covalently attached. The reporter group is usually an enzyme (alkaline phosphatase, peroxidase, etc.), which then reacts with a substrate to produce a color, a chemiluminescent, or a fluorescent response. Thus, indirect techniques can be used to produce fluorescent responses. Direct detection involves the incorporation of the reporter group directly into the DNA probe or primer. Since indirect detection procedures have been treated extensively in the other chapters, this review will concentrate on direct fluorescent labels that are either covalently bound to a probe or primer or noncovalently associated via intercalation or electrostatic binding.

Direct Labeling of Oligonucleotide Probes and Primers

The direct labeling of oligonucleotide probes and PCR primers is achieved by reacting a functionalized form of the oligonucleotide with an activated form of the fluorophore. While oligonucleotides can be functionalized with a number of different groups including primary amines, sulfhydryl, and aldehydes, the primary amine groups are probably the most useful. Table 11.1 lists some of the ways oligonucleotides have been functionalized and directly labeled with a variety of reporter groups. A recent general review of this subject has been given by Goodchild (1990).

Synthesis and functionalization of oligonucleotide sequences with primary amine groups can be carried out using any of the presently

TABLE 11.1. Functionalization of oligonucleotides and subsequent labeling with various reporter groups.

Functionalization	Reporter	Reference
LAN[a]-amino	Biotin	Ruth (1984)
5'-Terminal amino	Fluorophore	Smith (1990)
LAN-amino	Enzyme	Jablonski et al. (1986)
5'-Terminal amino	Enzyme	Li et al. (1987)
5'-Terminal amino	Enzyme	Sproat et al. (1987)
Thiol group	Enzyme	Chu and Orgel (1988)
Biotin-nucleoside	Enzyme[b]	Cook et al. (1988)
LAN-amino	Enzyme	Urdea et al. (1988)
Phosphorothioates	Fluorophores	Hodges et al. (1989)
Polyamide	Fluorophores	Haralambidis et al. (1990)

[a]Linker arm nucleoside with protected primary amine.
[b]Streptavidin–peroxidase conjugate.

available automated DNA synthesizers and standard phosphoramidite chemistry (5'-dimethoxytrityl nucleoside b-cyanoethyl phosphoramidite reagents, controlled pore glass solid support synthesis columns, etc.). In addition to the "standard phosphoramidite chemistry" other chemistries including RNA, hydrogen phosphonate, and phosphorothioate may also be used. Modified oligonucleotides with both internal or terminal functional primary amine groups for subsequent labeling can be obtained in several ways. The two easiest and most useful methods to incorporate functional groups are LAN and 5'-Aminolink, described below.

Linker Arm Nucleoside (LAN): One or more functional primary amine groups can be incorporated at selected positions within a sequence, and at the 3'- and 5'-terminal positions as suitably protected linker arm nucleosides (5'-dimethoxytrityl-5[N-(7-trifluoroacetylaminoheptyl)-2'-deoxyuridine 3'-O-phosphoramidite). This linker arm nucleoside (supplied by Glen Research) can be easily incorporated during the automated synthesis procedure. At the end of each synthesis the finished oligonucleotide is released from the support, and blocking groups are removed by treatment with concentrated ammonium hydroxide for 12 hr at 55°C. Alternatively, the 5'-dimethoxytrityl group can be left on the oligonucleotide to aid in the purification by reverse-phase high-pressure liquid chromatography (HPLC). The purity of the functionalized oligonucleotide

product can be determined by analytical polyacrylamide gel electrophoresis. At this point the oligonucleotide containing the functional primary amine group(s) is ready for reaction with an appropriate activated fluorescent reagent.

5'-Aminolink: A primary amine functional group can also be incorporated at the 5'-terminal position by using Aminolink 2 (supplied by Applied Biosystems). Aminolink 2 is a phosphoramidite derivative with a six carbon chain arm and a protected amine group. This protected linker group can be incorporated at the 5'-terminal position only at the end of the automated synthesis procedure. After the final deprotection and cleavage of the oligonucleotide from the resin, it provides a primary amine group for subsequent coupling reactions with various activated fluorophores and chromophores. Fluorescent reagents that readily react with primary amines include derivatives of (1) isothiocyanates (example, fluorescein isothiocyanate), (2) succinimidyl esters (example, succinimidyl pyrene butyrate), and (3) sulfonyl halides (example, Texas Red or sulforhodamine sulfonyl chloride). A variety of these reagents are available from commercial suppliers; a particularly wide selection of reagents with supporting references is available from Molecular Probes (Haugland, 1989). Table 11.2 gives a list of some of the fluorescent reagents that can be reacted with functionalized oligonucleotides. The fluorescent proper-

TABLE 11.2. Fluorescent reagents useful for the direct covalent labeling of DNA probes, PCR primers, or PCR products.

Fluorophore	EX[a]	EM[b]	$(\epsilon \times 10^{-3})^c$	Q^d
Texas red	596	615	85	H
Rhodamine X isothiocyanate	578	604	80	H
Tetramethylrhodamine isothiocyanate	541	572	82	H
Fluorescein isothiocyanate	494	520	72	H
Lucifer yellow vinyl sulfone	426	530	13	M
Coumarin isothiocyanate	383	468	29	M
Succinimidyl pyrene butyric acid	340	395	40	H
Allophycocyanin pyridyldisulfide[e]	650	660	700	H
R-phycocyanin pyridyldisulfide[e]	565	578	1960	H
B-phycocyanin pyridyldisulfide[e]	545	755	2410	H

[a]EX, wavelength at the excitation or absorption maximum.

[b]EM, wavelength at the emission maximum.

[c]$(\epsilon \times 10^{-3})$, extinction coefficient multiplied by 1000. Units are $cm^{-1} M^{-1}$ (H or high, $>25,000$; M or medium, $10,000-25,000$; and L or low, $<10,000$).

[d]Q, quantum yield (H or high, $0.3-1.0$; M or medium, $0.1-0.3$; and L or low, <0.1).

[e]Coupled to amino functional groups with crosslinking reagents like succinimidyl maleimidylbenzoate (SMB).

ties of each of the fluorophores is included in Table 11.2.

The oligonucleotides functionalized with primary amines are easily reacted with fluorescent reagents, particularly those activated with isothiocyanate or sulfonyl chloride. For example, $0.1-0.2$ μmol of a purified oligonucleotide containing a primary amine group can be reacted with $\sim 0.5-1.0$ mg of either Texas Red (sulforhodamine 101 sulfonyl chloride) or fluorescein isothiocyanate (both available from Molecular Probes). The reaction is carried out in 50 μl volume of 0.1 M sodium bicarbonate (pH 8.5) for 2 hr at 20°C. After the reaction is complete, the excess reagent is removed by passing the solution through a Sephadex G-25 gel filtration column. The final purification of the fluorescent-labeled oligonucleotide from the unlabeled oligonucleotide can be carried out by preparative polyacrylamide gel electrophoresis or HPLC. The yields for these types of reactions are usually 50–80%.

Alternatively, RNA sequences, or DNA sequences to which a 3'-terminal ribonucleotide has been added, can be functionalized by periodate oxidation. Sodium periodate is used to oxidize the ribose ring diols to form reactive aldehydes groups that can be coupled with a variety of fluorophores and chromophores containing primary amino groups or hydrazide groups by the Schiff's base procedures (Lowe and Dean, 1974). In general, a wide variety of reagents and procedures exist for incorporating different fluorophores and chromophores into functionalized oligonucleotides (Goodchild, 1990; Symons, 1989; Keller and Manak, 1989).

All of the various functionalization and labeling procedures that were developed for DNA probe technology are of course applicable to PCR technology. In most cases they are useful for the direct fluorescent labeling of either the PCR primers or the probes for secondary verification of PCR products. The only exception would be the 3'-terminal labeled oligonucleotides, which would not function as PCR primers.

Fluorescent Intercalating Dyes for PCR Products

The easiest method for visualizing DNA fragments in agarose gels is the use of the fluorescent staining dye ethidium bromide (Sharp et al., 1973). As was stated previously, this method is used extensively by a large number of workers for detection of PCR products. Detailed procedures for preparing and using

TABLE 11.3. Fluorescent dyes useful for labeling PCR products by noncovalent binding and intercalation.

Fluorophore	EX[a]	EM[b]	$(\epsilon \times 10^{-3})^c$	Q^d
Propidium iodide	493	630	5.8	M
Ethidium bromide	482	616	5.5	M
Ethidium homodimer	492	627	8.9	M
Acridine orange	487	510	62	M
Hoechst 33258	343	480	46	—
TOTO[e]	510	530	—	—
YOYO[f]	490	510	—	—

[a]EX, wavelength at the excitation or absorption maximum.
[b]EM, wavelength at the emission maximum.
[c]$(\epsilon \times 10^{-3})$, extinction coefficient multiplied by 1000. Units are $cm^{-1} M^{-1}$ (H or high, >25,000; M or medium, 10,000–25,000; and L or low, <10,000).
[d]Q, quantum yield (H or high, 0.3–1.0; M or medium, 0.1–0.3; and L or low, <0.1).
[e]A dimer of thiazole orange.
[f]A dimer of oxazole yellow.

ethidium bromide for staining DNA in agarose gels are found in most molecular biology manuals (Sambrook et al., 1989). Ethidium bromide binds very strongly to double-stranded DNA by intercalation (Steiner and Kubota, 1983), a process where the planar ring structure of the ethidium molecule inserts between the stacked bases of DNA. The intercalation of the dye into the DNA causes a marked increase in the fluorescent yield compared to the free dye in solution. The UV irradiation absorbed by the DNA (260 nm) and/or irradiation absorbed by the molecule at 300 nm (transilluminators) causes strong fluorescence emission at ~590 nm. The normal excitation maximum and emission maximum for ethidium are 482 and 616 nm, respectively. Ethidium bromide allows for the detection of about 1–10 ng of DNA per band in an agarose gel. A number of other dyes are useful for fluorescent staining of DNA and RNA fragments in agarose and polyacrylamide gels (see Table 11.3). These include the intercalating dye propidium iodide (Ex 493, Em 630), and the nonintercalating dye Hoechst 33258 (Ex 342 nm, Em 480 nm), which are used less frequently than ethidium bromide for DNA staining. Acridine orange is used most often for staining single-stranded DNA or RNA.

While some of the DNA fluorescent staining dyes may not provide the best sensitivity for detecting PCR products, other dyes, including some relatively new ones, may prove to be very sensitive and useful. Ethidium homodimer (dimeric form of ethidium) has a much higher affinity for DNA than the "normal" ethidium, and is reported to produce a large fluorescent enhancement and improved detectability of DNA in gels (Markovits et al., 1979). Ethidium homodimer is reported to have a detection limit of ~60 pg of DNA per band (Glazer et al., 1990). More recently, ethidium homodimer was used as the fluorescent stain together with a confocal fluorescent gel scanner to carry out high sensitivity DNA sequencing applications (Quesada et al., 1991). Two new dyes called "TOTO" and "YOYO," which have very high binding affinities, are reported to be ultrasensitive fluorescent stains for DNA and RNA (see BioProbes 1991). TOTO is a dimer of thiazole orange (Ex 510 nm, Em 530 nm), and YOYO is a dimer of oxazole yellow (Ex 490 nm, Ex 510 nm). Detection of as little as 4 pg of DNA in gel bands is reported for the TOTO dye, and YOYO may be even more sensitive. These dyes are mixed directly with the DNA sample before application to the gel. They require somewhat more effort to use than ethidium bromide, but may prove very useful for PCR product analysis on gels because of their very high sensitivity.

Fluorescent PCR Applications

It becomes very obvious that most of the procedures and technology that have been developed for the analysis of DNA and RNA during the last decade can be, and are in many cases being applied to the analysis and/or the verification of PCR products. These procedures and technologies include (1) the labeling of oligonucleotides with reporter groups, (2) the utilization of many of the DNA probe hybridization schemes (solid phase sandwich assay systems, etc.), (3) methods for improved detection of DNA on agarose and polyacrylamide gels, (4) methods and instrumentation for DNA sequencing, and (5) technology for the automation of these types of assays. The major difference between the requirements of PCR and classical probe technology is that PCR being a target amplification system does not press the detection technologies for ultimate sensitivity. Thus, requirements and criteria for PCR detection technology will be concerned more with speed, ease of use, reproducibility, and probably cost effectiveness.

A special application of fluorescent detection technology unique to PCR has been developed (Chehab and Kan, 1989). These workers have developed a color complementation PCR-based assay that allows rapid screening of specific genomic sequences, including point mutations (Cheb and Kan, 1990). The assay is based on the simultaneous amplification of two or more DNA segments with fluorescent oligonucleotide primers such that the generation of a color, or a combination of colors can be readily visualized and used for diagnosis. The fluorescent primers are oligonucleotides functionalized with Aminolink 2, and then reacted with four fluorescent reagents used in DNA sequencing applications. The color complementation assay obviates the need for gel electrophoresis, and lends itself readily to automation.

Another application to PCR product analysis combines time-resolved fluorescent detection with a solid phase sandwich type assay system (Dahlen et al., 1991). In this system the first DNA segment to be detected is amplified according to the standard PCR procedures. Then a pair of europium (Eu^{3+}) and biotin-labeled primers nested within the amplified fragment is incorporated in the last few PCR cycles. The amplified fragments contain both a biotin (affinity label) and a europium (reporter label). The double-labeled fragments are collected onto streptavidin-coated microtitration strips and the bound europium is measured in a time-resolved fluorometer. The method is reported to be sensitive (as few as five copies of HIV-1 target DNA were detected), rapid, and easy to employ. This system also lends itself readily to automation.

There are several other solid phase or affinity type PCR assay systems utilizing colorimetric detection that might be used with fluorescent reporter groups. These include the affinity-based hybrid collection system utilizing 5′-terminal labeled biotin primers (Syvanen et al., 1988), and an enzyme-based colorimetric detection system designed for mass screening (Kemp et al., 1989).

Summary and Future Directions

PCR, as befits a truly revolutionary technology, is catalyzing advances in many other areas. Development of synergistic nonisotopic detection systems is just one example of this effect. Fluorescence may ultimately play its strongest role as the detection technology of choice in future automated PCR systems for research and clinical use. The important role that fluorescent detection is playing in automated DNA sequencing may be prophetic of PCR automation. One of the newest and most exciting applications that requires less instrumentation and should be examined further is the new intercalating dyes. These dyes may significantly improve the detection range for PCR analysis on agarose gels, and certainly will lessen toxic waste concerns about the copious amounts of ethidium bromide that are common in most laboratories today.

References

BioProbes (1991): Molecular Probes, Eugene, Oregon, #14, pp. 11.

Chehab FF, Kan YW (1989): Detection of specific DNA sequences by fluorescent amplification—A color complementation assay. *Proc Natl Acad Sci USA* 86:9178–9182.

Chehab FF, Kan YW (1990): Detection of sickle cell anaemia mutation by colour DNA amplification. *Lancet* 335:15–17.

Chu ECF, Orgel LE (1988): Ligation of oligonucleotides to nucleic acids or proteins via disulfide bonds. *Nucl Acids Res* 16:3671–3691.

Connell C et al. (1987): Automated DNA sequence analysis. *BioTechniques* 5:342–348.

Cook AF, Vuocolo E, Brackel C (1988): Synthesis of a series of biotinylated oligonucleotides. *Nucl Acids Res* 16:4077–4095.

Dahlen P, Litia A, Mukkala VM, Hurskainen P, Kwiatkowski M (1991): The use of europium (Eu^{3+}) labelled primers in PCR amplification of specific target DNA. *Mol Cell Probes* 5:143–149.

Glazer AN, Peck K, Mathies RA (1990): A stable double-stranded DNA ethidium homodimer complex—Application to picogram fluorescent detection of DNA in agarose gels. *Proc Natl Acad Sci USA* 87:3851–3855.

Goodchild J (1990): Conjugates of oligonucleotides and modified oligonucleotides: A review of their synthesis and properties. *Bioconjugate Chem* 1:165–187.

Haralambidis J et al. (1990): The preparation of polyamide oligonucleotide probes containing multiple non-radiative labels. *Nucl Acids Res* 18:501–505.

Haugland RP (1989): *Molecular Probes—Handbook of Fluorescent Probes and Research Chemicals.* Eugene, OR: Molecular Probes, Inc.

Heller MJ, Morrison LE (1985): Chemiluminescent and fluorescent probes for DNA hybridization systems. In: *Rapid Detection and Identification of Infectious Agents.* Kingsbury DT, Falkow S, eds. New York: Academic Press.

Hodges RR, Conway NE, McLaughlin LW (1989): Post assay covalent labelling of phosphorothioate containing nucleic acids with multiple fluorophores. *Biochemistry* 28:261–267.

Jablonski E, Moomaw EW, Tullis R, Ruth JL (1986): Preparation of oligodeoxynucleotide-alkaline phosphatase conjugates and their use as hybridization probes. *Nucl Acids Res* 14:6115–6128.

Keller GH, Manak MM (1989): *DNA Probes.* New York: Stockton Press.

Kemp DJ, Smith DB, Foote SJ, Samaras N, Gregory Peterson M (1989): Colorimetric detection of specific DNA segments amplified by polymerase chain reaction. *Proc Natl Acad Sci USA* 86:2423–2427.

Li P, Medon P, Skingle DC, Lanser JA, Symons RH (1987): Enzyme-linked synthetic oligonucleotide probes: Non-radioactive detection of E. coli in faecal specimens. *Nucl Acids Res* 15:5275–5287.

Lowe CR, Dean PDG (1974): *Affinity Chromatography.* New York: John Wiley.

Luckey JA et al. (1990): High speed DNA sequencing by capillary electrophoresis. *Nucl Acids Res* 18:4417–4421.

Markovits J et al. (1979): Ethidium dimer—A new reagent for the fluorimetric determination of nucleic acids. *Anal Biochem* 94:259.

Mullis KB, Faloona FA (1987): Specific synthesis of DNA in vitro via a polymerse-catalyzed chain reaction. *Methods Enzymol* 155:335–351.

Mullis KB, Faloona FA, Scharf SJ, Saiki RK, Horn GT, Erlich HA (1986): Specific enzymatic amplification of DNA in vitro: The polymerase chain reaction. *Cold Spring Harbor Symp Quant Biol* 51:263–273.

Nguyen DC, Keller RA, Jett JC, and Martin JC (1987): Detection of single molecules of phycoerythrin in hydrodynamically focused flows by laser-induced fluorescence. *Anal Chem* 59:2158–2161.

Prober JM et al. (1987): A system for rapid DNA sequencing with fluorescent chain-terminating dideoxynucleotides. *Science* 238:336–341.

Quesada MA, Rye HS, Gingrich JC, Glazer AN, Mathies RA (1991): High sensitivity DNA Detection with laser excited confocal fluorescence gel scanner. *BioTechniques* 10:616–625.

Ruth JL (1984): Chemical synthesis of non-radioactively-labeled DNA hybridization probes. *DNA* 3:123.

Saiki RK, Gelfand DH, Stoffel S, Scharf SJ, Higuchi R, Horn GT, Mullis KB, Erlich HA (1988): Primer-directed enzymatic amplification of DNA with a thermostable DNA polymerase. *Science* 239:487–491.

Sambrook J, Fritsch EF, Maniatis T (1989): *Molecular Cloning: A Laboratory Manual,* 2nd ed., Part 1. New York: Cold Spring Harbor Press.

Sharp PA, Sugden B, Sambrook (1973): Detection of two restriction endonuclease activities in

Haemophilus parainfluenza using analytical agarose. *Biochemistry* 12:3055.

Smith LM (1990): Automated DNA sequencing and analysis of the human genome. *Genome* 31:929–937.

Sproat BS, Beijer B, Rider P (1987): The synthesis of protected 5′-amino-2′,5′dideoxyribonucleoside-3′-O phosphoramidites; applications of 5′-amino oligodeoxyribonucleotides. *Nucl Acids Res* 15:6181–6196.

Steiner RF, Kubota Y (1983): Fluorescent dye—nucleic acid complexes. In: *Excited States of Biopolymers.* Steiner RF, ed. New York: Plenum Press, 203–254.

Symons RH (1989): *Nucleic Acid Probes.* Boca Raton: CRC Press.

Syvanen AC, Bengtstrom M, Tenhunen J, Soderlund H (1988): Quantification of the polymerase chain reaction products by affinity based hybrid collection. *Nucl Acids Res* 16:11327–11338.

Taylor DL, Waggoner AS, Murphy RF, Lanni F, Birge RR (1986): *Applications of Fluorescence in Biomedical Sciences.* New York: A. R. Liss.

Urdea MS, Warner BD, Running JA, Stempien M, Clyne J, Horn T (1988): A comparison of non-radioisotopic hybridization assay methods using fluorescent, chemiluminescent, and enzyme-labelled synthetic oligodeoxyribonucleotide probes. *Nucl Acids Res* 16:4937–4956.

Wilson RK et al. (1990): Development of an automated procedure for fluorescent DNA sequencing. *Genomics* 6:626–634.

12

Enzyme-Labeled Oligonucleotides

Eugene Tu and Edward Jablonski

Introduction

Investigators using the polymerase chain reaction as an analytical method or for developing clinical applications can envision a number of ways to detect amplified target nucleic acid sequences by hybridization to a specific oligonucleotide probe. The nonisotopic detection method of interest for this article is the use of enzyme labels.

Enzyme labels were first used indirectly to detect hybridization between target DNA bound to a filter membrane and a complementary probe through an avidin–biotin bridge. Biotin is incorporated into long cloned probes as a modified base (Langer et al., 1981). The hybridization reaction occurs over a relatively long time under stringent conditions. The incorporated biotin survives this process and is detected on the filter by the addition of an avidin–enzyme conjugate under conditions favoring the maintenance of enzyme activity. The complex is visualized by allowing the enzyme to catalyze the formation of a highly colored dye product (Leary et al., 1981; Brigati et al., 1983).

The properties of synthetic oligonucleotide probes permit target nucleic acid to be hybridized under rapid and mild conditions. This allows the use of enzymes as direct, as well as indirect labels. The indirect oligonucleotide systems still favor the use of biotin as the primary label (Leary and Ruth, 1989), with digoxigenin as a viable alternative (Kessler, 1991). Either biotin or digoxigenin can be incorporated into synthetic oligonucleotides by reaction with their respective analogues. The biotin labels are detected after hybridization with enzyme–avidin complexes, while digoxigenin is determined by binding to antibody-enzyme conjugates.

Oligonucleotides labeled directly with enzymes have been shown to be specific, sensitive, and very stable (Jablonski et al., 1986). The enzyme label retains its catalytic activity and does not affect the hybridization characteristics of the oligonucleotide probe. The direct labeled systems eliminate the extra steps of reagent addition and washing, necessary for the detection of a secondary label, and avoids the nonspecific binding and consequent background signal that frequently accompanies avidin or antibody–enzyme conjugate reagents. The enzymes and direct labeled oligonucleo-

The Polymerase Chain Reaction
K.B. Mullis, F. Ferré, R.A. Gibbs, editors
© 1994 Birkhauser Boston

tide methods available to detect PCR amplified target were first developed to analyze and quantitate unamplified target with greater sensitivity than ^{32}P labels. The result is a choice of systems where speed and simplicity may be more relevant than sensitivity, unless the investigator wishes to limit the number of thermal cycles of the PCR. Nevertheless, direct enzyme-labeled oligonucleotides are hybridized and detected rapidly, with sensitivities of 10^5 to 10^6 copies of target nucleic acid for colorimetric formats and one or more orders of magnitude less for luminometric methods (Bronstein et al., 1989a,b; Geiger et al., 1989). Issues more relevant to the investigator wishing or needing to use a nonisotopic detection method for PCR products are the availability of reagents and instruments, the number of assays to perform, the desire for some aspect of automation, and experience or understanding of the different modes of signal generation, such as colorimetric, fluorescence, or chemiluminescence.

Direct Enzyme Labeling of Oligonucleotides

The first formulation of an oligonucleotide–enzyme conjugate and demonstration of the hybridization characteristics has been reported by Jablonski et al. (1986). These conjugates are formed by a 1:1 association of calf intestine alkaline phosphatase and an internally modified amine linker-arm probe. These conjugates have been successfully introduced into a number of clinical and forensics assay kits, and are available for custom applications under the trade name SNAP® (Syngene Inc., La Jolla, CA). The linker arm probes are synthesized using standard automated phosphoramidite chemistry with the incorporation of a modified thymidine base into the chain. The modification consists of a six carbon atom linker arm attached to the C-5 position and terminating in a protected primary amine (Ruth, 1984). The linker-arm phosphoramidite is available from Glen Research (Sterling, VA). The linker arm can serve as an attachment

point for a multitude of nonisotopic labels such as fluorophores, haptens, biotin, and enzymes. These probes can also be end labeled with ^{32}P by standard procedures.

The enzymes most commonly used for probe labels are alkaline phosphatase and horseradish peroxidase. Recent papers describe the use of glucose-6-phosphate dehydrogenase (Balaguer et al., 1989, 1991). These particular enzymes exhibit excellent stability, high catalytic activity, low cost, availability, and ability to be conjugated without significant loss of specific activity. These enzymes also utilize a variety of substrate systems for different detection modes. A procedure for labeling amine containing linker-arm probes is outlined from a previous report (Ruth, 1991).

The linker arm probe prepared by automated synthesis is purified by reverse-phase HPLC, eluting from a Perkin Elmer C_8 column with a linear gradient of acetonitrile from 5 to 40% over 30 min. The eluted probe is detritilated in 80% acetic acid for 45 min at room temperature, evaporated to dryness, and resuspended in 200 mM sodium acetate. The probe is desalted over a G-25 spun column, ethanol precipitated, and dissolved at 5 mg/ml in 1 mM EDTA, pH 8.0. The probe may be stored at $-70°C$ for several years without loss of hybridization specificity or labeling efficiency.

The linker arm probe is made alkaline by the addition of two-tenths volume of 1 M sodium bicarbonate. The amine function is activated with the homobifunctional reagent, disuccidimidyl suberate (Pierce, Rockland, IL) at 10 mg/ml in anhydrous dimethyl sulfoxide added to the probe solution in a ratio of 1:1 (v/v). The reaction is allowed to proceed for 1 min at room temperature. Excess reagent is removed by FPLC chromatography employing a Sephadex G-25 column equilibrated in 1.0 mM sodium acetate, pH 5.0, eluting at 1.0 ml/min. The first eluted peak is collected and rapidly concentrated in a Centricon C-10 (Amicon, Beverly, MA) by centrifugation at 4°C. The activated probe is reduced in volume to a few hundred microliters and quickly added to a concentrated solution of alkaline phosphatase (100 mg/ml), prepared by dialyses against 3 M sodium chloride, 0.1 M sodium bicarbonate,

1 mM magnesium chloride, and 0.05% azide, pH 8.25. The enzyme is present in a 2-fold molar excess over probe in the coupling reaction, which develops for 4 hr to overnight at room temperature. The reaction solution is partially desalted by dilution with water and reconcentrated in a Centricon C-30. The conjugate is purified free of excess enzyme and unreacted probe by FPLC ion-exchange chromatography on a MONO Q 5/5 column using a linear gradient of sodium chloride from 0 to 1.0 M in 0.2 M Tris-HCl, pH 8.0, over 30 min. The three major peaks correspond, in order of elution, to free enzyme, probe conjugate, and unreacted probe. These conjugates have full enzyme activity, and unaltered DNA hybridization properties, compared to ^{32}P-labeled probes. The probe conjugate may be stored in a high salt buffer with azide at 4°C for more than 2 years without loss of enzyme activity or hybridization efficiency. SNAP® probes have been labeled with several enzymes, including horseradish peroxidase, by similar methods. These enzyme labels have retained full specific activity on coupling.

Other methods have since appeared in the literature for preparing enzyme-labeled oligonucleotides. A paper from the University of Adelaide describes the use of a 30 atom spacer arm, consisting of 4 extraneous bases on the 3′-terminus of a synthetic probe for enterotoxigenic *Escherichia coli* (Li et al., 1987). The last base is an aminoalkyl derivatized cytosine, functionalized with a sulfhydryl group. Conjugates are formed in a 1:1 stoichiometry by reaction with bromacetyl derivatized phosphatase. The enzymatic activity of the conjugate is reduced 40% by the process, but the reagent functions well in the colorimetric detection of nitrocellulose bound target DNA.

A hydrazone-based conjugation method provides enzyme-probe conjugates in yields of 80–85% (Ghosh et al., 1989). Oligonucleotides are derivatized on the 5′-end with hydrazine and reacted with alkaline phosphatase or horseradish peroxidase modified with aldehyde groups. The authors report a detection sensitivity of 7 amol of plasmid target DNA with a 1-hr colorimetric development for the alkaline phosphatase conjugate. The horserad-

ish peroxidase-labeled probes are 40-fold less sensitive.

The method described by Murakami et al. (1989) uses a probe derivitized with cystamine, introduced at the 5′-phosphate site via a water-soluble carbodiimide. The adduct is purified by HPLC and activated by treatment with DTT. Alkaline phosphatase is modified with *N*-succinimidyl-3-(2-pyridyldithio)propionate (SPDP), and purified by gel filtration chromatography. The free sulfhydryl probe and SPDP activated enzyme are reacted to form conjugates of 2:1 probe to enzyme stoichiometry. No direct assessment of specific activity is available, but the conjugates function well in detecting phage target DNA in both colorimetric and fluorometric filter hybridization formats.

Commercial kits have now appeared that make labeling probes with enzymes convenient for small scale or research oriented applications. A group at ICI previewed the E-link-labeling system with a note that appeared in *Nucleic Acids Research* (Alves et al., 1988). This system contains reagents to convert a 5′-amino link probe (an oligonucleotide synthesized with an additional amino phosphoramidite at the 5′-end, available from Applied Biosystems Inc., Foster City, CA) to a 5′-sulfhydryl modified probe. Alkaline phosphatase is supplied as a dry reagent preactivated with *m*-maleimidobenzoyl *N*-hydroxysuccinimide ester. The maleimide function reacts with the free sulfhydryl on the probe to form a 1:1 conjugate. Columns and elution buffers are supplied to purify the intermediates and final product.

A similar direct labeling system is marketed by Amersham. The label in this case is horseradish peroxidase. A cyanoethyl phosphoramidite containing a protected SH group is added directly to the 5′-end of the probe, eliminating the need to convert the amino function. The amino function is, however, more stable with time. Horseradish peroxidase, which has been modified with a reagent specific for coupling to sulfhydryl groups, is supplied. The resulting horseradish peroxidase–probe conjugates are not as sensitive as the alkaline phosphatase–probe conjugates, but this is usually not an issue with PCR-generated targets. Amersham recommends detection by enhanced chemiluminescence, hence the name "ECL" labeling system.

Hybridization and Detection of Enzyme-Labeled Oligonucleotide Probes

Filter Hybridization

Filter hybridization is the most common format for detecting a target sequence by nucleic acid probes, including directly labeled enzyme–probe conjugates. This format has also been used to detect amplified targets (Olive, 1989; Dallas et al., 1989; Cai et al., 1989). Target nucleic acid is denatured by treatment with sodium hydroxide, then "blotted" onto a nylon or nitrocellulose membrane by vacuum filtration through a manifold (Sambrook et al., 1989). Similarly, DNA fragments that have been separated by electrophoresis can be Southern transferred to membranes by wicking the samples within the gel onto a membrane. The conditions for applying and fixing the target are determined by the nature of the membrane. Methods that work well for detection by ^{32}P or biotin-labeled probes are usually appropriate for direct enzyme-labeled probes.

The filter bound target is hybridized by exposing the filter membrane to a solution of probe–enzyme conjugate at a temperature and ionic strength largely dictated by the length and base composition of the oligonucleotide sequence (Wetmur, 1991). A typical hybridization reaction mixture includes probe at 1–10 nM in 6× SSC, 5× Denhardt's solution and 0.5–1% SDS. The hybridization temperature should not have to exceed 50–55°C for longer than 30 min. Both alkaline phosphatase and horseradish peroxidase will retain specific activity under these conditions. Excess, unhybridized probe is removed by washing the hybridized membrane in 1× SSC with SDS, followed by buffer alone. This final wash removes residual SDS, which can interfere with color dye deposition. Substrate solution is added and

the immobilized enzyme catalyzes the formation of insoluble color product that deposits on the membrane.

The color visualization system for alkaline phosphatase labels uses 5-bromo-4-chloro-3-indolyl phosphate (BCIP) as the substrate. The formation of the indolyl product provides reducing equivalents to convert soluble nitro blue tetrazolium (NBT) to an insoluble formazan dye (McGadey, 1970). A reaction mixture consists of 0.33 mg/ml NBT, 0.17 mg/ml BCIP, 0.33% dimethylformamide in 0.1 M Tris-HCl, pH 9.5, 0.1 M sodium chloride, and 5 mM magnesium chloride. The time of appearance of a purple color is dependent on target concentration.

Horseradish peroxidase labels are developed by equilibrating the hybridized filter in 0.1 mg/ml 3,3′,5,5′-tetramethylbenzidine in 0.1 M sodium citrate, pH 5.0, followed by transfer to 0.0015% hydrogen peroxide in the TMB-citrate solution (Saiki et al., 1988).

Substrates are also available that become fluorescent or chemiluminescent when acted on by the enzyme labels (Murakami et al., 1989; Bronstein et al., 1989a). Filters hybridized with alkaline phosphatase-labeled probes can be incubated in a minimal volume of 0.1 mM 4-methylumbelliferyl phosphate (4-MUBP) in a high pH-buffered medium. The fluorescent product, 4-methylumbelliferone, is soluble. The reaction solution is usually pipetted into a cuvette for fluorescence analyses at an excitation of 363 nm and emission of 447 nm. This detection method is more quantitative than dye deposition, but because of the manipulations involved in developing the signal, is better suited for use in nonfilter sandwich type assays. A luminometric method for alkaline phosphatase-labeled probes more compatible with a filter dot blot or Southern transfer hybridization uses an enzyme triggerable dioxetane phenyl phosphate. The substrate is available under the trade names AMPPD (Tropix, Bedford, MA) and PPD (Lumigen, Detroit, MI). Alkaline phosphatase catalyzes a dephosphorylation, generating a moderately stable anion, which breaks down to form an excited state methyl meta-oxy benzoate anion. The decay of the excited state produces visible light, which can be detected by exposing the filter to X-ray or high speed film. The chemiluminescent method is significantly more sensitive than the corresponding dye deposition technique, but can be somewhat unfriendly as additional blocking treatments are needed to prevent background emission (Bronstein et al., 1989b). An uncharged neutral membrane is recommended for chemiluminescent detection. A typical procedure involves treating a hybridized and washed membrane with a blocking agent (0.2% casein, 0.1% Tween in PBS) for 30 min at room temperature. The filter is rinsed and incubated with 0.25 mM substrate in a carbonate or 2-amino-2-methyl-1-propanol buffer for a few minutes. The saturated membrane is sealed in a transparent detection folder or seal-a-meal bag and exposed to X-ray film. Kits and instructions are available for detecting target sequences by this method. Horseradish peroxidase labels can also be detected with chemiluminescence. The method of enhanced chemiluminescence is the catalyzed oxidation of luminol by hydrogen peroxide in the presence of an enhancer molecule, p-benzoquinone. This process, described by Kricka and co-workers, is embodied in the ECL DNA kits sold by Amersham (Matthews et al., 1985).

Sandwich Hybridization

An alternative approach to membrane based assays is the sandwich assay as described by Ranki et al. (1983). The target DNA is removed from a crude sample by hybridization to a complementary sequence immobilized on a matrix (direct capture) or by hybridization with a probe labeled with a ligand, such as biotin, followed by capture onto an avidin affinity support (indirect capture). Bound target is detected by a second directly or indirectly labeled probe specific for a proximal sequence (Kemp et al., 1989). The addition of this second hybridization step enhances selectivity for the target and reduces the possibility of nonspecific interactions. This is one of the most applicable formats for routine diagnostics since it eliminates protracted sample preparation, purification, and nonspecific filter-based

target immobilization, and, above all, is clearly suited for instrumentation.

Direct capture sandwich hybridization supports are created by attaching nucleic acids through chemical modification, adsorption, or enzymatic processes to a myriad of solid phases including nitrocellulose (Ranki et al., 1983), cellulose (Goldkorn and Prockop, 1986), nylon (Van Ness et al., 1991), polystyrene (Ruth et al., 1987), teflon-acrylamide (Duncan et al., 1988), polypropylene (Polsky-Cynkin et al., 1985), agarose (Polsky-Cynkin et al., 1985), sephacryl (Langdale and Malcolm, 1985), latex (Wolf et al., 1987), and paramagnetic (Albretsen et al., 1990; Lund et al., 1988). Such supports are difficult to make and exhibit relatively poor loading capacities. Mixed-phase direct capture hybridizations are also limited kinetically and may be inefficient due to the inaccessibility of immobilized DNA (Bunemann, 1982).

In contrast, indirect capture supports are more efficient because hybridization occurs in solution, which is virtually complete (Podell et al., 1991), and significantly faster than hybridizations on solid supports (Bunemann, 1982; Gingeras et al., 1987; Wolf et al., 1987). Furthermore, the ligand/ligand interaction is less sensitive to steric constraints than mixed phase hybridizations. Streptavidin–biotin is the most widely used affinity pair because of its specificity and high affinity (Harju et al., 1990; Syvanen et al., 1986; Yehle et al., 1987). Other haptens have been used with anti-hapten antibodies such as digoxigenin and biotin (Kessler, 1991; Newman et al., 1989).

Automated DNA assays have been developed that incorporate the advantage of sandwich hybridization using biotin and enzyme-labeled oligonucleotide probe pairs, with capture on avidinylated paramagnetic particles. This system consists of a robotic sample processor (RSP) such as the Tecan RSP5051 or Packard Probe 1000 on which is positioned a magnetic rack. The magnetic rack is thermally controlled at 37°C and consists of an array of 48 assay tubes capable of alternating clockwise/counterclockwise rotation. Each tube is positioned between a pair of permanent side mounted magnets that provide a field strength of approximately 1000 G at the center of the tube. When the tubes are stationary the particles are cleared to the sides of the tube. Addition and removal of liquids can then be accomplished by the sampling tip of the RSP without loss of paramagnetic particles. The particles are redispersed and maintained in homogeneous suspension when the tubes are agitated such that the physical action is sufficient to overcome the magnetic attraction. The on/off action of the tubes is controlled by photoswitches that are activated by the RSP sampling tip itself. This negates the need for any electronic interfaces, making the magnetic rack extremely versatile. The magnetic rack also contains reagent wells for probe solutions and wash buffers and an inset for a microtiter plate.

The paramagnetic particles contain a CrO_2 or Fe_3O_4 core, with a mean diameter of 0.5–1.5 μm and exhibit neither remanence nor hysteresis. The large surface area (40–100 m^2/g) permits protein loading capacities of up to 40 mg/g solid. Streptavidin is covalently linked to the magnetic particles through a 30 atom spacer with mixed hydrophilic/hydrophobic character. The linkage is stable in aqueous or mildly acidic or basic (pH 4–9) environments, unlike conventional glutaraldehyde, carbodiimide, or cyanogen bromide crosslinking. Streptavidin-derivatized magnetic particles produced by this method have a biotin-binding capacity of greater than 1.0 nmol of biotin per mg particles. Given these capacities, only 15 μg of streptavidin particles is necessary to perform a DNA assay. This is an important feature because it is impractical to use milligram amounts of particles in terms of cost and performance. Additionally, magnetic clearing cannot be accomplished with such quantities due to shielding.

This automated system is compatible with the detection of PCR-generated target. HIV in blood, for example, can be automatically amplified and detected when a thermocycler is added to the base of the RSP. Target preparation is performed in a sterile hood using positive displacement pipettes (Gilson, Villiers-le-bel, France) and sterile technique to prevent contamination problems. All reagents are made with tissue culture grade water (Sigma, St. Louis, MO) and ultrapure reagents. Buffers are prepared in a separate sterile hood, preferably in another room, in bulk, and partitioned into single use aliquots stored at $-70°C$.

Mononuclear cells from approximately 7 ml of blood are isolated from HIV seropositive and seronegative patients utilizing LeukoPrep cell separation tubes (Becton-Dickinson, Franklin Lakes, NJ). Alternate methods such as Ficoll-Hypaque and Sepracell-MN are suitable as well. The buffy coat containing monuclear cells is removed and 0.5-ml aliquots are transferred to 1.5-ml Eppendorf tubes, in duplicate. The cells are pelleted by centrifugation, the supernatant aspirated, and the pellet resuspended by vortexing in 0.5 ml lysis buffer (10 mM Tris-HCl, pH 8.3, 50 mM KCl, 2.5 mM MgCl$_2$, 0.1 mg/ml gelatin, 0.45% NP-40, 0.45% Tween-20, 5 mg/ml proteinase K). The reactions are incubated at 55°C for 1 hr followed by boiling for 20 min to inactivate the protease before addition to the PCR reaction mix.

Duplicate 0.6-ml tubes (Robbins Scientific, Sunnyvale, CA) are prepared, each tube containing 25 μl of cell lysate plus 75 μl amplification buffer (10 mM Tris-HCl, pH 8.3, 50 mM KCl, 1.5 mM MgCl$_2$, 0.1 mg/ml gelatin, 200 μM each dNTP, 0.25 μM biotinylated forward primer, 1.0 μM unmodified reverse primer, and 2.5 units AmpliTaq). The primers amplify a 115-bp region in the *gag* gene. Water blanks are set up as described, but 25 μl water is substituted for the cell lysate. The reactions are overlayed with 100 μl mineral oil and placed on a thermal cycler (Ericomp, San Diego, CA) positioned on the worktable of an RSP in still another room. The reactions are amplified as follows: 1 min denaturation at 94°C, 30 cycles of 1 min at 55°C and then 1 min at 94°C, 5 min extension at 72°C, and 5 min denaturation at 94°C.

After target amplification, the RSP automatically dispenses 200 μl chloroform and 50 μl water into each PCR reaction tube, which inverts the organic and aqueous layers. The RSP then aspirates 102 μl hybridization buffer containing 3 nM alkaline phosphatase–probe conjugate complementary to the biotinylated strand of the amplicon and 20 μl directly from the PCR reaction tubes. It dispenses the mix into assay tubes on the magnetic rack. The sampling tip performs an active and passive wash to eliminate the possibility of carryover between samples. Hybridization proceeds at 37°C for 30 min with agitation. The RSP then dispenses 15 μl of a homogeneous 1 mg/ml streptavidin particle suspension to each tube containing a 35-fold molar excess of biotin-binding sites relative to biotin primer input. Capture of the complex onto particles proceeds at 37°C for 30 min with agitation. The particles are washed 3 times with 200 μl wash buffer at 37°C for 5 min each. After the third wash the RSP adds 150 μl of 30 μM 4MUBP substrate. Incubation with substrate proceeds at 37°C for 30 min with agitation. The RSP then aspirates 110 μl of solution from the assay tubes and dispenses it with 40 μl of 100 mM EDTA buffer into a black microtiter plate (Dynatech, Chantilly, VA). The plate is read on a FCA fluorescent plate reader (Idexx, Portland, ME) that scans each well automatically (365 nm/450 nm). Alternatively, a single well fluorometer can be used manually. The samples can be read immediately or when convenient.

Twice the highest signal obtained from negative blood samples or PCR water blanks from an individual assay is taken as background. Since duplicates are performed at the sample preparation and amplification steps, four results are obtained from each patient sample. To be considered positive, at least three of four must be above background. Results from 97 clinical samples show sensitivities and specificities of 96 and 100%, respectively, relative to serology.

References

Albretsen C, Kalland K-H, Haukanes B-I, Havarstein L-S, Kleppe K (1990): Application of magnetic beads with covalently attached oligonucleotides in hybridization: Isolation and detection of specific measles virus mRNA from a crude cell lysate. *Anal Biochem* 189:40–50.

Alves AM, Holland D, Edge MD, Carr FJ (1988): Hybridization detection of single nucleotide changes with enzyme labeled oligonucleotides. *Nucl Acids Res* 16:8722.

Balaguer P, Terouanne B, Eliaou JF, Humbert M, Boussioux AM, Nicolas JC (1989): Use of glucose-6-phosphate dehydrogenase as a new label for nucleic acid hybridization reactions. *Anal Biochem* 180:50–54.

Balaguer P, Terouanne B, Boussioux AM, Nicolas JC (1991): Quantification of DNA sequences obtained by polymerase chain reaction using a bioluminescent adsorbant. *Anal Biochem* 195:105–110.

Brigati DJ, Myerson D, Leary JJ, Spalholz B, Travis SZ, Fong CKY, Hsiung GD, Ward DC (1983): Detection of viral genomes in cultured cells and paraffin-embedded tissue sections using biotin-labeled hybridization probes. *Virology* 126:32–50.

Bronstein I, Cate RL, Lazzari K, Ramachandram KL, Voyta JC (1989a): Chemiluminescent 1,2 dioxetane based substrates and their application in the detection of DNA. *Photochem Photobiol* 49:9–14.

Bronstein I, Voyta JC, Edwards B (1989b): A comparison of chemiluminescent and colorimetric substrates in a Hepatitus B virus DNA hybridization assay. *Anal Biochem* 180:95–98.

Bunemann H (1982): Immobilization of denatured DNA to macroporous supports: II. Steric and kinetic parameters of heterogeneous hybridization reactions. *Nucl Acids Res* 10:7181–7196.

Cai S-P, Chang CA, Zhang J-Z, Saiki RK, Erlich HA, Kan YW (1989): Rapid prenatal diagnosis of β thalassemia using DNA amplification and nonradioactive probes. *Blood* 73:372–374.

Dallas PB, Flanagan JL, Nightingale BN, Morris BJ (1989): Polymerase chain reaction for fast, nonradioactive detection of high- and low-risk papillomavirus types in routine cervical specimens and in biopsies. *J Med Virol* 27:105–111.

Duncan CH, Cavalier SL (1988): Affinity chromatography of a sequence-specific DNA binding protein using teflon-linked oligonucleotides. *Anal Biochem* 169:104–108.

Geiger R, Hauber R, Miska W (1989): New, bioluminescence-enhanced detection systems for use in enzyme activity tests, enzyme immunoassays, protein blotting and nucleic acid hybridization. *Mol Cell Probes* 3:309–328.

Ghosh SS, Kao PM, Kwoh DY (1989): Synthesis of 5′-oligonucleotide hydrazide derivatives and their use in preparation of enzyme-nucleic acid hybridization probes. *Anal Biochem* 178:43–51.

Gingeras TR, Kwoh DY, Davis GR (1987): Hybridization properties of immobilized nucleic acids. *Nucl Acids Res* 15:5373–5390.

Goldkorn T, Prockop DJ (1986): A simple and efficient enzymatic method for covalent attachment of DNA to cellulose. Application for hybridization-restriction analysis and for in vitro synthesis of DNA probes. *Nucl Acids Res* 14:9171–9191.

Harju L, Janne P, Kallio A, Laukkanen M-L, Lautenschlager I, Mattinen S, Ranki A, Ranki M, Soares VRX, Soderlund H, Syvanen A-C (1990): Affinity-based collection of amplified viral DNA: Application to the detection of human immunodeficiency virus type 1, human cytomegalovirus and human papillomavirus type 16. *Mol Cell Probes* 4:223–235.

Jablonski E, Moomaw EW, Tullis R, Ruth JL (1986): Preparation of oligonucleotide-alkaline phosphatase conjugates and their use as hybridization probes. *Nucl Acids Res* 14:6115–6128.

Kemp DJ, Smith DB, Foote SJ, Samaras N, Peterson MG (1989): Colorimetric detection of specific DNA segments amplified by polymerase chain reaction. *Proc Natl Acad Sci USA* 86:2423–2427.

Kessler C (1991): The digoxigenin:anti-digoxigenin (DIG) technology—a survey on the concept and realization of a novel bioanalytical indicator system. *Mol Cell Probes* 5:161–205.

Langdale J, Malcolm ADB (1985): A rapid method of gene detection using DNA bound to Sephacryl. *Gene* 36:201–210.

Langer PR, Waldrop AA, Ward DC (1981): Enzymatic synthesis of biotin-labeled polynucleotides: Novel nucleic acid affinity probes. *Proc Natl Acad Sci USA* 78:6633–6637.

Leary JJ, Ruth JL (1989): Nonradioactive labeling of nucleic acid probes. In: *Nucleic Acid and Monoclonal Antibody Probes; Applications in Diagnostic Microbiology.* Swaminathan B, Prakash G, eds. New York: Marcel Dekker.

Leary JJ, Brigati DJ, Ward DC (1983): Colorimetric method for visualizing biotin-labeled DNA probes hybridized to DNA or RNA immobilized on nitrocellulose: Bio-blots. *Proc Natl Acad Sci USA* 80:4045–4049.

Li P, Medon PP, Skingle DC, Lanser JA, Symons RH (1987): Enzyme-linked synthetic ologinucleotide probes: non-radioactive detection of enterotoxigenic *Escherichia coli* in faecal specimens. *Nucl Acids Res* 15:5275–5287.

Lund V, Schmid R, Rickwood D, Hornes E (1988): Assessment of methods for covalent binding of nucleic acids to magnetic beads, Dynabeads™,

and the characteristics of the bound nucleic acids in hybridization reactions. *Nucl Acids Res* 16:10861–10880.

Matthews JA, Batki A, Hynds C, Kricka LJ (1985): Enhanced chemiluminescent method for the detection of DNA dot-hybridization assays. *Anal Biochem* 151:205–209.

McGadey J (1970): A tetrazolium method for non-specific alkaline phosphatase. *Histochemie* 23:180–184.

Murakami A, Tada J, Yamagata K, Takano J (1989): Highly sensitive detection of DNA using enzyme-linked DNA-probe. 1. Colorimetric and fluorometric detection. *Nucl Acids Res* 14:5587–5595.

Newman CL, Modlin J, Yolken RH, Viscidi RP (1989): Solution hybridization and enzyme immunoassay for biotinylated DNA-RNA hybrids to detect enteroviral RNA in cell culture. *Mol Cell Probes* 3:375–382.

Olive M (1989): Detection of enterotoxigenic *Escherichia coli* after polymerase chain reaction amplification with a thermostable DNA polymerase. *J Clin Micro* 27:261–265.

Podell S, Maske W, Ibanez E, Jablonski E (1991): Comparison of solution hybridization efficiencies using alkaline phosphatase-labelled and ^{32}P-labelled oligodeoxynucleotide probes. *Mol Cell Probes* 5:117–124.

Polsky-Cynkin R, Parsons GH, Allerdt L, Landes G, Davis G, Rashtchian A (1985): Use of DNA immobilized on plastic and agarose supports to detect DNA by sandwich hybridization. *Clin Chem* 31:1438–1443.

Ranki M, Palva A, Virtanen M, Laaksonen M, Soderlund H (1983): Sandwich hybridization as a convenient method for the detection of nucleic acids in crude samples. *Gene* 21:77–85.

Ruth JL (1984): Chemical synthesis of non-radioactively-labeled DNA hybridization probes. *DNA* 3:123.

Ruth JL (1991): Oligodeoxynucleotides with reporter groups attached to the base. In: *Oligonucleotides and Analogues: A Practical Approach.* Eckstein F, ed. New York: Oxford University Press.

Ruth JL, Jablonski E, Lohrmann R, Tu E (1987): Biofluorescent detection of oligomer sandwich hybridizations. Conference of Therapeutic and Diagnostic Applications of Synthetic Nucleic Acids. Cambridge, U.K.

Saiki RK, Chang C-A, Levenson CH, Warren TC, Boehm CD, Kazazian HH, Erlich HA (1988): Diagnosis of sicule cell anemia and β-thalassemia with enzymatically amplified DNA and nonradioactive allele-specific oligonucleotide probes. *N Engl J Med* 319:537–541.

Sambrook J, Fritsch EF, Maniatis T (1989): *Molecular Cloning: A Laboratory Manual,* 2nd ed. New York: Cold Spring Harbor.

Syvanen A, Laaksonen M, Soderlund H (1986): Fast quantification of nucleic acid hybrids by affinity-based hybrid collection. *Nucl Acids Res* 14:5037–5048.

Van Ness J, Kalbfleisch S, Petrie CR, Reed MW, Tabone JC, Vermeulen NMJ (1991): A versatile solid support system for oligodeoxynucleotide probe-based hybridization assays. *Nucl Acids Res* 19:3345–3350.

Wetmur JG (1991): DNA probes: Applications of the principles of nucleic acid hybridization. *Crit Rev Biochem Mol Biol* 26:227–259.

Wolf SF, Haines L, Fisch J, Kremsky JN, Dougherty JP, Jacobs K (1987): Rapid hybridization kinetics of DNA attached to submicron latex particles. *Nucl Acids Res* 15:2911–2926.

Yehle CO, Patterson WL, Boguslawski SJ, Albarella JP, Yip KF, Carrico RJ (1987): A solution hybridization assay for ribosomal RNA from bacteria using biotinylated DNA probes and enzyme-labeled antibody to DNA:RNA. *Mol Cell Probes* 1:177–193.

13

Application of the Hybridization Protection Assay (HPA) to PCR

Norman C. Nelson and Sherrol H. McDonough

Introduction

The development of *in vitro* DNA amplification techniques has made detection of specific sequences more sensitive and rapid than ever before. The ability to amplify rare sequences has greatly improved our ability to detect chromosomal translocations, allelic variability, and infectious agents (Innis et al., 1990). Polymerase chain reaction (PCR) is a method of DNA amplification performed by repeatedly denaturing a DNA target, annealing specific oligonucleotide primers, and extending the primers with a DNA-dependent DNA polymerase (Mullis et al., 1986; Mullis and Faloona, 1987; Saiki et al., 1988b). Each cycle theoretically results in a doubling of the number of target sequences. Other amplification systems, such as the transcription-based amplification system, or TAS (Kwok et al., 1987), also give significant amplification of target sequences.

Because it often takes 2–10 times as long to detect amplified product as it does to perform the amplification reaction, rapid, simple, yet sensitive and specific detection systems are needed to allow researchers to take full advantage of the benefits of rapid target amplifica- tion, and to allow widespread use outside the research laboratory.

Methods for detection of amplification product generally fall into two categories: those that assay for extension of primers, and those that, by hybridization, assay for amplification of a sequence internal to the primers.

Primer Incorporation Methods

The most common method used to detect extension of primers is based on detection of a specific size fragment. This is accomplished by gel electrophoresis and ethidium bromide staining, with or without restriction endonuclease digestion. Although widely used, it is recognized that spurious incorporation of primers does occur and nonspecific bands equal in length to the expected fragment can be generated. This is particularly a problem for samples that contain a high level of nontarget DNA, such as cell lysates. The method is also somewhat insensitive, with limits of detection 10- to 100-fold lower than methods using hybridization.

Other methods for detection of primer incorporation have been described (Chehab and

The Polymerase Chain Reaction
K.B. Mullis, F. Ferré, R.A. Gibbs, editors
© 1994 Birkhäuser Boston

Kan, 1989; Hayashi et al., 1989; Kemp et al., 1989; Triglia et al., 1990). These methods all require a step or series of steps to separate extended from unextended primers. In addition, these methods are highly dependent on the specificity of the primer incorporation as nonspecific incorporation is difficult to distinguish from specific incorporation. For these reasons, hybridization of a probe to the internal region of the amplification product is still considered the method of choice for confirmation of amplification of specific sequences (Abbott et al., 1988; Larzul et al., 1989).

Radioactive Hybridization Detection Methods

A number of hybridization techniques have been used to confirm the identity of amplified products. By far the most common methods utilize ^{32}P-labeled DNA probes that can provide sensitive detection of amplified product. These probes must be used in assay formats that physically separate the unhybridized and hybridized probe. In one commonly used assay, the amplification product is attached to a membrane such as nylon either by direct blotting (dot blots) or by transfer after size fractionation by gel electrophoresis (Southern blots) (Keller and Manak, 1989). Blots are hybridized, washed to remove the unhybridized probe, and detected by autoradiography. Quantitation is done visually or by densitometry. This process takes from 1 to 3 days.

Other methods utilize more efficient solution hybridization of amplified product and detection probe. These methods differ in the method used to differentiate hybridized and unhybridized probe. In the detection method described by Kwok et al. (1987), the products were hybridized to a ^{32}P-labeled oligonucleotide in solution and then hybridized to a second oligonucleotide bound to Sephacryl beads. The beads were washed, centrifuged, and radioactivity measured in a scintillation counter. The authors reported that the method required about 4 hr to complete.

Syvanen and co-workers (1988) simplified this format by performing PCR with 5′-biotinylated primers. Following hybridization of the amplification product to a ^{32}P-labeled DNA probe, the hybrids were collected on avidin-coated polystyrene particles. Radioactivity was determined following extensive washing steps.

Alternatively, Kwok and co-workers (1987) described an assay in which probe hybridized to product was subjected to restriction endonuclease digestion. The resulting fragments were separated by polyacrylamide gel electrophoresis and the appearance of a specific cleavage product was monitored. Final detection was by autoradiography. This method required several hours to complete.

Nonradioactive Hybridization Methods

Nonisotopic detection systems are particularly attractive, as increased shelf-life and decreased biohazard are desirable. A number of hybridization formats utilizing nonradioactive detection probes have been reported. Both the Southern blot and dot blot formats have been modified to allow the use of detection probes labeled with digoxigenin (Carl et al., 1990), acetylaminofluorene (AAF) (Larzul et al., 1989), or horseradish peroxidase (Saiki et al., 1988a). In the latter, amplified DNA was attached to membranes and hybridized to oligonucleotide probes linked to horseradish peroxidase. This method has the advantage that the probes are already linked to the enzyme, but suffers from a lack of sensitivity. The authors reported that the nonisotopic method gave signals 1–10% of that observed with ^{32}P-labeled probes after a 15-min autoradiographic exposure. The procedure allowed allele-specific detection to be achieved and took about 3 hr to perform. A similar procedure was used by Bugawan and co-workers (1988) to detect amplified HLA DQ and globin sequences. These authors reported better results with horseradish peroxidase-labeled probes than psoralen-biotinylated probes.

Gregerson and co-workers (1989) describe the use of biotinylated oligonucleotide probes for the detection of amplified α_1-antitrypsin gene variant DNA attached to membranes. In a slightly different format, Keller and co-workers (1989) describe hybridization of the amplification product simultaneously to biotin-labeled detection probes and to capture probes attached to the surface of a microtiter dish. This latter method was used for the detection of amplified HIV-1 DNA sequences. Following hybridization and washing steps, hybrids were incubated with an enzyme conjugate and washed extensively prior to addition of the substrate, which allows color development to occur. Enzyme-labeled probes should theoretically give high sensitivity due to the accumulation of signal with time. However, backgrounds are also typically higher. Indeed, the authors mentioned difficulties finding conditions to completely inactivate nonspecific binding sites, which led to backgrounds higher than desired. In addition, lower sensitivity was observed with the nonisotopic probes compared to ^{32}P-labeled probes. It was necessary to compensate by amplifying product for a larger number of cycles to allow adequate signal detection. This method took more than a day to complete, but allowed allele-specific detection, and so should be useful for those situations when specificity is important and sufficient target sequences are available such that exquisite sensitivity is not required.

A "reverse dot blot" format has been described for analysis of the HLA DQA locus genes following amplification (Saiki et al., 1989). In this procedure, PCR reactions were performed with biotinylated primers. Following amplification, PCR products were hybridized to oligonucleotide probes immobilized on a membrane and streptavidin–horseradish peroxidase conjugate was simultaneously bound. Detection was accomplished by incubation of the membranes with substrate to allow color development. The technique requires 1 to 2 hr to complete and was particularly suited to situations where the number of probes exceeds that of the number of samples to be analyzed.

Another nonisotopic hybridization format, referred to as the hybridization protection assay (Arnold et al., 1989; Nelson et al., 1990; Tenover et al., 1990), has been developed that utilizes DNA oligonucleotide probes directly labeled with a chemiluminescent acridinium ester. This format is completely homogeneous, not requiring any physical separation steps to distinguish hybridized and unhybridized probe, thus greatly simplifying the assay. The system exhibits excellent sensitivity and specificity, and the hybridization and detection steps can be completed in about 30–40 min.

We describe here the application of this assay format to the detection of amplified sequences from viruses, chromosomal translocations, and bacteria.

Methods of Synthesis and Use of Acridinium Ester-Labeled Probes

Acridinium ester (AE) was synthesized as described previously (Weeks et al., 1983). Oligonucleotide probes were labeled by reacting the N-hydroxysuccinimide derivative of AE with a primary alkyl amine on a non-nucleotide-based phosphoramidite linker-arm (Arnold et al., 1988) introduced into the oligomer during DNA synthesis. The acridinium ester-labeled probe (AE probe) was then purified using high-performance liquid chromatography. Chemiluminescence was detected in a Leader I luminometer (Gen-Probe, San Diego, CA) by the automatic injection of 200 μl of 0.1% H_2O_2 in HNO_3 (5–400 mM), then 200 μl of 1 N NaOH (with or without surfactant). The measurement period was 2–5 sec; chemiluminescence was expressed as Relative Light Units, or RLU.

Amplifications were performed with Ampli-Taq polymerase (Perkin-Elmer/Cetus) using the conditions recommended by the manufacturer. Hybridizations with AE probes were performed at 60°C in 0.05–0.1 M lithium succinate buffer, pH 5.2, containing 1–10% lithium laurel sulfate, 2–10 mM EDTA, and 2–10 mM EGTA. Hybridization volumes ranged from 50 to 200 μl and incubation times ranged from 10 to 20 min. Differential hydrolysis was performed at 60°C in 0.15–0.20 M sodium tetraborate, 1–5% Triton X-100, pH 7.5–8.5.

Ester hydrolysis rates were determined as follows: AE probe (typically 0.1 pmol) was hybridized with an excess of target (typically 0.5–1 pmol). Aliquots of 15 μl containing approximately 100,000 RLU were placed in 100 μl of 0.2 M sodium tetraborate, pH 7.6, 5% Triton X-100, and incubated at 60°C. At various times, separate aliquots in individual tubes were removed and measured for chemiluminescence. The resulting data were plotted as log of percent initial chemiluminescence versus time; slopes and associated half-lives were determined by standard linear regression analysis.

The HPA procedure was as follows:

1. Denature—add target (typically in 10 μl) to the reaction tube and incubate at 95°C for 3–5 min.
2. Hybridize—add AE probe (typically in 50 μl) and incubate 10–20 min at 60°C.
3. Hydrolyze—add hydrolysis buffer (typically in 300 μl) and incubate 6 min at 60°C.
4. Detect—put reaction tube in luminometer and measure chemiluminescence for 2–5 sec.

Characteristics of the Hybridization Protection Assay

The hybridization protection assay (HPA) format is centered around the highly chemiluminescent acridinium ester (AE) shown in Figure 13.1. The AE reacts with hydrogen peroxide under alkaline conditions to rapidly (2–5 sec) produce light at 430 nm, which is easily detected in a standard, commercially available luminometer. Detection is very sensitive, with a limit of approximately 5×10^{-19} mol (3×10^5 molecules) of AE, and is linearly quantitative over a concentration range of more than 4 orders of magnitude. The rapid reaction kinetics of the AE improve sensitivity since the short read time limits the contribution of back-

ground noise, and allow reading a large number of samples within a short time.

To be utilized in a DNA probe-based hybridization assay, the AE is covalently attached directly to the DNA probe using standard N-hydroxysuccinimide (NHS) coupling chemistry (Weeks et al., 1983) (Fig. 13.1). Direct labels greatly simplify assay formats since the "capping," binding, and washing steps required for indirect labels (those attached through a biotin/avidin interaction, for example) are not necessary, and separate reagent additions for label coupling or substrate addition are not necessary. An additional, very important aspect of the AE label is that the acri-

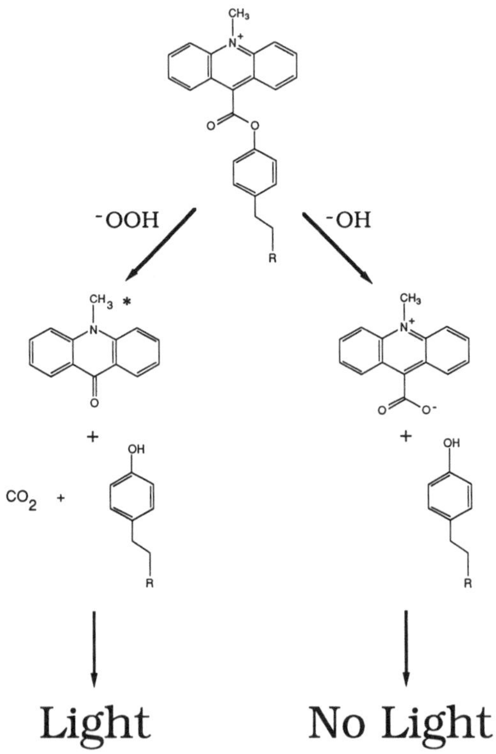

FIGURE 13.1. Structure and reaction pathways of acridinium ester. The N-methyl, phenyl acridinium ester reacts with alkaline peroxide to produce light, and with hydroxide to yield nonchemiluminescent ester hydrolysis products. The R group represents the N-hydroxysuccinimide (NHS) moiety, which reacts with primary amines, thus providing a means to specifically label DNA probes (see text); *electronically excited state.

dinium ring is cleaved from the DNA probe before light emission occurs (Fig. 13.1), thus minimizing intramolecular quenching (Weeks et al., 1983). To provide a site of attachment of the AE within a deoxyoligonucleotide probe, nonnucleotide based alkyl amine linker-arms have been developed, which can be incorporated at any location in the probe during standard phosphoramidite synthesis (Arnold et al., 1988). The amine is reacted with the NHS derivative of AE, yielding a DNA probe with a chemiluminescent AE directly attached through a covalent amide bond.

Acridinium ester attached to a DNA probe displays the same reaction kinetics as the free label, and is detected as sensitively and quantitatively as free chemiluminescent label (Fig. 13.2), demonstrating that performance is not compromised by attachment to the probe. Furthermore, AE probes display hybridization characteristics (thermal stability, rate and extent of hybridization, and specificity) essentially equivalent to their ^{32}P-labeled counterparts, demonstrating that attachment of the AE label does not compromise hybridization performance. Additionally, hybridization and detection of AE probes can also be performed in the presence of relatively large amounts of clinical specimen material.

Several rapid and simple formats have been developed that use AE probes for detecting target DNA or RNA sequences, and a number of these have been incorporated into commercially available assays (Gegg et al., 1990; Granato and Franz, 1989; Kranig-Brown et al., 1990; Rubin et al., 1990; Snider et al., 1990; Tenover et al., 1990; Watson et al., 1990). In these formats, the hybridization and detection reactions were performed in solution, which offers significant advantages compared to standard target immobilization techniques (Keller and Manak, 1989), including faster hybridization kinetics, availability of all the target molecules for hybridization, much better quantitation, fewer steps and less complexity, and much shorter time to result. This in-solution approach is particularly well suited to the analysis of PCR products, because a portion of the amplified sample can be analyzed directly with no further manipulations such as blotting, electrophoresis, binding, or washing steps, which are not only time consuming, but can also result in spread of amplification product throughout the laboratory.

The hybridization protection assay is a completely homogeneous format requiring no physical separation for the discrimination of hybridized and unhybridized AE probe. This format is based on differential chemical hydrolysis of the ester bond of the AE molecule (hydrolysis of this bond renders the AE permanently nonchemiluminescent, as shown in Fig. 13.1). The system is designed such that the rate of hydrolysis of the AE attached to unhybridized probe is rapid, whereas the rate of hydrolysis of AE attached to probe that is hybridized with its target nucleic acid is slow. By adjusting reaction chemistry, the chemiluminescence associated with unhybridized probe is rapidly reduced to low levels, whereas the chemiluminescence associated with hybridized probe is minimally affected. Thus, after this differential hydrolysis process, the

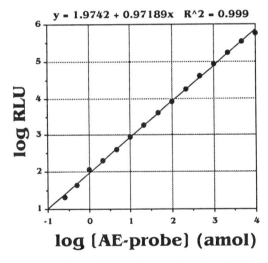

$$y = 1.9742 + 0.97189x \quad R^2 = 0.999$$

FIGURE 13.2. Sensitivity of detection of acridinium ester-labeled DNA probe. AE probe (see text) was serially diluted and measured for chemiluminescence as described in the text. Each point represents the average of four replicates: background was about 50 relative light units (RLUs) (subtracted from data before plotting). The equation of the line (obtained from regression analysis) appears above the graph.

remaining chemiluminescence is a direct measure of the amount of target present.

An example of differential hydrolysis of hybridized and unhybridized probe is shown in Figure 13.3, which illustrates loss of chemiluminescence with time due to ester hydrolysis. From linear regression analysis, the half-lives for hydrolysis were determined to be 53.6 and 0.96 min for hybridized and unhybridized probe, respectively. The theoretical percent remaining chemiluminescent label after a given hydrolysis time can be calculated using the equation

$$(0.5)^{T/t_{1/2}} \times 100 =$$
percent remaining chemiluminescence

where T is the elapsed time of differential hydrolysis, and $t_{1/2}$ is the half-life of loss of chemiluminescence. Using the half-life values given above, the calculated values for remaining chemiluminescence after a 20-min differential hydrolysis step would be 77% for hybridized probe and 0.00005% for unhybridized probe. This is greater than a one million-fold discrimination between hybridized

and unhybridized AE probe, in 20 min, with the addition of a single reagent and without any physical separation.

Application of HPA to the Detection of PCR-Amplified Products

The HPA format has been utilized to specifically detect a variety of PCR amplification products. In one application (Kacian et al., 1990), an overlapping pair of AE-labeled oligonucleotide probes (AE probes) specific for sequences within the *gag* gene of human immunodeficiency virus-1 (HIV-1) amplified by the SK38/SK39 primers described by Ou and co-workers (1988) were designed and synthesized. The performance characteristics of this AE probe pair in the HPA format were first evaluated utilizing known amounts of M13 cloned HIV target DNA (Fig. 13.4A). Detection was linearly quantitative over a concentration range of four orders of magnitude, with a limit of sensitivity of about 10^{-16} mol of target.

The detection of PCR-amplified HIV-1 DNA using the HPA format was next evaluated, the results of which are shown in Figure 13.4B. The assay detected serial dilutions of the final PCR product over a range of more than three orders of magnitude. In a separate experiment, an input of three genome equivalents of HIV-1 DNA was easily detected with a signal 22 times over background (data not shown). Ou and co-workers (1990) reported the detection of HIV-1 proviral DNA amplified in the presence of cell lysate containing a constant amount (1 fg) of human genomic DNA utilizing the HPA system described here. They observed a dynamic response over approximately three orders of magnitude of input HIV-1 DNA, with a sensitivity of about four copies. They compared the HPA detection format with a radioisotopic method utilizing a ^{32}P-labeled SK19 probe (solution hybridization, restriction enzyme digestion, gel electrophoresis, and autoradiography) and found the HPA format gave equivalent (if not more sensitive)

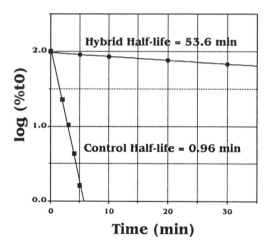

FIGURE 13.3. Differential hydrolysis of hybridized and unhybridized acridinium ester-labeled DNA probe. Rates of acridinium ester hydrolysis were measured for hybridized and unhybridized AE probe. Results were plotted as log of percent initial chemiluminescence versus time, and half-lives of hydrolysis were determined by standard linear regression analysis.

results to the ^{32}P method, and the HPA method was complete in less than an hour as compared to the full day required to complete the ^{32}P assay. They also performed a comparative study using PCR-amplified DNA from the peripheral blood mononuclear cells of HIV-seropositive and HIV-seronegative patients, and again found the HPA format to perform at least

equivalently to the ^{32}P method, yet take a small fraction of the time to complete.

In another application of the HPA format, the chromosomal translocation product known as the Philadelphia chromosome (Adams, 1985), which is associated with chronic myelogenous leukemia (CML), was amplified and detected (Arnold et al., 1989). In this study chimeric messenger RNA from K562 cells, which carry the Philadelphia chromosome, was converted to DNA and then amplified using PCR. Dilutions of the product were then detected with a DNA probe specific for the Philadelphia chromosome using either the HPA format with AE probe or a standard Southern analysis (Southern, 1985) with ^{32}P probe (Fig. 13.5). The Southern blot was sensitive to the 125-fold dilution after a 2.5-hr autoradiographic exposure (a band appeared at

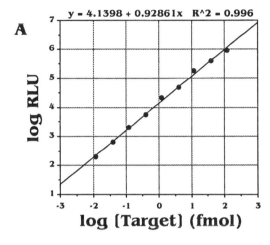

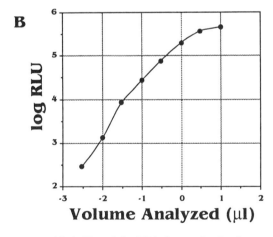

FIGURE 13.4. Use of the HPA format for the detection of PCR amplified HIV-1 DNA. AE probes specific for the *gag* region of HIV-1 (see text) were used to detect HIV-1 DNA. (A) Decreasing amounts of M13 cloned HIV-1 DNA were assayed directly using the HPA format. The equation of the line (obtained from regression analysis) appears above the graph. (B) HIV-1 DNA was PCR amplified (SK38/SK39 primer set; 30 cycles), and serial dilutions were then assayed using the HPA format as described in the text.

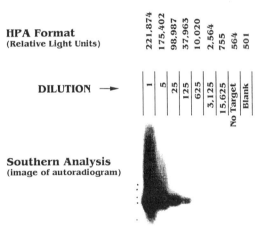

FIGURE 13.5. Comparison of the HPA and Southern blot formats for the detection of PCR amplified Philadelphia chromosome. The Philadelphia chromosome (which is associated with chronic myelogenous leukemia) was amplified from K562 cells and the product was serially diluted in 5-fold increments and detected using either an AE probe in the HPA format or a ^{32}P probe in a standard Southern blot format. The HPA format was performed as described in the text (3 min denaturation, 10 min hybridization). For the Southern analysis, probe was 5'-end-labeled with ^{32}P immediately before use (specific activity = 3.6×10^6 cpm/pmol) and 3×10^8 cpm/ml were used in the hybridization. Autoradiography was performed at $-80°C$ with intensifier screens for 2.5 hr.

the 625-fold dilution after overnight exposure). In the HPA format, the 3125-fold dilution gave a strong, positive signal, and the 15,625-fold dilution gave a significantly greater signal over blank (254 RLU) than the "No Target" sample over blank (63 RLU). Furthermore, the Southern analysis required 2 days to perform (prior to autoradiography) whereas the HPA was complete in less than 30 min.

The HPA has also been used to detect amplified hepatitis B virus (HBV) DNA. Dilutions of cloned HBV (serotype adw) as well as plasma positive for HBV surface antigen (sAg) were subjected to 30 rounds of PCR using the 109/585R primers (SAg region) described previously (Kaneko et al., 1989) and amplification product was assayed using the HPA format (Fig. 13.6). A wide dynamic response, good sensitivity (signal to background ratio of 26 at 6 genomes input), and the ability to perform the assay in the presence of clinical sample were again observed. Comparing these data with the results of PCR detection of HBV reported by Kaneko and co-workers (1989), the HPA format was equivalent in sensitivity to normal PCR coupled with Southern blot analysis or a "double-PCR" method coupled with ethidium-stained agarose gel detection, and 103-fold more sensitive than normal PCR coupled with ethidium staining of gels. Specificity was also equivalent in the HPA and Southern blot formats, whereas in the ethidium staining procedure specificity of amplified bands had to be confirmed by Southern blot analysis. Furthermore, the HPA format was more rapid and easier to perform.

Other PCR-amplified sequences that have been detected using the HPA format include segments of the genes that code for the 16 S ribosomal RNA (rRNA) subunit of *Neisseria gonorrhoeae* (Gegg et al., 1990) and the 23 S rRNA subunit of *Chlamydia trachomatis* (Kranig-Brown et al., 1990), the 7.5-kB cryptic plasmid of *Chlamydia trachomatis* known as pCHL1, the HIV-1 envelope region, and the HIV-2 viral protein X region. The HPA format has also been applied to other systems, including the targeting of rRNA, which provides a natural target amplification (each bacterial cell

contains up to 10,000 rRNA copies) as well as increased specificity since rRNA sequences are excellent phylogenetic markers (Enns, 1988; Kohne, 1986; Woese, 1987). Commercially available HPA applications utilizing rRNA targets include detection of *Campylobacter jejuni* (Tenover, 1990), *Haemophilus influenzae* (Snider et al., 1990), and several other organisms isolated in culture, detection

A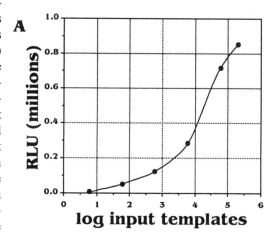

B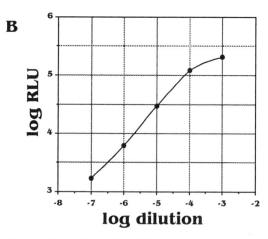

FIGURE 13.6. Use of the HPA format for the detection of PCR amplified HBV DNA. (**A**) HBV cloned DNA was amplified using PCR as described in the text in the absence of clinical sample. (**B**) Plasma positive for HBV surface antigen was diluted in normal serum, alkali treated, neutralized, and amplified by PCR. All products were analyzed by the HPA format utilizing a mix of 2 overlapping AE probes specific for the surface antigen region of HBV.

of bacteria and yeast in urine samples (Watson et al., 1990), and detection of sulfate-reducing bacteria and all bacteria in a research assay. The differential hydrolysis aspect of the HPA has also been combined with a rapid magnetic separation procedure (Arnold et al., 1989) for the detection of *Chlamydia trachomatis* (Kranig-Brown et al., 1990) and *Neisseria gonorrhoeae* (Gegg et al., 1990; Granato and Franz, 1989) directly in patient specimen (urogenital swab in this case). The HPA format has also been used to detect single site mismatches (Arnold et al., 1989).

The HPA format compares favorably with other methods for the detection of PCR amplification products. Sensitivity of the assay is comparable to or better than the other commonly used methods, including those utilizing ^{32}P. The HPA format exhibits the excellent specificity of detection afforded by other hybridization-based methods such as Southern blots, dot blots, and the ^{32}P-oligomer: restriction method (Kwok et al., 1989). One distinct advantage of the HPA format is the ease of use and short time to result. In all of the applications cited, the HPA format consisted of the same three steps: (1) solution hybridization (10–20 min; a brief heat denaturation step prior to hybridization is required in most PCR applications), (2) differential hydrolysis (6–10 min), and (3) detection (2–5 sec). This procedure is simpler and faster than any of the other techniques commonly in use, yet retains high sensitivity and the specificity of a hybridization-based procedure. Additionally, the procedure is nonisotopic, thus avoiding the biohazards associated with radioisotopes and does not include steps such as washing, which result in spread of target through the laboratory.

In conclusion, the HPA format is a simple, rapid, sensitive, and specific method for detection and quantitation of amplified DNA from a number of sources.

References

Abbott MA, Poiesz BJ, Byrne BC, Kwok S, Sninsky JJ, Ehrlich GD (1988): Enzymatic gene amplification: qualitative and quantitative methods for detecting proviral DNA amplified in vitro. *J Infec Dis* 158:1158–1169.

Adams JM (1985): Oncogene activation by fusion of chromosomes in leukemia. *Nature (London)* 315:542–543.

Arnold LJ Jr, Bhatt RS, Reynolds MA (1988): Non-nucleotide linking reagents for nucleotide probes. PCT/US88/03173.

Arnold LJ Jr, Hammond PW, Wiese WA, Nelson NC (1989): Assay formats involving acridinium-ester-labeled DNA probes. *Clin Chem* 35:1588–1594.

Bugawan TL, Saiki RK, Levenson CH, Watson RM, Erlich HA (1988): The use of non-radioactive oligonucleotide probes to analyze enzymatically amplified DNA for prenatal diagnosis and forensic HLA typing. *Bio/Technology* 6:943–947.

Carl M, Tibbs CW, Dobson ME, Paparello S, Dasch GA (1990): Diagnosis of acute typhus infection using the polymerase chain reaction. *J Infect Dis* 161:791–793.

Chehab FF, Kan YW (1989): Detection of specific DNA sequences by fluorescence amplification: A color complementation assay. *Proc Natl Acad Sci USA* 86:9178–9182.

Enns RK (1988): DNA probes: An overview and comparison with current methods. *Lab Med* 19:295–300.

Gegg C, Kranig-Brown D, Hussain J, McDonough S, Kohne D, Shaw S (1990): A clinical evaluation of a new DNA probe test for *Neisseria gonorrhoeae* that included analysis of specimens producing results discrepant with culture. Abstracts of the 90th Annual Meeting of the American Society for Microbiology 356.

Granato PA, Franz MR (1989): Evaluation of a prototype DNA probe test for the nonculture diagnosis of gonorrhea. *J Clin Microbiol* 27:632–635.

Gregerson N, Winter V, Petersen KB, Koch J, Kolvraa S, Rudiger N, Heinsvig E-M, Bolund L (1989): Detection of point mutations in amplified single copy genes by biotin-labeled oligonucleotides: Diagnosis of variants of alpha-1-antitrypsin. *Clin Chim Acta* 182:151–164.

Hayashi K, Orita M, Suzuki Y, Sekiya T (1989): Use of labeled primers in polymerase chain reaction (LP-PCR) for a rapid detection of the product. *Nucl Acids Res* 17:3605.

Innis MA, Gelfand DH, Sninsky JJ, White TJ (ed.) (1990): *PCR Protocols.* San Diego, CA: Academic Press.

Kaneko S, Feinstone SM, Miller RH (1989): Rapid and sensitive method for the detection of serum hepatitis B virus DNA using the polymerase chain reaction technique. *J Clin Microbiol* 27:1930–1933.

Keller GH, Manak MM (1989): *DNA Probes*. New York: Stockton Press.

Keller GH, Huang D-P, Manak MM (1989): A sensitive nonisotopic hybridization assay for HIV-1 DNA. *Anal Biochem* 177:27–32.

Kemp DJ, Smith DB, Foote SJ, Samaras N, Peterson MG (1989): Colorimetric detection of specific DNA segments amplified by polymerase chain reactions. *Proc Natl Acad Sci USA* 86:2423–2427.

Kohne DE (1986): Application of DNA probe tests to the diagnosis of infectious disease. *Am Clin Prod Rev* November:20–29.

Kranig-Brown D, Gegg C, Hussain J, Johnson R, Shaw S (1990): Use of PCR amplification and unlabeled probe competition for analysis of specimens producing results discrepant with culture in an evaluation of a DNA probe test for *Chlamydia trachomatis*. Abstracts of the 90th Annual Meeting of the American Society for Microbiology 356.

Kwok S, Mack DH, Mullis KB, Poiesz B, Ehrlich G, Blair D, Friedman-Kien A, Sninsky JJ (1987): Identification of human immunodeficiency virus sequences by using in vitro enzymatic amplification and oligomer cleavage detection. *J Virol* 61:1690–1694.

Kwok DY, Davis GR, Whitfield KM, Chappelle HL, DiMichele LJ, Gingeras TR (1989): Transcription-based amplification system and detection of amplified human immunodeficiency virus type 1 with a bead-based sandwich hybridization format. *Proc Natl Acad Sci USA* 86:1173–1177.

Larzul D, Chevrier D, Guesdon J-L (1989): A nonradioactive diagnostic test for the detection of HBV DNA sequences in serum at the single molecule level. *Mol Cell Probes* 3:45–57.

Laure F, Rouzioux C, Veber F, Jacomet C, Courgnaud V, Blanche S, Burgard M, Griscelli C, Brechot C (1988): Detection of HIV-1 DNA in infants and children by means of the polymerase chain reaction. *Lancet* 2(8610):538–540.

Mullis KB, Faloona FA (1987): Specific synthesis of DNA in vitro via a polymerase-catalyzed chain reaction. *Meth Enzymol* 155:335–350.

Mullis K, Faloona F, Scharf S, Saiki R, Horn G, Erlich H (1986): Specific enzymatic amplification of DNA in vitro: The polymerase chain reaction. *Cold Spring Harbor Symp Quant Biol* 51:263–273.

Nelson NC, Hammond PW, Wiese WA, Arnold LJ Jr (1990): Homogeneous and heterogeneous chemiluminescent DNA probe-based assay formats for the rapid and sensitive detection of target nucleic acids. In: *Luminescence Immunoassay and Molecular Applications*. van Dyke K, ed. Boca Raton, FL: CRC Press, 293–309.

Ou C-Y, Kwok S, Mitchell SW, Mack DH, Sninsky JJ, Krebs JW, Feorino P, Warfield D, Schochetman G (1988): DNA amplification for direct detection of HIV-1 in DNA of peripheral blood mononuclear cells. *Science* 239:295–297.

Ou C-Y, McDonough SH, Cabanas D, Ryder TB, Harper M, Moore J, Schochetman G (1990): Rapid and quantitative detection of enzymatically amplified HIV-1 DNA using chemiluminescence-labeled oligonucleotide probes. *AIDS Res Human Retrovirus* 6:1323–1329.

Rubin SM, Murphy-Clark KA, Bee GG, Gordon PC, Roberts SS, Johnson R (1990): Development of rapid non-isotopic DNA probe assays for fungi: *Blastomyces dermatitidis*. Abstracts of the 90th Annual Meeting of the American Society for Microbiology 409.

Saiki RK, Chang C-A, Levenson CH, Warren TC, Boehm CD, Kazazian HH Jr, Erlich HA (1988a): Diagnosis of sickle cell anemia and β-thalassemia with enzymatically amplified DNA and nonradioactive allele-specific oligonucleotide probes. *N Engl J Med* 319:537–541.

Saiki RK, Gelfand DH, Stoffel S, Scharf SJ, Higuchi R, Horn GT, Mullis KB, Erlich HA (1988b): Primer-directed enzymatic amplification of DNA with a thermostable DNA polymerase. *Science* 239:487–491.

Saiki RK, Walsh PS, Levenson CH, Erlich HA (1989): Genetic analysis of amplified DNA with immobilized sequence-specific oligonucleotide probes. *Proc Natl Acad Sci USA* 86:6230–6234.

Snider E, Gordon P, Dean E, Trainor D (1990): Development of a DNA probe culture confirmation test of *Haemophilus influenzae*. Abstracts of the 90th Annual Meeting of the American Society for Microbiology 398.

Southern E (1975): Detection of specific sequences among DNA fragments separated by gel electrophoresis. *J Mol Biol* 98:503–517.

Syvanen A-C, Bengstrom M, Tenhunen J, Soderlund H (1988): Quantification of polymerase chain reaction products by affinity-based hybrid collection. *Nucl Acids Res* 16:11327–11338.

Tenover FC, Carlson L, Barbagallo S, Nachamkin I (1990): DNA probe culture confirmation assay for identification of thermophilic *Campylobacter* species. *J Clin Microbiol* 28:1284–1287.

Triglia T, Argyropoulos VP, Davidson BE, Kemp DJ (1990): Colourimetric detection of PCR products using the DNA-binding protein TyrR. *Nucl Acids Res* 18:1080.

Watson M, Zepeda-Bakan M, Smith K, Alden M, Stolzenbach F, Johnson R (1990): Evaluation of a DNA probe assay for screening urinary tract in-fections. Abstracts of the 90th Annual Meeting of the American Society for Microbiology 392.

Weeks I, Beheshti I, McCapra F, Campbell AK, Woodhead JS (1983): Acridinium esters as high-specific-activity labels in immunoassay. *Clin Chem* 29:1474–1479.

Woese CR (1987): Bacterial evolution. *Microbiol Rev* 51:221–271.

PART ONE
Methodology

SECTION IV
Instrumentation

14

PCR Instrumentation: Where Do We Stand?

Christian C. Oste

Introduction

Like any major undertaking, this comprehensive book on PCR has gone through a rather long genesis. Needless to say, the situation on the PCR instrumentation front has evolved quite a bit since the time the concept of making this book crystallized. This chapter required several rewrites in an attempt to make it current at the time of publication, and to anticipate future directions for the field.

One of the most striking differences between even only a few years ago and today is that PCR, and, to a more limited extent, the existing alternative *in vitro* nucleic acid amplification methods, have shifted from being laboratory curiosities to becoming actual commodities. Those of us involved with PCR since the early days (about 1986), when the first attempts were made at developing instrumentation suited for automating the process, knew that this was going to happen sooner or later. The truth is that with this technique as well, we saw an expansion in adopting the technology first in the United States, besides few local exceptions in other countries around the world. It is fair to say that PCR had already

gone mainstream in the United States by 1989, when the rest of the world in fact started becoming interested in implementing the method.

We have now reached the point where PCR has become as common as the Southern blotting technique, which, in fact, it has partially displaced as a result. If you attend a few seminars and/or conferences per year, you will undoubtedly have noticed this trend: as a matter of fact, the use of PCR has become in many cases so implicit that it just receives a cursory mention in the Materials and Methods section of most recent papers or is simply mentioned matter-of-factly in the footnotes accompanying the figures.

So, why a chapter on PCR instrumentation at this point in time? The answer to this question is actually several-fold. As a result mostly of the feedback from PCR users, the instrumentation available early on has improved quite significantly. We have gone from a situation where the instrumentation was the rate-limiting step in rapidly obtaining PCR data, to a point where the emphasis has shifted toward improving the speed, accuracy, and reproducibility of the pre- and post-PCR processes involved in the analysis of the data. And this

The Polymerase Chain Reaction
K.B. Mullis, F. Ferré, R.A. Gibbs, editors
© 1994 Birkhäuser Boston

mostly because the devices assisting in performing the PCR process have become faster, more accurate with regard to temperature control, and more versatile with respect to formatting the sample. The last point is probably the most important since the users may not always have the luxury of preparing the sample in a fashion that would be compatible with the use of microcentrifuge tubes. The currently available format versatility is, after all, a logical development: as the PCR method became more and more popular, a growing number of scientists attempted to adapt the technique to different types of sample presentations.

One last comment before moving on: we deviated quite substantially from the original plan regarding the present chapter. Initially, the intention was for me to pool and summarize the contributions from a variety of sources, representing commercially available instrumentation options. However, along the way, it was decided to include the contributions from other sources as separate chapters, as the reader will notice from the table of contents.

Microtube versus Alternative Formats

By and large, the microtube format is still currently the most popular one, for its flexiblity and the variety of instruments available on the market. Initially, the PCR samples were routinely prepared in final volumes of up to 100 μl, typically in 0.5- to 0.7-ml tubes. It was soon discovered that the payoff with respect to the final amount of amplified product obtained was relatively limited when larger sample volumes were used, which pretty much limited the use of 1.5-ml microtubes to a marginal occurrence. It is worth mentioning that some instruments suppliers still continue to offer the possibility of using the larger microtubes, although apparatuses equipped with blocks compatible with the larger tubes represent a very small percentage of installed units.

As a matter of fact, the trend has been to substantially reduce the sample volume, even in those cases where the small microtube is being used. The majority of users relying on the 0.5- to 0.7-ml microtube are currently preparing their PCR samples in final volumes ranging from 20 to 50 μl, although I have heard of successful PCR reactions with that format, in final sample volumes as low as 5 μl.

Over the long run, the reduction in sample volume translates into significant savings for the user, mostly with regard to the most expensive reaction components such as thermostable DNA polymerases and synthetic primers. In addition, as described elsewhere in this volume, advanced reaction parameters optimization methods have also contributed to decreasing the final concentrations of those two reaction components, thereby further adding on to the savings.

Initially, microtubes came only in one flavor: thick walls. The downside of this microtube characteristic was their resulting high time constant. In layperson terms, regardless of how quickly the instrument block would reach the target temperature, and regardless of how quickly and uniformly the temperature would equilibrate across the block, the temperature within the sample would be lagging somewhat, probably on the order of 20–30 sec until the sample itself would equilibrate at the target temperature.

This important factor had to be taken into account when programming the instrument, in the sense that each of the incubation steps in the PCR protocol would have to include an amount of time, at temperature equilibrium, sufficient for the specific reaction to take place with the highest possible efficiency. This constraint certainly did not help when attempting to shorten cycle times, which, in the early days, were on the order of about 5–6 min, with probably less than one-third of that total time spent at temperature equilibrium, samplewise. It still amazes me that "Turbo-PCR" ever worked at the time, i.e., two-steps protocols (no marked pause for the elongation step), with thick wall microtubes and shortened incubation times. Then again, those fast PCR protocols worked mostly in the cases where the initial target copy number was high and the amplicon did not exceed a few hundreds base pairs.

Another seldom perceived problem has to deal with the geometry of the microtubes. Indeed, independent measurements in several laboratories uncovered the fact that the standard size microtubes (i.e., 0.5–0.7 ml), with sample volumes on the order of 50 to 100 μl, actually create a temperature gradient within the sample, even when the sample supposedly has reached temperature equilibrium. This quite intriguing fact was discovered initially by accident, when the K-type probe used to measure the temperature inside of the sample was not located "properly," i.e., all the way at the bottom of the sample, as would normally be done. The average temperature differential subsequently measured between the bottom of a 100-μl sample, in a standard microtube, and the sample–oil interface was as much as 10°C, even at temperature equilibrium. The reader will certainly be knowledgeable enough at this point to understand the consequences of this situation: the sample will feature "zones" where the temperature would be lower than the optimized annealing temperature, resulting in partial loss of specificity, lower than the ideal extension temperature, which will decrease the efficiency of the elongation step, and lower than the adequate denaturation temperature, which, in turn, will reduce the efficiency of the following annealing step.

However, and this is a definite tribute to the robustness of the PCR technique, the reaction kept on working, because only part of the sample is exposed to lower-than-programmed temperatures in the standard microtube format. Perhaps, we have grown content with the efficiencies obtained in microtubes, not knowing all along that yield and specificity can actually be higher with other sample configurations.

The redemption of the microtubes fortunately came along just in time for that format to remain competitive with the emerging alternatives. First, the thickness of the wall was reduced, which helped reduce the time constant and therefore speeded up the sample temperature equilibration. The reduction in wall thickness unfortunately affected the thin wall microtube sturdiness, which made it more prone to cracking when spun in a microcentrifuge. At any rate, this is a minor inconvenience

since most users would simply pipet directly through the oil overlay to obtain an aliquot for their gel analysis or other assays. In addition, it appears that the problem has been addressed by the various suppliers of 0.5- to 0.7-ml thin-wall microtubes, and that the microtubes currently available will successfully withstand centrifugation in a table-top microcentrifuge.

Second came a size reduction. Thin wall microtubes are now available in 0.2 ml size, suited for use in microtiter plate-like format. The samples prepared in this type of "mini" microtubes would still be amplified in a block-type instrument, and would be held in place by a specially designed holder that would provide actual sample coordinates identical to those used in classical 96-well plates. One of the major advantages of this configuration is that it allows for easy interfacing with automated pipetting stations, for pre- and post-PCR samples processing. In addition, 96-well plates are now available where the wells are shaped like 0.2-ml tubes; at least one commercially available cycler will accommodate both 0.2-ml tubes and this new type of plate, providing incremental flexibility in the samples formatting.

Finally came the "oil-free" PCR, not to be confused with "Hot Start" whose usefulness can still be argued about and would be limited to microtubes format, for the time being anyway. Several suppliers currently offer block-type instruments with a heated lid, whose major function is to prevent condensation from forming in the upper part of the microtube. The question of whether we were really looking at condensation forming in the upper part of the tube or whether we were dealing with a "spattering" effect due to the presence of a mix of an aqueous phase with oil is pretty much rhetorical at this point, since heated lids have preempted the requirement for oil overlay. The bottom line is that the temperature gradient effect within the sample in the microtube format has probably also been reduced significantly, due to the combination of the heated lid and smaller air volumes above the sample, at least in the case of the 0.2-ml microtube. The absence of an oil overlay also eliminates the need for a chloroform extraction, for those users who were accustomed to that step, and generally allows for cleaner pipetting of a sample aliquot, post-PCR.

So, in conclusion, it appears that the microtube format, in particular that 0.2-ml variant, with thin wall and heated lid, remains a valid contender, despite the emergence of alternative formats, which we will look at now.

The Alternative Formats

When referring to alternative formats, two aspects have to be considered: the type of instrument design and the sample presentation. I will first focus on the sample presentation.

In the last few years, microtiter plates have steadily gained ground over microtubes, although one of the major problems has been to encounter the right type of polymer from which to cast those plates. We all remember the very first microtiter plates that were promoted for preparing sequencing samples, and our bewilderment looking at the same plates irreversibly warped at the end of the last high temperature incubation step. Needless to say, those plates, regardless of the shape of their well bottoms, were absolutely unsuitable for PCR reactions. Progress has been made in the development of suitable plates, mainly by resorting to polycarbonate for casting the plates (instead of polystyrene). Although not completely devoid of problems of its own, so far, that polymer appears to be the best choice for the time being.

Block-type instruments are available, where the contact between the bottoms of the microtiter plate wells and the block has been improved considerably. Although it is no longer a standard recommendation, it might still be advisable to layer some thermal compound between the block and the plate, just to ensure a good heat (and cold) transfer to the samples. This recommendation would particularly apply to the currently available thermal cycler, where the plates are physically moved by a robotic arm, between the various incubation stations. The improved plate resistance to warping has also resolved one of the major problems that appeared early, namely the fact that the lid of the plate would not be exposed to the same temperature variations as the plate itself, thereby not warping as much and eventually not covering the plate adequately, which potentially led to sample-to-sample cross-contamination.

The major benefit of using microtiter plates for PCR, as mentioned earlier, is the possibility of interfacing simply the corresponding thermal cycler and an automated pipetting station (also known as robots), both during sample preparation and in post-PCR processes, such as dot-blotting and even agarose gel loading. Several additional applications, such as, perhaps, capillary gels array loading, are currently in development in various laboratories, and, hopefully, will eventually become available commercially.

The next major level in throughput increase will come from the suitable automation of PCR in high-density microtiter plates. Although not very popular yet, microtiter plates featuring 384 wells (4 × 96 wells) and even 864 wells (9 × 96 wells) are now becoming commercially available. These new plates provide a truly remarkable throughput, although there are, in my opinion, two remaining problem areas. First, the type of thermal cycling instrument currently used with those plates (i.e., programmable oven), although probably adequate, significantly lacks in performance.

Second, most currently available robots use 8 (or 12) channels "tools," which will therefore require a lot of iterative operations in order to, for instance, fill the wells of the high-density plates with the PCR reaction mix, then add the DNA template, or to dot-blot the amplification product at the end of the reaction. Nevertheless, the mythical barrier of performing 10,000 individual PCR reactions in a day has already been trespassed in several laboratories, emphasizing the need for major improvements in the other traditional bottleneck areas, such as sample DNA preparation and mass-screening by probe hybridization, to name just a few.

The previous comment brings up an interesting question: Is there a way of offsetting high throughput in a relatively slow piece of hardware by simply speeding up the PCR reaction itself, and running smaller batches of samples?

The answer is probably. This leads me to comment for a moment about one of my favorite format for PCR samples: capillary vessels. Currently, two variants of that exciting new format are commercially available: one uses glass capillaries, whereas the other one uses the same tips that are used with a popular type of positive displacement pipets.

I should first explain why I find this format so exciting. One of the reasons, again, is the geometry of the sample. In capillary PCR, the sample is presented as a cylinder, and the sample vessel is completely "buried" inside the instrument block. Regardless of the vessel's reduced cross section and of its nature (glass or plastic), the heat (and cold) transfer is practically instantaneous and the sample temperature equilibrates within seconds of the block reaching the programmed temperature.

In addition, since the mass of the block is so much lower (at least in the case of the "crown" or circular block design) than in a conventional thermal cycler, ramping rates, both for heating and cooling, reach respectable values of approximately 5°C/sec, vs., at best, up to 2.5°C/sec (heating only) in more common designs. Overshoot and undershoot, traditionally somewhat of a problem with the classical, heavier blocks, are practically nonexistent with the circular block instrument.

Finally, still because of the geometry of the vessel, the problem of temperature gradient observed with the microtube simply does not exist with the capillary format, since the diameter of the sample "cylinder" is constant over the few mm the sample actually occupies within the vessel.

For all practical purposes, I feel that the capillary system that relies upon pipet tips (Fig. 14.1) as the reaction vessel is somewhat superior to the glass design for the following two reasons. First, sealing the plastic tips is a lot more straightforward than sealing the glass capillaries. Second, the manufacturer of the tips also supplies a programmable automated pipetting station that allows the reaction mix and the DNA template to be sequentially pipetted, directly into the tip. As a matter of fact, we have performed even more sophisticated experiments with that system, pipetting suc-

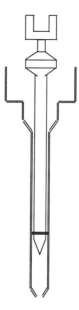

FIGURE 14.1. Representation of the pipet tip used both with positive displacement pipets and with the circular block thermocycler design. Those tips are available in two sizes: 0–25 and 0–250 μl, although only the 0–25 μl size is used as the vessel for capillary PCR. The tips come preassembled (with plunger already engaged) in racks of 96, and are autoclavable.

cessively, the reaction mix, the template, a small air bubble, and finally an aliquot of isopsoralen solution for post-PCR amplified product "sterilization" (Fig. 14.2; Bataller et al., 1994), a method that has proved at least as efficient as the UNG approach, in our and others' (e.g., Rys and Persing, 1993) hands.

The capillary approach is particularly appropriate for the laboratory that requires quick production of relevant data. PCR sample preparation usually requires on the order of 15 min for multiple samples, starting from scratch up to loading the capillaries, whereas the PCR reaction itself with those instruments takes no more than about 30 min, even when running as many as 35 cycles and a final extension step (Fig. 14.3). In fact, running the gel is now the rate-limiting step in obtaining the data. In all, providing the sample DNA was available (and there are now preparation protocols that take less than 1/2 hr from raw sample to amplifiable DNA), it is possible to go all the way from

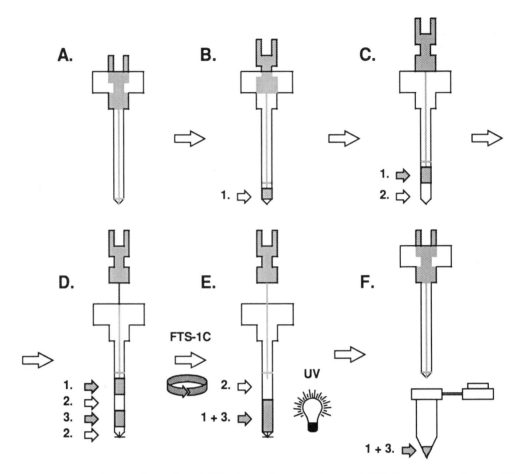

FIGURE 14.2. The six steps in capillary PCR using positive displacement pipet tips. (**A**) Pick up the tip using the automated pipet, driven by the programmable unit (not shown). (**B**) After programming the control unit, plunge the end of the tip in the complete (including the DNA template) reaction mix (1) and depress the key on the body of the pipet for the first step: the programmed volume of reaction mix will be picked up into the tip. (**C**) Next, remove the tip from the reaction mix vial and simply hold the pipet in the air: depress the key again, and the programmed volume of air (2) will be pipetted into the tip. (**D**) Dip the end of the tip into the isopsoralen solution, and depress the same key again: the programmed volume of isopsoralen solution (3) will be loaded into the tip. When this is done, remove the tip from the isopsoralen vial and repeat step **C** to introduce an additional air bubble. Heat-seal the end of the tip using the accessory provided with the circular block thermocycler, or by inserting a one-use plastic pin. (They come preloaded in specially designed racks.) (**E**) Perform the PCR reaction in the circular block thermocycler. Typical "hold"

times are 5 sec at 94°C, 2 sec at annealing, and 2 sec at 72°C. Ramping rates both for heating and cooling are approximately 5°C/sec. At the end of the PCR reaction, remove the tips from the block, place them in empty microtubes (0.5–0.7 ml), and spin them for a few seconds. The two phases that remained separated by the air bubble during the PCR reaction will now mix together near the end of the tip. Irradiate the samples for 10–15 min at room temperature using a broad-band UV source, but making sure that no radiation below 300 nm will be transmitted. (The plastic of the tip itself will help screening the <300 nm radiations.) *Caution:* Please make sure to wear goggles for this step. (**F**) After the UV irradiation step is completed, remove the sealing pin or simply cut the end of the tip with the provided special cutting tool, and collect the "sterilized" PCR product in a microtube by pushing the plunger down, using the conventional positive displacement pipet. The PCR product is ready for gel analysis, hybridization assays, and/or sequencing with nonthermostable DNA polymerases, but is no longer (further) amplifiable.

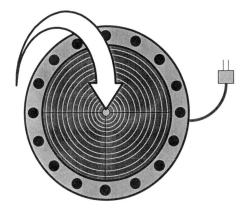

FIGURE 14.3. View from the top of the circular block. Actual sample capacity is for 40 0–25 µl pipet tips. Block diameter is approximately 12 cm, including the "crown" (sample holder). Heating elements are embedded into the block, as well as a temperature probe connected to the control processor. The arrow indicates the movement of the air used for cooling the block: the air is aspirated downward through the hollow center (equipped with fins) of the block by a fan located under the block. (The fan is actuated only during the down ramps.)

preparing the sample mix to having a picture of the gel in less than 1 and 1/4 hr, using the capillary approach and analyzing as many as 40 samples (circular block design), including controls.

So, why hasn't the capillary format become more popular? For a number of reasons, some dealing with market forces, some dealing with users' habits, and some other dealing with reaction components problems. We have known for quite some time that all thermostable DNA polymerases are not equivalent when it comes to efficiency in PCR. The capillary format simply exacerbates the differences, not only at the level of the different thermostable DNA polymerases available, but also with respect to the combination of enzyme and reaction buffer. Kary Mullis, for one, and among many others, has long recommended using "robust" reaction buffers for the PCR reaction. Because of the faster ramping rates (both heating and cooling) in the capillary format, it is essential to use "robust" reaction buffers, i.e., buffers that

are not susceptible to significant pH changes over wide temperature ranges, simply because, in my opinion, the buffer's pH will not have enough time to equilibrate at any temperature, even during the very short "holds," as the cycles proceed.

This statement may be somewhat misleading, since we should actually consider, as mentioned above, the combination of enzyme and buffer. Perhaps, some commercially available thermostable DNA polymerases recover more thoroughly and rapidly from fast and substantial temperature transitions than others; at least, that is how it appeared in our hands, provided they were used in conjunction with robust reaction buffers.

Finally, with respect to alternative formats, I would like to mention *in situ* PCR, which has been unfortunately plagued with a series of apparent "false starts." I recall that *in situ* PCR was claimed to be operational as far back as 1989, at the UCLA symposium held in Keystone, CO. The first "real" paper describing in details *in situ* PCR was most likely the one published by Haase et al. in 1990 (see Chapter 5, this volume). And slow progress has been made since, in spite of the tremendously promising aspects of this new flavor of PCR; the most promising (and colorful) results I have seen so far were reported recently by Gosden and Hanratty (1993).

The problems affecting *in situ* PCR are of a somewhat different nature, namely, making sure that the PCR product does not "escape." Since a significant percentage of *in situ* PCR experiments, for the time being, are aimed at locating the site where mRNA is encountered within a tissue section, it is important to be able to detect the accumulation of the PCR product on top of the initial template. I will leave to the expert(s) in this particular field the task of discussing more in depth the details of the methodology (see Chapter 5, this volume), but would like to conclude by mentioning that it appears that no dedicated instrumentation, except perhaps for a plain, flat block, will be required to efficiently perform *in situ* PCR, at least for now.

The Hardware

As mentioned earlier in this chapter, the PCR technology has really become a commodity, and, to a certain extent, the same thing has happened with the hardware used to perform the process.

By and large, the block configuration still remains the most relied on design, with some notable exceptions, which will be examined. Block designs are a natural for the microtube format, still favored by the vast majority of users. Blocks are also used for the microtiter plate format, which represents only a variation of the typical vessel used in PCR.

Heated lids have become standard on a number of commercially available instruments, the same way that Peltier elements used in cooling have finally become more reliable, in some cases, by simply keeping them physically away from the high temperature range. Performances, across the board, have become more uniform over time, since the user's requirements dictated significant mechanical improvements in some of the initially lesser competitive instruments. By now, the user's purchasing decision will be based on a number of criteria, including quality/price ratio, extent of product support on the part of the manufacturer, and, in final analysis, actual performance in PCR.

I do not believe there would be any purpose in my continuing to expound on the compared merits of the various commercial offerings. I also do believe that the average user had matured enough during the expansion years of the technology to understand that, in most cases, the success or failure of a PCR experiment cannot be blamed exclusively on the hardware used. Performing PCR using an automated thermal cycling device is very much like many other things in real life: one has to adjust to the idiosyncrasies of the surrounding mechanical devices.

Even the capillary devices mentioned in the previous section fall into that category; after all, there are just much faster block designs. The type of device that, however, falls into a category of its own is the convection oven. Al-though significantly underperforming by the accepted standards, the convection oven may develop into a device worth considering, in particular if the same user wishes to use a variety of formats. Microtubes, microtiter plates, capillaries, even slides: they will all fit inside the convection oven. Ramping rates are slow, relative to the performance of a capillary block in particular; undershoot and overshoot appear to be under control, but nevertheless more significant than with block formats.

The real question is, should the user be concerned about slow cooling rates, since we know all about the competition between amplified product reannealing and primers hybridizing to the target? The truth is that PCR reactions performed in the convection oven appear to reach approximately the same yields as in the microtube format: yet another mystery to solve. Sample-to-sample contamination, due to air movement, especially with microtiter plates does not seem to be a problem, in particular with polycarbonate plates where the lid keeps providing an adequate seal throughout the process, or with the newly available adhesive film which tightly seals the top edge of the wells.

If nothing else, the convection oven will deserve an honorable mention in the books of the future, that will relate the fascinating story of PCR: it is indeed in one of those devices that the threshold of 10,000 individual PCR reactions in a day was reached and surpassed. Furthermore, it is actually the most versatile of the currently available thermal cycling instruments: I still have only limited faith in the reliability and performance reproducibility of the instruments that feature "interchangeable" blocks. Due to the mechanical and engineering constraints in those devices, that aim at pleasing all types of users, it is likely that they will not handle any of the available formats as well as comparable dedicated instruments.

The Next Level

Is the PCR instrumentation market losing steam? Not by a long shot. Laboratories will continue to acquire the equipment best suited for their needs, which will most likely mean that increased output will be obtained by adding on more devices in any given laboratory. It comes as no surprise that the PCR instruments market has matured so rapidly: we have observed the same phenomenon with DNA synthesizers. After all, PCR is an extremely powerful and versatile technique, whose advent came at a time where the scientific community was in dire need of any technology that could improve the sensitivity in nucleic acid analysis.

Incidently, it will be quite interesting to determine whether PCR (and sequencing, for that matter) will go the way DNA synthesis has gone recently. I am thereby referring to the rapid proliferation of commercial operations, which, for a fee, will provide those services perceived as tedious, boring, and time-consuming by the scientific community. My guess, at this point: DNA sequencing, probably; PCR, not very likely.

The next level of sophistication in PCR instrumentation will probably come as a breakthrough in improving the throughput, rather than the speed of the process itself. I believe that the basics have already been established with regard to performing PCR reactions within very short times; the challenge will be to combine that capability with the type of throughput required by routine diagnostics and genetic analysis, rather than by the huge number of samples handled by laboratories associated, for instance, with the Human Genome project.

In the meantime, as mentioned earlier, the emphasis on the part of instruments manufacturers is being put on attempting to eliminate the other traditional bottlenecks, namely the sample preparation steps as well as the post-PCR sample analysis. Rapid protocols, involving minimum hardware, are now available for sample preparation, although it appears that, after all, robots might be the way to go.

In post-PCR analysis, increasingly sophisticated detection methods are being implemented, among which I should mention capillary electrophoresis coupled with fluorescence detection, for its rapidity, sensitivity, and automation potential. In addition, CE requires a minuscule amount of sample to complete the analysis. Indeed, what good would it do to reduce the PCR sample volume to 10 or even 5 μl, as would be the case with capillary PCR, and still have to load the whole sample on a submarine agarose gel, just to see the product band?

So, in conclusion, just as in the current economic climate, we are well on our way to achieving the task: doing more with less—smaller samples volumes, reduced process times, and faster analysis methods requiring steadily less material.

References

Bataller A, Oste C (1994): *Biotechniques*. In preparation.

Gosden J, Hanratty D (1993): *Biotechniques* 15: 78–80.

Haase AT, Retzel EF, Staskus KA (1990): Amplification and detection of lentiviral DNA inside cells. *Proc Natl Acad Sci USA* 87:4971–4975.

Rys, Persing (1993): *ASM Annual Meeting Program Abstract* C2.22.

15

Rapid Cycle DNA Amplification

Carl T. Wittwer, Gudrun B. Reed, and Kirk M. Ririe

DNA amplification requires temperature cycling of the sample. From the viewpoint of the sample, the only relevant characteristics of a temperature cycler are its speed and homogeneity. How fast the sample temperature can be changed largely determines the cycle time. How uniform the sample temperature is affects reproducibility. As cycle speed increases, it becomes harder to maintain homogeneous temperatures within and between samples. Standard commercial instrumentation usually completes 30 cycles (94, 55, 74°C) in about 2–4 hr. A new "high-performance" system requires about half as much time and is reported to run two temperature profiles (60, 94°C) in a little over an hour (Haff et al., 1991). "Rapid cycle DNA amplification" as used here refers to completion of 30 cycles of amplification in 10–30 min. The physical (denaturation and annealing) and enzymatic (elongation) reactions of DNA amplification occur very quickly; with the proper instrumentation, amplification times can be reduced an order of magnitude from prevailing protocols.

Initial Development

Before commercial temperature cycling instrumentation was available, we started work on a thermal cycling system using capillary tubes with hot air temperature control (Wittwer et al., 1989). Our original instrument was designed to approximate the temperature profile and amplification of 100-μl samples in microfuge tubes transferred between water baths. Because of the low heat capacity of air, the thin walls and high surface area of capillary tubes, we realized that small volume samples could be cycled much faster than this if high velocity air were blown past the tubes. What effect rapid cycling would have on amplification was not known.

We modified our instrument for faster cycling of 10-μl samples (Wittwer et al., 1990). Total amplification times for 30 cycles were reduced to 10 min, and still specific amplified product was observed on ethidium bromide stained gels. Since there are six temperature/time variables in a typical three-temperature amplification protocol, what is the effect of changing each variable systematically? This

The Polymerase Chain Reaction
K.B. Mullis, F. Ferré, R.A. Gibbs, editors
© 1994 Birkhauser Boston

was difficult to determine previously because of long transition times between temperatures in other instruments.

Cycle Optimization

The optimal times and temperatures for the amplification of a 536-bp fragment of β-globin from genomic DNA were determined (Wittwer and Garling, 1991). Amplification yield and product specificity were optimal when denaturation (93°C) and annealing (55°C) times were less than 1 sec. There was no advantage to longer denaturation or annealing times, as long as the DNA was heat denatured before temperature cycling. Yield increased with longer elongation times, although there was little change above 10–20 sec. These results may be surprising, but merely reflect the poor match between most commercial instrumentation for DNA amplification and the physical/enzymatic requirements of the reaction.

Figure 15.1 compares four different sample temperature/time profiles and their resultant amplification products after 30 cycles. Profiles A and B were obtained on a standard heating block/microfuge tube system. The transitions between temperatures are slow and many nonspecific bands are present. Some of the nonspecific bands can be eliminated by limiting the time at each temperature (A vs B) within the limits of the instrument. Profiles C and D were obtained with the rapid air cycler. Amplification is specific, and although yield is maximal in C (60 sec elongation), it is entirely adequate in D (10 sec elongation).

The importance of annealing time on product specificity is systematically studied in Figure 15.2A. As annealing time increases, so do spurious, undesired amplification products. Not only is the time spent at annealing important, but long transition times (25 vs 9 sec) also increase nonspecific amplification, probably because of more time spent near the annealing temperature.

We have now amplified over 50 primer pairs by rapid cycling and the method seems generally applicable. We have never observed any advantage to extending denaturation times be-

yond the minimum possible, as long as template DNA is denatured before cycling. The best specificity is obtained with minimal annealing times, although in some amplifications there appears to be a tradeoff between specificity and yield. Using minimal denaturation and annealing times is convenient because it reduces the total number of temperature cycling variables for optimization from six to four. If a constant denaturation temperature of 94°C is used (DMSO may be needed for high GC sequences), only three variables remain. In most cases, an elongation temperature of 70–74°C works well. The exceptions in our hands are certain VNTR areas (Boerwinkle et al., 1989) and DNA extracted from paraffin blocks, both of which seem to amplify better at 65–70°C. Two variables remain, the elongation time and the annealing temperature. The elongation time seems loosely determined by the product length. Fragments around 100 bp usually require no specific elongation time; extension is apparently adequate during the transition from annealing to denaturation, even with rapid cycling (Fig. 15.2B). This extension during transition explains the recent popularity of two-temperature amplification; slower conventional cycling would provide more than enough time for the extension of much larger fragments. Elongation times of 5–20 sec are usually appropriate for fragments up to 500 bp, while up to 30 sec may be needed for a 1-kb amplification. Algorithms for the prediction of the remaining variable (annealing temperature) have been published (Rychlik et al., 1990), although their application to rapid cycling has not been thoroughly tested.

Amplification Additives

DNA amplification is robust and a variety of buffers and additives can be used without serious effect. These include Ficoll and electrophoresis indicator dyes to simplify gel loading directly out of capillary tubes (Wittwer and Garling, 1991). Bovine serum albumin seems to be most effective in preventing surface denaturation of the polymerase on glass capillary walls. Ethidium bromide can also be included

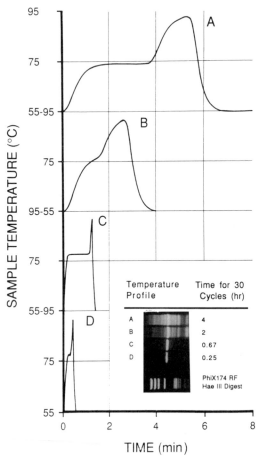

at concentrations used for staining gels (0.5 μg/ml) without apparent change in yield or specificity (Fig. 15.2C). This is surprising because of the known influence of ethidium bromide on DNA melting (Maeda et al., 1990). The potential for using ethidium bromide fluorescence during amplification as a monitor of double stranded DNA production is attractive. Figure 15.2D shows the relative fluorescence of reactions in capillary tubes before and after amplification. The capillary tubes were directly placed on a standard UV transilluminator. Although viral and plasmid amplifications can be monitored this way (with <5 ng starting DNA/10 μl reaction), background fluorescence from the larger amounts of DNA used in genomic amplifications (50–100 ng/10 μl) is quite high. With DNA nearly doubling each elongation step, direct measurement of the efficiency of each cycle might be possible. The end of elongation might even be triggered dynamically after a certain efficiency was achieved. Fluorescence monitoring could also control the number of cycles needed to achieve the fluorescence level for a particular yield. The effect of ethidium bromide on base incorporation error rate during DNA amplification has not been studied.

FIGURE 15.1. Comparison of standard heat block instrument (**A** and **B**) to rapid cycling instrumentation (**C** and **D**). Temperature–time profiles and amplification products obtained after 30 cycles of amplification of a 536-bp β-globin fragment from genomic DNA. Ten-microliter samples were electrophoresed through 1.5% agarose and stained with ethidium bromide. Sample temperature was monitored with a 0.2-mm-diameter thermocouple probe (IT-23, Sensortek, Clifton, NJ). Profiles **A** and **B** were obtained with 100-μl samples in microfuge tubes overlaid with 60 μl of mineral oil as recommended by the manufacturer (Perkin-Elmer Cetus DNA Thermal Cycler, Norwalk, CT). In **A**, a typical protocol is shown (heating block at 93°C for 1 min, 55°C for 2 min, and 74°C for 3 min). In **B**, the times were reduced so that the sample just momentarily reached denaturation and annealing temperatures (block at 55°C for 35 sec, 77°C for 45 sec, and 92°C for 35 sec). Profiles **C** (1 min elongation) and **D** (10 sec elongation) were obtained on 10-μl samples in capillary tubes in a custom rapid air cycler (Wittwer et al., 1990). Reprinted with permission of Eaton Publishing from *BioTechniques* (Wittwer and Garling, 1991).

Capillary Tubes versus Microfuge Tubes

The microfuge tube is the standard small container in molecular biology. However, it is a poor container for rapid temperature cycling. This is only partly because of wall thickness: GeneAmp™ tubes have a wall thickness of 0.51 mm, MicroAmp™ tubes, 0.30 mm, and standard glass capillary tubes, 0.20 mm. Just as important, the geometry of samples in conical tubes limits the available surface area for heating. The rate of heat transfer at any surface is directly proportional to the surface area. The sample geometry in microfuge tubes is not easily described, but it approaches a cone with its tip truncated by a hemisphere. For any given volume, a sphere has the lowest surface area. In contrast, both cylinders and sheets can

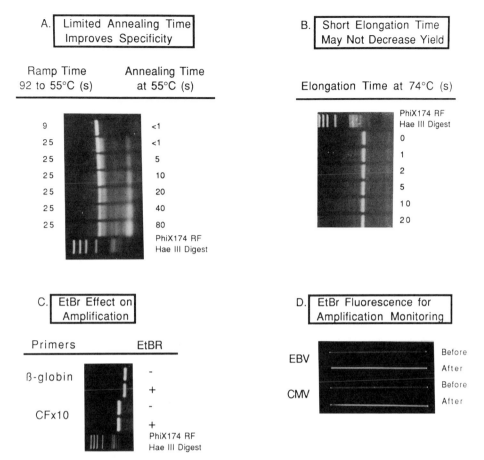

FIGURE 15.2. Amplification by rapid cycling: parameter optimization and use of ethidium bromide. (A) The effect of annealing time on the specificity of a β-globin fragment (536 bp) amplified from primers RS42 and KM29. Reprinted with permission of Eaton Publishing from *BioTechniques* (Wittwer and Garling, 1991). (B) The effect of varying elongation time on the yield of product (149 bp) from primers Y1.1 and Y1.2 (Kogan et al., 1987). Thirty cycles of amplification from 50 ng genomic DNA were performed with settings of 0 sec at 94°C, 0 sec at 55°C, and the time indicated at 74°C. At 0 sec elongation, the total amplification time was 9.8 min. (C) The presence of 0.5 μg/ml ethidium bromide in the amplification reaction does not seem to alter specificity or yield. The β-globin fragment was amplified from 50 ng genomic DNA and primers PC03 and PC04 (Saiki et al., 1985) by

35 cycles of 0 sec at 94°C, 0 sec at 55°C, and 10 sec at 74°C. Exon 10 of the cystic fibrosis gene (Riordan et al., 1989) was amplified from 50 ng genomic DNA and primers GACTTCACTTCTAATGATGA and CTCTTCTAGTTGGCATGCTT) by 40 cycles of 0 sec at 94°C, 0 sec at 45°C, and 10 sec at 74°C. (D) Photograph of UV transilluminated reaction mixtures containing 0.5 μg/ml ethidium bromide in capillary tubes before and after amplification. Five nanograms of DNA isolated from Epstein–Barr virus (EBV) or cytomegalovirus (CMV) cultures was cycled 30 times at 0 sec at 94°C, 0 sec at 50°C, and 10 sec at 74°C. A custom rapid hot air cycler (Wittwer et al., 1990) was used in A, with reactant concentrations as given previously (Wittwer and Garling, 1991). The Idaho Technology 1605 thermal cycler (Idaho Falls, ID) was used for all other amplifications.

be made to have an arbitrarily high surface area for any given volume if there is no restriction on the long dimension(s). A planar configuration would be appropriate for *in situ* amplification, for instance, between two microscope slide covers. A long cylinder (capillary tube) is more attractive for ease of sample addition and removal in routine DNA amplification.

The new "high-performance" amplification system (Haff et al., 1991) is probably the ultimate in heat-block, conical-tube amplification instruments. Its engineering is exquisite, but the technology is not well matched to rapid cycling as described here. A 10-μl sample in a MicroAmp^{TM} tube has less than 25% of the surface area of a 10-μl capillary tube (Fig. 15.3A vs D). Although the conical portion of the tube is in direct contact with the heating block, the hemispherical tip appears insulated from it by a pocket of still air. With the small sample volumes optimal for rapid cycling, much of the sample surface area is insulated rather than heated. It is also more difficult to predict the temperature of small samples because of a lower "thermal time constant" (Haff et al., 1991). Samples are said to be rapidly mixed by convection. Convection is caused by temperature differences within the sample, a problem seldom discussed but sure to affect amplification, at least rapid cycle amplification. Temperature gradients become more difficult to control and more important as the cycle time decreases. The temperature variation throughout a 10-μl sample in a commercial rapid air cycler (1605 Air Thermo-cycler, Idaho Technology, Idaho Falls, ID) is $\pm 1\,°C$ at all time points of a 30-sec cycle, measured by moving a 0.2-mm-diameter thermocouple through the sample in a 0.5-mm-diameter i.d. capillary tube. We do not know the within-sample temperature variation in other systems. It is not easy to measure because of the small volumes involved. Nevertheless, temperature gradients significant enough for "rapid mixing by convection" apparently occur. Finally, the realization that denaturation and annealing times can be reduced to a minimum is not widely recognized. Sophisticated control algorithms have been developed to carefully approach and hold these temperatures without

overshoot. Since denaturation and annealing temperatures do not need to be held, the transition to these temperatures can be at the maximal heating or cooling rate of the system. The next heating or cooling step can be triggered immediately when the target temperature is reached. This significantly speeds up cycle time by turning the denaturation and annealing "plateaus" into temperature "spikes" (Fig. 15.1).

Figure 15.3 compares the scale of different tubes and their obtainable temperature/time profiles with a 10-μl sample. A custom air cycler (Wittwer et al., 1990) was adjusted for temperatures of 93, 55, and 75°C with a 10 sec hold at elongation for each tube type. As the diameter of the tube increases, transition times and the total cycle time also increase. Although we cannot easily monitor conical tubes in our air cycler, some idea of the deterioration in temperature response with more globular samples is apparent.

Even though capillary tubes have many advantages for rapid cycling, many people initially have difficulty using them. Accessories for holding, handling, and labeling capillary tubes are not as developed as for microfuge tubes. Samples are best mixed in microtiter plates with U-shaped wells and can be quantitatively loaded by capillary action, assisted by tilting the plates. Although yield may sometimes be increased by siliconizing the tubes (SigmaCote^{TM} or others), this eliminates capillary action and is not routinely necessary. Capillary tubes holding up to 20 μl are available precut to length and are made of soft glass that can be readily sealed, not only with a torch or Bunsen burner, but with a cigarette lighter or candle. A candle is most convenient, although shielding from room air turbulence is necessary. Labeling, ordering, and handling the tubes have been problems. A simple device that holds eight capillary tubes at once at microtiter spacing is very useful. With this device, eight samples can be simultaneously loaded from a microtiter tray by capillary action, sealed, and cycled. After cycling, the ends of the tubes can be scored with a file and individually emptied into the wells of an analysis gel with a microaspirator. Sapphire or ce-

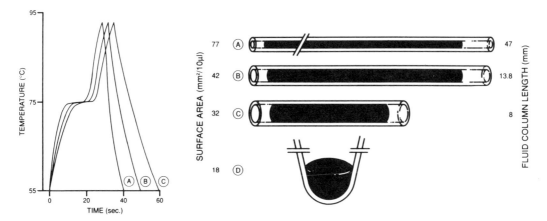

FIGURE 15.3. Effect of sample container on temperature response. Temperature–time tracings and scale drawings of 10-μl samples in three different capillary tubes. The tubes were Kimble KIMAX (Vineland, NJ) #46485-1 (**A**, 10 μl volume at 4.7 cm), #46485-15 (**B**, 34 μl volume at 4.7 cm), and #34500-99 (**C**, 59 μl volume at 4.7 cm). A scale drawing of a 10-μl sample in a MicroAmp™ tube of the Perkin-Elmer Cetus GeneAmp PCR System 9600 (Haff et al., 1991) is shown for comparison (**D**).

ramic glass cutters last longer than diamond-coated triangular files that tend to lose their edge. All of these items mentioned, as well as prescored capillary tubes are now commercially available (Idaho Technology).

Rapid Cycle Instrumentation

Early custom-made hot air cyclers have been previously described (Wittwer et al., 1989, 1990). They can be envisioned as temperature-controlled recirculating hair dryers. For rapid cooling, the circular air path is broken and room temperature air introduced. Air is unique as a heat transfer medium; it is inexpensive, readily available, easily mixed, and never makes a mess. If it is rapidly blown past a high surface area-to-volume sample, heat transfer is rapid. For rapid cycling, air velocities of about 1000 m/min are used. This is in contrast to the convection oven design of some "stirred air" thermal cyclers that actually have slower cycle times than heat block instruments.

The commercial rapid cycling instrument (Fig. 15.4) has several unique features that distinguish it from earlier custom rapid cyclers. The sample temperature is no longer moni-tored by a delicate miniature thermocouple in a mock sample (that tends to evaporate). A permanent tubular thermocouple probe is precisely matched in temperature response to the sample in a capillary tube that can hold up to 20 μl. Although instrument settings can be modified to amplify higher volumes in larger diameter tubes, temperature transition rates increase and the advantage of rapid cycling decreases (Fig. 15.3). With larger tubes, denaturation and annealing times must be held for several seconds to allow the sample temperature to catch up to the air temperature. This is similar to the problem of matching the sample and block temperatures in heat block instruments; we do not recommend larger tubes. Instead of a nichrome wire coil as a heat source, a 500-W halogen light bulb is used. The bulb irradiates the surface of a cylindrical sample chamber that is lined with a light-absorbing, heat-stable foam, that in turn heats the circulating air and the sample tubes (Fig. 15.4). The air flow pattern in the commercial instrument has also been modified for more uniform air speed and temperature.

Besides DNA amplification, rapid cycling should also be useful in cycle sequencing, and other amplification protocols such as the ligase

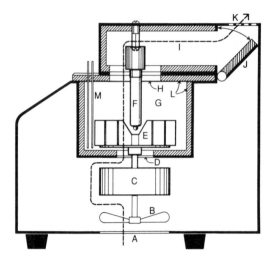

FIGURE 15.4. Schematic cross section of the Idaho Technology 1605 thermocycler. Samples in capillaries M are placed in cyclindrical air chamber G with turbulence created by fan blades E. Halogen lamp F irradiates the surface of chamber G, which is lined by light-absorbing foam L. Foam L heats the turbulent air, which in turn heats the samples in the capillaries. Room temperature air enters the instrument through vent A propelled by blade B. When the solenoid-operated door J is closed during heating, air exits through vent K without entering the sample chamber G or top chamber I. The top of chamber G contains top vent H of larger radius than bottom vent D, tending to draw air up through the sample chamber. However, no significant air can flow up through the chamber while door J is closed. The dotted line indicates the air flow path during cooling, initiated by opening door J. Cooling air flows around the fan motor C, through vent D, sample chamber G, vent H, top chamber I, and out through vent K. Rapid mixing of the air in chamber G by the fan blade E ensures spatial temperature homogeneity. All elements in the sample chamber are symmetric around the central vertical heating element (patents pending University of Utah/Idaho Technology).

chain reaction. Required times can be significantly reduced and specificity increased with rapid cycling. It is clear from Figure 15.2B that even current rapid cycle instrumentation may be too slow for the reactions comprising DNA amplification. Cycle times can be decreased further. More compact instruments can be built. Direct coupling to sensitive anal-

ysis systems is feasible. Rapid cycling only requires that the time-revered icons of heating blocks and conical tubes be left behind.

Note added in proof: After submission of this chapter, reports utilizing ethidium bromide for simultaneous amplification and detection in PCR have appeared (Higuchi et al., 1992, 1993). Others have since described gel loading dyes compatible with PCR (Hoppe et al., 1992). Rapid cycle DNA amplification has recently been used to increase the yield of long product amplifications (Gustafson et al., 1993), improve single base discrimination in allele specific PCR (Wittwer et al., 1993), reduce sequencing ambiguities in cycle sequencing (Swerdlow et al., 1993), minimize "shadow banding" in dinucleotide repeat amplifications (Odelberg and White, 1993), and improve quantitative PCR (Tan and Weis, 1992).

References

Boerwinkle E, Xiong W, Fourest E, Chan L (1989): Rapid typing of tandemly repeated hypervariable loci by the polymerase chain reaction: Application to the apolipoprotein B 3' hypervariable region. *Proc Natl Acad Sci USA* 86:212–216.

Gustafson CE, Alm RA, Trust TJ (1993): Effect of heat denaturation of target DNA on the PCR amplification. *Gene* 123:241–244.

Haff L, Atwood JG, DiCesare J, Katz E, Picozza E, Williams JF, Woudenberg T (1991): A high-performance system for automation of the polymerase chain reaction. *BioTechniques* 10:102–112.

Higuchi R, Dollinger G, Walsh PS, Griffith R (1992): Simultaneous amplification and detection of specific DNA sequences. *Bio/Technology* 10:413–417.

Higuchi R, Fockler C, Dollinger G, Watson R (1993): Kinetic PCR analysis: real time monitoring of DNA amplification reactions. *Bio/Technology* 11:1026–1030.

Hoppe BL, Conti-Tronconi BM, Horten RM (1992): Gel-loading dyes compatible with PCR. *BioTechniques* 12:679–680.

Kogan SC, Marie Doherty BS, Gitschier J (1987): An improved method for prenatal diagnosis of genetic diseases by analysis of amplified DNA sequences. *N Eng J Med* 317:985–990.

Maeda Y, Nunomura K, Ohtsubo E (1990): Differential scanning calorimetric study of the effect of intercalators and other kinds of DNA-binding drugs on the stepwise melting of plasmid DNA. *J Mol Biol* 215:321–329.

Odelberg SJ, White R (1993): A method for accurate amplification of polymorphic CA-repeat sequences. *PCR Meth Appl* 3:7–12.

Riordan JR, Rommens JM, Kerem BS, Alon N, Rozmahel R, Grzelczak Z, Zielenski J, Lok S, Plavsic N, Chou JL, Drumm ML, Iannuzzi MC, Collins FS, Tsui LC (1989): Identification of the cystic fibrosis gene: Cloning and characterization of complementary DNA. *Science* 245:1066–1073.

Rychlik W, Spencer WJ, Rhoads RE (1990): Optimization of the annealing temperature for DNA amplification in vitro. *Nucl Acids Res* 18:6409–6412.

Saiki RK, Scharf S, Faloona F, Mullis KB, Horn GT, Erlich HA, Chang CA (1985): Enzymatic amplification of β-globin genomic sequences and restriction site analysis for diagnosis of sickle cell anemia. *Science* 230:1350–1354.

Swerdlow H, Dew-Jager K, Gesteland RF (1993): Rapid cycle sequencing in an air thermal cycler. *BioTechniques* 15:512–519.

Tan ST, Weis JH (1992): Development of a sensitive reverse transcriptase PCR assay, RT-RPCR, utilizing rapid cycle times. *PCR Meth Appl* 2:137–143.

Wittwer CT, Garling DJ (1991): Rapid cycle DNA amplification: Time and temperature optimization. *BioTechniques* 10:76–83.

Wittwer CT, Fillmore GC, Hillyard DR (1989): Automated polymerase chain reaction in capillary tubes with hot air. *Nucleic Acids Res* 17:4353–4357.

Wittwer CT, Fillmore GC, Garling DJ (1990): Minimizing the time required for DNA amplification by efficient heat transfer to small samples. *Anal Biochem* 186:328–331.

Wittwer CT, Marshall BC, Reed GB, Cherry JL (1993): Rapid cycle allele-specific amplification: studies with the cystic fibrosis delta F508 locus. *Clin Chem* 39:804–809.

16

Automating the PCR Process

H.R. Garner

Introduction

The general diagnostic applicability of the PCR process, coupled with the needs of certain research programs or businesses that require the analysis of a massive number of samples, has introduced new challenges for the user and developers of PCR related technology (Mullis and Faloona, 1987). Specific program examples include the screening of various DNA libraries (in a variety of hosts) for the Human Genome Project, animal paternity testing, hybrid seed/animal research, and the genetic screening for genetic diseases or disease carriers in the clinical setting. As an example, yeast artificial chromosome (YAC) libraries (thousands of members) and cosmid libraries (tens of thousands of members) have been made from the 150 megabases (mb) chromosome 11 (libraries also exist for many of the chromosomes) (Yager et al., 1991; Landegren et al., 1988). The screening of a YAC library for positive cosmid clones corresponding to specific sequence tagged site (STS) sequences would require on the order of one million PCR reactions. In order to successfully use PCR as an analysis method for the Human Genome Project or other large scale screening efforts (drug development screening, blood bank screening) techniques must be developed to quickly process more samples than is typical today. The objective of this chapter is to discuss the problems encountered when a scale-up of the PCR process is to be done to obtain high-throughput and the solutions to those problems that are currently in place. For each of the examples just cited, many of the components of the PCR-based analysis and their scale-up to high sample throughput are the same. This chapter will use the PCR-based mapping component of the Human Genome Project as the example of note (see Fig. 16.1).

To obtain high sample analysis throughput several areas require work: (1) upstream reaction set-up, (2) thermal cycling, (3) downstream product detection, (4) cost control, and (5) computer analysis (product detection analysis and databasing, primer selection). Solutions in each of these areas were required because, although there are many hardware options available, either they do not match the needs, or, taken by themselves, transfer the sample analysis bottlenecks to one of the other areas.

The Polymerase Chain Reaction
K.B. Mullis, F. Ferré, R.A. Gibbs, editors
© 1994 Birkhauser Boston

FIGURE 16.1. As an example where sustained high-throughput PCR is required, the flow chart for the screening of YAC and cosmid libraries for positive clones, of which PCR is a major component of the work, is shown. Note that there are upstream processes (primer design from an STS sequence fragment, primer testing for specificity, etc.) and downstream processes (finished data entry into a database, analysis for consistency and map assembly).

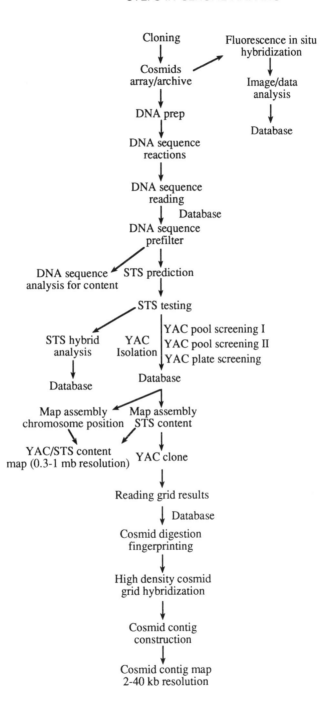

STEPS IN GENOME MAPPING

There are a few key concepts, some nonobvious, that emerge from the scale-up process:

1. Integrated automation, computer sample tracking and databasing are required.
2. The bottlenecks are sample assembly and detection, not thermal cycling.
3. There are tradeoffs among detection accuracy, speed, and cost.
4. Reaction volumes should be minimized to that of the detection or manipulation (pipetting) limit to control cost.
5. There are many myths (black art) about PCR; some have relevance and some do not. The general concept is that if the protocol requires very specific and touchy elements, it is probably not robust enough for scale-up for routine practice.
6. Different levels of laboratory throughput and purpose have different solutions.

It should also be noted that there is a difference between high-throughput and sustained high-throughput. To attain true, sustained high-throughput it is essential to develop an integrated approach with all processes upstream and downstream of thermal cycling. These should be seamless and in general require a minimum of human intervention or decision making. For example, if a particular run fails, which can be due to a host of reasons (failed equipment, bad reagents, poor quality target DNA, variation in the design of production of primers, etc.), then an automatic decision tree should be followed. In a production environment, fault analysis prior to beginning sustained production must be done. In general this means that with a sufficient number of positive and negative controls integrated into each step, process fault can be revealed, giving the technician immediate indications as to what must be adjusted prior to attempting the run again. What cannot be done in this environment is the inclusion of a large number of specific tests and adjustments into the process, which would bring sustained operation to a halt.

In the process of scaling up for high sample throughput, cost per sample becomes an important constraint. We have found that labor, amortization of capital equipment (robotics,

computers, scanners, cameras), and plasticware consumables become minor compared to reagent cost, specifically polymerase and synthetic oligonucleotides. The minimum amount of primers that can typically be manufactured or ordered is sufficient for complete screening of pooled libraries, which ultimately requires over 1000 PCR reactions per screening of a library. Much of the scaling up process involves reducing the reaction volume to minimize the amount of polymerase required. The minimum reaction volume (typically $5-10$ μl) is set by pipetting accuracy, minimum sustaining volumes during thermal cycling, and detection sensitivity limits. Even so, $0.10-$0.15 per sample is obtained, but this still leads to $1000+ per day operations cost to screen 10,000 samples a day (typical for laboratories performing $10-20$ library screening passes per day).

In the special case of screening libraries, cost is further controlled by minimizing the number of samples to be processed, maximizing the amount of information determined per pass, and maximizing the reliability of the primers used. The total number of samples is minimized by pooling the libraries to be searched prior to reaction assembly. We and others have performed statistical studies to determine the optimal pooling strategy (B. Miller, private communication; Evans, 1991). The optimal strategy is a function of several factors: the size of the starting library, the depth of the library (the number of hits expected per screening pass), the final number of pools that are assembled, and the number of screening passes to eliminate ambiguous hits (positives) to obtain the final answer. Complex multidimensional pooling strategies and complex remapping of samples to be assembled have been used to minimize the total number of pools, to represent a library and minimize the number of second and third pass screenings required to eliminate ambiguities. These also require more sophisticated analysis routines, but this is not significant once conversion to computerized automation has been implemented. The thermal cycling of several thousand samples at once usually consists of several actual experiments (many primer pairs, each used to independently screen the library). This is possible only if the thermal cycling condition (primer binding temperature) for the primers is the same. A primer design program is used to select the primers for the screen and also calculate the binding temperature. The use of these primer design programs has greatly increased our success rate. As an example, the program used in our lab is PRIMER, developed in the Human Genome Center at MIT. Using this program also minimizes the number of total failed screenings due to nonoptimized primer conditions. It should be emphasized that sometimes primers cannot be used reliably even if they are predicted to do so. This then requires a second experiment at a new binding temperature or the complete redesign of the primer pair from the original sequence from which the primer sequence was first generated. Primer design is still not completely understood.

Components of a High-Throughput Laboratory—A Human Genome Example

Just as the advent of the automated sequencing gel reader enabled the sequencing component of the international Human Genome Project to be begun, the PCR process has enabled the genome to be mapped, indeed a precursor to sequencing. Currently PCR-based and hybridization grid-based screening of the large clone libraries are the workhorses of the physical mapping effort, i.e., ordering the clone libraries to ultimately construct a contiguous and minimum set of clones that spans entire genomes. One of the most useful and ultimately long-lived approaches is based on the use of sequence tagged sites (STS), especially since this approach is based on a unique sequence, making it a permanent map marker and independent of the clone library on which it was derived or on which it is to be used to screen for clones. Construction of an STS requires the acquisition of some sequence from which PCR primers can be designed to pro-

duce a product of known length, and the testing of those primers for valid functionality. The essential beauty of the STS concept (Olson et al., 1989) comes from the ease in defining the site, permanence, and ease of use as a library screening starting point. The automatability of the PCR process is making it the process of choice (if not the only true choice at this level) for scaling up for completing the genome maps.

As mentioned earlier, there are several identifiable components required for a PCR-based screening analysis and each therefore requires special attention when scaling up. Those are DNA preparation, oligonucleotide production, reaction assembly, thermal cycling, product detection, and process clean-up.

DNA Preparation

The first and often time-consuming step required to perform multiple PCR-based screenings of a template library is preparation (extraction and purification) of template DNA from a clone library. Since typical clone libraries for Human Genome labs can contain between 3000 and 100,000 members (plasmids, cosmids, YACs, etc.), this can require considerable work. Typically, to reduce the total number of PCRs required to completely screen a library, pooling of the DNA is required, adding additional up-front work in assembling the pools, but this greatly reduces the time and cost of the subsequent screening passes.

The steps required in preparing the DNA templates are (1) a series of decisions must be made as to how the library will be stored and manipulated, (2) a pooling strategy must be determined, (3) calculations of the required culture volume (based on the total number of screenings to be conducted, clone copy number per cell, and yield) must be made, (4) sufficient consumables must be acquired, (5) cultures of each member in the clone library must be made, (6) the cultures must be pooled, (7) DNA usually must be extracted and purified from the pooled cultures, (8) these DNA pools must be stored and arranged for most efficient use during screening, and (9) positive, negative, and other controls must be integrated into the pool storage medium.

To attain true, efficient high-throughput, analysis samples must be contained in a storage medium (plasticware) that can be manipulated robotically. This means some type of microwell plate is used; there are several choices, and each may be appropriate at different steps in the process—96-well, 96-deep well (1–2 ml volume) 384-well, and 864-well. In our case, clone stocks are stored in both 96-well and 864-well plates—864-well for preservation and 96-well for daily use. A Beckman Biomek 1000 with a side loader (additional storage for plates and pipette tips) is used to dispense growth media into 96-well plates of either 1 or 2 ml volume. These are inoculated from the stock clone storage (warmed, glycerol stock solution) using a 96-pin transfer tool designed to transfer 10 to 100 nl. Cultures are grown overnight in incubators with or without shaking. We have found that shaking and oxygenation affect the ultimate yield by roughly a factor of two, not enough to justify additional work (shaking or oxygenation) that is not easily automated, requires additional instrumentation, or risk of cross-contamination. There are many formulations for growth media known and these are commercially available that can also affect the cell density (yield) also by factors of approximately 2.

Each library member is cultured independently because of the various growth rates of each clone and competition among each clone. The DNA cloned into them affect their vitality.

Following culturing, a decision must be made whether to pool cultures or extract the DNA first. We choose to extract the DNA first. The disadvantage is that there are a larger number of DNA minipreps that must be done. The advantages are that individual DNA stocks from cultures are saved and are available for testing or verification of "hits" from the PCR analysis of the pools. The cultures grown in 96-well deep-well plates are ready for robotic processing using a dedicated DNA extraction system named Prepper, PhD. This extraction robot is centrifuge-based, can process viral, bacterial, or yeast cultures, and operates autonomously at a rate of 48 samples per hour (Garner et al., 1992; Armstrong and Garner, 1992).

Pooling involves a mapping of samples within a group to condense a library so that positive members can be found with less work (B. Miller, private communications; Evans, 1991). This simplest pooling scheme would be to sum (add) all the members of a given row and column. In the case of a single positive its coordinate within a rectangular array can be determined from the intersection of its X and Y coordinates, i.e., from two positive pools. The amount of work to discover this positive is reduced from X times Y to X plus Y PCR-based tests. Pooling schemes can be highly dimensional and complex. There is a tradeoff between reducing the number of pools to be analyzed and the amount of information that must be maintained to obtain unambiguous answers (see Fig. 16.2 for a description of how unambiguous answers occur and see Fig. 16.3 for a summary of the performance of some example pooling schemes).

In our case, after miniprepping, the DNA extracts (or in other cases, before miniprepping, the cultures) still in 96-well plates are pooled in one of two ways, robotically or using specially designed pooling systems. Again, each has advantages and disadvantages, and there are also functions of the size of the library, library depth (redundancy, coverage), and pooling strategy. The advantages of using robotic pooling are they can be programmed for any pooling scheme and plasticware, the programs can be changed, robots can usually run autonomously, and if programmed correctly they do not make mistakes. The disadvantages are they are costly, can be slow, and can be hard to program. We have used the Beckman Biomek 1000 SL running under the Windows-based Nemisis and Biomek Quick Basic control software to perform pooling (Biomek robot; S. Reifel, private communication). Scientists at the Salk Institute for Biological Studies have recently produced a set to Teflon pooling manifolds designed to pool the rows, columns, and diagonals of 96-well plates using a 96-tip pipettor tool (J. Quackenbush, private communication). The advantages of

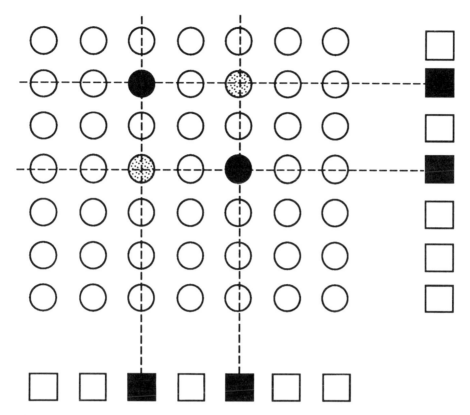

FIGURE 16.2. More than one hit can result in ambiguous information that cannot be resolved without a second tier of screenings of all the possible combinations resulting from the positives found in the pooled data. There are two true positive hits (black dots) within this array of 49 possible wells. There are a total of 14 horizontal and vertical pools (squares). The two positives generate 4 "hits" (positives) within the pools as shown by the black squares. Note that because there are 2 hits within this array, there are 4 possible combinations derived from the 4 positives in the pools. Therefore there are 2 nonpositives (dashed dots) that can be detected only by an additional round of screening for this simple pooling scheme.

this approach are that it is quite fast, inexpensive, and reliable. The disadvantage is that it works only for a fixed plate geometry and pooling scheme, neither of which is a real hinderance. The 96-well format is a standard and the pooling scheme with rows, columns, and diagonals appears to strike a good balance between the total number of pools that need be made and the unresolvable hits that occur during a screen that would then require a second tier of screenings to complete the analysis.

Oligonucleotide Production

For some applications of PCR in a high-throughput mode the number of oligonucleotides required is not an issue. Genetic screening done repeatedly on multiple samples using the same primer sets is an example. However, for screening libraries as is done in mapping projects associated with the Human Genome Project, large numbers of unique oligonucleotide primers are required. This introduces a need to investigate not only the science

Pooling Scheme	Number of 'Hits' (N-hit)								
	2	3	4	5	6	7	8	9	10
Array and recorded array	0.	0.	0.025	0.11	0.28	0.51	0.74	0.89	0.97
Array broken into 4 small arrays	0.22	0.55	0.83	0.96	0.99	1.	1.	1.	1.
Array only	0.93	1.	1.	1.	1.	1.	1.	1.	1.

FIGURE 16.3. The fraction of ambiguities (uncertain calls) as a function of the pooling scheme. Since all pooling schemes result in some lost information, random events such as hits in adjacent pooled columns, rows, and diagonals (or other remapping geometries) can be modeled statistically using numerical simulation techniques because they cannot always be determined in a closed algorithmic form. The advantage of different mapping reordering of the samples within a pooling scheme compared to the simplest pooling scheme, i.e., pooling of rows and columns (array only) is shown. Dividing the array into 4 subsets somewhat reduces the number of unresolvable solutions without a further screening pass. A pooling scheme (array and reordered array) with a minimum data loss reordering such as pooling rows, columns, and diagonals has the smallest number of unresolvable redundancies. N-hit is the total number of true positives found in the library in the first pass of the screen. This simulation is for a 29 × 29 member library interrogated by 10,000 random arrays of possible hits.

and development issues, but also business issues. Oligonucleotides can be ordered from commercial vendors that simply provide the service of synthesis using commercially available hardware. The cost is typically approximately $3.00 per base, however, for large bulk orders or guaranteed regular orders of a large number of oligonucleotides, there are very significant discounts available. Recent competition has made discounting so competitive that one must seriously consider these options before establishing oligonucleotides synthesis in-house.

Currently, there are a number of vendors that offer multicolumn synthesis machines for sale. However, for labs that consume 50 to 100 custom oligonucleotides a week, this implies that several machines are necessary, along with the cost of reagents, servicing, and operations personnel. There are several groups that have recently demonstrated or are near demonstrating very high-volume (96-column equivalent) machines (M. Melnick, private communication; J. Jaklevic, private communication). These devices are still based on the standard phosphoramadide chemistry, but have introduced new geometries that avoid the need for use-once, throw-away columns with enclosed beads. One of these new devices uses beads attached to a set of small tubes that are dipped into the various synthesis fluids. Another device uses frit-bottomed microwell plates (96 well) in which fluids are systematically added and vacuumed away. Beads on which the oligonucleotides are attached are added to the wells, and the final product is liberated from the beads and recovered for use in the last step. A unique oligonucleotide is synthesized in each well, and the order of the bases is determined by the sequence of the fluids being added in each round of synthesis. The fluids are added from a set of nozzles. The wells of the plate are moved beneath the appropriate nozzle on an X–Y motion table. These or similar devices are in the prototype stage, but should be available commercially in 1994.

Reaction Assembly

To assemble the PCR reaction components (Taq, dNTPs, primers, buffers) in a high-throughput mode, a robotic pipetting station is essential. Currently, the Beckman Biomek 1000 can do this quite well and with all the available types of plasticware. Custom robotic stations that incorporate the assembly function with the thermal cycling and detection functions are also in construction (see Fig. 16.9).

The characteristics of the Biomek workstation that make it the machine of choice now is that it can, using an 8 channel pipettor transfer fluids with submicroliter accuracy, address the various plasticware (including the 864-well, 20 μl/well plate) and it now operates using an icon-based (Nemisis and Biomek QuickBasic) user interface with all the necessary controls.

To assemble reactions in the 864-well plate, master mixes of the PCR components minus the template DNA are dispensed from a common reservoir using a modified MP 20 pipetting tool that is of higher precision and accepts the smaller Rainin P-10 pipetting tips that work well with the 2-mm-diameter wells of the 864-well plate. Following the distribution of the master mixes, the template DNA can be added to the wells in two ways. Using an 864-pin replicator tool (10 nl transfer volume) and a master plate (also 864 well) containing the pooled DNA, the template can be transferred in-mass in a single motion. For template DNA of insufficient concentration or storage in another type of plasticware, standard pipetting is done again using the modified MP-20 tool or modified P-20 (single tip) tool (see Fig. 16.4).

The final remaining issue is the sealing technique. There are two options that work equally well and each has certain advantages. First, an oil overlay can be added to the top of the assembled PCR reaction. This is usually followed by a short, low-speed centrifugation to guarantee a sealed oil overlay and eliminate bubbles in the reaction that will expand and contract during thermal cycling, possible forcing the reaction fluids from the 20-μl well. The other method of sealing is simply to use tape. The tape must have an adhesive that works to temperatures above 100°C, does not interfere with the PCR process, and seals reliably. We have found that some commercial plastic book tapes that are 3 in. wide work well. Beckman has recently developed a metal tape and adhesive that is designed for this process (J. Quint, private communication). The advantage of metal tape is that it need not be removed after thermal cycling, thus possibly introducing cross-contamination. The metal tape can be punctured by a standard pipettor or the pipettor tools on the Biomek 1000. The air thermal cycling oven allows one to easily use this tape sealing method because the lid (tape), plate, and liquid are all at uniform temperature, thus eliminating condensation on the tape. Elimi-

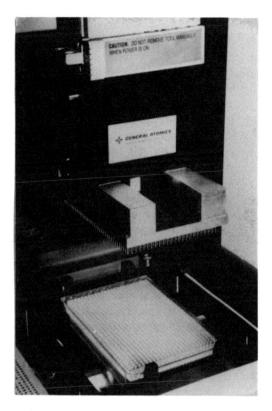

FIGURE 16.4. A new class of special new robotic tools (pipettors, detectors, automatic gel loaders) is required to work with these large sample numbers and small volumes. Shown is a custom Beckman Biomek tool that is used to transfer 10 nl volumes using pins that can simultaneously transfer from one 864-well plate to another. This tool is used to transfer template DNA from a pooled source plate to the plate in which the thermal cycling will be done. This tool is also useful to spot hybridization grid samples on membranes.

nating the oil overlay is very beneficial; sample handling and separation of the oil and sample for downstream processes are simplified.

Thermal Cycling

DNA amplification has been demonstrated in a number of sample formats: microfuge tubes, capillaries, and microwell plates (Wittwer et al., 1990; Haff et al., 1990; Garner and Armstrong, 1993). Of these, only microwell plates are readily amenable to automation—robot handling, storage, and sample tracking. A number of types of temperature-resistive polycarbonate plates are available, ranging from thin-wall 96-well vac-u-formed plates to 864-well injection molded plates. These plates can be thermal cycled in various commercial and prototype thermal cyclers. To attain our objective of sustained, high-throughput operations of 10,000 PCR samples per day, it was necessary to use 864-well plates that have a 9-fold higher well density than standard microwell plates. In this way only 12 plates need be manipulated to achieve our throughput objective.

There are only a few options for thermal cycling machines that can process samples in the plate format. First, there are commercially available thermal cycling machines with heated and cooled blocks on which thin-walled 96-well plates can be processed. These offer a substantial increase in processing speed above the typical machines that process only microfuge tubes. At the next level of throughput are a couple prototype devices (E. Lander, private communication; J. Jaklevic, private communication). The first device is a "waffle iron" machine used at the Human Genome Center at MIT. That machine is basically an assembly of 16 heating blocks that can accept 96-well plates and cycle them rapidly (~ 2 min cycle time). This device has also been interfaced with a linear robot that also assembles the reactions. The second device, operational at Lawrence Berkeley Laboratories, again processes 96-well, thin-wall plates. This device can currently handle only one plate, but the cycle time is shorter, approximately 1 min. That machine functions by switching water from four different temperature reservoirs and forcing the water past the bottom of the plate that is sealed to a manifold. There are plans for that device to be interfaced with a robot system as well. The third type of device is the air thermal cycler, for example, the BioTherm BioOven II. This is the device that is used to process samples in the 864-well format. That device functions by forcing heated air past up to 6 plates held in a rotisserie in the machine. The function of the rotisserie is to guarantee plate-to-plate and well-to-well temperature uniformity. The advantages of this oven is the ease in which it can be interfaced to a robot, the uniform temperature achievable at the top and bottom of each plate well (thus eliminating

the need for an oil overlay to control condensation), it is inexpensive ($< \$5,000$), the temperature feedback sensor is not imbedded in a sample (it is in a mock sample plate with identical thermal properties as the plate and sample being processed), and any plate geometry can be immediately processed in the machine. Programming this type of machine is very similar to the standard block thermal cycler (see Fig. 16.5). The major disadvantage is that the machine has a long cycle time set by the plasticware, not the properties of the machine, 10–12 min, for the 864-well plate. This cycle time is long because the thermal mass of the 864-well plate is high. A long cycle time ensures temperature uniformity from sample to sample within a plate. Since it is possible to process 10,000 samples per day with a single machine, this long cycle time is not prohibitive.

Product Detection

With robotics like the Beckman Biomek 1000, air oven thermal cyclers like the BioTherm BioOven II, and unique plasticware like the Helix 864-well microwell plate it is possible to assemble and thermal cycle thousands of samples per day; however, without a suitable detection scheme this throughput is wasted. The primary method for detection of PCR products is electrophoresis gels. However, even with robot-assisted gel loading and computer-assisted gel reading it is still difficult to efficiently measure the results from 10,000 PCRs per day using electrophoresis gels. Other alternatives include Oligo-ligation assays (OLA) and ELISA-based methods (Nickersion et al., 1990). Although these methods are very specific, they can add additional cost and work to a library screening effort because they require additional oligonucleotides to be manufactured and additional chemistry to be performed. We have developed a scheme applicable to library screening and genetic disease screening. The essence of our high throughput detection system is to prescreen the PCR reactions for the production of dsDNA. This prescreen is done directly in the plate in which the PCRs were assembled and thermal cycled by the addition of ethidium bromide and subsequent detection

Step	Function
1	controls active
2	flag 1 off 0:00:00
3	asurd soak discrete 1
4	flag 1 on 0:00:05
5	tuneset 2
6	time seg 0:00:01 sp 92
7	time seg 0:01:00 sp 92
8	label 1
9	tuneset 2
10	time set 0:00:01 sp 92
11	time seg 0:01:00 sp 92
12	tuneset 2
13	time seg 0:00:01 sp 55
14	time seg 0:01:00 sp 55
15	tuneset 2
16	time seg 0:00:01 sp 72
17	time seg 0:01:00 sp 72
18	loop count 30 label 1
19	tuneset 2
20	time seg 0:00:01 sp 72
21	time seg 0:01:00 sp 72
22	tuneset 2
23	time seg 0:00:01 sp 30
24	time seg 0:01:00 sp 30
25	flag 1 off 0:00:00
26	controls off
27	end

FIGURE 16.5. This program is utilized to perform up to 5184 PCR reactions at a time (six 864-well plates with a 10 μl reaction volume). This program is for the Biotherm II Oven, an air-based oven, and the only one currently available that can immediately be used to process large numbers of samples. The program above is in the "language" of the controller used by the system, however, recently a new version of the oven with a modern menu-driven controller has become available. Specifically note that the feedback parameters (temperature ramp speed, overshoot control, etc.) are contained within the parameter, "tuneset." In this case because of the large thermal mass of the 864-well plate, a conservative (slow ramp rate) tune set of level 2 is used.

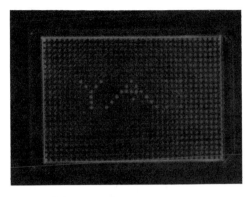

FIGURE 16.6. The basis for sustained high-throughput operations is that all PCR-based operations are done within a microwell plate: reaction assembly, library (template) storage, thermal cycling, and detection. This is a photograph of an 864-well microplate that dramatically shows the ability to detect positive PCR reactions via dsDNA detection. In this case, the first two letters of "YAC" and 4 dots defining the "C" are positive and the remaining dots in the "C" are negative.

on a UV light box. In our case, this includes a video camera and document scanner for computer-aided positive and negative selection (see Fig. 16.6 for a view of the appearance of positive and negative samples identified by dsDNA–ethidium bromide stain detection and Fig. 16.7 for a description of the HelixBlot software used to automate the detection and archival of the resulting data). This greatly reduces the number of necessary gel runs. For library screenings, the number of resulting gel runs scales with the depth (redundancy) of the library divided by the total number of pools involved in the screen. This can be a factor of 10 to 100. To guarantee that there are no false positives (which are much more detrimental than false negatives when screening libraries), after detection and cataloging all the positives based on dsDNA content, these data are downloaded to the Biomek robot for automatic loading of the appropriate putative positive PCR reactions on gels for verification of product size.

For this scheme to be robust (work for a variety of primers and libraries being screened) it was necessary to optimize the components of the PCR mixture and the amount of ethidium bromide added to the reaction mixture. For our case the total reaction volume in the 864-well plates is 10 μl. Two microliters of ethidium bromide dye is added after thermal cycling (see Fig. 16.8 for a graph showing the effect on sensitivity for various concentrations of ethidium bromide added to the PCR reaction volume). Starting from the standard conditions specified within the Perkin-Elmer PCR kit, we found that decreas-

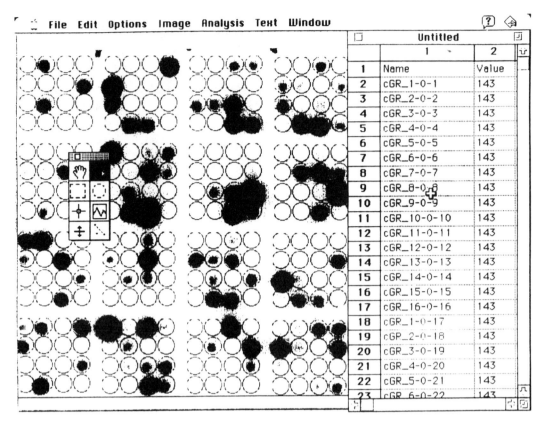

FIGURE 16.7. HelixBlot, a Macintosh-based software package designed to perform hybridization grid analysis and microplate reading. In this example, a hybridization grid (autorad) has been scanned into the computer, saved as a TIFF file, and is being evaluated. A variety of densitometry tests are conducted and the results entered into a spreadsheet that can be exported to databases or used as the basis of subsequent robot control (selection of positives for subsequent gel-based product verification). This dedicated hardware has all the standard Macintosh features that lead to enhanced productivity: menu-driven operation, multiple windows, automatic positive/negative (and flagged maybe) calls with final operator editing. Premade analysis grids for microplates are first aligned by the operator before evaluation is begun; the entire operation requires only 1 min with a few minutes for inspection of the calls by the operator. The results are held in a standard spreadsheet table that can be exported to a variety of standard commercial databases.

ing the recommended amount of primers (250–500 nM), increasing the amount of *Taq* slightly (~2× or 0.05 units/μl PCR volume) and increasing the amount of template can greatly reduce the competing processes that contribute the background. Background limits the dynamic range of the detection and thus the intensity-based separation between a positive and negative. Those competing processes are primer dimer formation and nonspecific amplification. After adjusting the component concentrations, we find that we can typically achieve an intensity difference of 5 to 10 times between a positive and negative, quite easily measured visually or with computer vision systems. The one complication that applies specifically to using this technique for screening libraries with a variety of primer pairs is that the difference between positives and negatives changes slightly from primer to primer. The overall offset value for the intensity varies, making it necessary to adjust the detection threshold for making the call for each primer pair being used. However, in the software we

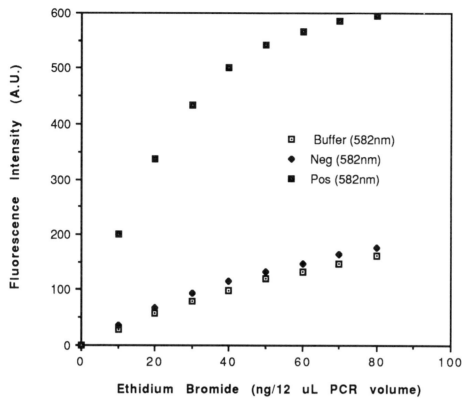

FIGURE 16.8. The first pass detection following thermal cycling is done by measuring the presence or absence of dsDNA. For this step, robust conditions that minimize the sample-to-sample variations not only within a particular run, but from run to run, are developed. To obtain the largest difference between a true positive and a true negative, parametric studies of the target concentration, primer concentration, polymerase concentration, and ethidium bromide concentration were made. Shown here is the fluorescence intensity for a true positive and true negative and fluorescence of the buffer/ethidium bromide mixture only. It is important to obtain not only the maximum fluorescence intensity, but also minimize the intensity variation due to dye pipetting error; therefore, an ethidium bromide concentration of 5–7 ng/μl is used.

use to make the calls (HelixBlot), this can easily be adjusted and thus it is easy to achieve sustained high-throughput detection.

Process Clean-up

In any production line environment there is always a component to the process that involves handling the irregularities, data finishing, and quality assurance. This is a challenging part of any analysis because it is difficult to anticipate the types of problems that can arise. There certainly are a few that can be provided for from the onset: (1) PCR failure can occur for a number of reasons, including bad chemicals and bad thermal cycling conditions. In each screen there are positive and negative controls built in as additional samples. If these fail, we know that the entire run is unreliable. In that case the entire screening for a given set of primers is repeated, with fresh chemicals. Primers are chosen and tested prior to screening in a separate set of reactions against possible library contaminants (mouse, yeast) and total human DNA to select the best conditions for the thermal cycling (annealing temperature). (2) The second type of error is detected after the data have been taken, i.e., the final results of the screening are inconsistent or conflicting. This is usually an indication of an excessive false-positive rate or to some extent an excessive false-negative rate. It can also indicate, for example, that the clones within a library are not intact, i.e., they contain rearrangements, chimeras, or microdeletions. There are a number of ways this is resolved; first the original screening results (raw data) can be viewed again for computer or reader error, and second, the library members in question can be reevaluated (rescreened).

It is apparent from the above failure modes that considerable effort must be allotted to handle these problems. Although the primary data screening of libraries can be very quick, a considerable fraction of time can be consumed in resolving difficulties, thus slowing the effective screening rate. For experiments or diagnostics that do not involve a continual stream of new primers, genetic screening for example, some of these problems will not arise, so the effective throughput can be quite high.

Dispelling Some Myths

Trial-and-error and black magic are often components of a PCR analysis in the lab, however, high-throughput automated labs require a high degree of first time successes in the experimental conditions and therefore must be based on rugged, flexible protocols. One consequence of developing a high-throughput PCR-based screening process—adapting existing protocols to make them automation friendly, performing systematic tests, and developing methods to control cost and simplify PCR product detection—is that a number of interesting facts (to some, opinions) have surfaced. Several groups involved in similar research have also made observations. Since we are talking about myths here, I am certain some researchers and some manufacturers will debate these comments, so I suggest researchers reading this section think about them and then make their own decision.

Some myths:

1. Thermal cycler cycle time and ramp rate are important. Perhaps for the typical researcher that sets up an experiment and needs immediate results, these parameters may be valid measures. For high-throughput labs, the reaction set up, analysis of results, and smooth, seamless operation play a more important role. There are three important things to be realized about thermal cycling: first, the plasticware plays the major role in setting the ramp rate for temperature changes. Measurements of the thermal transport diffusion times and the plasticware geometry determine the maximum ramp rate without sacrificing uniformity. Second, if it is possible to complete the thermal cycling of 5000 samples in 6 hr, what does it matter if another machine with a faster cycle time can do 30 samples in 1 or 2 hr. Third, tests of the efficacy of *Taq* polymerase show that there is no significant degradation in functionality in going to plasticware geometries that require longer cycle times, provided that the time spent above 90°C is minimized. Further, 35 cycles are possible without significant loss of fidelity or gain, thus increasing the sensitivity of screening experiments.

2. Advertisements would lead you to believe that there are large differences in thermal stable polymerases. In our hands and those of others, no major differences in the functionality of various brands have been observed. However, there are differences that can be of importance; for example, buffer solutions provided with polymerases vary. Promega's buffer contains Triton-X as a wetting agent. The presence of this chemical is ordinarily not important for amplification action (but Promega thinks it is important for something), however, for our detection scheme, it is a disaster. Triton-X, even unbound, fluoresces heavily for the combination of excitation and emission wavelengths (300 and 500 nm) used to detect bound ethidium bromide. At the concentrations used in the buffer, the signal from this component dominates by over an order of magnitude, making it impossible to use fluorescent-based bulk detection with this buffer. Also, because many manufacturers in this competitive market devise proprietary formulations for their polymerase so-

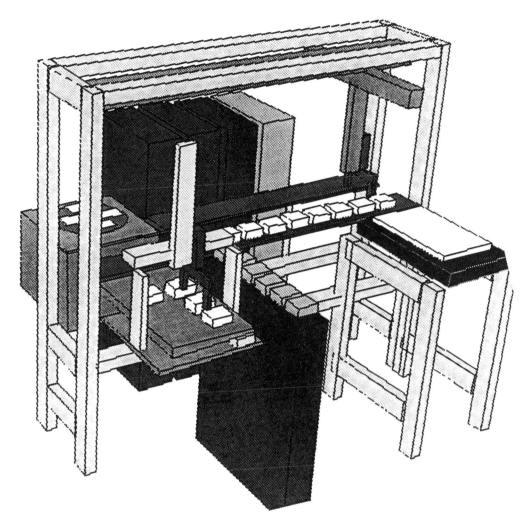

FIGURE 16.9. This is a 3-D rendering of the Genome Automation System, a dedicated high-throughput robot for the screening of genomic libraries via PCR and the assembly and thermal cycling of sequencing reactions prior to sample measurement on an automated gel-based reader (Applied Biosystems Inc. 373A sequencer). This system has modules for complete independent operation: sample storage, sample incubation, thermal cycling, precision pipetting station, centrifuge, scanner, and video detection subsystem. This system is an integration of modules that have demonstrated high-throughput operations independently.

lutions and buffers, often complications can arise that are difficult or time consuming to track down. It would help all involved if suppliers gave more information to the users, but proprietary restrictions preclude this. We have noted two other things of interest with regard to polymerases. First, there appears to sometimes be a noticeable batch-to-batch variation in polymerases/ buffers that affect functionality (yield). In general, it is recommended that large batches be bought and then tested against a known standard once delivered. Second, one important variable we have found that can often improve the sensitivity (product gain vs. background gain) is the polymerase concentration. Although the polymerase is the single most costly item in high-throughput experiments, we use up to double the concentration recommended in amplification kits.

3. The reaction storage temperature after thermal cycling is important. This is not true. The provision for low temperature storage (4°C) is apparently a carryover from the initial design descriptions for the original thermal cycling machines at Cetus, prior to knowing all the details of how PCR functions and how it would be used (K. Mullis, private communication). Manufacturers of all the various thermal cyclers confirm this because some have subroom temperature cooling, and some do not. This is particularly true for the class of thermal cycling systems based on an air oven. Our experiments using this type of air oven confirm that a postcycling holding temperature of 25°C (room temperature) is adequate for sustaining the products and reaction such that it can be detected hours or days following thermal cycling. It is now routine in a lab that is operating in a sustained high-throughput fashion to set up reactions and begin thermal cycling in the evening. Air ovens with longer cycle times (set by the thermal transport through plasticware) typically take 10 to 12 min/cycle, i.e., approximately 6 hr to complete cycling. So it is efficient to process samples at night, unattended. Product detection is done the next day, after typically 12 hr at room temperature with no change in the product integrity or detection sensitivity.

4. Reaction assembly must be done just prior to thermal cycling. This is not true. It is most efficient to run a high-throughput lab as a factory in an assembly-line fashion. So, typically, reaction assembly is done just prior to thermal cycling. However, we conducted a sensitivity study for the time between assembling all the reaction components (*Taq*, template, primers, dNTPs, buffer) and thermal cycling. We have found that samples can be stored at 4°C for months (3 months was the longest time studied) prior to thermal cycling with no noticeable change in the amount or quality of the product or any other aspect of the

PCR analysis. It should also be noted that current robotics used to assemble the PCR reaction components cannot keep up with the thermal cycling of samples in an air oven, so again it is not anticipated that assembled reactions will need extensive storage. However, some labs that do most of the work manually may not have the necessary thermal cycler capacity and may want to store samples ready for cycling.

5. Special precautions such as aerosol filter tips are required to eliminate cross-contamination. Not true, other things are much more important. There are many places in assembling PCR reactions where cross-contamination can occur—DNA extraction/purification, DNA template pooling, and template distribution to the PCR reaction mixture. Since PCR is a very sensitive assay, it is important to minimize this cross-contamination. The precautions we take are periodic decontamination of robotic tools, design of robotic manipulations to minimize splashing or aerosol generation, plasticware is never cleaned and reused, and the areas where master mixes of PCR reaction components (everything minus the template) are kept sterile (clean, air flow control, or in a biological hood).

6. Not all thermal cyclers were created equal. Now, this is indeed true. There are many suppliers of thermal cyclers that work on a number of different heating/cooling principles (block machines, air ovens, Peltier heaters/coolers, circulating fluids). Other publications have pointed out the differences in these machines (Linz, 1990). I submit that since all these machines can be used to do PCR, these variations are minor. What is important is the accuracy of the programmed target temperatures and that the variations from one brand to another are known so that conditions for experiments can be reliably exchanged. Just prior to purchasing a new block type device that we use for primer characterization, supplies checking, and secondary screening, we evaluated all the leading brands with a calibrated thermal couple and chart recorder and found (1) there were wide variations in the actual

temperatures reached for given programmed temperatures, enough to require
adjustments in programmed experimental
conditions from machine to machine, (2) we
noticed variations from device-to-device
within a brand of cyclers, (3) price was no
indicator of temperature accuracy, and (4)
overshoot conditions also varied. Let the
buyer beware. We bought an MJ Research
block thermal cycler.

7. High quality/purity DNA templates are required for reliable amplification. This is not
true. Some users of PCR, forensic scientists, for example, require many cycles or a
second round of amplification to have the
necessary sensitivity (without sacrificing
selectivity). Some users performing library
screening have found that one can make
very simple, crude DNA preparations prior
to amplification with regular success. Simple cell lysis to release the DNA is sufficient
(R. Drmanac, private communication).
Sometimes this is not even required; for
example, phage DNA that is normally ex-
truded from the cell can be amplified directly from diluted aliquotes of the growth
media. The one important sensitive parameter in these approaches is control of the
amount (concentration) of the DNA that is
transferred to the reaction mixture for amplification. Failure can occur from both too
little or too much template DNA (or possibly too much interfering debris). To minimize problems, it is imporatnt to reproducibly grow the cultures to be used in the
screening process.

Acknowledgments. Much of the work summarized here was funded either internally by General Atomics or by the National Institutes of
Health—National Center for Human Genome
Research. The author specifically wishes to
thank Dr. Glen Evans at the Salk Institute for
Biological Studies who contributed much, including Figure 16.1. Mary Petrowski, Dan
Kramarsky, and Barbara Armstrong conducted
much of the at-the-bench work involving scaling up the PCR process and now its utilization.

Figures 16.2 and 16.3 were produced with Dr.
Bob Miller, a theoretical physicist at General
Atomics.

References

Armstrong B, Garner HR (1992): Analysis of protocol variations on DNA yield. *GATA* 9(5–6):
134–139.

Biomek robot is available from Beckman Instruments.

Drmanac R, Private communication, Argonne
National Laboratories.

Evans G (1991): Combinatoric strategies for
genome mapping. *BioEssays* 13:39–44.

Garner HR, Armstrong B, Kramarsky D (1992):
High-throughput DNA prep system. *GATA* 9(5–
6):127–133.

Garner HR, Armstrong B (1993): High-throughput
PCR. *BioTechniques* 14(1):112–115.

Haff L, Atwood JG, DiCesare J, Katz E, Picozza E,
Williams JF, Woudenberg T (1990): A high-performance system for automation of the polymerase chain reaction. *BioTechniques* 10:102–
112.

Jaklevic J: Private communication, Lawrence
Berkeley Laboratories.

Jaklevic J, Pollard M: Private communication,
Lawrence Berkeley Laboratories.

Landegren U, Kaiser R, Caskey C, Hood L (1988):
DNA diagnostics—molecular techniques and automation. *Science* 242:229–237.

Lander E: Private communication, available as a
product through Intelligent Automation.

Linz U (1990): Thermocycler temperature variation
invalidates PCR results. *BioTechniques* 9:286–
293.

Melnick M: Private communication, Harvard University.

Miller B: Private communication, General Atomics.

Mullis K: Private communication, Consultant, La
Jolla, California.

Mullis KB, Faloona FA (1987): Specific synthesis
of DNA in vitro via a polymerase-catalyzed chain
reaction. *Methods Enzymol* 155:335–350.

Nickersion DA, Kaiser R, Lappin S, Stewart J,
Hood L, Landegren U (1990): Automated DNA
diagnostics using an ELISA-based oligonucleotide ligation assay. *Proc Natl Acad Sci USA*
87:8923–8927.

Quackenbush J: Private communication, The Salk
Institute.

Olson M, Hood L, Cantor C, Botstein D (1989): A common language for physical mapping of the human genome. *Science* 245:1434–1435.

Quint J: Private communication, Beckman Instruments.

Reifel S: Private communication, Software is available from Stan Reifel, Inc.

Wittwer CT, Fillmore GC, Garling DJ (1990): Minimizing the time required for DNA amplification by efficient heat transfer to small samples. *Anal Biochem* 186:328–331.

Yager TD, Nickerson DA, Hood LE (1991): The Human Genome Project: Creating an infrastructure for biology and medicine. *TIBS* 16:454–461, and Evans G, private communication.

PART ONE
Methodology

SECTION V
Sequencing

17

PCR and DNA Sequencing

Bjorn Andersson and Richard A. Gibbs

Introduction

The development of protocols for the direct DNA sequence analysis of PCR products and the use of PCR to facilitate conventional sequencing strategies have been the focus of investigators since 1986. Direct PCR sequencing enables rapid and precise determination of sequence identity and variation, which is useful in most aspects of molecular biology and for diagnostic genetic applications. In a more general way, PCR improves the ease and capacity of all DNA sequencing activities, by simplifying the screening, preparation, and manipulation of DNA templates.

Many different variations of the integration of sequencing and PCR amplification have therefore been described. This chapter provides a general overview of issues and methods, and the subsequent chapters describe some particular approaches in detail, to illustrate both procedural aspects and the situations in which individual protocols may be favored. Interested readers may also refer to previous reviews on this subject (Gibbs et al., 1991; Gyllensten, 1989; Bevan et al., 1992).

Direct DNA Sequencing versus Cloning and Sequencing

"Direct DNA sequencing" refers to the analysis of unfractionated PCR amplified DNA molecules, which contrasts to the process of molecularly cloning fragments prior to the sequence determination (Fig. 17.1). The two procedures are similar to carry out, and offer similar results; however there are several important distinctions. The foremost of these is that direct sequencing simultaneously views an entire mixture of PCR amplified DNA molecules in a single assay. If the sequences to be analyzed are homogeneous, then a single unambiguous sequence results. However, if a mixture of similar sequences is present then a direct sequence analysis will reveal ambiguous signals at the mixed positions. For example, a PCR-amplified human DNA sample that is heterozygous for a single DNA base substitution will yield a mixture of two kinds of DNA fragments. The data will contain unambiguous sequences at the homozygous positions, but an equal representation of the two bases at the polymorphic position.

The Polymerase Chain Reaction
K.B. Mullis, F. Ferré, R.A. Gibbs, editors
© 1994 Birkhauser Boston

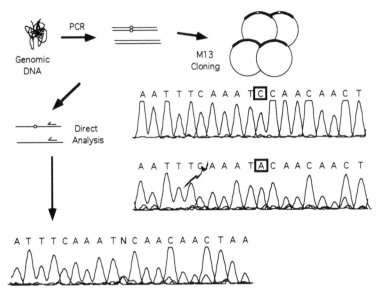

Cloning PCR products allows DNA sequence variants to be separated before the sequencing (see Chapter 2 for details of PCR cloning procedures). In the example of a human heterozygous mutation, an equal number of clones is expected to be recovered with each of the base substitutions. When each separate clone is sequenced, the results are unambiguous, but when different clones are compared about one-half will contain one of the polymorphic bases, and the other half the different base. In theory, the identification of these mixed bases is a simple statistical problem, and provided a sufficient number of clones is examined it is highly likely that polymorphic base postions will be correctly identified.

When more complex mixtures of bases are to be analyzed a larger number of individual clones can be sequenced. In these experiments the cloning of PCR products has an additional advantage compared to direct sequencing, as the relative linkage of multiple base differences can be determined. For example, if DNA base differences were to result from the presence of two bases at two positions in an amplified fragment, direct sequencing would not show which of the alternate bases at each position were to be found on the same molecule. By cloning the DNA prior to sequencing the individual molecules are separated and so the linkage is identified.

The Effect of Polymerase Errors on Sequencing Strategy

Polymerase errors introduced during PCR amplification are of concern primarily when cloning is used prior to the DNA sequencing, but can also influence direct sequencing (Keohavong and Thilly, 1989; Eckert and Kunkel, 1991). In either case, when the abundance of the initial template DNA is very low, such as when single molecules or cells are amplified, then a polymerase error that occurs early in the amplification will result in a significant fraction of the molecules containing a misincorporated base. In an extreme case, an error in the first cycle of a PCR can result in 25% of all amplified molecules being in error. This would be identified by either cloning or direct PCR sequencing strategies.

These are unlikely scenarios, however, and the vast majority of amplifications begin with larger numbers of template molecules. For example, amplification of a single copy gene from a nanogram of total human DNA involves approximately 500 starting template molecules. Assuming that at least 10% of the templates are copied in early PCR cycles, even if there was a "first cycle error," the representation of PCR errors in the final product would still be masked in a direct sequencing assay by the more than 99% representation of faithful copies at any one site. When cloning is used the probability of a single base being incorrectly identified when 99% of the molecules are correct is just 1 in 100, and the consensus, or majority sequence, will be revealed by the analysis of just a few clones.

In practice the effect of polymerase errors on final results is minimal when templates are simple and abundant, such as unique human sequences. When assaying rare templates, or when fidelity is particularly important such as when products are to be cloned for expression studies, then attention must be given to the problem.

Cloning and Sequencing

Aside from statistical considerations there are practical aspects of cloning and sequencing strategies that influence the choice of experimental protocol. A particular concern when cloning PCR products is the recovery of spurious amplification products, including primers in single or concatanated form, misprimed target sequences, and primed sequences unrelated to the desired target. The recovery of these can occur even when the presence of spurious amplification products is not apparent from agarose gel electrophoresis of reaction products due to their low individual representation. The bacterial growth phase of the protocol can also favor the propagation of particular clones among a mixture of transformants, leading to higher representation of unwanted fragments. When the target of amplification is homogeneous then the spurious cloned material may be easily distinguished from the desired products. However, if the initial population is a complex mixture of molecules then it can be very difficult to determine which products are artifactual and which properly represent the template molecules. Although these ambiguities can be minimized by careful, optimal amplifications, and by repetition of assays, they are very difficult to eliminate entirely, and can be regarded as an intrinsic disadvantage of cloning PCR products prior to sequencing.

An additional source of confusion when trying to interpret cloned PCR sequence results is the phenomenon of strand-swapping during amplification, where incomplete polymerization products prime one another to form chimeric molecules. This type of error can cause two previously unlinked mutations to be recovered on the same molecule and give the appearance of a "double heterozygote." In general this artifact is more common when there are excessive cycles of amplification, or where some factor limits the completion of full synthesis of each strand in a single cycle. Trial assays with control templates can define conditions that avoid this problem.

Analysis of PCR fragments by cloning and DNA sequencing creates considerable demands on data management. In practice the requirement to catalogue the large amounts of raw sequence data can quickly dominate a project. Currently there are no specialized computer programs for organizing and analyzing data generated by diagnostic DNA sequencing studies, and most manipulations are performed by adapting software developed for large-scale DNA sequencing projects. While these programs have the utility to perform the basic functions needed to compare sequences from different samples, they lack the ability to easily manage genetic data, or to clearly identify and annotate sites that represent differences between samples, or base mixtures in heterozygotes. This area is under active development by different investigators, and is therefore a likely area for future improvement (Jia-Hsu et al., 1993).

Direct Sequencing Methods

Generating direct sequences from PCR products is technically more difficult than the analysis of cloned single-stranded DNA template preparations, as the PCRs generate complementary strands that can compete with a sequencing primer to bind to the template, and also contain salt and other reagents that can influence the sequencing chemistry. The reactions may also contain spurious products that have incorporated the recognition sites for the sequencing primers. These contaminants can lead to artifacts including completely failed reactions, "stops" in every lane, and mixtures of faint sequences. Sequence reactions are complex mixtures, however, and it is often difficult to trace the precise source of a sequencing problem. For example, accidental omission of any single ingredient can yield the same "null" result as mutation of a primer site or trace amounts of organic solvents that might inhibit the activity of the sequence enzyme. Fortunately, the converse is not true and it is possible to consistently generate artifacts by certain approaches, which in turn yield some insight into the usual source of problems. There are a few common difficulties associated with particular situations:

1. *Too much salt:* Sequence reactions that contain too much salt, carried over from the PCR or subsequent manipulations, often fail completely, are faint, or yield strong stops distributed along their entire length. These artifacts are best distinguished by the overall products being substandard, as opposed to the presence of a few discrete stops within the ladders. The salt carried over from amplification steps can in extreme cases cause a diagnostic change in the electrophoretic pattern of the dye front.

2. *Presence of unrelated fragments with priming sites:* When a mixed sequence ladder is seen, then amplification of fragments unrelated to the primary template may have occurred. These DNA molecules will be sequenced at the same time as the intended fragment if the DNA sequencing primer is the same used for amplification. In extreme cases the complexity of the mixtures may prevent any of the true sequence signals from being distinguished. Often the visualization of the amplified material on an agarose gel prior to the sequencing will show if more than one band is present. In this case the PCRs should be optimized until the agarose gel profiles are homogeneous.

3. *Presence of related fragments with priming sites:* Prominent stop sequences that appear after a certain length of unambiguous sequence usually indicate the presence of secondary PCR priming sites in the amplified fragments. These may arise from the generation of shorter fragments that are from spurious internal priming of the anticipated fragment. In these cases the mixture yields an identical pattern until the shorter molecules are "run off." As the majority of the fragments that are primed in any sequence reactions are extended for their full length, even a small amount of these contaminating smaller molecules can yield prominent stops.

In general the use of labeled sequencing primers that are nested within PCR fragment is preferred for direct DNA sequencing. When attempting to perform the reactions with either dye-labeled terminators or with the use of a radiolabeled nucleotide that is incorporated into the growing DNA chain during the synthesis, then all fragments that are extended during the reaction will be labeled. Therefore, any primers that are left over following the amplification reaction will be seen in the final sequencing ladders.

Several different approaches that have been developed to overcome problems associated with direct DNA sequencing are summarized in Table 17.1. In general the approaches improve sequence data by reducing the effect of competition between the template and complementary strands of DNA that can occur during annealing. In addition, the techniques aim to remove the salt, oligonucleotide, and short primed contaminants that might interfere with efficient primer binding and extension (Table 17.1). The principle of each method represents different ways to achieve these common aims. Some are adaptations of standard molecular biology procedures, and others represent novel approaches to the problem.

The very first description of direct PCR sequencing relied on gel electrophoresis to purify the PCR products (Engelke et al., 1988). Later asymmetric priming was described by Gyllensten and Ehrlich (1988) for the amplification and sequencing of fragments of the human DQ-α locus. The PCRs were carried out with one primer in excess, and the other in limiting concentrations. As a consequence the

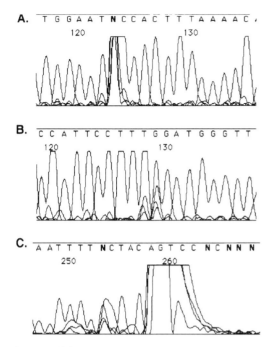
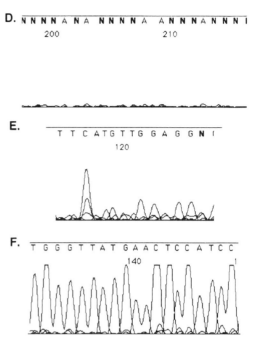

FIGURE 17.2. Common gel artifacts from direct sequencing. (A) Stop caused by the presence of a "runoff" in an otherwise unambiguous sequence. (B) High background, caused by reaction contaminants or by unrelated fragments containing sequencing primer sites. (C) Peaks caused by "runoff" at the end of a linear template. (D, E) Failed extension due to inhibition of the DNA polymerase used for sequencing. (F) Unambiguous sequence data.

reactions proceeded until the supply of the limiting primer was exhausted, so that the products of subsequent cycles were predominantly single-stranded DNA. This is an elegant method that has enjoyed widespread use; however, careful optimization of the primer ratios is required to ensure the reliable generation of the sequenceable templates. Single-stranded DNA and double-stranded DNA can be distinguished by agarose gel electrophoresis, which is generally the method used to decide that the asymmetric amplification is optimal. Unfortunately the agarose gel patterns can be complex, and often do not correlate with the final sequence result. The need to use the final sequence as the single criteria for quality control is a practical disadvantage when many different fragments are to be analyzed, as more effort is spent in establishing the different conditions than in the final sequence determinations.

We previously described a slight modification of the asymmetric amplification protocol that affords greater reliability but adds an extra step (Gibbs et al., 1989). In the modification a regular, double-stranded PCR was performed. Next a second single-strand producing reaction (SSPR) was performed using a dilution containing 1% of the first reaction, one of the original primers, and ingredients that are otherwise identical to the usual PCR. The thermocycling conditions are identical for SSPRs as for the PCRs, except that the annealing and extension times are doubled. The two-step protocol probably is more reliable because the critical asymmetric phase of the procedure utilizes a higher concentration of the specific template than the usual one-step method, and is not influenced by variation in the efficiency of the initial cycles of single asymmetric PCRs.

Other reports describe methods that improve the sequencing by use of rapid annealing temperatures to prevent incorrect hybridizations, nuclease digestion of one DNA strand, or the addition of organics to the PCR/sequencing

TABLE 17.1. Approaches to direct DNA sequencing.

Method	Reference	Principle
Asymmetric PCR	Gyllensten and Erlich (1988)	Single-stranded DNA is generated by PCR using an excess of one PCR primer, and a limited amount of an opposing primer
Modified asymmetric PCR	Gibbs et al. (1991)	Similar to asymmetric PCR except two sequential reactions are performed, using first balanced and then nonbalanced ratios of primers, to give more reliability
Quick temperature drop annealings	Kusakawa et al. (1990)	Rapid annealing allows the highly concentrated primer to bind to a template, but minimizes the possibility of less abundant competing template strands from binding
Addition of organics (DMSO or detergents)	Winship (1989)	DNA hybridization stringency is raised, favoring rapid oligonucleotide binding but limiting template reannealing to other strand
Exonuclease three	Higuchi and Ochman (1989)	One strand of the DNA template is removed, leaving single-stranded material
Chemical sequencing	Rosenthal and Jones (1990)	Specific labeling of the PCR fragment is combined with Maxam–Gilbert sequencing
In vitro transcription	Stoflet et al. (1988), Sarkar and Sommers (1988)	Tails attached to oligonucleotide primers allow *in vitro* transcription to generate an excess of single-stranded RNA template
Native gel purification	Engelke et al. (1988)	Double-strand PCR fragments are purified by gel electrophoresis to remove unwanted PCR products and reagents
Denaturing gel purification	Andersson (1992)	Single-strand PCR fragments are purified to remove unwanted PCR products, reagents, and the strand complementary to the DNA template
Binding to solid phase	Mitchell and Merril (1989)	Fragments are biotinylated and bound to a column
Biotin bead binding	Hultman et al. (1990)	Biotinylated fragments are bound to streptavidin-coated beads
Cycle sequencing	Murray (1989)	Repetitive thermocycling
Coupled amplification and sequencing	Ruano and Kidd (1991)	PCR and sequencing are performed simultaneously

mixture (summarized in Table 17.1). Each of these methods works well when optimized and the data reported from the original laboratories are of high quality. Some investigators swear by their favorite method, while others anecdotally report no success with some, and excellent results with others. As with the majority of techniques in molecular biology, the unifying explanation is that all the methods can be made to work in all situations, with sufficient careful optimization.

Solid-Phase (Bead) Sequencing

One method that represents both a dramatic departure from previous approaches, and a great improvement in quality is solid-phase DNA sequencing. An early report of this methodology utilized streptavidin coupled to agarose beads, so that a biotinylated DNA template could be captured by column chromatography (Mitchell and Merril, 1989). Mild alkaline treatment then separated the biotinylated strand from its complement. DNA sequence from this method was of high quality.

Although functional, the agarose solid support is clumsy relative to a popular magnetic bead support system. In the current version of this system, biotin is introduced into a DNA fragment via the 5′-terminus of an oligonucleotide used in PCR, and then the PCR fragments are mixed with magnetic beads coated with streptavidin. The beads are washed in alkaline solution and then added to the sequencing reaction. Finally the DNA produced in the sequencing reactions is eluted from the beads in formamide and loaded onto an acrylamide gel.

The success of the method is to a large extent due to the commercial availability of beads that are coated with streptavidin. The original supplier of these, Dynal, takes advantage of the technology developed by Dr. John Ugelstad to generate the particles that have the property of being monodispersed in solution, yet easily captured and concentrated by placing a magnet adjacent to the reaction tube. Since the captured material can be washed quite vigorously it is a simple matter to remove the sale proteins and other PCR leftovers that are in solution.

As long as high quality biotinylated oligonucleotide primers are available and high quality PCRs are achieved the bead sequencing generally is trouble free. Some investigators report that while PCR fragments less than 500–600 nucleotides in length are easily sequenced, longer fragments can produce variable results. The reason for this problem is uncertain, but does not appear to be a physical or steric phenomena, and may be related to the total charge accumulation on the surface of the beads. In general this difficulty can be overcome by simply using more DNA and beads for each preparation.

Many different applications of the bead sequencing methodology have been reported, with the focus of these developments in the laboratory of Dr. Mathias Uhlen at the Royal Institute of Technology in Stockholm. The use of direct PCR sequencing to explore human mutations and for subtyping of various human pathogens has been explored. In our hands bead sequencing has become the preferred method for diagnostic DNA sequencing, where human gene mutations and HIV-1 subtypes are to be analyzed. This is because the method allows the reliable production of fluorescent DNA sequencing results that have a low overall background signal, that in turn allows clear differentiation of naturally occurring mixtures of DNA bases from artifactual mixed signals. These studies are described further below.

Fluorescent versus Radioactive Sequencing

PCR products can be sequenced by radioactive conventional methods, or by fluorescent automated DNA sequencing (Smith et al., 1988; Voss et al., 1989). Most of the advantages or disadvantages of each are not peculiar to the analysis of PCR products, but are generally true of each approach. For example, the fluorescent methods are well suited for relatively high throughput studies, with direct computer entry of the final data. Manual methods are inexpensive and somewhat more time consuming. However, the radioactive direct sequencing can generally be successful using templates of poor quality, while the fluorescent methods generally require more stringent control of variation of the reagents. This is particularly true of the fluorescent methodologies that mix four different fluorescent dye colors for analsyis in a single channel, as the chemistry of each sequence reaction must be carefully balanced. In contrast, fluorescent sequencing chemistries that utilize a single dye color, but analyze the sequence reaction products from each base-specific reaction in separate channels, in an analogous fashion to radioactive sequencing, are somewhat more robust.

The current fluorescent DNA sequencing strategies work most favorably with oligonucleotides with dyes attached at the 5'-terminus, which can require the production of custom dye-labeled primers for each new fragment to be analyzed. PCR provides a simple alternative, and fragments can be amplified by primers that have a universal sequencing primer recognition site at the 5'-terminus. This site is incorporated into the amplified fragment via one PCR primer and then commercially available fluorescent primers are used for the sequencing (McBride et al., 1989).

An intrinsic advantage of fluorescent assays is that the detection of the primary signal offers a linear response to the amount of material that is present over a wider range than is found for radioactive alternatives. Consequently the prospects for the use of fluorescent DNA sequencing methods for the accurate quantitation of DNA base mixtures via PCR are favorable.

Direct Sequencing and Molecular Diagnostics

The prospect of using direct DNA sequencing as a routine diagnostic tool is an attractive one because the method provides definitive information about the fragment being examined. Bases that are altered as a result of a disease-causing mutation are easily seen and the "normal" sequence serves as a definitive control. As noted above, carriers of genetic disease can be identified by the mixture of DNA bases at the position of individual mutations.

We previously showed that DNA sequencing could provide comprehensive diagnostics for the rare X-linked genetic disease, the Lesch–Nyhan syndrome (LNS) (Gibbs et al., 1990). Male patients with LNS have mutations in the hypoxanthine phosphoribosyltransferase (HPRT) gene while female carriers of the disease are heterozygous for altered sequences. Diagnosis is now by PCR amplification of each of the nine HPRT exonic fragments followed by DNA sequencing. Nine exons are amplified simultaneously (see Chapter 3) and each fragment is sequenced using a modification of the methods of Hultman et al. (1989). Data from these sequencing reactions are transferred to a computer for comparison with normal sequences, allowing molecular diagnosis of LNS within a single day. In the past 2 years we have provided diagnosis for members of over 60 LNS families, correctly genotyping all individuals tested and detecting a variety of mutations. The HPRT studies therefore demonstrate that a DNA sequencing assay can be routinely used to analyze an entire gene when it is essential to determine if the complete sequence is either normal or altered in any way. The power of this assay contrasts strongly with other methods where either the precise DNA base changes must be known a priori, or the possibility that some mutations might be missed in the analysis must be tolerated.

One limitation of this method of diagnosis is that the existing DNA base calling software provided by the manufacturers of the automated DNA sequencer cannot reliably identify DNA base mixtures that occur in genetic carriers. In about one-half of cases the 50 : 50 mixtures at single positions that result from heterozygosity are represented as "N" by the computer, while in the remaining cases one or the other base is recognized as predominant. Therefore the automatic comparison of the sequence text data output from the machine with the normal sequence does not provide a reliable basis for sample diagnosis. Currently the individual sequence traces are examined by eye to identify these mixed bases that the computer has not distinguished from normal sequences. This manual procedure is reliable but both labor intensive and difficult to record and report in a concise and systematic fashion. The different kinds of base calling are illustrated in Figure 17.3 (Jia Hsu et al., 1993).

Sequencing AZT-Resistant HIV-1 Isolates

We have also studied mutations that arise in the human immunodeficiency virus (HIV-1) that lead to resistance to the drug AZT. Acquired resistance to AZT is an important limitation of the application of this drug in AIDS therapy. Previously four individual codon changes in the proviral *pol* gene of HIV-1 have been demonstrated to be additive contributors to viral resistance (Larder and Kemp, 1989). A facile assay that could monitor the emergence of these alterations has the potential for providing early detection of resistance, and an indication for alternative drug therapies. We have shown that the individual mutations can be readily identified by PCR fluorescent solid-phase sequencing. Correlations have been established between clinical outcome of patients treated with AZT over time and the emergence of the specific DNA motifs within the *pol* gene.

In these experiments, and in other epidemiological studies that we have performed, the signal from the strongest DNA base has been

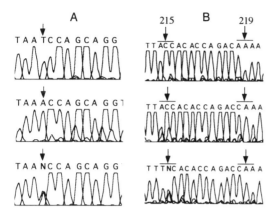

FIGURE 17.3. Visualizing DNA base mixtures by direct DNA sequencing. (**A**) Amplified human DNA representing normal, mutant, and heterozygous individuals. (**B**) Sequence from the HIV-1 pol gene, amplified from proviral sequences from patients treated with the antiviral drug AZT. Variation at codons 215 and 219 is detected.

used to determine the consensus sequence for each individual population (Burger et al., 1991). In the samples exhibiting drug resistance the emergence of the resistant codons cannot yet be quantitated because the available DNA sequence analysis software does not yield the quantities of the signal from each of the four bases at each postion in the sequencer output. So far we have relied on the time consuming and subjective identification of the mixed bases by manual examination of the sequence chromatogram.

Combining Direct Sequencing with Other Techniques

The power of direct DNA sequencing for the analysis of homogeneous fragments and simple mixtures of related DNAs can be extended by combining the methods with physical techniques for DNA fractionation. We have used this approach for the analysis of HIV-1 sequences by denaturing gradient gel electrophoresis (DGGE), a gel technique that resolves DNA fragments that differ by as little as a single nucleotide, on the basis of their melting properties (Andersson et al., 1993). Samples are first amplified using oligonucleotides that define a region that has been chosen because

the normal base sequence offers a profile of DNA melting behavior that is favorable for DGGE analysis. The amplified material is then electrophoresed in a gradient of denaturants so that samples of different sequence migrate to different positions on the gel.

In addition to initial sample preparation, PCR can also be used to analyze samples following gel electrophoresis. The preferred procedure is to visualize individual bands by minimal ethidium bromide staining and UV light exposure, and then to extract a small sample for reamplification and sequencing. Numerous molecules can be easily obtained from each gel slice, so that the influence of possible PCR errors on the studies is not significant. This general approach incorporating other physical separation techniques has been used by others for the analysis of human gene mutations (see Chapter 1).

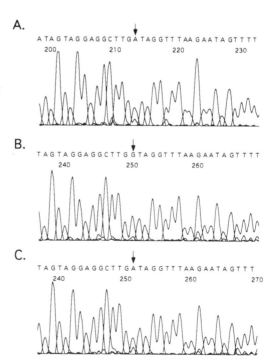

FIGURE 17.4. Separation of PCR product from the HIV-1 envelope gene from patient samples via DGGE, followed by direct DNA sequencing. (**A**) Direct sequence from the original HIV-1 PCR product. (**B**, **C**) Sequence variants found after DGGE separation.

We have combined DGGE with direct DNA sequencing to analyze complex mixtures of PCR-amplified HIV-1 provirus from AIDS patients. In these samples there can be many forms of the target sequence, with varying abundance. The complexity of the populations can complicate the alternative approach of cloning and sequencing the amplified materials, because natural molecular variants can be difficult to distinguish from artifacts of the amplification and cloning. Direct sequencing can be difficult because the diversity of the mixture can lead to such complicated sequence patterns that the composition cannot be deciphered. The application of DGGE provides an initial overview of the mixture of molecules, and allows major viral forms to be isolated as homogeneous populations for the final sequence study.

The sequence results from the material that has been resolved by the DGGE are usually unambiguous. In some cases small amounts of contamination from other forms in the mixture are present, although this occurs only when the particular band is a minor one, relative to the other material. In these cases the purity of the isolated fragment can be improved by increased separation via larger gels.

DNA versus RNA

Another issue that arises in planning an experiment for the direct sequence analysis of a particular gene is whether to use genomic DNA or cDNA made from the mRNA of the target gene via reverse transcription as the template for the PCR. Several methods for the rapid synthesis of the first strand cDNA from preparations of total cellular RNA, followed by PCR amplification, have been described. The cDNA can be synthesized using either oligo(dT)priming or a primer specific for the target mRNA for the reverse transcriptase reaction.

The utilization of genomic DNA has the disadvantage that several PCR products need to be produced and sequenced in order to characterize all exons of a gene. If cDNA is used the entire coding sequence can often be amplified in a single PCR product. However, the use of cDNA is dependent on the availability of a tar-

get tissue in which the gene is expressed. In addition, to obtain cDNA in a sufficient amount, it is usually necessary to obtain high-quality mRNA preparations. In addition, the RNA preparations require more fastidious handling than their DNA counterparts. In contrast, DNA from any tissue can be used, and the preparations require little effort, so that high-quality PCR products can be obtained on a routine basis.

PCR Sequencing in the Genome Project

PCR is being used extensively for the execution of the human genome project. Current and future applications range from physical and genetic mapping, to the initial sequencing and then the comparison of sequences from different organisms. Some details of these studies have been discussed elsewhere as the techniques have been applied to coarse levels of gene mapping, and for pilot large-scale sequencing studies.

PCR will continue to be used to prepare some of the DNA templates required for the DNA sequence reactions used to initially generate sequences from each species. It is not clear which specific technique will be favored for the majority of the sequencing, however, and therefore it is possible that PCR will not be the ideal method. Possible scenarios include the predominance of fluorescent DNA sequencing methods where the superior quality of the sequence generated from microbially prepared templates may outweigh advantages provided by the convenience of PCR. Alternatively, new methods might utilize templates that are longer than can be easily amplified, such as lambda clone inserts or cosmids. In developing optimal strategies the PCR process is usually incorporated where possible.

One PCR application that has been discussed less frequently is the comparative analysis of closely related sequences. Once a genomic sequence is obtained then insight into the functional role of encoded genes, the significance of specific sequence motifs, and the evolutionary origins of the fragments can each be better analyzed if information from homologous DNAs is known. For example, the conservation of exonic coding regions in genomic DNA that has been isolated from syntenic regions of human and murine DNA is a powerful tool for the identification of genes within noncoding or intronic regions. Similarly, the identification of alterations in a human gene that is a candidate for a genetic disease can reveal that mutations at this locus are the cause of the abnormality. In these contexts, the initial step of generating a "normal" sequence provides the basis for the design of PCR primers to direct subsequent sequencing efforts to the related organisms.

The power of this approach has been shown by the identification of mutations in human genes that were candidates for genetic disease. For example, alterations in the superoxide dismutase gene have linked that locus to Lou Gehrig's disease (Rosen et al., 1993). This example illustrates that a gene that was characterized and sequenced at one time can later be found to have a central role in human disease using the technique of PCR direct DNA sequencing. In experiments where the sequence of a gene is compared in populations of individuals with genetic disease and normals, the clue that has led the investigator to the locus has usually been generated by prior genetic mapping studies. As the possibility of directly assigning function to the products of newly sequenced genes increases, then the criteria of putative function may be increasingly important.

In our studies of the evolution of the human CD4 locus, we have also illustrated how the generation of a normal or reference DNA sequence can be used to construct PCR primers that are used for direct DNA sequencing to reveal unexpected evolutionary relationships. Sequence characterization of a 14-kb fragment of the gene showed the presence of a medium reiteration frequency (MER) repeat element that, in one clone, contained an inserted human Alu repeat element. Subsequent studies showed that the Alu insertion was dimorphic, with about 70% of chromosomes in a North American Caucasian population having the insertion. The fine structure of this region was subsequently examined in individuals with and without the insertion using PCR direct DNA sequencing and primers designed to be complementary to the normal sequence. To our surprise the Alu minus site was characterized by the presence of a remnant of the Alu sequence. In combination with further evidence generated from PCR/hybridization experiments, we concluded that the sequence of events at this locus was that the Alu had been lost from one allelic form to generate the dimorphism. This is different from the sequence assumed by other investigators who have examined different diomorphic Alu insertions, but not examined the fine structure of the loci by the approach of PCR and direct DNA sequencing (Edwards and Gibbs, 1992).

The Future of PCR Sequencing

In the short term the combination of PCR and DNA sequencing methods will continue to be developed to provide greater convenience to the user, with an overall increased reliability. Already several manufacturers offer simple "kit" forms of reagents that allow the use of different approaches and standardized reagents. Our experience with some of these has shown them to be reliable, but not a substitute for the stringent quality control that must accompany the preparation of the PCR products and their sequencing using home-prepared reagents.

Currently PCR direct DNA sequencing is just one of several options that might be applied for comparative DNA studies. Where alternatives such as SSCP (see Chapter 1) or heteroduplex analysis, denaturing gradient gel electrophoresis (Fischer and Lerman, 1983), or chemical cleavage of mismatch studies (Cotton et al., 1988) are used, it is generally with the rationale that the chosen approach is technically easier than sequencing. One consequence of the evolution of the sequencing procedures to the point where "kits" are available is therefore that the method will be increasingly favored above the alternatives.

This change will be initially most apparent where the objective is for genetic diagnosis. In that type of application there is very often a preference for methods where, all else being equal, the maximum amount of information can be obtained. In that case, in addition to providing a means to characterize positions where predictable genetic alterations might occur, then a broader survey that confirms the normal structure of surrounding bases is possible. The application of direct PCR sequencing may therefore be extended to the routine detection of mixed DNA sequences in a variety of genetic diseases. In that case individuals may present for the comprehensive testing of many loci for alterations where there is a small but finite chance of a mutation.

A key development needed for the widespread implementation of these methods is the creation of specialized computer software that deals with the comparative analysis of DNA fragments from different individuals or species. Customizable data analysis packages are required to provide both data storage and retrieval functions and the means to perform structural comparisons that can be automatically interpreted to show significant genetic differences.

Conclusions

Combinations of PCR and DNA sequencing are now standard items in the tool kit of the molecular biologist, and are likely to remain so for the near and distant future. The investigator has a wide range of choices including cloning and sequencing, direct DNA sequencing, and various methodological approaches. The range of applications now includes diagnostic and basic molecular biology studies. In the future PCR and direct DNA sequencing is likely to become even more frequently used.

References

Andersson B, He SM, Lambert B (1992): Mutations causing defective splicing in the human HPRT gene. *Environ Molec Mutagenesis*, 89–95.

Andersson B, Jia-Hsu Y, Lewis DE, Gibbs RA (1993): Rapid characterization of HIV-1 sequence diversity using denaturing gradient gel electrophoresis and direct automated DNA sequencing of PCR products. *PCR Methods Applic* 2:293–300.

Bevan IS, Rapley R, Walker MR (1992): Sequencing of PCR amplified DNA. *PCR Methods Applic* 1:222–228.

Burger H, Weiser B, Flaherty K, Gulla J, Nguyen PN, Gibbs RA (1991): Evolution of human immunodeficiency virus type 1 nucleotide sequence diversity among close contacts. *Proc Natl Acad Sci USA* 88:11236–11240.

Cotton RGH, Rodrigues NR, Campbell RD (1988): Reactivity of cytosine and thymine in single-base-pair mismatches with hydroxylamine and osmium tetraoxide and its application to the study of mutations. *Proc Natl Acad Sci USA* 85:4397–4401.

Eckert KA, Kunkel TA (1991): DNA polymerase fidelity and the polymerase chain reaction. *PCR Methods Appl* 1:17–24.

Edwards MC, Gibbs RA (1992): A human dimorphism resulting from loss of an *Alu*. *Genomics* 14:590–597.

Engelke DR, Hoener PA, Collins FS (1988): Direct sequencing of enzymatically amplified human genomic DNA. *Proc Natl Acad Sci USA* 85:544–548.

Fischer S, Lerman L (1983): DNA fragments by single base par substitution are separated in denaturing gradient gels: Correspondence with melting theory. *Proc Natl Acad Sci USA* 80:1579–1583.

Gibbs RA, Nguyen PN, McBride LJ, Koepf SM, Caskey CT (1989): Identification of mutations leading to the Lesch-Nyhan syndrome by automated direct DNA sequencing of in vitro amplified cDNA. *Proc Natl Acad Sci USA* 86:1919–1923.

Gibbs RA, Nguyen PN, Edwards A, Civitello AB, Caskey CT (1990): Multiplex DNA deletion detection and exon sequencing of the hypoxanthine phosphoribosyltransferase gene in Lesch-Nyhan families. *Genomics* 7:235–244.

Gibbs RA, Nguyen PN, Caskey CT (1991): Direct DNA sequencing of complementary DNA amplified by the polymerase chain reaction. In: *Methods in Molecular Biology*, Vol 9, *Protocols in Human Molecular Genetics*. Mathew C, ed. Clifton, NJ: Humana Press.

Gyllensten UB (1989): PCR and DNA sequencing. *Biotechniques* 7:700–708.

Gyllensten UB, Ehrlich HA (1988): Generation of single stranded DNA by the polymerase chain reaction and its application to direct sequencing of the HLA DQa locus. *Proc Natl Acad Sci USA* 85:7652–7656.

Higuchi RG, Ochman H (1989): Production of single-stranded DNA templates by exonuclease digestion following the polymerase chain reaction. *Nucl Acids Res* 17:5865.

Hultman T, Stahl S, Hornes E, Uhlen M (1989): Direct solid phase sequencing of genomic and plasmid DNA using magnetic beads as solid support. *Nucl Acids Res* 17:4937–4946.

Jia-Hsu Y, Gilson H, Long K, Gibbs RA (1993): Data management for re-sequencing DNA. Proceedings of the Supercomputer Computations Research Institute Second International Conference, Lim et al. eds. Singapore: World Scientific (Publ.), 207–218.

Keohavong P, Thilly WG (1989): Fidelity of DNA polymerases in DNA amplification. *Proc Natl Acad Sci USA* 86:9253–9257.

Kusakawa H, Uemori T, Asada K, Kato I (1990): Rapid and reliable protocol for direct sequencing of material amplified by the polymerase chain reaction. *Biotechniques* 9:66–72.

Larder BA, Kemp SD (1989): Multiple mutations in HIV-1 reverse transcriptase confer high-level resistance to zidovudine (AZT). *Science* 246:1155–1158.

McBride LJ, Koepf SM, Gibbs RA, Salser W, Mayrand PE, Hunkapiller MW, Kronick MN (1989): Automated DNA sequencing methods involving polymerase chain reaction. *Clin Chem* 35:2196–2201.

Mitchell LG, Merril CR (1989): Affinity generation of single-stranded DNA for dideoxy sequencing following the polymerase chain reaction. *Anal Biochem* 178:239–242.

Murray V (1989): Improved double stranded DNA sequencing using the linear polymerase chain reaction. *Nucleic Acids Res* 17:8889.

Rosen DR et al. (1993): Mutations in the Cu/Zn superoxide dismutase gene are associated with familial amyotrophic lateral sclerosis. *Nature (London)* 362:59–62.

Rosenthal A, Jones DS (1990): Genomic walking and sequencing by oligo-cassette mediated polymerase chain reaction. *Nucleic Acids Res* 18:3095–3096.

Ruano G, Kidd KK (1991): Coupled amplification and sequencing of genomic DNA. *Proc Natl Acad Sci USA* 88:2815–2819.

Sarkar G, Sommer SS (1988): RNA amplification with transcript sequencing (RAWTS). *Nucl Acids Res* 16:5197.

Sheffield VC, Cox DR, Lerman LS, Myers RM (1998): Attachment of a 40 base pair G+C rich sequence (GC clamp) to genomic DNA fragments by the polymerase chain reaction results in improved detection of single base changes. *Proc Natl Acad Sci USA* 86:232–236.

Smith L et al. (1986): Fluorescence detection in automated DNA sequence analysis. *Nature* 321:674.

Stoflet ES, Koeberl DD, Sarkar G, Sommer SS (1988): Genomic amplification with transcript sequencing. *Science* 239:491–494.

Voss H, Schwager C, Wirkner U, Sproat B, Zimmermann J, Rosenthal A, Erfle H, Stegemann J, Ansorge W (1989): Direct genomic fluorescent on-line sequencing and analysis using *in vitro* amplification of DNA. *Nucl Acids Res* 17:2517–2517.

Wilson RK, Chen C, Hood L (1990): Optimization of asymmetric polymerase chain reaction for rapid fluorescent DNA sequencing. *Biotechniques* 8:184–189.

18

Phage Promoter-Based Methods for Sequencing and Screening for Mutations

Steve S. Sommer and Erica L. Vielhaber

Introduction

Genomic amplification with transcript sequencing (GAWTS) (Stoflet et al., 1988; Sommer et al., 1990) is a generally applicable method for direct sequencing of PCR material. GAWTS is centered around the attachment of a phage promoter sequence (T7, SP6, or T3) to the 5'-end of one or both PCR primers. The phage promoter sequence allows the PCR product to be transcribed into RNA. Subsequently, the RNA is utilized as a single-stranded template for dideoxynucleotide sequencing with reverse transcriptase (Figure 18.1).

GAWTS has several advantages over other direct sequencing methods: (1) the transcription step provides a subsequent amplification of the region of interest, which eliminates further purification following the PCR, (2) the additional amplification at the transcriptional level compensates for suboptimal PCR, and (3) a single-stranded template provides increased sequence reproducibility over a double-stranded template. GAWTS lends itself to automation with a robotic device because cumbersome methods such as ethanol precipitation or centrifugation are not required. These advantages make GAWTS a "forgiving" and technically robust method. The disadvantages of GAWTS versus other methods include limited choice of sequencing enzyme and the additional expense of synthesizing oligonucleotides with 23-bp promoter sequences. **Degradation of RNA is *not* a problem;** a great abundance of template RNA is generated in an essentially nuclease-free environment. This is in contrast to mRNA, which is often unstable because it is present at low levels and is isolated from cells that contain large amounts of nucleases.

In our laboratory, GAWTS has been the method utilized for determining the causative mutation in 350 hemophilia B patients. Sequence data have also been obtained for other human genes such as p53, transthyretin, and the dopamine D_2 receptor (Sommer et al., 1992; Ii et al., 1991; Sarkar et al., 1991). In total, almost one megabase of genomic sequence has been generated with GAWTS. Sequence has also been obtained from mRNA by generating one strand of cDNA and diluting the sample in the PCR reaction (Sarkar and Sommer, 1988).

Two phage promoter-based PCR methods have been developed for rapid screening for the

The Polymerase Chain Reaction
K.B. Mullis, F. Ferré, R.A. Gibbs, editors
© 1994 Birkhäuser Boston

GAWTS

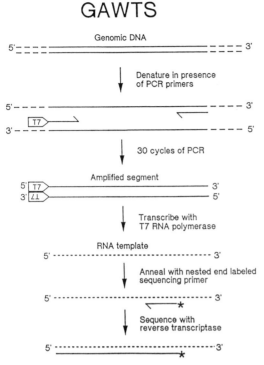

FIGURE 18.1. Schematic of GAWTS. GAWTS consists of the following three steps: (1) PCR, in which one or both oligonucleotides contain a phage promoter in addition to a sequence targeting the primer to the region to be amplified, (2) transcription with the phage promoter, and (3) dideoxy sequencing of the transcript with reverse transcriptase that is primed with a nested (internal) oligonucleotide. Reprinted with permission of Academic Press from Sommer et al. (1990).

presence of mutations. One method, RNA single-strand conformation polymorphism (rSSCP) (Sarkar et al., 1992a; Danenberg et al., 1992), is a modification of single-strand conformation polymorphism (SSCP) (Orita et al., 1989). A direct comparison between the methods indicates that rSSCP is significantly more efficient than SSCP at detecting mutations, but not as good as direct sequencing. The other method, dideoxy fingerprinting (ddF) (Sarkar et al., 1992b), is a hybrid of SSCP and GAWTS in which one lane of a dideoxy sequencing reaction is electrophoresed through a *non*denaturing gel. ddF detected 100% of a group of 84 mutations, which included a blinded comparison with direct sequencing for the analysis of the regions of functional significance in the factor IX gene of 30 patients with hemophilia B.

The protocols for GAWTS, rSSCP, and ddF are given below. In addition, the reader is referred to protocols on four related methods. GAWTS is used to sequence DNA segments when at least some of the segment sequence is previously available. Cellular RNA can be sequenced by RNA amplification with transcript sequencing (RAWTS) (Sarkar and Sommer, 1988). GAWTS and RAWTS are used to determine the sequence of DNA from an individual when at least part of the sequence has been previously determined. Novel DNA sequence can be obtained on an unlimited number of isolates from a cDNA or genomic library by an extension of GAWTS known as promoter ligation and transcript sequencing (PLATS) (Schowalter et al., 1990) (Fig. 18.2). With PLATS, an unlimited amount of DNA sequence can be obtained in both directions with a few generic oligonucleotides. Finally, any desired segment of a protein can be translated *in vitro* by attaching a Kozak translation initiation sequence 3' to the phage promoter sequence of an oligonucleotide (Sarkar and Sommer, 1989). The protein may be full length or any desired segment or a mutated segment generated by the megaprimer method of *in vitro* mutagenesis (Sarkar and Sommer, 1990).

Protocols

GAWTS, rSSCP, and ddF (Fig. 18.3A–C) are all phage promoter-based methods for mutation detection; however, they follow slightly different protocols. The points of divergence among the protocols are indicated as appropriate.

PCR

Genomic DNA (250 ng) was added to 25 μl of 50 mM KCl, 10 mM Tris-HCl (pH 8.3), 1.5–3.5 mM MgCl$_2$ (empirically determined for each set of primers), 200 μM each dNTP, 0.03–0.1 μM each primer (modified Perkin-Elmer Cetus protocol), and 0.5 unit of *Taq* polymerase. Thirty cycles of PCR were performed (denaturation: 1 min at 94°C; annealing: 2 min at 50°C; elongation: 3 min at 72°C) with the Perkin-Elmer Cetus automated thermal cycler. After the last cycle of PCR, a final 10-min elongation was performed.

Promoter Ligation and Transcript Sequencing (PLATS)

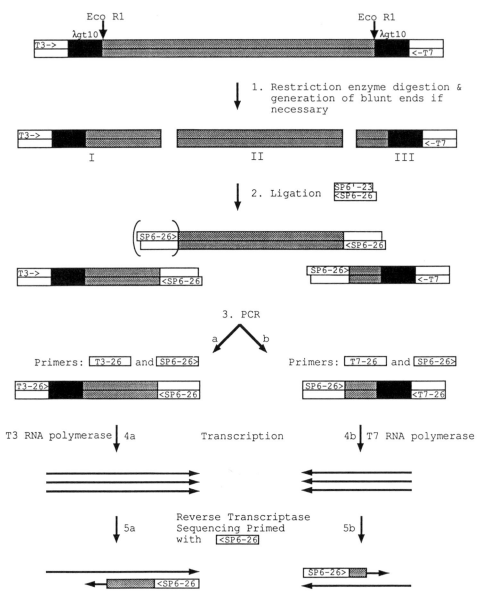

FIGURE 18.2. Schematic of promoter ligation and transcript sequencing (PLATS). A segment of DNA (here a clone in λgt10) is amplified by means of PCR with a pair of oligonucleotide primers, each containing a different phage promoter sequence. Digestion of the segment with an appropriate restriction enzyme (step 1) yields fragments that can be ligated to a third promoter (step 2). Additional PCR amplification with appropriate primers (step 3a or 3b) results in smaller segments which, following transcription (step 4a or 4b), are sequenced with reverse transcriptase (step 5a or 5b). For details, see Schowalter et al., 1990. Reprinted with permission of Academic Press from Schowalter et al. (1990): A method of sequencing without subcloning and its application to the identification of a novel ORF with a sequence suggestive of a transcriptional regulator in the water mold Achlya ambisexualis. *Genomics* 6:23–32.

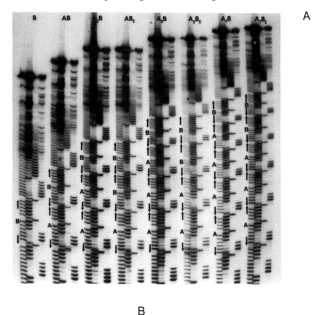

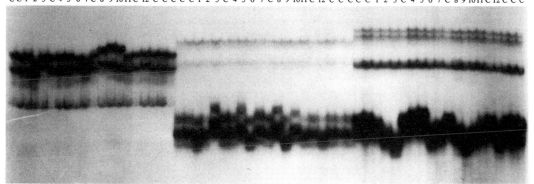

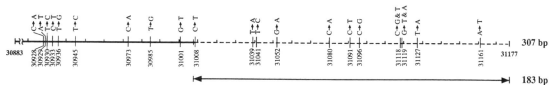

FIGURE 18.3. (A) Sequence of the eight polymorphic ($A_{0-4}B$ and $A_{1-3}B_2$) alleles of a cryptic RY(i) in intron 1 of the factor IX gene utilizing GAWTS. Reprinted with permission of American Journal of Human Genetics from Jacobson et al. (1993). (B) Comparison of SSCP and rSSCP (T7 and SP6) of 12 different mutations contained in a 183-bp segment of the factor IX gene. Of the mutations, 92% were detected with SSCP, 100% with T7 rSSCP, and 92% with SP6 rSSCP. Panels A, SSCP; B, T7-rSSCP; and C, SP6-rSSCP. Lanes labeled C, normal control sample from one individual (each loading taken from the same transcription reaction). Lanes labeled C', normal control samples from three different normal individuals. Lanes labeled 1–12, templates containing mutations 1–12. The 12 mutations all lie in the region indicated by the broken lines (183 bp). The lane numbers above (1–12) correspond to the mutations in this region, from left to right. The numbering is from Yoshitake et al. (1985). Reprinted with permission of Oxford University Press from Sarkar et al. (1992a). (C) (See next page.) Identification of 12 different mutations in the factor IX gene by ddF. The mutations are shown at the top. The corresponding ddF patterns are shown below. Arrows in each lane indicate the first aberrant (informative) band. Lanes C, wild type; lanes 1–12, mutants. Reprinted with permission of Oxford University Press from Sarkar et al. (1992b).

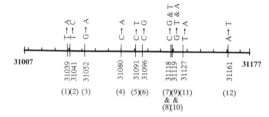

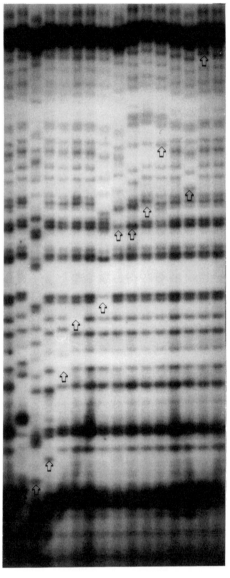

FIGURE 18.3. *Continued*

In Vitro Transcription

GAWTS and ddF: A 3-μl sample of the amplified material was added to 17 μl of RNA transcription mixture. The final mixture contains 40 mM Tris-HCl (pH 7.5), 6 mM MgCl$_2$, 2 mM spermidine, 10 mM sodium chloride, 0.5 mM of the four ribonucleoside triphosphates, RNasin (1 U/μl), 10 mM DTT, and 1.0 U of T7 or SP6 RNA polymerase. Samples were incubated for 1–2 hr at 37°C, and the reaction was stopped by freezing the sample.

rSSCP: A 1.5 μl sample of the amplified material was added to a 9 μl reaction containing 2 μCi of [α-^{32}P]UTP and all of the aforementioned reagents in equimolar concentrations. Following incubation, 50 μl of stop buffer (95% formamide, 20 mM EDTA, 0.05% bromophenol blue, and 0.05% xylene cyanol) was added. Samples were incubated at 94°C for 4 min and chilled in ice water for 10 min. A 1-μl sample was loaded on a 48-cm, 0.35-mm-thick nondenaturing polyacrylamide gel (5.6% acrylamide) and electrophoresed 5–7 hr at 30 W constant power with cooling provided by a fan, water jacket, or cold room. Subsequently, the gel was dried for 1 hr and autoradiography was performed.

End Labeling

A 0.1-μg sample of oligonucleotide was incubated in a 13-μl reaction volume containing 50 mM Tris-HCl (pH 7.4), 10 mM MgCl$_2$, 5 mM spermidine, 100 μCi [γ-^{32}P]ATP (5000 Ci/mmol), and 10 units of T4 polynucleotide kinase for 30 min at 37°C. The reaction was heated to 65°C for 5 min, and 7 μl of water was added for a final concentration of 5 ng of oligonucleotide per microliter.

Sequencing Protocols

GAWTS: A 2-μl sample of the transcription reaction and 1 μl of ^{32}P end-labeled sequencing primer were added to 10 μl of annealing buffer [250 mM KCl, 10 mM Tris-HCl (pH 8.3)]. The samples were denatured at 80°C for 3 min and then annealed at 45°C for 30–45 min (approximately 5°C below the Wallace temperature [4°C × (G+C) + 2°C × (A+T)] of the oligonucleotide). Microfuge tubes were labeled with A, C, G, and T. The following reagents were added: 3.3 μl of reverse transcriptase buffer [24 mM Tris-HCl (pH 8.3), 16 mM MgCl₂, 8 mM DTT, 0.8 mM dATP, 0.4 mM dCTP, 0.8 mM dGTP, and 1.2 mM dTTP] containing 100 μg/ml actinomycin D, one unit of AMV reverse transcriptase, 1 μl of a dideoxyribonucleoside triphosphate (1 mM ddTTP, ddATP, ddGTP, and 0.25 mM ddCTP) and, finally, 2 μl of the primer RNA template solution. The sample was incubated at 55°C for 45 min and the reaction was stopped by adding 2.5 μl of stop buffer (85% formamide, 25 mM EDTA, 0.1% bromophenol blue, and xylene cyanol FF). Samples were incubated at 94°C for 3 min, placed in ice water, and 1.5 μl was loaded onto a 48-cm, 0.2–0.4 mm wedged sequencing gel (6% polyacrylamide). The samples were electrophoresed for 2 hr at 50 W constant power. Subsequently, the gel was dried for 1 hr, and autoradiography was performed.

ddF

Two protocols are used in the laboratory. Each protocol is described separately below. The advantages and disadvantages of each protocol are examined in the "Discussion."

Protocol 1. A 0.5-μl sample of the transcription reaction and 0.5 μl of the ³²P end-labeled primer were added to 3 μl of the annealing buffer (concentrations as above). The samples were denatured at 80°C for 3 min and annealed at 45°C for 15 min. Subsequently, 4 μl of a "mixture" containing the following reagents were added to the primer/RNA template solution: 4 μl of reverse transcriptase buffer (concentrations as above) containing 100 μg/ml actinomycin D, 1 unit of AMV reverse transcriptase, and 1 μl of 0.25–1.0 mM ddNTP (for selection of the appropriate ddNTP and concentration to utilize, see "Discussion"). This mixture was incubated at 55°C for 30 min and the reaction was stopped by adding 20–100μl of stop buffer (40% formamide, 25 mM EDTA, 0.1% bromophenol blue and xylene cyanol FF) (see "Discussion" for selection of an appropriate stop buffer volume). Samples were incubated at 94°C for 3 min and placed in ice water for 10 min. Subsequently, 1.5 μl of sample was loaded onto a 48-cm, 0.40-mm thick nondenaturing sequencing gel (5.6% polyacrylamide with 10% glycerol

at 20°C or without glycerol at 4°C or 25% MDE gel at 20°C) with square sample wells, formed on utilizing a W comb. The samples were electrophoresed at room temperature for 2.5–3 hr at 13 watts constant power. After electrophoresis, the gel was dried for 1 hr and autoradiography was performed.

Protocol 2. A 1-μl sample of the transcription reaction and 1 μl of the ³²P end-labeled primer were added to 10 μl of annealing buffer (concentrations as above). The samples were denatured at 80°C for 5 min and annealed at 45°C for 45 min. Subsequently, 1 μl of the primer/RNA template solution was added to a mixture of the following reagents: 3.3 μl reverse transcriptase buffer (concentrations as above) containing 100 μg/ml actinomycin D and 2 units of AMV reverse transcriptase, 1 μl of 0.25–1.0 mM ddNTP (for the selection of the appropriate ddNTP and concentration to utilize, see "Discussion"). This reaction was incubated at 55°C for 45 min, and the reaction was stopped by adding 20–500 μl of stop buffer (40% formamide, 2 mM NaOH, 0.5 mM EDTA, 0.1% bromophenol blue and xylene cyanol FF) (see "Discussion" for selection of an appropriate stop buffer volume). Samples were incubated at 94°C for 3 min and placed in ice water for 10 min. Subsequently, a 1.5-μl sample was loaded onto a 48-cm, 0.40-mm thick nondenaturing sequencing gel (25% MDE) with square sample wells, formed by utilizing a W comb. The sample were electrophoresed at 4°C for 4 hr at 13 watts constant power. After electrophoresis, the gel was dried for 1 hr and autoradiography was performed.

Discussion

The great majority of our experience has been with a 29-base T7 phage promoter sequence. This sequence contains the 23 base canonical T7 phage promoter sequence (TAA TAC GAC TCA CTA TAG GGA GA), and an additional 6 bp (GGT ACC) 5′ of the 23 base sequence, which places the promoter sequence a short distance from the end of the PCR product. However, further experiments have shown the 23-bp promoter sequence works equally as well as the 29-bp sequence.

Additional phage promoter sequences, such as SP6 or T3, may be attached to the second PCR primer for the purpose of sequencing the opposite strand. For many applications, sequence of one strand is sufficient. However, faint shadow bands may occasionally interfere with the identification of mutations in which heterozygosity occurs at a particular position. Uncertainty concerning heterozygosity can be eliminated by sequencing the other strand of DNA. Performing rSSCP and ddF on both strands can help to identify mutations that may have been difficult to detect by analyzing only one strand.

The SP6 and T3 phage promoter sequences are as follows:

SP6: 5' AAT TAG GTG ACA CTA TAG AAT AG 3'

T3: 5' AAT TAA CCC TCA CTA AAG GGA AG 3'

Extensive experience with GAWTS, rSSCP, and ddF has resulted in the identification of certain problems that may lead to suboptimal results. Often these problems can be easily remedied. For example, with GAWTS, a smearing of the sequence is observed at the top of the sequencing gel when an abundance of transcript is utilized in the sequencing reaction. Smearing can be eliminated by diluting the transcript tenfold, or by stopping the sequencing reactions with a sixfold to eightfold excess of stop buffer (15–20 μl). Also, occasional shadow bands are observed on a GAWTS sequencing autoradiogram when the sequence contains T followed by G. A reduction in the concentration of transcript or reverse transcriptase, or the use of terminal deoxytransferase (DeBorde et al., 1986) may help to eliminate the "T shadow bands." Segments of high G + C can be sequenced but a high ratio of dNTP to ddNTP may be required in the "G" and "C" reactions.

For rSSCP, the intensity of the signal on the autoradiogram may at times be suboptimal. The signal intensity can be increased by decreasing the amount of stop buffer added to the reaction by 10-fold. Also, for electrophoresis of the rSSCP (or SSCP) and ddF samples, it is absolutely critical that the polyacrylamide gel be polymerized evenly throughout, and the sample wells be perfectly level and free of debris. Both of these criteria can be met in one of two ways: (1) use of large amounts of the polymerization catalysts, APS (10%) and TE-

MED (800 and 80 μl, respectively) results in rapid, even polymerization of the gel, and wells that are less susceptible to tearing; (2) substitution of MDE gel solution for the standard acrylamide solution produces sample wells that are level and resistant to tearing.

In order to maximize detection of mutations with ddF, there are several parameters that must initially be optimized. However, these parameters are specific for a particular region of DNA, and thus can vary from gene to gene and within a particular gene itself. For example, the single ddNTP utilized in ddF is determined by analyzing the dideoxy sequence of the region of interest and choosing the ddNTP that is most evenly spaced throughout the sequence. In addition, the concentration of the ddNTP utilized in the ddF reaction is chosen to be the concentration of ddNTP that produces equal band intensity between the upper and lower portions of a dideoxy sequencing gel. Once the ddF reaction is completed in a particular region for the first time, a varying amount of stop buffer can be added to the reactions in order to determine the volume of stop buffer that maximizes the signal intensity without producing a smearing of the bands at the top of the gel.

The two ddF protocols described in the "Methods" section are only slightly different, however, there are advantages and disadvantages to each protocol (Liu and Sommer, in preparation). For example, Protocol 1 is simpler than Protocol 2 since the entire reaction can be performed in one tube. However, Protocol 2 tends to produce ddF gels with sharper bands. By performing the electrophoresis at room temperature, the ddF reactions are less susceptible to smearing than the ddF reactions electrophoresed at 4°C. However, ddF gels that have been electrophoresed at 4°C on average show greater mobility shifts than gels electrophoresed at room temperature. Finally, although MDE gels produce slightly sharper bands and greater band separation on the lower portion of the gel, the resolution at the top of an MDE gel (electrophoresed at room temperature) is somewhat decreased over acrylamide. In contrast, for gels electrophoresed at 4°C, the MDE gels have all the advantages over acrylamide as stated above and, in addition, produced greater band separation near the top of the gel. No condition is ideal for optimal gel quality and convenience, but *all* detect virtually 100% of mutations. For routine screening, 25% MDE at 20°C is most often used.

A direct comparison of the rapidity, accuracy, and informativeness of the three methods for mutation detection (GAWTS, rSSCP, and ddF) indicates that each method has certain advantages and disadvantages. GAWTS accurately detects the presence of a sequence change essentially 100% of the time while also providing precise information about the location of the sequence change. However, this method is labor intensive compared to rSSCP and ddF. rSSCP is the most rapid of the techniques, since it requires only the PCR and transcription steps. However, this method does not detect all sequence changes and provides no information about the location of the sequence change. ddF requires about 50% more effort than SSCP when performed under *one* condition and can be performed with 3-fold greater rapidity than GAWTS. When SSCP is performed with small segment size, or under multiple conditions, ddF is substantially faster. The main advantage of ddF is the ability to detect virtually 100% of sequence changes. Finally, ddF is able to provide some information as to the location of the sequence change. Once a sequence change is detected with rSSCP or ddF, GAWTS can be used to identify the precise sequence change within the particular region.

Acknowledgements. This work was supported by a grant from the Share Foundation.

References

Danenberg PV, Horikoshi T, Volkenandt M, Danenberg K, Lenz H-J, Shea LCC, Dicker AP, Simoneau A, Jones PA, Bertino JR (1992): Detection of point mutations in human DNA by analysis of RNA conformation polymorphism(s). *Nucl Acids Res* 20:573–579.

DeBorde DC, Naeve CW, Herlocher ML, Maassab HF (1986): Resolution of a common RNA sequencing ambiguity by terminal deoxynucleotidyl transferase. *Anal Biochem* 157:275–282.

Ii S, Minnerath S, Ii K, Dyck PJ, Sommer SS (1991): Two tiered DNA-based diagnosis of transthyretin amyloidosis reveals two novel point mutations. *Neurology* 41:893–898.

Jacobson DP, Schmeling P, Sommer SS (1993): Characterization of the patterns of polymorphism in a "cryptic repeat" reveals a novel type of hypervariable sequence. *Am J Hum Genet* 53: 443–450.

Orita M, Suzuki Y, Sekiya T, Hayashi K (1989): Rapid and sensitive detection of point mutations and DNA polymorphisms using the polymerase chain reaction. *Genomics* 5:874–879.

Sarkar G, Kapelner S, Grandy DK, Marchionni M, Civelli O, Sobell J, Heston L, Sommer SS (1991): Direct sequencing of the dopamine D_2 receptor (DRD2) in schizophrenics reveals three polymorphisms but no structural change in the receptor. *Genomics* 11:8–14.

Sarkar G, Sommer SS (1988): RNA amplification with transcript sequencing (RAWTS). *Nucl Acids Res* 16:5197.

Sarkar G, Sommer SS (1989): Access to an mRNA sequence or its protein product is not limited by tissue or species specificity. *Science* 244:331–334.

Sarkar G, Sommer SS (1990): The "mega primer" method of site-directed mutagenesis. *BioTechniques* 8:404–407.

Sarkar G, Yoon H-S, Sommer SS (1992a): Screening for mutations by RNA single-strand conformation polymorphism (rSSCP): Comparison with DNA-SSCP. *Nucl Acids Res* 20:871–878.

Sarkar G, Yoon H-S, Sommer SS (1992b): Dideoxy fingerprinting (ddF): A rapid and efficient screen for the presence of mutations. *Genomics* 13:441–443.

Schowalter DB, Toft DO, Sommer SS (1990): A method of sequencing without subcloning and its application to the identification of a novel ORF with a sequence suggestive of a transcriptional regulator in the water mold, *Achlya ambisexualis*. *Genomics* 6:23–32.

Sommer SS, Sarkar G, Koeberl DD, Bottema CDK, Buerstedde J-M, Schowalter DB, Cassday JD (1990): Direct sequencing with the aid of phage promoters. In: *PCR Protocols: A Guide to Methods and Applications*. Innis MA, Gelfand DH, Sninsky JJ, White TJ, eds. New York: Academic Press, pp. 197–205.

Sommer SS, Cunningham J, McGovern RM, Saitoh S, Schroeder JJ, Wold LE, Kovach JS (1992): Pattern of p53 gene mutations in breast cancers of women of the Midwestern United States. *J. Natl Cancer Inst* 84:246–252.

Stoflet ES, Koeberl DD, Sarkar G, Sommer SS (1988): Genomic amplification with transcript sequencing. *Science* 239:491–494.

Yoshitake S, Schach BG, Foster DC, Davie EW, Kurachi K (1985): Nucleotide sequence of the gene for human factor IX (anti-hemophilic factor B). *Biochemistry* 24:3736–3750.

19

Capture PCR: An Efficient Method for Walking Along Chromosomal DNA and cDNA

André Rosenthal, Matthias Platzer, and D. Stephen Charnock-Jones

Introduction

The polymerase chain reaction (PCR) is an enzymatic process that allows the generation of millions of identical DNA molecules *in vitro* in a few hours, starting with as little as one copy of DNA (Mullis et al., 1986; Mullis and Faloona, 1987; Saiki et al., 1988). In contrast to conventional cloning, this *in vitro* amplification process is quick, efficient, and can easily be automated. In addition to its enormous potential for clinical diagnosis PCR has found numerous applications in all fields of biology and medicine (Innis et al., 1990; Erlich, 1989; Erlich et al., 1991).

In a typical PCR reaction two short oligonucleotide primers are hybridized to opposite strands of a target DNA molecule. A thermostable DNA polymerase catalyzes the strand-copying reaction by extending the primers in the presence of all four deoxynucleoside triphosphates. The primers are oriented in such a way that elongation proceeds across the region between the two primers. Repetitive cycles consisting of denaturing the newly synthesized strands, annealing the primers, and enzymatically synthesizing the DNA lead to an exponential amplification of the target DNA molecule.

PCR has dramatically changed the way in which experiments in molecular biology and molecular genetics are designed. However, its application to the field of genome analysis is limited because of two problems present in the original concept. Due to the enzymatic nature of the strand-copying process only relatively small pieces of DNA with a length of up to a few kilobases can be efficiently amplified. The second limitation of conventional PCR is the fact that there is a general requirement for sequence information in order to design the two primers. In fact, in most cases the DNA molecule to be amplified has already been cloned and sequenced and PCR is only used as a convenient tool to produce known ("old") DNA in large amounts. Thus, the original PCR method cannot be used to amplify an unknown DNA fragment adjacent to a known sequence and sequential walking along chromosomal DNA is impossible.

During the past 5 years several new amplification schemes have been developed to address this problem (for a review see Rosenthal, 1992). They fall into three classes: inverse PCR (Triglia et al., 1988; Ochman et al.,

The Polymerase Chain Reaction
K.B. Mullis, F. Ferré, R.A. Gibbs, editors
© 1994 Birkhauser Boston

1988; Silverman et al., 1989; Ochman et al., 1990; Earp et al., 1990; Huckaby et al., 1991; Arveiler and Porteous, 1991), cassette-based PCR (Mueller and Wold, 1989; Pfeifer et al., 1989; Shyamala and Ames, 1989; Kalman et al., 1990; Riley et al., 1990; Roux and Dhanarajan, 1990; Fors et al., 1990; Copley et al., 1991; Mueller and Wold, 1991; Pfeifer, 1992; Garrity and Wold, 1992; Jones and Winistorfer, 1992, 1993; Palittapongarnpim et al., 1993), and biotin capture PCR (Rosenthal and Jones, 1990; Rosenthal et al., 1991; Lagerström et al., 1991; Espelund and Jakobsen, 1992; Törmänen et al., 1992). In all these methods, genomic DNA is first digested with a suitable restriction enzyme to generate fragments with staggered ends. Importantly, the enzyme must cut the genomic template near to the known sequence.

Inverse PCR involves a ligation step in which circular molecules are formed and the unknown DNA is bounded by the known sequence. Amplification is then carried out with two primers that hybridize to the ends of the known sequence, but are reversed in their direction with respect to their normal orientation in PCR. In cassette-based techniques, synthetic oligonucleotide cassettes are ligated to all ends of the restriction fragments. Therefore, during this step one fragment is being formed that contains the known sequence, the adjacent unknown segment of interest and the synthetic oligo cassette. Amplification is then carried out using a primer complementary to the known sequence and a second primer complementary to the cassette. Since all restriction fragments have a cassette at each end, nonspecific amplification can occur due to the use of the cassette-specific primer.

To avoid this, special cassettes named "vectorettes" or "bubbles" (Riley et al., 1990; Copley et al., 1991) or "panhandles" (Jones and Winistorfer, 1992, 1993) have been constructed. These cassettes possess single-stranded portions to which a special cassette-specific primer cannot initially hybridize. Only after the primer complementary to the known genomic sequence has been extended in the first linear PCR cycle, can the cassette-

specific primer bind and take part in the subsequent PCR cycles.

Capture PCR: Principles

We have recently developed another amplification strategy that is named biotin capture PCR (Rosenthal and Jones, 1990; Rosenthal et al., 1991) based on the use of the biotin/streptavidin system. A biotinylated primer complementary to the known sequence region is first extended by linear amplification. Consequently, the biotinylated extension products, comprising the last portion of the known sequence and the adjacent unknown segment, are selectively captured on a streptavidin-coated solid support. Several supports including paramagnetic beads, microtiter plate wells, or a 96-pin manifold (Lagerström et al., 1991) have been successfully used to process many samples in parallel. The support is then washed several times to remove all unbiotinylated DNA present. During this purification step, the originally highly complex mixture of genomic or cDNA fragments is reduced to one of much lower complexity before exponential amplification is carried out. Hence, the background of nonspecific amplification is reduced.

Capture PCR has many interesting applications including:

1. identifying and characterizing sequences adjacent to a known locus;
2. identifying exon/intron boundaries within genes;
3. isolation of unclonable loci;
4. isolating YAC ends for physical mapping; and
5. extension incomplete cDNAs.

Walking Along Chromosomal DNA by Capture PCR

Figure 19.1 illustrates three ways to amplify an unknown DNA segment adjacent to a known locus. In our original procedure (Fig. 19.1A), synthetic oligo cassettes are ligated to all ends of genomic restriction fragments before linear

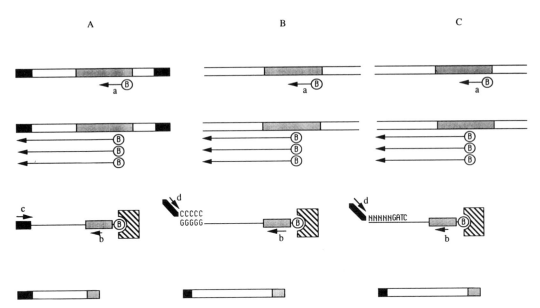

FIGURE 19.1. PCR walking along chromosomal DNA using biotin capture. Amplification of flanking genomic regions using (A) oligo cassettes ligated to all restriction fragments; (B) homopolymeric tailing; and (C) anchored degenerate primers. Open boxes illustrate genomic DNA fragments. Solid boxes represent synthetic oligo cassettes attached to the ends of these fragments. The hatched area within the open box is the known locus. The circled B describes the biotin moiety. The striped box is the solid support coated with streptavidin. (a) Biotinylated locus-specific primer; (b) nested locus-specific primer; (c) cassette-specific primer; (d) tail-specific primer.

amplification using a biotinylated locus-specific primer "a" is performed. The cassettes contain the M13 (-20) universal primer sequence facilitating subsequent fluorescent sequencing of product. After purification on the streptavidin-coated solid support system, the captured fragment can be exponentially amplified using nested locus-specific primer "b" and a primer "c" complementary to the cassette. We have used this method extensively to walk within total genomic DNA of yeast, nematode, shark, and human.

There is a need for more universal PCR amplification schemes that do not rely on initial manipulation of genomic DNA (such as restriction enzyme cleavage and ligation), since PCR walking might be difficult or impossible in regions of the genome totally resistant to restriction-enzyme digestions, or if a given set of enzymes does not cut in the region of interest at a suitable distance from the known locus. To overcome these difficulties, we have devel-

oped two new amplification schemes based on biotin capture. Both methods shown in Figure 19.1B and C do not involve any initial digestion of genomic DNA. A locus-specific biotinylated primer "a" is extended from the known locus into the adjacent unknown region by linear amplification. Afterward, the heterogeneous extension products are captured using a streptavidin-coated support and purified from the genomic DNA and the other reaction components.

In the scheme shown in Figure 19.1B the captured locus-specific fragments are then tailed with terminal transferase and dGTP. Consequently, further washings of the support are performed to remove the enzyme and the reaction components. An oligo(dC)$_{15}$ primer containing a specific tail sequence at its 5'-end is then hybridized to the homopolymeric region and is extended using Sequenase 2.0. After the extension reaction, excess of the oligo(dC)$_{15}$ primer is removed by washing the support several times. Then exponential amplification is performed using a nested locus-specific primer "b" and the tail primer "d."

In the scheme shown in Figure 19.1C a universal semirandom primer, 5' M13(-20)-NNN-NNNNNNNNNGATC 3', is hybridized to the captured locus-specific fragments. It contains a specific M13 (-20) tail sequence at its 5'-end followed by 8 to 12 degenerated bases plus four specific nucleotides, e.g., GATC at its 3'-end. These four 3' bases should anchor the primer at *Sau*3AI sites and therefore occur approximately every 256 bases. If the primer contains five specific bases at its 3'-end, it will anchor approximately every thousand basepairs.

Next, the primer is extended using Sequenase 2.0. Excess primer is then removed and exponential amplification is performed using a nested locus-specific primer "b" and the tail primer "d." The use of a universal semirandom primer together with a locus-specific primer is very attractive as it allows for significant reduction in the number of steps necessary for amplifying flanking regions.

Recently, a similar design for the universal semirandom primer has been reported for DNA sequencing (Verhasselt et al., 1992) and PCR walking (Sarkar et al., 1993). However, neither method includes a biotin capture step.

In Vitro Extension of Incomplete cDNAs Using Capture PCR

One of the major goals of the human genome project is the isolation of all human genes, yet only about 100 disease genes have so far been identified, using either biochemical knowledge of the disease and the enzyme involved or positional cloning methods. In principle, genomic sequencing could be used for finding genes in large chromosome segments. However, this approach is still too slow and expensive and only a few labs have the experience and resources required for such large-scale sequencing projects. Therefore, emphasis has now shifted toward rapid identification of a large number of genes by partial cDNA sequencing. In the last 2 years thousands of new partial

cDNAs or expressed sequence tags (ESTs) have been identified by single pass sequencing methods (for review see: Sikela and Auffray, 1993). It is expected that this number will further increase while the search continues for all human genes. Yet, the scientific value of partial cDNA fragments is limited unless they can be used as tools for isolating and sequencing the full length of their parent molecules. Full-length sequence is obviously needed to permit expression of recombinant proteins, aiding in the understanding of their biology. As conventional library screening methods are tedious and not very effective at achieving this goal, there is an increasing need for an *in vitro* method to extend partial cDNA clones.

In 1988, an *in vitro* method for the rapid amplification of cDNA ends (RACE) was proposed (Frohman et al., 1988; Frohman, 1990) and since has been widely used to obtain and sequence 3' and 5' cDNA ends when some sequence from the internal portion of the gene is known. Various modifications and improvements on the RACE procedure have also been developed and successfully employed (Dumas et al., 1991; Fritz et al., 1991; Jain et al., 1992; Borson et al., 1992).

However, as there are several shortcomings with the original RACE technique, it might not be suitable for processing many incomplete cDNAs in parallel. Capture PCR, on the other hand, using the biotin/streptavidin system can also be applied for walking along cDNAs. It can be performed in microtiter plates and has therefore the potential for high throughput and automation.

In Figure 19.2 we present modifications on this system that permit the extension of the 5'-ends of incomplete cDNAs. Either mRNA or double-stranded cDNA can be used as the starting material for extension. In both cases, a biotinylated locus-specific primer "a" is extended using an appropriate DNA polymerase. When RNA is the template reverse transcriptase must be used. The utilization of double-stranded cDNA permits repetitive linear amplification in a manner similar to that used in genomic walking. The extended product is then captured, washed, tailed, and exponentially amplified as already described.

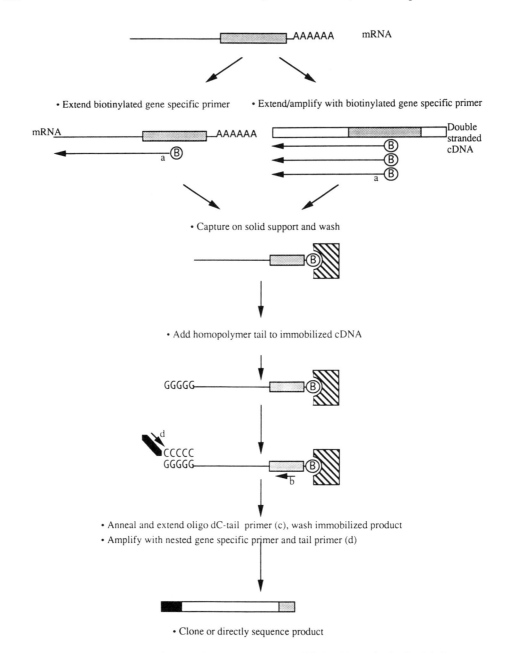

FIGURE 19.2. 5'-Extension of incomplete cDNAs by a modified PCR method using biotin capture and homopolymeric tailing.

Extension to the 3'-end of the cDNA is less complex (Fig. 19.3). The first strand cDNA is synthesized with an oligo(dT) primer containing a specific tail at its 5'-end. A primer "c" that is complementary to this tail, together with a nested locus-specific primer "b", is subsequently used during exponential amplification of the immobilized template.

Our method has several advantages over the RACE technique: it is very specific and often allows direct final product sequencing without subcloning. We have been able to show that

FIGURE 19.3. 3'-Extension of incomplete cDNAs by a modified
PCR method using biotin capture.

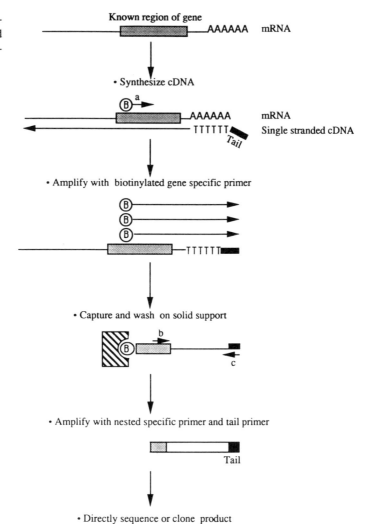

cDNA walks can be obtained from locus-specific sequences as short as 26 bp (Charnock-
Jones et al., 1993).

Sequencing of PCR Products

To prepare template DNA from PCR products,
obtained by the capture PCR walking methods
described in this article, we routinely use three
techniques.

Method 1: For single specific PCR products
the aqueous supernatant is removed from beneath the oil into a new tube. The PCR DNA is
recovered by precipitation with polyethylene
glycol (PEG). A special 26.2% PEG 8000 solution at pH 5.2 containing 6.6 mM MgCl$_2$ and
0.6 M NaOAc is used that removes efficiently
the excess of primer, nucleotides and low-
molecular-weight truncated PCR fragments
(Rosenthal et al., 1993).

Method 2: If the PCR product is not highly
specific the mixture is first separated on a 1%
agarose gel. DNA is then recovered from the
agarose by adsorption to glass beads.

Method 3: PCR products are cloned directly
into a commercial TA-vector system, or after
end-repairing with T$_4$ DNA polymerase are
cloned into the *Eco*RV site of BluescriptII. Recombinant colonies are picked into a microtiter

dish containing TB broth and the appropriate antibiotic. After overnight grow, the templates are prepared in a microtiter dish by PCR using a 96-pin hedgehog device. Excess primers, nucleotides, and small-molecular-weight products are removed by PEG precipitation as just described.

All PCR templates are cycle sequenced in 0.5-ml test tubes or in microtiter dishes using *Taq* dye terminator chemistry and the ABI 373A sequencer. Up to 96 templates can easily be sequenced in a single dish. Excess dye terminators are removed 24, 36, or 48 samples at a time by gravity chromatography using special perspex blocks of microcolumns scaled down to microtiter format (Rosenthal and Charnock-Jones, 1992). Highly accurate reads routinely yielding up to 400 bp of sequence usually result. Furthermore, both ends of the PCR product can easily be sequenced.

References

Arveiler B, Porteous DJ (1991): Amplification of end fragments of YAC recombinants by inverse-polymerase chain reaction. *Technique* 3:24–28.

Borson ND, Salo WL, Drewes LR (1992): A lock-docking oligo(dT) primer for 5' and 3' RACE PCR. *PCR Methods Applic* 2:144–148.

Charnock-Jones DS, Platzer M, Rosenthal A (1993): Extension of incomplete cDNAs (EST's) by biotin/streptavidin mediated walking using the polymerase chain reaction. *J Biotechnol,* in press.

Copley CG, Boot C, Bundell K, McPheat WL (1991): Unknown sequence amplification: Application to *in vitro* genome walking in *Chlamydia trachomatis* L2. *Bio/Technology* 9:74–79.

Dumas JB, Edwards M, Delort J, Mallet J (1991): Oligodeoxyribonucleotide ligation to single-stranded cDNA's: A new tool for cloning 5' ends of mRNA and for constructing cDNA libraries by *in vitro* amplification. *Nucl Acids Res* 19:5227–5232.

Earp DJ, Lowe B, Baker B (1990): Amplification of genomic sequences flanking transposable elements in host and heterologous plants: A tool for transposon tagging and genome characterization. *Nucl Acids Res* 18:3271–3279.

Erlich HA (ed) (1989): *PCR Technology—Principles and Applications for DNA Amplification.* New York: Stockton Press.

Erlich HA, Gelfand D, Sninsky JJ (1991): Recent advantages in the polymerase chain reaction. *Science* 252:1643–1651.

Espelund M, Jakobsen KS (1992): Cloning and direct sequencing of plant promotors using primer-adapter mediated PCR on DNA coupled to a magnetic solid phase. *BioTechniques* 13:74–81.

Fors L, Saavedra RA, Hood L (1990): Cloning of the shark Po promotor using a genomic walking technique based on the polymerase chain reaction. *Nucl Acids Res* 18:2793–2799.

Fritz JD, Greaser ML, Wolff JA (1991): A novel 3' extension technique using random primers in RNA-PCR. *Nucl Acids Res* 19:3747.

Frohman MA (1990): RACE: Rapid amplification of cDNA ends. In: *PCR Protocols—A Guide to Methods and Applications.* Innis MA, Gelfand DH, Sninsky JJ, White TJ, eds. San Diego: Academic Press.

Frohman MA, Dush MK, Martin GR (1988): Rapid production of full-length cDNA from rare transcripts: Amplification using a single gene-specific oligonucleotide primer. *Proc Natl Acad Sci USA* 85:8998–9002.

Garrity PA, Wold BJ (1992): Effects of different DNA polymerases in ligation-mediated PCR: Enhanced genomic sequencing and *in vivo* footprinting. *Proc Natl Acad Sci USA* 89:1021–1025.

Huckaby CS, Kouri RE, Lane MJ, Peshick SM, Carroll WT, Henderson SM, Faldasz BD, Waterbury PG, Vournakis JN (1991): An efficient technique for obtaining sequences flanking inserted retroviruses. *GATA* 8:151–158.

Innis MA, Gelfand DH, Sninsky JJ, White TJ (eds) (1990): *PCR Protocols—A Guide to Methods and Applications.* San Diego: Academic Press.

Jain R, Gomer RH, Murtagh JJ (1992): Increasing specificity from PCR-RACE technique. *BioTechniques* 12:58–59.

Jones D, Winistorfer SC (1992): Sequence specific generation of a DNA panhandle permits PCR amplification of unknown flanking DNA. *Nucl Acids Res* 20:595–600.

Jones DH, Winistorfer SC (1993): Genome walking with 2- to 4-kb steps using panhandle PCR. *PCR Methods Applic* 2:197–203.

Kalman M, Kalman ET, Cashel M (1990): Polymerase chain reaction (PCR) amplification with a single specific primer. *Biochem Biophys Res Commun* 167:504–506.

Lagerström M, Parik J, Malmgren H, Stewart J, Petterson U, Landegren U (1991): Capture PCR: Efficient amplification of DNA fragments adjacent to known sequences in human and YAC DNA. *PCR Methods Applic* 1:111–119.

Mueller PR, Wold B (1989): *In vivo* footprinting of a muscle specific enhancer by ligation mediated PCR. *Science* 246:780–786.

Mueller PR, Wold B (1991): Ligation-mediated PCR: Applications to genomic footprinting. *Methods: Companion Methods Enzymol* 2:20–31.

Mullis KB, Faloona FA (1987): Specific synthesis of DNA in vitro via a polymerase catalyzed chain reaction. *Methods Enzymol* 155:335–350.

Mullis KB, Faloona FA, Scharf SJ, Saiki RK, Horn GT, Erlich HA (1986): Specific enzymatic amplification of DNA in vitro: The polymerase chain reaction. *Cold Spring Harbor Symp Quant Biol* 51:263–273.

Ochman H, Gerber AS, Hartl DL (1988): Genetic applications of an inverse polymerase chain reaction. *Genetics* 120:621–623.

Ochman H, Medhora MM, Garza D, Hartl DL (1990): Amplifications of flanking sequences by inverse PCR. In: *PCR Protocols—A Guide to Methods and Applications*. Innis MA, Gelfand DH, Sninsky JJ, White TJ, eds. San Diego: Academic Press.

Palittapongarnpim P, Chomyc S, Fanning A, Kunimoto D (1993): DNA fingerprinting of *Mycobacterium tuberculosis* isolates by ligation-mediated polymerase chain reaction. *Nucl Acids Res* 21:761–762.

Pfeifer GP (1992): Analysis of chromatin structure by ligation-mediated PCR. *PCR Methods Applic* 2:107–111.

Pfeifer GP, Steigerwald SD, Mueller PR, Wold B, Riggs AD (1989): Genomic sequencing and methylation analysis by ligation mediated PCR. *Science* 246:810–813.

Riley J, Butler R, Ogilvie D, Finniear R, Jenner D, Powell S, Anand R, Smith JC, Markham AF (1990): A novel, rapid method for the isolation of terminal sequence from yeast artificial chromosome (YAC) clones. *Nucl Acids Res* 18:2887–2890.

Rosenthal A (1992): PCR amplification techniques for chromosome walking. *Trends Biotechnol* 10:44–48.

Rosenthal A, Jones DSC (1990): Genomic walking and sequencing by oligo-cassette mediated polymerase chain reaction. *Nucl Acids Res* 18:3095–3096.

Rosenthal A, MacKinnon RN, Jones DSC (1991): PCR walking from microdissection clone M54 identifies three exons from the human gene for the neural cell adhesion molecule L1 (CAM-L1). *Nucl Acids Res* 19:5395–5401.

Rosenthal A, Charnock-Jones DS (1992): New protocols for DNA sequencing with dye terminators. *DNA Sequence—DNA Sequencing Mapping* 3:61–64.

Rosenthal A, Coutelle O, Craxton M (1993): Large-scale production of DNA sequencing templates by microtitre format PCR. *Nucl Acids Res* 21:173–174.

Roux KH, Dhanarajan P (1990): A strategy for single site PCR amplification of ds DNA: Priming digested cloned or genomic DNA from an anchor-modified restriction site and a short internal sequence. *BioTechniques* 8:48–57.

Saiki RK, Gelfand DH, Stoffel S, Scharf SJ, Higuchi R, Horn GT, Mullis KB, Erlich HA (1988): Primer-directed enzymatic amplification of DNA with a thermostable DNA polymerase. *Science* 239:487–491.

Sarkar G, Turner RT, Bolander ME (1993): Restriction-site PCR: A direct method of unknown sequence retrieval adjacent to a known locus by using universal primers. *PCR Methods Applic* 2:318–322.

Shyamala V, Ames FL (1989): Genome walking by single-specific-primer polymerase chain reaction: SSP-PCR. *Gene* 84:1–8.

Silverman GA, Ye RD, Pollock KM, Sadler JE, Korsmeyer SJ (1989): Use of yeast artificial chromosome clones for mapping and walking within human chromosome segment 18q21.3. *Proc Natl Acad Sci USA* 86:7485–7489.

Sikela JM, Auffray C (1993): Finding new genes faster than ever. *Nature Genet* 3:189–191.

Törmänen YT, Swiderski PM, Kaplan BE, Pfeifer GP, Riggs AD (1992): Extension product capture improves genomic sequencing and DNase I footprinting by ligation-mediated PCR. *Nucl Acids Res* 20:5487–5488.

Triglia T, Peterson MG, Kemp DJ (1988): A procedure for in vitro amplification of DNA segments that lie outside the boundaries of known sequences. *Nucl Acids Res* 16:8186.

Verhasselt P, Voet M, Volckaert G (1992): DNA sequencing by a subcloning-walking strategy using a specific and a semi-random primer in the polymerase chain reaction. *DNA Sequence* 2:281–287.

PART TWO
Applications

SECTION I
General Applications

20

In Vitro Evolution of Functional Nucleic Acids: High-Affinity RNA Ligands of the HIV-1 *rev* Protein

Craig Tuerk, Sheela MacDougal-Waugh, Gerald Z. Hertz, and Larry Gold

Introduction

Naturally occurring nucleic acids are primarily viewed as information-bearing macromolecules. In addition to encoding protein gene products, genomic DNA (or RNA) contains sequences that serve as recognition sites for the binding of various regulatory and catalytic proteins as well as RNA structural information crucial to a variety of biochemical functions. Thus, any nucleic acid sequence found in nature may be composed of tiers of information whose evolved function is revealed at discrete points in the cellular biochemistry and life cycle of the organism from which it is derived. One of the tasks facing a molecular biologist is to distinguish at what level each piece of sequence information is relevant. One level of information is the sequence-specific contributions of nucleic acids to protein–nucleic acid interactions. It was during investigations into such contributions of RNA sequence to affinity for T_4 DNA polymerase that we developed a system we call SELEX (for Systematic Evolution of Ligands by EXponential enrichment).

SELEX is a protocol for isolating from a pool of variant nucleic acid sequences high af-finity ligands to a target protein (Tuerk and Gold, 1990). Basically this procedure involves cycles of affinity selection by a target molecule from a heterogeneous population of nucleic acids, replication of the bound species (the ligands), and *in vitro* transcription to generate an enriched pool of RNA (if the ligand is to be an RNA) (see Fig. 20.1). To begin, oligonucleotide templates for *in vitro* transcription by T_7 RNA polymerase are created with a random region flanked by two regions of fixed sequence. *Selection* requires physical separation of bound RNAs from unbound RNA. Selected RNAs from this population can be replicated by annealing the *3' primer* to the 3' fixed region and extending with reverse transcriptase (*cDNA synthesis*). The *5' primer*, which is annealed to the cDNA in the first cycle of *PCR*, adds the T_7 promoter sequence required for *in vitro* transcription to start the next round. In experiments in which DNA is the ligand, there is no need for an added promoter sequence or for the steps of *in vitro* transcription and cDNA synthesis.

The term "*in vitro* evolution" is appropriately applied to SELEX. Evolution can be simply defined as a process by which selection is applied to a population of nonidentical replica-

The Polymerase Chain Reaction
K.B. Mullis, F. Ferré, R.A. Gibbs, editors
© 1994 Birkhäuser Boston

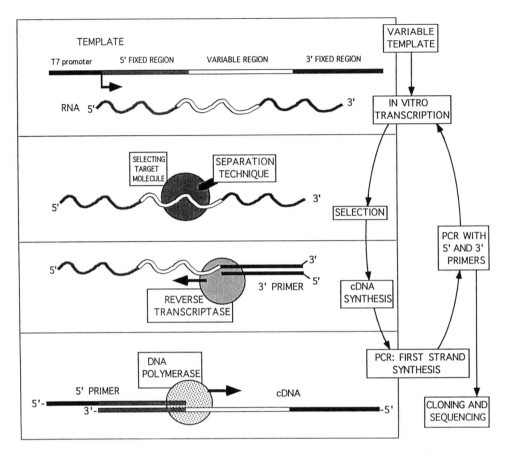

FIGURE 20.1. SELEX. Illustrated are the various nucleic acid species and enzymatic processes used during cycles of SELEX (see text).

ble units so that subsets of the population survive to reproduce. Subsequent variation and selection further alter the character of the population by enriching for adaptive traits. In nature, variation is serially introduced mainly through (necessarily) infrequent errors in replication so that new sequence combinations are incompletely tested. *In vitro* evolution systems make use of the relatively vast sequence potential provided by random incorporation during the synthesis of oligonucleotides; in addition, the enzymatic processes used for replication also introduce some variation at each round. Natural selection is a process that encompasses a host of adaptive and accidental biases that in sum determine evolutionary outcomes. *In vitro* evolution seeks to apply one or few

selective criteria, which is affinity for a target molecule in SELEX.

The original SELEX experiment was used to provide an expanded phylogeny of RNAs that interact with bacteriophage T$_4$ DNA polymerase. T$_4$ DNA polymerase regulates its own synthesis by binding a 36-nucleotide sequence that overlaps its ribosome binding site; phylogenetic comparisons to other related bacteriophages highlighted an RNA hairpin with an absolutely conserved eight nucleotide loop sequence within this translational operator (Andrake et al., 1988; Tuerk et al., 1990). Tuerk and Gold (1990) constructed templates in which the 8 nucleotides of that conserved loop were varied by random incorporation at those positions during oligonucleotide synthesis.

In vitro transcription from these templates yielded a library of variant sequences with 65,536 potential species. Four rounds of selection by T_4 DNA polymerase on nitrocellulose filters followed by replicative and *in vitro* transcription steps yielded a pool of high-affinity RNA sequences that was composed of essentially two major sequences. One sequence was the wild-type sequence, AAUAACUC, found in the bacteriophage mRNA. The other sequence was a variant, AGCAACCU, that differed as underlined from the wild type at four positions, formed a different secondary structure by extending the operator hairpin by two more base pairs, and bound to T_4 DNA polymerase equivalently well. Single nucleotide variants of each of these two species were recovered and found to bind with 2- to 5-fold lower affinity. This simple experimental result suggested that (1) SELEX could precisely discriminate against ligands of slightly less affinity for the target molecule, (2) optimal ligand/target interactions can be achieved through unique sequences that may defy attempts to rationalize their equivalence based on structure or common atomic group presentation, and (3) arriving at one unique sequence from another unique sequence (e.g., from the wild-type sequence to the major variant sequence) by serial single-point mutations (as probably occurs in nature) would be discriminated against by the resultant lower affinities encountered at the intermediate steps; or, to put it in other words, it is unlikely that natural evolution can find all possible sequence solutions to a stringent selective pressure. Our earlier work with T_4 DNA polymerase (Tuerk et al., 1990) established that association with its RNA recognition site inhibited the polymerase function of this enzyme. We thus imagined one could evolve functional nucleic acid ligands that inhibit many target proteins (including those for which there is no biological precedent of binding nucleic acids). We have since isolated RNA pseudoknot inhibitors of HIV-1 reverse transcriptase using SELEX (Tuerk et al., 1992).

Here we describe the collection of RNA ligands we have isolated against the HIV-1 *rev* protein. The *rev* protein is essential for produc-tive infection of the HIV-1 virus (Sodroski et al., 1986; Feinberg et al., 1986; Heaphy et al., 1990). Its role is involved in the appearance of *gag-pol* and *env* mRNAs during the viral cycle (Malim et al., 1990; Felber et al., 1989; Emerman et al., 1989: Hammarskjold et al., 1989) and presumably its function is mediated by its interaction with those messages at a specific site in the HIV genome referred to as the *rev*-responsive element or RRE (Malim et al., 1990; Heaphy et al., 1990; Kjems et al., 1991) (Fig. 20.2). Because the sequences of the RRE are also coding sequences for the HIV-1 surface protein gp120, there is an overlapping biological constraint that limits the natural variability of RNA sequences that interact with *rev* protein. We thus decided to test the capacity of SELEX to provide a consensus of RNA sequences, unbiased by biological precedence and constraints for the HIV-1 *rev* protein, both to see how related that consensus would be to the wild-type recognition site and to find RNA ligands of higher affinity than the wild-type sequence.

Materials and Methods

SELEX (Systematic Evolution of Ligands by EXponential Enrichment)

Initial templates for *in vitro* transcription were assembled by ligation as described (Tuerk and Gold, 1990) using the oligos listed in Table 20.1. Purified template (500 pmol, containing approximately 10^{14} of the possible 10^{19} sequences that could be expected from the randomization at 32 positions) was transcribed with T_7 RNA polymerase as described (Tuerk and Gold, 1990). The typical RNA concentration for rounds of SELEX was approximately $3 \times 10^{-5} M$. For SELEX with HIV-1 *rev* protein the concentration of protein was $1.8 \times 10^{-7} M$ in the first round and $2.5 \times 10^{-8} M$ in all subsequent rounds. Because we had found that sequences could arise during SELEX that are significantly retained by nitrocellulose filters (Tuerk et al., 1992), the initial pool of RNAs was prefiltered through nitrocellulose before the first, third, sixth, and ninth rounds

TABLE 20.1. Oligonucleotide primers used in this work with the function of each in template construction, PCR, and cloning identified.[a]

1. 5'-taatacgactcactatagggagccaacaccacaattccaatcaag-3'
   (bridging oligo for 5' construction and 5' PCR oligo)
2. 5'-atctatgaaagaattttatatctc-3'
   (bridging oligo for 3' ligation)
3. 5'-gaattgtggtgttggctccctatagtgagtcgtatta-3'
   (template construction oligo)
4. 5'-tttcatagatnnnnnnnnnnnnnnnnnnnnnnnnnnnnnnnnncttgattg-3'
   (template construction oligo)
5. 5'-ccggatccgtttcaatagagatataaaattc-3'
   (3' cloning oligo and template construction oligo)
6. 5'-gtttcaatagagatataaaattctttcatag-3'
   (3' primer for PCR)
7. 5'-ccgaagcttctaatacgactcactatagggag-3'
   (5' cloning primer)
8. 5'-TAATACGACTCACTATA-3'
   (T_7 promoter oligo)
9. 5'-GCACTATACCAGACAATAATTGTCTGGCCTGTACCGTCAGCGTCATTGACGCTGCGCCCATAGTGCTCCC-
   TATAGTGAGTCGTATTA-3'
   (oligo template for in vitro transcription of wild-type RRE)
10. 5'-GAGACCCGAGTCCACGGCCGAAGCCGTGTATCTCAAGGGTCCCTATAGTGAGTCGTATTA-3'
    (oligo template for in vitro transcription of consensus motif I)

[a]All oligos were prepared as described in Gauss et al. (1987).

of selection. At every third round of selection we purified the cDNA product to avoid anomalously sized species which typically appear during multiple rounds of SELEX. All RNA-protein binding reactions were done in a buffer of 200 mM KOAc, 50 mM Tris-HCl, pH 7.7, 10 mM dithiothreitol. RNA and protein dilutions were mixed, stored on ice for 30 min, and incubated at 37°C for 5 min. (In binding assays the reaction volume was 60 μl of which 50 μl was assayed; in SELEX rounds the reaction volume was 100 μl). Each reaction was suctioned through a prewet (with binding buffer) nitrocellulose filter and rinsed with 3 ml of binding buffer after which it was dried and counted for assays or subjected to elution as part of the SELEX protocol (Tuerk and Gold, 1990; Tuerk et al., 1990).

Information Content Analysis

The sequences were aligned to optimize the information content within a subregion of the alignment by a modification of the procedure described in Stormo and Hartzell (1989) and Hertz et al. (1990). After the best subalignment was determined, the sequences were re-

aligned to find the best alignment excluding the subregion of each sequence that was contained in the first alignment. The alignment of each of the subregions was summarized in a matrix whose elements were the number of times each base was observed at each position of the alignment. The cloned sequences were scored according to how closely they matched the matrix patterns as described in Stormo and Hartzell (1989).

Results

Sequence Analysis of *rev* Protein Ligands

To create a consensus of relatively small high-affinity RNA ligands for a variety of proteins, we created template populations (see Materials and Methods and Table 20.1) with a 32-nucleotide-long random region flanked by fixed regions necessary for replicability in SELEX. After 10 rounds of SELEX using *rev* protein as the target, the sequence in the variable region of the RNA population was nonrandom. We cloned and sequenced 53 isolates from this

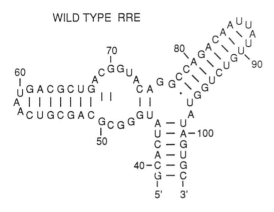

FIGURE 20.2. The computer program: predicted secondary structure of the wild-type RRE RNA. Shown is the optimal folding devised from a program developed by Zuker and colleagues (Zuker, 1989; Jaeger et al., 1989a,b).

population. The sequences are listed in Figure 20.3. Potential RNA secondary structures were examined using computer programs obtained from Zuker and colleagues (Zuker, 1989; Jaeger et al., 1989a,b). We allowed suboptimal foldings to discover (by eye) any consensus structures by which sequences could be grouped. We used information content analyses (Hertz et al., 1990; Stormo and Hartzell, 1989) to search for similarities in the primary sequence of the *rev* protein ligands. By these criteria of primary sequence and secondary structure homology, all sequences were classified into three motifs (I, II, III) as shown in Figures 20.3 and 20.4.

Motif I exhibits an internal bulge closed at each end by a helix as shown in Figure 20.3. The information content analysis identified two coexistent, significant regions of primary sequence similarity. The most common primary sequence patterns found in the Motif I isolates, UUGAGAUACA (Sequence I) and UGGACUC (Sequence II), are positioned opposite each other in the internal bulge. These sequences are boxed in Figure 20.3. The CA of Sequence I can be base paired to the UG of Sequence II; there are two sequences in which the A:U pair is replaced by a C:G (Sequence 12) or a U:A (Sequence 11). There is also potential base pairing of the GAG of Sequence

I across the bulge-loop to the CUC of Sequence II as indicated in Figure 20.4.

Motif II is similar to Motif I in that the subsequence -GAUACA predominates in a loop opposite -UGGACA- (both boxed in Fig. 20.4) with a similar pairing of -CA- to UG-. Motif II differs from Motif I in the size of the bulged loops and in the reduced base pairing across the bulge. The wild type *rev*-responsive element (RRE) (Malim et al., 1990; Heaphy et al., 1990) was also folded by the structure prediction program (Fig. 20.2). One domain of the folded wild-type RRE resembles Motifs I and II as shown in Figure 20.4. As shown, there are within this domain some significant sequence identities to the corresponding positions within the Motif I and II isolates.

Motif III is the least like all the other sequences, although it is characterized by two bulged Us immediately 5' to base paired -GA-:-UC- as in Motif I (Fig. 20.4). Unfortunately, further comparisons are complicated because the folding pattern of Motif III involves the 3' fixed sequence region in critical secondary structures; because these sequences are invariant there is no way to determine by sequence comparison the importance of any one nucleotide position. However, it is notable that each of the Motif III clones involves this fixed region in an identical fashion.

The ΔG of folding of each of the Motif I and II RNA isolates (including the fixed flanking sequences) as predicted by the folding program is shown in Table 20.2, along with the lowest energy competing secondary structure. Also shown in Table 20.2 are scores for evaluating the match of each Motif I and II sequence to the two consensus elements Sequence I and Sequence II.

Affinity Assays of RNA Ligands for *rev* Protein

The sequences were further analyzed for their affinity to the *rev* protein. Labeled *in vitro* transcripts were prepared and individually assayed for their ability to bind to *rev* protein (Tuerk and Gold, 1990; Tuerk et al., 1990). We also synthesized and tested labeled transcripts cor-

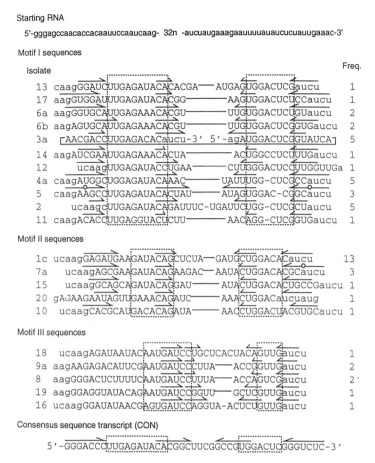

Starting RNA

5'-gggagccaacaccacaauuccaaucaag- 32n -aucuaugaaagaauuuuauaucucuauugaaac-3'

FIGURE 20.3. Listed in upper case letters are the sequences of the variable regions (flanked by some of the 5' and 3' fixed sequence shown in lower case letters) of 53 isolates cloned after 10 rounds of SELEX with HIV-1 *rev* protein. The sequences are grouped into three general motifs. Each sequence is followed by the number of isolates found in the population having that sequence [some with minor differences (mostly single base changes) that can be attributed to mutation during SELEX]. The criteria for these groupings are both secondary structure and primary sequence similarities. The secondary structures as predicted by the Zuker program (Zuker, 1989; Jaeger et al., 1989a,b) are shown with overlined arrows that highlight the inverted repeats indicative of base pairing. Similar sequences within each motif that are identified by the information content analysis (Hertz et al., 1990; Stormo and Hartzell, 1989) are boxed with a dotted line. Also shown at the top is the starting RNA with the complete sequence of 5' and 3' flanking sequences, and at the bottom the consensus sequence transcript whose values are shown in Table 20.2.

responding to the wild-type RRE (WT in Table 20.2) and to the consensus motif in a highly stable conformation (Fig. 20.3, Tuerk et al., 1988). To control for experimental variations (especially in protein dilutions), the highest affinity ligand, 6a, was assayed as a standard in every binding experiment. The best fit of the data to a bimolecular binding curve was obtained (Unnithan et al., 1990) and the ratio of the calculated K_a of each ligand to that of ligand 6a is presented in Table 20.2. The average K_a for ligand 6a was $8.26 \pm 0.25 \times 10^8 \, M^{-1}$.

In general, the affinity data confirm that Motif I defines the highest affinity ligands to *rev*

FIGURE 20.4. Schematic diagram of the consensus Motifs I, II, and III, and of a portion of the wild-type RRE (see Fig. 20.2). The lines between bases across the bulged loop indicate additional base pairs predicted by the computer program (see text). Regions of Motifs II and III and of the wild-type RRE that are identical to Motif I are boxed. Xs indicate lack of strong primary sequence consensus at that position and base pair to Xs.

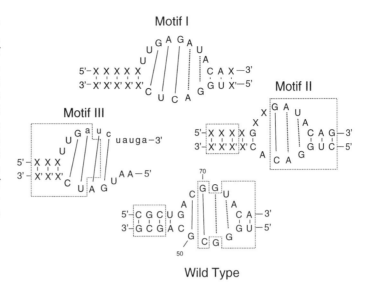

Discussion

protein. This consensus is composed of both primary sequence information and secondary structure. Changes in secondary structure have a dramatic effect on binding. Ligands 6a and 6b are identical in the regions of high primary sequence information content (Sequences I and II), but are quite different at the level of secondary structure resulting from differences at three nucleotide positions (Fig. 20.3). These differences, which predict the elimination of the bulged -UU- portion of Loop 1 by extending the base pairing of the adjacent stem, lower the affinity of 6b by 24-fold. Ligand 17 contains the maximum information score as shown in Table 20.2. However, there is an extra bulged U at the 5'-end of Sequence I that may explain ligand 17's reduced affinity for *rev* protein as compared to other sequences of Motif I. In contrast, single nucleotide deletions of the opposing loop sequences within Sequence II (as in sequences 5 and 4a), even those that diminish the prospect of cross-bulge base pairing (sequence 5), are well tolerated by the *rev* protein interaction. In addition, competing secondary structures (or lack of them) may be factors in other isolates' affinities for *rev* protein as suggested by the ΔGs of Table 20.2 for ligand Sequences 2 and 12.

These experiments highlight a specific region of the wild-type RRE that may be important for *rev* protein binding. This region has been identified by others (Heaphy et al., 1991; Karn et al., 1991; Cook et al., 1991; Bartel et al., 1991) as sufficient for high-affinity binding to *rev* protein. We show in Figure 20.4 a comparison of this wild-type region and the three Motifs exhibited by the *rev* protein ligands we have isolated. Because Motif I represents the highest affinity consensus for RNA interactions with *rev* protein, we have boxed the nucleotide positions and base pairings at which the other two motifs and the wild-type sequence are identical. Motifs I and II and the wild type feature a highly structured bulge flanked by two helices. Our results suggest that the most significant nucleotides identified in the wild type site are those boxed in Figure 20.4.

Bartel et al. (1991) performed a similar SE-LEX experiment on the *rev* protein, but with notable differences. Our experiment was unbiased for 32 nucleotides. Their experiment started with a randomized template that was biased toward the wild-type sequence (covering 66 nucleotides of the wild type RRE) and

TABLE 20.2. Characteristics of each of the isolates studied with comparisons to other species.[a]

Motif	Clone	Frequency	ΔG_f consensus structure	ΔG_f competing structure	Information score Sequence I	Information score Sequence II	Total information score	K_a / K_a^{6a}
I	6a	2	−11.6	−9.9	16.38	12.74	29.12	1.000
	13	1	−9.9	−9.7	18.25	12.74	30.99	0.576
	5	3	−10.4	−10.8	18.25	7.83	26.08	0.567
	4a	5	−14.2	−15.6	17.40	7.46	24.86	0.564
	3a	5	−9.5	−8.8	14.79	12.74	27.53	0.405
	12	1	−8.9	−10.2	15.79	10.74	26.53	0.298
	17	1	−14.8	−12.0	18.25	12.74	30.99	0.247
	2	5	−8.5	−9.1	18.25	3.87	22.12	0.114
	6b	2	−	−11.5	16.38	12.74	29.12	0.042
	14	1	−10.1	−10.2	16.38	10.16	26.54	−
	11	1	−8.6	−10.9	13.21	6.93	20.14	−
II	15	1	−11.1	−10.4	12.62	11.42	24.04	0.455
	20	1	−4.8	−6.4	7.39	4.91	12.30	0.191
	1c	13	−10.0	−13.2	15.67	11.42	27.09	0.154
	7a	3	−6.4	−5.6	13.21	11.42	24.63	−
	10	1	−10.2	−8.6	6.60	10.16	16.76	−
III	8	2	−	−	−	−	−	0.292
	18	1	−	−	−	−	−	0.149
	9a	2	−	−	−	−	−	0.106
	Evol. pop.	−	−	−	−	−	−	0.435
	CON	−	−21.1	−19.7	18.25	12.74	30.99	0.429
	WT	−	−27.0	−26.3	9.38	6.83	16.21	0.180
	32n	−	−	−	−	−	−	0.015

[a]The first and second columns list the isolate and the representation in the clonal population. The third column lists the energies of secondary structure formation assigned by the Zuker program to the folded RNA, which contains the consensus conformation shown in Figure 20.4. (Note that no foldings of 6b can achieve the consensus conformation that would require pairing an A to a G. As a consequence there is no value listed here. Note also that although ligand 17 has an extra bulged U, the energy listed is for the consensus conformation with that extra bulged U.) The fourth column lists the energy associated with the most probable competing conformation as predicted by the program. The fifth and sixth columns show the scores indicating how well each sequence matched the matrix patterns corresponding to the conserved subsequences Sequence I (UUGAGAUACA) and II (UGGACUC) as described in Materials and Methods. The scores are totaled in column seven. The eighth column lists the ratio of the K_as determined by a best-fit program written by (Unnithan et al., 1990) between each species and species 6a with which each isolate was experimentally compared for its affinity to *rev* protein. "CON" refers to the consensus sequence transcript shown in Figure 20.3; "WT" to the wild-type sequence shown in Figure 20.2.

was conducted for only three rounds of SE-LEX. As a result, only a limited sequence space was explored in a rigidly defined primary sequence and secondary structure framework, and the search was terminated so that only "neutral" changes would be detected. Nonetheless, their experiment confirmed the primary site of *rev* protein interaction through the invariability of many of those nucleotides at the bulge demarked by wild-type nucleotides U45 through G53 and C65 through A75, and by extension of the two base stem (U45, G46 paired to A75, C74) that closes the one end of the bulge in the wild-type sequence.

They also identified an unusual base pairing of G48–G70 by its interchangeability with a potentially isosteric A–A. The evolved ligands of Motifs I and II utilized the A–A pairing at this position frequently (see Fig. 20.3) although deletion of the A at the position that corresponds to wild-type G48 is allowed; the A at the position that corresponds to wild-type G70 is invariant. Whether the frequent occurrence of this A–A pair instead of G–G is indicative of the subtly higher affinity reported by Bartel et al. (1991) for this substitution or some other selective pressure such as replicative competence (see below) is not yet clear. Bartel et al.

(1991) also suggest that the invariance of A73 opposed to G47, combined with the commonality of such oppositions in other studies, argues for another unusual base pairing between them. Invariance of opposing nucleotides in a bulge is not a valid criterion for postulating that there is unusual base pairing between them. Those positions could be invariant because each represents a significant contact with *rev* protein. We find that the U that corresponds to wild-type U72 is preferred for the ligands we isolated, although substitution is allowable without significantly reducing affinity to *rev* protein. Without additional data, it is not reasonable to postulate the unusual base pairing of G47 to A73 instead of G47 to U72 that we have indicated. Bartel et al. (1991) also propose that the base pairing of G50 and C69 is not essential for wild-type *rev* protein binding, which we confirm with the lack of base pairing found at the corresponding position in the Motif II sequences.

The SELEX experiments that we conducted also provided a set of ligands (Motif I) that bind with higher affinity than wild type. The interaction of *rev* protein with the various subdomains of these ligands may be additive. Motifs II and III resemble Motif I at two adjacent subdomains as shown in Figure 20.4. We speculate that this is indicative of two *rev* protein-interacting sites that exist together in Motif I and separately in Motifs II and III and that the sum of these interactions can account for the generally higher affinities of the Motif I isolates. The interactive site on the *rev* protein for Motif II isolates is probably the same site that interacts with the wild-type RRE. The addition of the interaction utilizing the two bulged Us increases the affinity of Motif I isolates up to 6-fold. It is interesting that the highest affinity ligand to *rev* protein isolated by Bartel et al. (1991) also contained two bulged Us at approximately this site.

The abundance of individual *rev* protein ligand sequences in the cloned population is not strictly correlated with affinity to *rev* protein. The concentration of *rev* protein used during selection was sufficient to bind a significant percentage of all of these isolates and thus there may have been selection for replicability superimposed on a relatively low stringency selection for binding to *rev* protein (Irvine et al., 1991). There may have been some additional selection during the steps of cloning and screening. The mutagenicity of the replicative components of SELEX may produce higher affinity ligands in later rounds of SELEX so that representation in the population is not only a reflection of higher affinity to *rev* protein. Such possibilities necessitate careful assays of the affinity of the SELEX ligands for their target, in order to properly weight individual contributions to the perceived consensus.

SELEX Applications

There are few effective antiviral treatments. Because viruses recruit the intracellular machinery of the host to reproduce, there are far fewer targets for intervention than for pathogenic bacteria. However, many of the virally encoded proteins crucial to the progress of the viral life cycle involve specific nucleic acid recognition. Successful "intracellular immunization" (Baltimore, 1988; Sanford, 1988; Sanford and Johnston, 1985) has been achieved against HIV-1 infection in cultured cells by overexpressing a natural RNA recognition sequence for the tat protein (Sullenger et al., 1990). Incomplete inhibition of HIV-1 replication was accomplished by similar overexpression of a truncated RRE sequence (Lee et al., 1992). The use of these natural sequences as "decoys" may be problematic because they may also inhibit important cellular factors with which they specifically interact (Lee et al., 1992). Even more efficient immunization should be obtained with the ligands we describe that bind *rev* protein with higher affinity than wild-type sequences.

We have also used SELEX to isolate RNA pseudoknot inhibitors of HIV-1 reverse transcriptase that have no semblance to known natural RNA sequences (Tuerk et al., 1992). In developing nucleic acid ligand strategies against viral diseases, SELEX procedures will be invaluable in rapidly identifying the most promising sequences, especially for target proteins for which there is no described biological ligand. When the presently emerging strategies for functional nucleic acid delivery to cellular compartments become more routine (Malone et al., 1989; Sioud et al., 1992), these and related ligands may be developed as drugs to treat a variety of diseases. In addition, such RNAs, or model compounds based on their sequence and structure, may be useful against serum targets as is illustrated by the evolved DNA ligands inhibitory to thrombin (Bock et al., 1992).

Acknowledgments. The HIV-1 *rev* protein was a generous gift from Maria Zapp and Michael Green. We thank Sean Eddy, David Parma, Bruce Beutel, Matt Wecker, and Diane Tasset for critical reading of the manuscript. We also thank Catherine Conway Rucker for her excellent technical assistance early in this work, and Kathy Piekarski for her help. We thank Robin Gutell for his expert assistance and advice in formatting 2-D structures for presentation and in the computer-aided folding of RNA. The work was supported by NIH Grants GM28685 and GM19963 and, in the later stages, by NeXagen, Inc. We also thank the W.M. Keck Foundation for their generous support of RNA science on the Boulder campus.

References

Andrake M, Guild N, Hsu T, Gold L, Tuerk C, Karam J (1988): DNA polymerase of bacteriophage T4 is an autogenous translational repressor. *Proc Natl Acad Sci USA* 85:7942–7946.

Baltimore D (1988): Gene therapy: Intracellular immunization. *Nature (London)* 335:395–396.

Bartel D, Zapp ML, Green MR, Szostak JW (1991): HIV-1 *rev* regulation involves recognition of non-Watson-Crick base pairs in viral RNA. *Cell* 67:529–536.

Bock LC, Griffin LC, Latham JA, Vermass EM, Toole JJ (1992): Selection of single-stranded DNA molecules that bind and inhibit human thrombin. *Nature* 355:564–566.

Cook KS, Fisk GJ, Hauber J, Usman N, Daly TJ, Rusche JR (1991): Characterization of HIV-1 *rev* protein: Binding stoichiometry and minimal RNA substrate. *Nucl Acids Res* 19:1577–1583.

Emerman M, Vazeux R, Peden K (1989): The *rev* gene product of the human immunodeficiency virus affects envelope-specific RNA localization. *Cell* 57:1155–1165.

Feinberg MB, Jarrett RF, Aldovini A, Gallo RC, Wong-Staal F (1986): HTLV-III expression and production involve complex regulation at the levels of splicing and translation of viral RNA. *Cell* 46:807–817.

Felber BK, Hadzopoulou-Cladaras M, Cladaras C, Copeland T, Pavlakis BN (1989): *rev* protein of human immunodeficiency virus type 1 affects the stability and transport of the viral mRNA. *Proc Natl Acad Sci USA* 86:1495–1499.

Hammarskjold M-L, Heimer J, Hammarskjold B, Sangwan I, Albert L, Rekosh D (1989): Regulation of human immunodeficiency virus env expression by the *rev* gene product. *J. Virol* 63:1959–1966.

Heaphy S, Dingwall CI, Ernberg I, Gait MJ, Green SM, Karn J, Lowe AD, Singh M, Skinner MA (1990): HIV-1 regulator of virion expression (*rev*) protein binds to an RNA stem-loop structure located within the *rev* response element region. *Cell* 60:685–693.

Heaphy S, Finch JT, Gait MJ, Karn J, Singh M (1991): Human immunodeficiency virus type 1 regulator of virion expression, *rev*, forms nucleoprotein filaments after binding to a purine-rich "bubble" located within the *rev*-responsive region of viral mRNA. *Proc Natl Acad Sci USA* 88:7366–7370.

Hertz GZ, Hartzell GW III, Stormo GD (1990): Identification of consensus patterns in unaligned DNA sequences known to be functionally related. *Comput Appl Biosci* 6:81–92.

Irvine D, Tuerk C, Gold L (1991): SELEXION: Systematic evolution of ligands by exponential enrichment with integrated optimization by nonlinear analysis. *J Mol Biol* 222:739–761.

Jaeger JA, Turner DH, Zuker M (1989a): Improved predictions of secondary structures for RNA. *Proc Natl Acad Sci USA* 86:7706–7710.

Jaeger JA, Turner DH, Zuker M (1989b): Molecular evolution: Computer analysis of protein and nucleic acid sequences. *Methods Enzymol* 183:281–306.

Karn J, Dingwall C, Finch JT, Heaphy S, Gait MJ (1991): RNA binding by the tat and *rev* proteins of HIV-1. *Biochimie* 73:9–16.

Kjems J, Brown M, Chang DD, Sharp PA (1991): Structural analysis of the interaction between the human immunodeficiency virus *rev* protein and the *rev* response element. *Proc Natl Acad Sci USA* 88:683–687.

Lee TC, Sullenger BA, Gallardo HF, Ungers GE, Gilboa E (1992): Overexpression of RRE-derived sequences inhibits HIV-1 replication in CEM cells. *New Biologist* 4:66–74.

Malim MH, Tiley LS, McCarn DF, Rusche JR, Hauber J, Cullen BR (1990): HIV-1 Structural gene expression requires binding of the *rev* transactivator to its RNA target sequence. *Cell* 60: 675–683.

Malone WR, Felgner PL, Verma IM (1989): Cationic liposome-mediated RNA transfection. *Proc Nat Acad Sci USA* 86:6077–6081.

Sanford JC (1988): Applying the PDR Principle to AIDS. *J Theor Biol* 130:469–480.

Sanford JC, Johnston SA (1985): The concept of parasite-derived resistance-deriving resistance genes from the parasite's own genome. *J Theor Biol* 113:395–405.

Sioud M, Natvig JB, Førre Ø (1992): Preformed ribozyme destroys tumour necrosis factor mRNA in human cells. *J Mol Biol* 223:831–835.

Sodroski J, Goh WC, Rosen C, Dayton A, Terwilliger E, Haseltine WA (1986): A second post-transcriptional transactivator gene required for HTLV-III replication. *Nature (London)* 321:412–417.

Stormo GD, Hartzell GW III (1989): Identifying protein-binding sites from unaligned DNA fragments. *Proc Natl Acad Sci USA* 86:1183–1187.

Sullenger BA, Gallardo HF, Ungers GE, Gilboa E (1990): Overexpression of TAR sequences renders cells resistant to human immunodeficiency virus replication. *Cell* 63:601–608.

Tuerk C, Gold L (1990): Systematic Evolution of Ligands by Exponential Enrichment: RNA ligands to bacteriophage T4 DNA polymerase. *Science* 249:505–510.

Tuerk C, Gauss P, Thermes C, Groebe DR, Gayle M, Guild N, Stormo G, d'Aubenton-Carafa Y, Uhlenbeck OC, Tinoco I Jr, Brody EN, Gold L (1988): CUUCGG hairpins: Extraordinarily stable RNA secondary structures associated with various biochemical processes. *Proc Natl Acad Sci USA* 85:1364–1368.

Tuerk C, Eddy S, Parma D, Gold L (1990): Autogenous translational operator recognized by bacteriophage T4 DNA Polymerase. *J Mol Biol* 213: 749–761.

Tuerk C, MacDougal S, Gold L (1992): RNA pseudoknots that inhibit HIV-1 reverse transcriptase. *Proc Natl Acad Sci USA* 89:6988–6992.

Unnithan S, Green L, Morrisey L, Binkley J, Singer B, Karam J, Gold L (1990): Binding of the bacteriophage T4 regA protein to mRNA targets: An initiator AUG is required. *Nucl Acids Res* 18: 7083–7092.

Zuker M (1989): On finding all suboptimal foldings of an RNA molecule. *Science* 244:48–52.

21

The Application of PCR to Forensic Science

Bruce Budowle, Antti Sajantila, Manfred N. Hochmeister, and
Catherine T. Comey

Introduction

Genetic characterization of biological materials for forensic purposes is being performed increasingly at the DNA level. Presently, the molecular biology approach generally used for individualization is the typing of variable number of tandem repeat (VNTR) loci (Nakamura et al., 1987) by restriction fragment length polymorphism (RFLP) analysis via Southern blotting (Southern, 1975). Although this approach is valid and reliable for forensic and paternity testing (Adams et al., 1991; Budowle et al., 1991c; Devlin et al., 1992; Giusti et al., 1986; Kanter et al., 1986), it has certain limitations. These include (1) a sufficient quantity of high molecular weight DNA (usually at least 50 ng) is required for RFLP analysis (Budowle and Baechtel, 1990); (2) isotopically labeled probes are required to obtain a high level of sensitivity of detection. The requirement of radioactive materials can impede the transfer of RFLP technology to some application-oriented laboratories; (3) RFLP analysis is laborious as well as time-consuming, requiring 4 to 8 weeks to obtain results on four VNTR loci; and (4) the RFLP technique cannot re-solve unequivocally the alleles of most VNTR loci.

An alternative strategy for forensic testing at the DNA level is the use of polymerase chain reaction (PCR)-based assays (Saiki et al., 1985). The advantages a PCR-based technology affords, compared with the presently employed RFLP approach, are augmented sensitivity and specificity, decreased assay time and labor, and no need for an isotopic label. Additionally, many degraded DNA samples can be amplified by PCR and subsequently typed because alleles are much smaller in size compared with alleles detected by RFLP analysis. These qualities combine to make PCR an extremely useful tool for analyzing biological material found at crime scenes.

For purposes of applying PCR-based technology for characterizing forensic evidence, defined polymorphic loci and relatively simple analytical techniques are required, population studies on various genetic markers are needed, and validation studies, particularly environmental insult studies, have to be performed. While the advent of PCR is more recent than other genetic marker tests, the literature is becoming replete with DNA markers that are amenable to PCR. In addition, significant data

The Polymerase Chain Reaction
K.B. Mullis, F. Ferré, R.A. Gibbs, editors
© 1994 Birkhäuser Boston

already exist to support the utility of the PCR for forensic analyses. This chapter provides a discussion of a portion of those data that suggest that PCR-based techniques will provide valid and reliable approaches for characterizing biological evidence found at crime scenes.

Analytical Approaches and Marker Systems

PCR is nothing more than a sample preparation technique. It allows for the amplification of subanalytical quantities of DNA to a level such that routine analytical methods can be used to type the sample. (The theory and particulars of PCR are described elsewhere in this book and, therefore, will not be discussed here.) Once the sample has been amplified by PCR, there are three general approaches for analyzing the product, each dictated by the genetic marker and its particular type of polymorphism. The analytical methods that have been and are being evaluated for characterization of forensic materials are (1) dot blot assays using allele-specific oligonucleotide (ASO) probes to detect sequence polymorphisms; (2) electrophoretic separations in agarose and polyacrylamide gels to resolve size variants; and (3) sequencing.

Historically, first PCR-related approach used for forensic purposes was detection of sequence polymorphisms by use of ASO hybridization probes in a dot-blot format. Under appropriate conditions, ASO probes hybridize only to DNA sequences that contain their exact complement. Thus, a different ASO probe is required for each allele that will be detected for a DNA marker system. The reverse dot-blot format has become the method of choice (Saiki et al., 1989). In this situation, the ASO probes that detect each allele of a particular locus are fixed to a nylon membrane strip, and the amplified alleles of the sample are identified, via an identifier molecular (or tag) on the 5′-end of one of the primer sequences after hybridization to the immobilized ASO probes. The cumbersome nature of a test with a number of probes is greatly reduced because the amplified material is hybridized with all the probes in a single hybridization.

HLA-DQ-α is the most characterized PCR-based system using the reverse dot-blot format for the analysis of forensic specimens (Saiki et al., 1989). The HLA-DQ molecule is a heterodimer composed of one α-chain (encoded by the HLA-DQ α locus) and one β-chain. It is expressed in B-lymphocytes, macrophages, thymic epithelium, and activated T cells (Saiki et al., 1989). The HLA-DQ protein serves as an integral membrane protein for binding as well as presenting antigen peptide fragments to the T cell receptor of CD4$^+$ T lymphocytes (Saiki et al., 1989). The polymorphism that determines the alleles of this class II HLA gene is located in a 242-bp region (or 239 bp length for alleles 2 and 4) in the second exon of the HLA-DQ-α gene. Eight alleles have been identified; they are designated 1.1, 1.2, 1.3, 2, 3, 4.1, 4.2, and 4.3. A kit is commercially available (AmpliType, Cetus Corporation, Emeryville, CA) for typing six of the alleles (Fig. 21.1). Four of the probes are designed to detect alleles 1, 2, 3, and 4, and the 1 allele can be subtyped further as a 1.1, 1.2, or 1.3 allele by using a second set of ASO probes contained on the same typing strip (Fig. 21.1). Thus, one nylon strip permits phenotyping of the HLA-DQ-α locus for an individual. The reverse dot-blot format approach uses biotin-labeled primers in the PCR. During hybridization, a streptavidin–horseradish peroxide complex is added so that duplex formation between the amplified DNA and immobilized ASO probe can be detected by subsequent oxidation of tetramethylbenzidine resulting in a blue dot. Thus, there is no need for an isotopic label.

At present, polymorphic loci whose alleles are the result of VNTRs are the most informative genetic markers for attempting to individualize biological material. The size of the amplified fragment (or allele) is dictated by the number and size of the repeat sequences contained within it. With appropriate VNTR loci and high-resolution electrophoretic systems, amplification by PCR of specific VNTR sequences could prove useful for identity testing purposes. In forensics, several VNTR loci are being evaluated which include D1S80 (Bu-

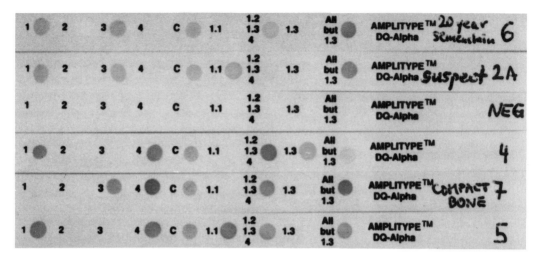

FIGURE 21.1. Typing strips for HLA-DQ-α displaying DNA types characterizing forensic evidence. The HLA-DQ-α types from top to bottom are 6, 1.2, 3; 2A, 1.1, 3; NEG, negative control; 4, 1.3, 4; 7, 3, 4; and 5 (a positive control), 1.1, 4.

dowle et al., 1991b; Kasai et al., 1990), D17S5 [or (D17S30)] (Horn et al., 1989), D19S20 (Odelberg et al., 1989), 3′-hypervariable region of the apolipoprotein B gene (Boerwinkle et al., 1989; Ludwig et al., 1989), HUMTH01 (Edwards et al., 1991), SE33 (Polymeropolous, personal communication), and Col2A1 (Wu et al., 1990), as well as sex-typing markers (Akane et al., 1991; Nakahori et al., 1991; Pascal et al., 1991).

The general approach for the analysis of PCR-amplified VNTR polymorphisms (or AMP-FLPs for amplified fragment length polymorphisms) (Allen et al., 1989; Budowle et al., 1991b) has been separation of the amplified products in agarose gels with subsequent ethidium bromide staining or separation in polyacrylamide sequencing gels with isotopic detection either by incorporation into the amplified product or by hybridization. Agarose gel electrophoresis, although generally employed, does not provide the resolution necessary to separate some VNTR alleles into discrete entities. Although sequencing gels provide high resolution of DNA fragments, they can be cumbersome to cast. Moreover, while short tandem repeat (STR) loci are of a size amenable for sequencing gel format analysis, AMP-FLPs with larger repeats may not

be easily typed with this electrophoretic approach. Furthermore, ethidium bromide and radioisotopes are hazardous materials that require special handling and disposal with the latter particularly hampering technology transfer.

Allen et al. (1989), Budowle and Allen (1991), and Budowle et al. (1991b) described a simple high-resolution, discontinuous buffer, horizontal polyacrylamide gel system that renders AMP-FLP analysis relatively easy and inexpensive (see Appendix). Ultrathin-layer polyacrylamide gels can be cast by the flap technique (Allen, 1980). Thus, no specialized gel casting equipment is required, and there is a high success rate for producing usable gels. Alternatively, rehydratable polyacrylamide gels can be used (Allen and Lack, 1987; Allen et al., 1989). These essentially are dried, empty gels that can be conveniently rehydrated with any separation buffer. Thus, rehydratable gels can be stored at ambient temperature for long periods of time and be used to conveniently prepare a gel within 30 min. Both types of gels are bound to Mylar films to facilitate manipulation. The discontinuous buffer system permits manipulation of the resolution potential by changing the ionic strength and viscosity of the resolving gel buffer, by adjusting the pH of the buffers, by altering the trailing ion, or by adjusting acrylamide concentration. Therefore, a wide variety of AMP-FLP loci can be accommodated with one general analytical system. Sample loading onto the horizontal gels is facilitated by surface application via fiberglass tabs (Budowle and Allen, 1991). Alternatively, vertical polyacrylamide gel systems can be employed with results comparable to those obtained with horizontal gels (Sajantila et al., 1992) (see Appendix). Visualization of the separated AMP-FLPs is achieved by silver staining (see Appendix) which is an inexpensive and nonmutagenic assay. Finally, a permanent record is obtained by subsequent drying of the gel that is backed on mylar.

AMP-FLP analysis, with appropriate VNTR loci, offers additional advantages over the typing of other highly polymorphic VNTR loci (e.g., D2S44, D17S79, D1S7, D4S139) by RFLP analysis. With RFLP typing, the resolution of VNTR alleles that differ by one to a few repeat units may not be possible. Therefore, the distribution of allele sizes in a population sample is quasicontinuous (Budowle et al., 1991c). However, since the sizes of fragments of VNTR loci amenable to PCR are small (generally less than 2 kb), high-resolution electrophoretic systems enable alleles to be resolved more effectively (Fig. 21.2). Thus, AMP-FLP analysis will reduce the level of measurement error encountered with RFLP analysis. Furthermore, with the AMP-FLP approach alleles can be designated specifically without determining base pair size. An unknown sample can be compared with an allelic ladder consisting of a composite of the common alleles of a particular VNTR (Fig. 21.2), and the alleles can be named generally based on repeat sequence number or with an arbitrary nomenclature.

An alternative approach to high-resolution, discontinuous polyacrylamide gel electrophoresis and silver staining is automated analysis of fluorescently tagged AMP-FLPs (Robertson et al., 1991). To detect AMP-FLPs the primers for PCR are tagged with fluorescein derivatives. The amplified product is loaded into a 2% agarose submarine gel, which has the capacity to resolve 15-bp repeats. Electrophoresis is carried out in an Applied Biosystems 362 Gene Scanner (Foster City, CA), which is a real-time fluorescent detection instrument. The labeled AMP-FLPs are detected by argon laser excitation as they migrate, during electrophoresis, past a designated window. The emissions, between 540 and 610 nm depending on the dye, are filtered through 10-nm band pass filters and collected by a photomultiplier tube. The signal is digitized and analyzed by computer, which assigns fragment size and, if desired, can quantify fluorescence. As few as 50 αmol of DNA fragments per band can be detected (Robertson et al., 1991).

This automated approach can provide some conveniences compared with the more routine manual approach. An internal standard, for example, labeled with a red dye, can be placed in every gel lane. This standard can serve as an internal electrophoretic lane control to evaluate lane-to-lane differences and thus obviate the need to subject a known and evidentiary sample to a coelectrophoresis experiment to confirm whether or not their AMP-FLP types, for example, labeled with a blue dye, are operationally the same. Additionally, multiple samples, each labeled with a different colored dye, can be typed for the same AMP-FLP marker within a single electrophoresis lane. Also, multiplexing of several VNTR loci amplified together in one PCR sample application can be achieved. One limitation of the automated approach, at present, is that the agarose gels employed do not have the resolving capacity of the discontinuous polyacrylamide gel electrophoresis system described by Allen et al. (1989). It is anticipated that future improvements in gel technology will overcome this limitation. Regardless, Robertson et al. (1991) have found concordance of AMP-FLP results for D1S80 with both the automated and manual approaches.

The PCR is an effective means for producing template for DNA sequencing. Sequencing was not considered a practical alternative method for revealing genetic variation for forensic purposes until instruments that provide automated analysis of fluorescently labeled sequence reaction products were made available. Using the Sanger method (Sanger et al., 1977), primer

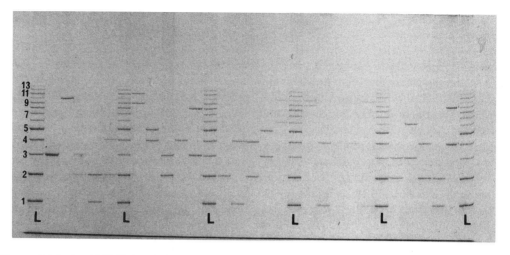

FIGURE 21.2. An AMP-FLP gel displaying D17S5 types. The lanes marked "L" are allelic ladders. Each step of the ladder differs in size by 70 bp. The smallest allele (designated "1" because it contains only one repeat sequence) is at the bottom. All alleles from 1 to 13 are contained within the allelic ladder. The sample types from left to right are 3, 10, 2-3, 1-2, 2-4, 9-11, 4-5, 2-3, 4, 3-8, 2, 1-4, 2-4, 3-5, 6-10, 9-10, 1-4, blank lane, 4, 1-10, 2-3, 3-6, 2-4, 1-2, and 4-9. Approximately 2 ng of genomic DNA was used for the PCR.

(Smith et al., 1985) or terminator dideoxynucleotide analogs (Prober et al., 1987) are tagged with fluorescent labels. Subsequently the sequence reaction products are separated in polyacrylamide gels and detected in real-time in a manner similar to that described above with the Gene Scanner. This approach permits automation of a cumbersome portion of the assay, which is sequence interpretation, eliminates the need for radioactivity, and because different fluorescent dyes are used in each chain termination reaction allows an entire analysis to be run in one lane instead of four lanes of a gel as done with conventional Sanger sequencing.

Nuclear genes, with the possible exception of those on the Y chromosome, may not be the most practical candidates for a sequencing approach in forensic analyses because the presence of two copies of each gene makes interpretation more complicated. This will be confounded further when the evidence contains fluids from multiple individuals, which is encountered frequently during acts of violent crimes. However, it was first suggested by Merril (1984) that mitochondrial DNA

(mtDNA) could serve as a useful genetic marker(s) for the characterization of evidentiary material. The mtDNA is an extrachromosomal, circular piece of DNA that has been sequenced completely and has had all genes mapped. The features that make mtDNA desirable for forensic analyses are (1) mtDNA can occur in greater than 5000 copies per cell, which, in essence, is an amplification process in itself, (2) it is maternally inherited and, therefore, monoclonal, (3) it generally appears to be homogeneous within different tissues of an individual, which facilitates comparisons of DNA derived from different body tissues such as blood and semen, and (4) portions of the noncoding D-loop region are highly polymorphic. In fact, sequencing of amplified mtDNA has been sought and been found successful on such items as 7000-year-old brain tissue (Paabo et al., 1988), 5500-year-old bone (Paabo et al., 1989), and 4000-year-old mummified tissue (Paabo, 1989). Besides bones an important potential application of mtDNA sequencing in forensics is the analysis of hair. Since individual hairs contain very small quantities of DNA, mtDNA sequence analysis may be the only viable technique for analysis. In fact, Higuchi et al. (1988) sequenced amplified mtDNA from a single hair root.

A single-stranded mtDNA sequence template can be generated by modifying the amplification process and using asymmetric PCR (Gyllensten and Erlich, 1988). In asymmetric PCR one of the primers is in excess so that one of the strands of the duplex will be amplified preferentially. Sullivan et al. (1991, 1992) recently described a two-round PCR procedure for preparing single-stranded mtDNA in which the first round was a hypervariable region of the D-loop amplified by standard PCR. In the second round unequal concentrations of nested primers were used during PCR. The DNA then was sequenced via the Sanger method (Sanger et al., 1977) using a fluorescently labeled universal sequencing primer. Automated sequence analysis enabled a 403-bp region of the D-loop to be sequenced in a single electrophoresis lane. Sullivan et al. (1991, 1992), using this approach, have been able to type successfully hair, bone fragments, and necrotic skin.

Population Genetics Issues

Criminal investigators collect biological evidence left at a crime scene in order to identify the perpetrator. DNA typing is a powerful tool for assisting in the inculpation or exculpation of an individual as source of biological evidence left at a crime scene. There are three interpretations of DNA profile comparisons between a known (e.g., a suspect) and an evidentiary (e.g., a vaginal swab containing semen) sample. These are (1) inconclusive—because there is insufficient information to render an interpretation, (2) exclusion—the two DNA profiles are sufficiently different such that the samples could not have originated from the same source, and (3) inclusion (or match)—the two DNA profiles are similar operationally and potentially could have originated from the same source. Population genetics issues do not arise with the first two interpretations. However, with an inclusion, it is desirable to convey a valid estimate as a guideline of how common or rare the DNA

profile is in the general population of potential perpetrators.

Before considering what the proper approach is for assessing the significance of a match, the legal question must be defined. The typical scenario is that the suspect's (or victim's) DNA profile matches the DNA profile derived from the evidentiary material and the suspect claims not to be the source of the biological material. Legally, the suspect is innocent until proven guilty. Therefore, the forensic scientist must determine the likelihood of another individual, carrying the same DNA type(s), contributing the sample found at the crime scene. While some critics (Lander, 1989; Lewontin and Hartl, 1991) have argued that the ethnic background of the suspect should determine the population database used as a reference for estimating a likelihood of observing a particular DNA profile, it is obvious, by framing the issue in the proper legal context, that the reference population should include anyone having access to the crime scene. Therefore, the suspect's ethnic background is irrelevant.

Chakraborty and Kidd (1991), Budowle and Stafford (1991a,b), Evett and Gill (1991), and Devlin et al. (1992) have demonstrated the validity of applying the multiplication rule, based on the assumptions of Hardy–Weinberg equilibrium and gametic phase equilibrium, using allele frequencies of highly polymorphic VNTR loci from general population databases to estimate multilocus genotype frequencies. In addition, some of the data that support the application of the multiplication rule for VNTR loci have been generated by analysis with PCR-based genetic marker systems (Budowle et al., 1991b; Edwards et al., 1991; Deka et al., 1991; Sajantila et al., 1991; Comey and Budowle, 1991).

PCR-based technology affords the capability of generating population data rapidly and easily. Therefore, a more refined picture of population structure based on DNA markers can be made. Examples of population data for HLA-DQ-α and D1S80 are shown in Table 21.1 and Figure 21.3. The HLA-DQ-α data fail to show any significant differences among any of the Caucasian samples ($p = 0.1830 \pm 0.0122$,

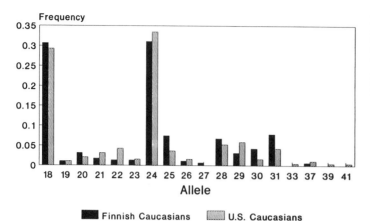

FIGURE 21.3. A histogram comparison of D1S80 allele frequencies between Finnish and United States Caucasians. Reprinted with permission of Sajantila et al. (1992).

χ^2 test, and $p = 0.1330 \pm 0.0107$, G statistic). In contrast, the frequency distribution of HLA-DA-α types varies significantly between racial groups (Table 21.1). In addition, Figure 21.3 shows histogram comparisons between United States and Finnish Caucasians for D1S80. Again, there is no significant difference between the two samples ($p = 0.1860 \pm 0.0123$, χ^2 test, and $p = 0.2180 \pm 0.0131$, G statistic). Lander (1991) asserted that the differences among ethnic groups within a racial group are greater than between racial groups. PCR-based data, protein markers, and RFLP markers (see Chakraborty and Kidd, 1991) fail to support Lander's assertion and demonstrate rather that the differences between racial groups are greater than differences among ethnic groups within the same race. It is anticipated, because of the ease of the PCR-based assays, that a large amount of population data for a variety of DNA markers will be developed for forensic uses. This data should shed additional light on the current population genetics controversies.

One of the advantages afforded by using PCR-based systems is an increased ease of performing interlaboratory comparisons of DNA profiles. The nature of RFLP analysis is such that changes in the technical procedure could result in slightly different size determinations of bands from the same DNA. In contrast, using the more discrete allelic data generated with PCR-based techniques standardization can be based on the result instead of the

method (Budowle et al., 1991a). Therefore, methodological variation can be tolerated for interlaboratory comparison purposes such as identifying a potential serial rapist or the establishment of a DNA database identification system. However, since electrophoretic systems with different resolving capabilities may be employed among laboratories, a degree of standardization will be essential. The use of standard allelic ladders is one approach being considered for standardization.

Validation

It is important to evaluate typing systems to understand the limitations of an analytical technique so that when the technique is applied in a forensic context proper interpretations can be made. A number of general issues need to be addressed to determine the validity of PCR-based assays for forensic analyses. These include the impact of environmental insults on DNA typing (Adams et al., 1991; Comey and Budowle, 1991) and laboratory contamination. These issues can be addressed in a straightforward manner within the laboratory; therefore, for the purpose of interest the issue of allele dropout only will be considered here.

For typing purposes it is important to minimize the possibility of detecting only one of the two alleles of a heterozygous individual. When DNA isolated from blood was amplified in a TC-1 Perkin-Elmer Cetus DNA Thermal

TABLE 21.1. Observed percentages of HLA-DQ alpha genotypes in various sample populations.

Genotype	USA Caucasian[a] (N = 150)	USA Caucasian[b] (N = 413)	Finnish Caucasian[c] (N = 122)	Australia Caucasian[d] (N = 280)	Swiss Caucasian[e] (N = 262)	USA Black[a] (N = 193)	Japanese[b] (N = 92)
1.1, 1.1	0.020	0.022	0.045	0.011	0.023	0.021	0
1.1, 1.2	0.060	0.036	0.063	0.046	0.065	0.078	0.011
1.1, 1.3	0.020	0.029	0.027	0.032	0.015	0.010	0.065
1.1, 2	0.053	0.019	0.027	0.046	0.050	0.031	0
1.1, 3	0.013	0.053	0.027	0.054	0.046	0.026	0.076
1.1, 4	0.060	0.092	0.134	0.100	0.069	0.088	0.022
1.2, 1.2	0.033	0.046	0.027	0.039	0.023	0.047	0.011
1.2, 1.3	0.020	0.034	0.036	0.032	0.034	0.016	0.033
1.2, 2	0.060	0.046	0.027	0.043	0.038	0.057	0
1.2, 3	0.040	0.082	0.071	0.071	0.073	0.062	0.012
1.2, 4	0.113	0.104	0.152	0.118	0.107	0.207	0.054
1.3, 1.3	0.007	0.012	0	0.011	0.004	0.005	0.044
1.3, 2	0.020	0.015	0	0.029	0.027	0.026	0.011
1.3, 3	0.027	0.017	0.036	0.032	0.034	0.010	0.217
1.3, 4	0.073	0.051	0.054	0.025	0.053	0.016	0.044
2, 2	0.013	0.022	0.009	0.021	0.031	0.010	0
2, 3	0.047	0.048	0.009	0.064	0.042	0.010	0
2, 4	0.087	0.046	0.036	0.068	0.082	0.088	0
3, 3	0.047	0.044	0.036	0.014	0.027	0.005	0.196
3, 4	0.080	0.114	0.116	0.075	0.111	0.083	0.087
4, 4	0.098	0.068	0.071	0.068	0.046	0.119	0.011

[a]Data from Comey and Budowle (1991).
[b]Data from Helmuth et al. (1990b).
[c]Data from Sajantila et al. (1991).
[d]Data from Harrington et al. (1991).
[e]Manuscript in preparation.

Cycler (Norwalk, CT) and typed for HLA-DQ-α using reverse dot-blot strips, sometimes there was failure to detect one of the alleles of a heterozygous individual (Comey et al., 1991). Dropout was observed with the 1.1, 1.2, and 1.3 alleles and was attributed to insufficient denaturation during PCR. Since the 1 alleles are more G/C rich than alleles 2, 3, and 4 (Gyllensten and Erlich, 1988), the duplex DNA of the 1 alleles could be more difficult to denature. If the wells of a thermal cycler do not reach the prescribed denaturation temperature during PCR, a HLA-DQ-α heterozygote (carrying the 1 allele) may appear as a homozygote. Fortunately, avoidance of placing samples in the front two rows of the TC-1 thermal cycler or using later Perkin-Elmer thermal cycler models, the 480 and 9600, which are more efficient at heat exchange,

obviates the problem of allele dropout for HLA-DQ-α.

Alternatively, Comey et al. (1991) reported that the use of the DNA denaturant formamide facilitates the amplification of the more G/C rich 1 allele of the HLA-DQ-α locus even when the desired denaturing temperature is not achieved. The presence of 5% formamide in the PCR permits effective denaturation of all HLA-DQ-α alleles even at 90°C. All samples type correctly and *Taq* polymerase does not appear to be inhibited.

Recently, Erlich et al. (1991) expressed concern regarding the preferential amplification of the smaller allelic PCR product of an AMP-FLP heterozygous profile. Additionally, Horn et al. (1989) observed for the D17S30 locus that larger alleles could be amplified to a significantly less extent than smaller alleles. This suggests that there is a potential of dropout of the larger allele of a heterozygous profile. However, Budowle (manuscript in preparation) demonstrated that using the Perkin-Elmer 9600 thermal cycler (Haff et al., 1991) for PCR and reducing the quantity of template DNA in the PCR can reduce the effect of preferential amplification.

Currently, there is an ongoing effort to validate the use of AMP-FLP markers for forensic analyses. While the studies are still underway, there is good evidence that AMP-FLP systems will prove valid and reliable for characterization of biological evidence. Various sources of DNA have been typed successfully with PCR-based systems, which include hair (Higuchi et al., 1988), sperm (Sajantila et al., 1992), bloodstains (Jinks et al., 1989; Williams et al., 1988; Sajantila et al., 1992), urine (Gasparini et al., 1989), bone (Hochmeister et al., 1991a); Hagelberg et al., 1989; Sullivan et al., 1992), saliva (Hochmeister et al., 1991b), and formalin-fixed paraffin-embedded tissues (Impraim et al., 1987). Notably, Hochmeister et al. (1991a) demonstrated the reliability of AMP-FLP typing of DNA extracted from compact bone of decomposed human remains. Additionally, Sajantila et al. (1991a) showed that DNA extracted from muscle tissue, bone marrow, and blood of severely burned bodies can be typed for HLA-DQ-α and D1S80. Both these studies, as well as that of Hagelberg et al. (1989) support the reliability of AMP-FLP and HLA-DQ-α typing by demonstrating concordance of Mendelian inheritance of the victims with family members. The utility of PCR-based systems in forensics is demonstrated further by a study described by Hochmeister et al. (1991b) in which DNA was extracted from cigarette butts. Only limited genetic information can be obtained from saliva typed by conventional serological means and, in general, saliva samples yield insufficient quantities of DNA for RFLP analysis. DNA isolated from 100 cigarettes smoked by 10 different individuals (10 cigarettes per individual) and three cigarettes recovered from two crime scenes were analyzed for D1S80, as well as HLA-DQ-α. The DNA from 99 out of 100 samples as well as the casework cigarette butts could be amplified and were consistent with control samples. Finally, Sajantila et al. (1992) described the utility of AMP-FLP analysis of the D1S80 locus in 36 forensic cases consisting of 18 rapes, 14 homicides, and 4 other violent crimes. Of the semen samples 88.2% were typable and 72.1% of the bloodstains were typable. In no case was there evidence of false positive or false negative results.

Conclusion

In conclusion, PCR-based techniques can provide a means for characterizing DNA for identity testing purposes. The technology is straightforward, sensitive, and specific, as well as can provide data in an expeditious manner. The technique makes it possible to obtain discrete allelic data and to correctly genotype DNA profiles. The PCR appears relatively resistant to a variety of environmental insults and false results do not appear to occur. As advances in PCR continue, it can be anticipated that PCR-based technology will become more applicable to the analysis of forensic situations.

This is publication number 92-03 of the Laboratory Division of the Federal Bureau of Investigation. Names of commercial manufacturers are provided for identification only, and inclusion does not imply endorsement by the Federal Bureau of Investigation.

Protocol

An example of an experimental protocol for typing the D17S5 AMP-FLP.

   I. DNA extraction either by organic method (Budowle and Baechtel, 1990) or by chelex 100 (Jung et al., 1991, Singer-Sam et al., 1990; Walsh et al., 1991).

  II. DNA quantitation by slot blot and hybridization with a human-specific alphoid probe (Waye et al., 1989).

 III. PCR primers (Wolff et al., 1988)

        5′—AAA CTG CAG AGA GAA AGG TCG AAG AGT GAA GTG—3′
        3′—AAA GGA TCC CCC ACA TCC GCT CCC CAA GTT—5′

 IV. PCR components

DNA template	5 ng
GeneAmp Buffer (Perkin-Elmer Cetus)	5 μl
Each dNTP	275 μM
Each primer	500 nM
AmpliTaq™	2.5 units
qs with sterile water to	50 μl

  V. Amplification conditions using TC-9600 (Perkin Elmer)

95°C	10 sec
63°C	10 sec
72°C	30 sec

      for 27 cycles followed by 15°C soak

 VI. Polyacrylamide gel recipe (Allen et al., 1989; Budowle and Allen, 1991)

    A. Horizontal gels (0.4 mm thick) cast by the flap technique (Allen, 1980).

       9%T, 3%C (acrylamide with piperazine diacrylamide)

       Gel buffer, 84 mM Tris-formate, pH 9.0

       Plug buffer, 0.28 M Tris-Borate, pH 9.0

    B. Vertical gels (0.75 mm thick) (Sajantila et al., 1992)

       3% T, 1.6% C stacking gel (4 cm in length) (acrylamide with bisacrylamide)

       10% T, 1.6% C resolving gel (10 cm in length) (acrylamide with bisacrylamide)

       Gel buffer, 33 mM Tris-sulfate, pH 9.0 and 7% w/v glycerol

       Electrode buffer, 1 × Tris-borate-EDTA, pH 9.0

 VII. Sample application for horizontal gels (Budowle and Allen, 1991; Budowle et al., 1991b)

      Surface loading via fiberglass tabs

VIII. Electrophoresis run conditions

    A. 600 V, 20 mA, 15 W

       15°C cooling temperature

    B. 200 V constant voltage

       Ambient temperature for cooling

       Stop run when bromophenol blue tracking dye contained within cathodal plug reaches anodal plug

IX. Silver staining (Budowle et al., 1991b)

Rinse gel in dH$_2$O	few seconds
Oxidize in 1% nitric acid solution	3 min
Rinse gel in dH$_2$O	few seconds
Place gel in 0.012 *M* silver nitrate solution	20 min
Rinse gel in dH$_2$O	few seconds
Reduce gel in a solution containing 0.28 *M* sodium carbonate (anhydrous) and 0.019% formalin	visually observe image
Stop reduction process with 10% glacial acetic acid	2 min
Wash gel in 5% glycerol solution	5 min
Air dry gel for permanent record	

References

Adams DE, Presley LA, Baumstark AL, Hensley KW, Hill AL, Anoe KS, Campbell PA, McLaughlin CM, Budowle B, Giusti AM, Smerick JB, Baechtel FS (1991): DNA analysis by restriction polymorphisms of blood and other body fluids stains subjected to contamination and environmental insults. *J Forens Sci* 36:1284–1298.

Akane A, Shiono H, Matsubara K, Nakahori Y, Seki S, Nagafuchi S, Yamada M, Nakagome Y (1991): Sex identification of forensic specimens by polymerase chain reaction (PCR): two alternative methods. *For Sci Int* 49:81–88.

Allen RC (1980): Rapid isoelectric focusing and detection of nanogram amounts of proteins from body tissues and fluids. *Electrophoresis* 1:32–37.

Allen RC, Lack M (1987): Standardization in isoelectric focusing on ultrathin-layer rehydratable polyacrylamide gels. In: *New Directions in Electrophoretic Methods.* Jorgensen JW, Phillips M, eds. Washington, D.C.: American Chemical Society.

Allen RC, Graves G, Budowle B (1989): Polymerase chain reaction amplification products separated on rehydratable polyacrylamide gels and stained with silver. *Biotechniques* 7:736–744.

Boerwinkle E, Xiong W, Fourest E, Chan L (1989): Rapid typing of tandemly repeated hypervariable loci by the polymerase chain reaction: Application to the apolipoprotein B 3′ hypervariable region. *Proc Natl Acad Sci USA* 86:212–216.

Budowle B, Allen RC (1991): Discontinuous polyacrylamide gel electrophoresis of DNA fragments. In: *Protocols in Human Molecular Genetics—Methods in Molecular Biology, Vol. 9,* Mathew CG, ed. Clifton, NJ: Human Press.

Budowle B, Baechtel FS (1990): Modifications to improve the effectiveness of restriction fragment length polymorphism typing. *Appl Theor Electrophoresis* 1:181–187.

Budowle B, Stafford J (1991a): Response to expert report by D. L. Hartl submitted in the case of the United States versus Yee. *Crime Lab Dig* 18(3):101–108.

Budowle B, Stafford J (1991b): Response to "population genetic problems in the forensic use of DNA profiles" by R.C. Lewontin submitted in the case of United States versus Yee. *Crime Lab Dig* 18(3):109–112.

Budowle B, Baechtel FS, Comey CT (1991a): Some considerations for use of AMP-FLPs for identity testing. *Adv Forens Haemogenet* 4, Rittner C, Schneider PM, eds. Berlin: Springer-Verlag, pp. 11–17, 1992.

Budowle B, Chakraborty R, Giusti AM, Eisenberg AJ, Allen RC (1991b): Analysis of the VNTR locus D1S80 by the PCR followed by high-resolution PAGE. *Am J Hum Genet* 48:137–144.

Budowle B, Giusti AM, Waye JS, Baechtel FS, Fourney RM, Adams DE, Presley LA, Deadman HA, Monson KL (1991c): Fixed bin analysis for statistical evaluation of continuous distributions of allelic data from VNTR loci for use in forensic comparisons. *Am J Hum Genet* 48:841–855.

Chakraborty R, Kidd KK (1991): The utility of DNA typing in forensic work. *Science* 254:1735–1739.

Comey CT, Budowle B (1991): Validation studies on the analysis of the HLA-DQ alpha locus using the polymerase chain reaction. *J Forens Sci* 36:1633–1648.

Comey CT, Jung JM, Budowle B (1991): Use of formamide to improve PCR amplification of

HLA-DQ alpha sequences. *Biotechniques* 10:60–61.

Deka R, Chakraborty R, Ferrell RE (1991): A population genetic study of six VNTR loci in three ethnically defined populations. *Genomics* 11:83–92.

Devlin B, Risch N, Roeder K (1992): Forensic inference from DNA fingerprints. *J Am Stat Assoc* 87:337–350.

Edwards A, Civitello A, Hammon HA, Caskey CT (1991): DNA typing and genetic mapping with trimeric and tetrameric tandem repeats. *Am J Hum Genet* 49:746–756.

Erlich HA, Gelfand D, Sninsky JJ (1991): Recent advances in the polymerase chain reaction. *Science* 252:1643–1651.

Evett IW, Gill P (1991): A discussion of the robustness of methods for assessing the evidential value of DNA single locus profiles in crime investigations. *Electrophoresis* 12:226–230.

Gasparini P, Savoia A, Pignatti PF, Dallapiccola B, Novelli G (1989): Amplification of DNA from epithelial cells in urine. *N Engl J Med* 320:809.

Giusti AM, Baird M, Pasquale S, Balazs I, Glassberg J (1986): Application of DNA polymorphisms to the analysis of DNA recovered from sperm. *J Forens Sci* 31:409–417.

Gyllensten UB, Erlich HA (1988): Generation of single-stranded DNA by the polymerase chain reaction and its application to direct sequencing of the HLA-DQ alpha locus. *Proc Natl Acad Sci USA* 85:7652–7656.

Haff L, Atwood JG, DiCesare J, Katz E, Picozza E, Williams JF, Woudenberg T (1991): A high-performance system for automation of the polymerase chain reaction. *Biotechniques* 10:102–112.

Hagelberg E, Sykes B, Hedges R (1989): Ancient bone DNA amplified. *Nature (London)* 342:485.

Harrington CS, Dunaiski V, Williams KE, Fowler C (1991): HLA-DQ alpha typing of forensic specimens by amplification restriction fragment polymorphism (ARFP) analysis. *For Sci Int* 51:147–157.

Helmuth R, Fildes N, Blake E, Luce MC, Chimera J, Madej R, Gorodezky C, Stoneking M, Schmill N, Klitz W, Higuchi R, Erlich HA (1990): HLA-DQ alpha allele and genotype frequencies in various human populations, determined by using enzymatic amplification and oligonucleotide probes. *Am J Hum Genet* 47:515–523.

Higuchi R, Von Beroldingen CH, Sensabaugh GF, Erlich HA (1988): DNA typing from single hairs. *Nature (London)* 332:543–546.

Hochmeister MN, Budowle B, Borer UV, Eggmann UT, Comey CT, Dirnhofer R (1991a): Typing of DNA extracted from compact bone tissue from human remains. *J Forens Sci* 36:1649–1661.

Hochmeister MN, Budowle B, Jung J, Borer UV, Comey CT, Dirnhofer R (1991b): PCR-based typing of DNA extracted from cigarette butts. *Int J Leg Med* 104:229–233.

Horn GT, Richards B, Klinger KW (1989): Amplification of a highly polymorphic VNTR segment by the polymerase chain reaction. *Nucl Acids Res* 17:2140.

Impraim CC, Saiki RK, Erlich HA, Teplitz RL (1987): Analysis of DNA extracted from formalin-fixed, paraffin-embedded tissues by enzymatic amplification and hybridization with sequence-specific oligonucleotides. *Biochem Biophys Res Commun* 142:710–716.

Jung JM, Comey CT, Baer DB, Budowle B (1991): Extraction strategy for obtaining DNA from bloodstains for PCR amplification and typing of the HLA-DQ alpha gene. *Int J Leg Med* 104:145–148.

Kanter E, Baird M, Shaler R, Balazs I (1986): Analysis of restriction fragment length polymorphisms in DNA recovered from dried bloodstains. *J Forens Sci* 31:403–408.

Jinks DC, Minter M, Tarver DA, Vanderford M, Hejtmancik JF, McCabe ERB (1989): Molecular genetic diagnosis of sickle cell disease using dried blood specimens on blotters used for newborn screening. *Hum Genet* 81:363–366.

Kasai K, Nakamura Y, White R (1990): Amplification of a variable number of tandem repeat (VNTR) locus (pMCT118) by the polymerase chain reaction (PCR) and its application to forensic science. *J Forens Sci* 35:1196–1200.

Lander ES (1989): DNA fingerprinting on trial. *Nature (London)* 339:501–505.

Lander ES (1991): Invited editorial: Research on DNA typing catching up with courtroom application. *Am J Hum Genet* 48:819–823.

Lewontin RC, Hartl DL (1991): Population genetics in forensic DNA typing. *Science* 254:1745–1750.

Ludwig EH, Friedl W, McCarthy BJ (1989): High-resolution analysis of a hypervariable region in the human apolipoprotein B gene. *Am J Hum Genet* 48:458–464.

Merril CR (1984): Genetics, forensics and electrophoresis. In: *Proceedings of the International Symposium on the Forensic Applications of Electrophoresis*. Washington, D.C.: US Government Printing Office.

Nakamura Y, Leppert M, O'Connell P, Wolff R, Holm T, Culver M, Martin C, et al (1987): Variable number of tandem repeat markers for human gene mapping. *Science* 235:1616-1622.

Nakahori Y, Hamono K, Iwaya M, Nakagome Y (1991): Sex identification by polymerase chain reaction using X-Y homologous primer. *Am J Med Genet* 39:472-473.

Odelberg SJ, Plaetke R, Eldridge JR, Ballard P, O'Connell P, Nakamura Y, Leppert M, et al. (1989): Characterization of eight VNTR loci by agarose gel electrophoresis. *Genomics* 5:915-924.

Paabo S (1989): Ancient DNA: extraction, characterization, molecular cloning, and enzymatic amplification. *Proc Natl Acad Sci USA* 86:6196-6200.

Paabo S, Gifford JA, Wilson AC (1988): Mitochondrial DNA sequences from a 7000-year-old brain. *Nucl Acids Res* 16:9775-9778.

Paabo S, Higuchi R, Wilson AC (1989): Ancient DNA and the polymerase chain reaction. The emerging field of molecular archaeology. *J Biol Chem* 264:9707-9712.

Pascal O, Aubert D, Gilbert E, Moisan JP (1991): Sexing of forensic samples using PCR. *Int J Leg Med* 104:205-207.

Prober JM, Trainor GL, Dam RJ, Hobbs FW, Robertson CE, Zagursky RJ, Cocuzza AJ, Jensen MA, Baumeister K (1987): A system for rapid DNA sequencing with fluorescent chain-terminating dideoxynucleotides. *Science* 238:336-341.

Robertson J, Schaefer T, Kronick M, Budowle B (1991): Automated analysis of fluorescent amplified fragment length polymorphism for DNA typing. *Adv Forens Haemogenet* 4, Rittner C, Schneider PM, eds. Berlin: Springer-Verlag, pp. 35-37, 1992.

Saiki RK, Scharf S, Faloona F, Mullis KB, Horn GT, Erlich HA, Arnheim N (1985): Enzymatic amplification of beta-globin genomic sequences and restriction analysis for diagnosis of sickle cell anemia. *Science* 230:1350-1354.

Saiki RK, Walsh PS, Levenson CH, Erlich HA (1989): Genetic analysis of amplified DNA with immobilized sequence-specific oligonucleotide probes. *Proc Natl Acad Sci USA* 86:6230-6234.

Sajantila A, Strom M, Budowle B, Karhunen PJ, Peltonen L (1991a): The polymerase chain reaction and post-mortem forensic identity testing: application of amplified D1S80 and HLA-DQ alpha loci to the identification of fire victims. *For Sci Int* 51:23-24.

Sajantila A, Strom M, Budowle B, Tienari PJ, Ehnholm C, Peltonen L (1991b): The distribution of the HLA-DQ alpha alleles and genotypes in the Finnish population as determined by the use of DNA amplification and allele specific oligonucleotides. *Int J Leg Med* 104:181-184.

Sajantila A, Budowle B, Strom M, Johnson V, Lukka M, Peltonen L, Enholm C (1992): Amplification of alleles at the D1S80 locus by the polymerase chain reaction: Comparison of a Finnish and a North American Caucasian population sample, and forensic casework evaluation. *Am J Hum Genet* 50:816-825.

Sanger F, Nicklen S, Coulson AR (1977): DNA sequencing with chain-terminating inhibitors. *Proc Natl Acad Sci USA* 74:5463-5468.

Singer-Sam J, Tanguary RL, Riggs AD (1990): Use of chelex to improve the PCR signal from a small number of cells. *Amplifications* 3:11.

Smith LM, Sanders JZ, Kaiser RJ, Hughes P, Dodd C, Connell CR, Heiner C, Kent SBH, Hood LE (1985): Fluorescence detection in automated DNA sequence analysis. *Nature (London)* 321:674-679.

Southern EM (1975): Detection of specific sequences among DNA fragments separated by gel electrophoresis. *J Mol Biol* 98:503-517.

Sullivan KM, Hopgood R, Lang B, Gill P (1991): Automated amplification and sequencing of human mitochondrial DNA. *Electrophoresis* 12:17-21.

Sullivan KM, Hopgood R, Gill P (1992): Identification of human remains by amplification and automated sequencing of mitochondrial DNA. *Int J Leg Med* 105:83-86.

Walsh PS, Metzger DA, Higuchi R (1991): Chelex 100 as a medium for simple extraction of DNA for PCR-based typing from forensic material. *Biotechniques* 10:506-513.

Waye JS, Presley L, Budowle B, Shutler GG, Fourney RM (1989): A simple method for quantifying human genomic DNA in forensic specimen extracts. *Biotechniques* 7:852-855.

Williams C, Weber L, Williamson R, Hjelm M (1988): Guthrie spots for DNA based carrier testing in cystic fibrosis. *Lancet* ii:693.

Wolff RK, Nakamura Y, White R (1988): Molecular characterization of a spontaneously generated new allele at a VNTR locus: No exchange of flanking DNA sequence. *Genomics* 3:347-351.

Wu S, Senio S, Bell GI (1990): Human collagen, type II, alpha 1 (Col2A1) gene: VNTR polymorphism detected by gene amplification. *Nucl Acids Res* 18:3102.

22

Recreating the Past by PCR

Matthias Höss, Oliva Handt, and Svante Pääbo

Evolutionists are driven by a desire to find out when and how past populations and species lived and how they were related to each other. Morphologically inclined evolutionists can satisfy this desire by studying fossils. Molecular evolutionists on the other hand, who tend to get the most satisfaction out of nucleic acid sequences, have access only to contemporary sequences and can only indirectly infer what the ancestral sequences may have looked like. To achieve this, phylogenetics has developed into a dynamic and confrontational field. However, when all the analyses is done, molecular evolutionists are left with a gnawing sense of insecurity since what they are left with is only the "most parsimonious" or "most likely" tree. It seems we will never be able to obtain certain knowledge of the past.

This sense of being "time trapped" has led to the desire among molecular evolutionists to attempt to do what paleontologists do, go back in time and directly approach the ancestors. The advent of the polymerase chain reaction has made this possible and thus opened up a new field of study, molecular archaeology. It is the joys, frustrations, and self-doubts of this young field that we wish to describe on the following pages.

The Pre-PCR Era

Inspired by the realization that subcellular details can be observed in, for example, insects of 40-million-year-old amber (Poinar and Hess, 1982), many previous attempts have been made to study macromolecules in ancient remains. Early studies showed that the peptide bond may survive up to 10^8 years in fossil shells and bones (Wyckoff, 1972). However, it has also been shown that proteins are highly modified, even in tissue remains that are preserved under exceptionally good conditions, such as a 40,000-year-old mammoth found in permafrost. Only about 2% of mammoth albumin was dissolvable in water and a majority of the dissolved protein was modified in charge, size and antigenicity (Prager et al., 1980).

Nevertheless, when antibodies were used to study albumin from mammoth remains, it was shown by microcomplement fixation that enough structural information was present to allow its phylogentic association with contemporary elephants to be demonstrated (Prager et al., 1980). Also, mammoth hair contains α-keratin which is partially native as judged

The Polymerase Chain Reaction
K.B. Mullis, F. Ferré, R.A. Gibbs, editors
© 1994 Birkhäuser Boston

by X-ray diffraction (Gillespie, 1970). By immunological methods, it was also possible to place the marsupial wolf within the tree for extant carnivorous marsupials and Stellar's sea cow within the radiation of present sea cows (Lowenstein et al., 1981).

Substantial efforts have also gone into determining polymorphic antigens in ancient human populations. The ABO system has been much studied as well as the HLA system. For example, an indirect method was used to show that two Pharaohs of the Eighteenth Dynasty were of the same blood group (Harrison et al., 1969). More recently, hemoglobin has been detected in Roman bones that are up to 4500 years old (Ascenzi et al., 1985).

However, immunological studies of ancient protein and carbohydrate remains are susceptible to a number of pitfalls due to chemical modifications and degradation of the antigens as well as the existence of related antigens on microorganisms giving rise to false-positive reactions (e.g., Flaherty and Haigh, 1986). The fundamental problem is that no method allows the selection of partially or completely undamaged molecules.

The same problem also pertained to pre-PCR studies of DNA from archaeological remains. Higuchi et al. in 1984 published the first sequences from an old specimen (Higuchi et al., 1984). Among bacterial clones of DNA extracted from a dried quagga skin kept in a museum for 120 years, they managed to identify two mitochondrial sequences. These revealed that the quagga, an extinct African member of the horse family, was closely related to the plains zebra. However, two sequence positions appeared dubious in that they differed from all other vertebrates tested. Since the cloning efficiency of ancient DNA is extremely low it was not feasible to verify the sequences by isolating independent clones from the quagga skin. Similarly, the first cloning of older DNA—a 2300-year-old Egyptian mummy (Pääbo, 1985)—could not be verified by reproduction of the experiments. Thus, early work on ancient DNA suffered from the same problems as the protein work—that the vast excess of damaged and modified molecules might perturb the results and that

there was no way of verifying and reproducing the results.

The Polymerase Chain Reaction

The advent of the polymerase chain reaction (Mullis and Faloona, 1987) changed the dismal situation in which molecular evolutionists keen on time travel found themselves. The PCR offered a technique by which the few intact molecules that exist in an extract of an ancient tissue could be amplified and studied without gross interference from the vast excess of damaged molecules. Even more important was that the efficiency of the PCR allowed the results to be repeated *ad libidum*. The first demonstration that this was possible was the amplification of DNA sequences from the same quagga skin that had previously been used by Higuchi et al. for cloning (Pääbo and Wilson, 1988). The amplified sequences showed that the positions in which the cloned quagga sequences were unique with respect to other vertebrates were cloning artifacts, presumably caused by damaged template molecules that had been corrected by error-prone repair mechanisms in the bacteria.

This result could be repeated many times from one extract and also reproduced from other extracts prepared from the same skin. Furthermore, the direct sequencing (Wrischnik et al., 1987) of PCR products offers additional advantages. One single directly determined sequence reaction represents the consensus of initial amplification events from many ancient template molecules. It is therefore more reliable than a molecular clone, which is derived from one single molecule in a tissue extract.

It was soon realized that a general feature of amplifications from old DNA is that only short pieces of DNA can be amplified, generally no longer than 100 to 150 bp. This is presumably due to the large amount of chemical modifications that exist in old DNA (Pääbo, 1989). More substantial sequences have to be reconstructed by the use of several overlapping amplifications. However, it also became clear that even the short products amplified from ancient remains may not always stem from intact template molecules but rather be reconstructed *in vitro* during the PCR (Pääbo et al., 1990). This reconstruction activity is particularly seen when no molecules exist that are long enough to carry both primer sites. During the first few cycles of PCR, the primers are then extended on shorter templates and can in subsequent cycles with their extended 3'-ends anneal to other template molecules lacking the initial primer site. Several such jumping events may be necessary before a sufficient number of primers have been extended from both sides so that their 3'-ends overlap and an exponential amplification can ensue. The result is *in vitro* recombination products that carry a large number of substitutions where adenosine and thymidine residues are gained due to the tendency of *Taq* polymerase to add an adenine at the end of a template. For mitochondrial or chloroplast amplifications this cause no problem since only one type of template molecules is at hand and in the direct sequencing reaction the randomly inserted substitutions are not detected. For nuclear genes, which have to be cloned in order to distinguish the alleles, the jumping between templates cause a substantial number of cloned amplification products to be recombinant (Lawlor et al., 1991; Goloubinoff et al., 1992). Furthermore, if contaminating DNA molecules are present in an extract, jumping PCR may cause recombinant molecules between ancient and modern sequences to be generated. However, when this is not the case, the net effect of the jumping PCR phenomenon is a positive one. It allows us to actually amplify products that are longer than the longest template molecule present in an extract.

Molecular Archaeology

The PCR and direct sequencing made possible not only the retrieval of DNA sequences from museum skins but from archaeological finds as well. A 7000-year-old human brain from a peat bog in Florida was shown to yield amplifiable mitochondrial DNA sequences (Pääbo et al., 1988). This bog as well as other similar sites in Florida are unusual in that neutral and anoxic water condition allow particular good preservation of brain substance. Subsequent work has shown that also nuclear genes of the MHC can be retrieved from such finds (Lawlor et al., 1991).

Other early work (Thomas et al., 1989) verified that the extinct marsupial wolf was closely related to the extant marsupial carnivours in Australia and that numerous morphological traits, such as tooth characters, which this animal had in common with extinct marsupials of South America were convergencies, produced by adaptations to similar ecological nisches in the two areas of the world. Recently, the cytochrome *b* sequences determined in the original work has been determined from another marsupial wolf specimen (Krajewski et al., 1992) and found to be identical except at two positions that may represent intraspecies variation. This is an important result since it shows that ancient sequences can be reproducibly determined in different laboratories.

Several workers demonstrated that the PCR can retrieve sequences from bones of different ages (Hagelberg et al., 1989; Horai et al., 1989; Hänni et al., 1990). Furthermore, dried plant remains seem often to be well preserved. Notably, RNA as well as DNA exist in the extracts of archaeological maize specimens (Rollo, 1991) and Peruvian maize samples that are 4500 years old allow single copy chromosomal sequences to be amplified (Goloubinoff et al., 1992). One report even documents that Southern blotting can be used to visualize single copy sequences in 500-year-old maize found in desert conditions (Helentjaris, 1989), thus indicating that under some circumstances DNA fragments of substantial length may survive.

An unexpected result was achieved when skins and bones of the extinct moas of New Zealand were studied (Cooper et al., 1992). These giant flightless birds belonged to a group of birds that lack a keeled breastbone and have an archaic palate. They include the kiwis, which still live on New Zealand, the emus and cassuaries of Australia, and the rheas and ostriches of South America and Africa, respectively. To obtain enough sequences to construct a reliable phylogenetic tree, five sets of primers were used to amplify a total of 370 bp of the mitochondrial 12 S rRNA gene, which was thus "puzzled together" from shorter overlapping amplifications. The sequencing results were verified in 4 of the 11 paleontologically identified species of moas. The moas formed a clearly defined group within the radiation of flightless birds of the Southern Hemisphere, thus lending credit to the sequences determined. However, contrary to expectation, the moas were not the closest relatives of the kiwis. Rather, the latter were more closely related to the Australian emus and casuaries than to their extinct New Zealand compatriots. Thus the molecular phylogeny for the moas support the notion that the ancestors of kiwis and moas came independently to New Zealand and that the kiwi ancestor arrived later and from Australia. Thus it may have been a flying bird and only later become flightless. The notion that the common ancestor of flightless birds had the ability to fly is controversial but not without support among a minority of students of bird evolution (Houde, 1988).

Fossil DNA

DNA sequences have also been amplified from fossils that are millions of years old (Golenberg et al., 1990). Such findings represent the ultimate dream of the evolutionist—to be able to go back over geological time periods and truly follow the process of mutations becoming fixed in a species. The two reports on "fossil" DNA sequences thus stand in a class of their own in the field. They both stem from 17-million-year-old plant compression fossils from the Clarkia site in Idaho. That site contains large amounts of leaves that show extraordinary preservation (Niklas and Brown, 1981). About 10% of extracts were reported to contain high-molecular-weight DNA and from one of these extracts, Golenberg et al. (1990) were able to amplify an 800-bp-long chloroplast sequence that was compatible with being of Magnolia origin. We have felt some concern about

this finding since the water that is present in the Clarkia fossils should, according to known rates of depurination (Lindahl and Nyberg, 1972), have destroyed all DNA fragments of >800 bp in a mere 5000 years (Pääbo and Wilson, 1991). The age of the Clarkia fossils not only exceeds that number by more than three orders of magnitude, they are also different in that they allow amplification of DNA segments that are around 10 times longer than specimens which are only a few hundred years old. Furthermore, the high-molecular-weight DNA that is seen in ethidium-stained gels of Clarkia extracts is of bacterial origin (Sidow et al., 1991). However, recently another group has repeated the initial work, this time by the amplification of a 1200-bp-long piece of DNA from a *Taxodium* species (Soltis et al., 1992). These sequences are very closely related to the extant *Taxodium* sequenced by the authors and thus may confirm that the Clarkia site somehow defeats the rules of chemistry. Further work will have to address how that is so.

Another promising place to look for fossil sequences could be amber. Since amber is hygroscopic, conditions inside the amber are dry and, provided the amber has been deposited at a place sealed by stone formations, it may have been protected from oxygen. Thus the DNA in insects and pollen found in amber is protected from the two agents that are the most damaging to DNA, water and oxygen. Work in this direction is underway (Cano et al., 1992) and may come up with fascinating results in the future.

Museums as Genetic Reposatories

Other work has exploited the possibility to follow populations over time. The kangaroo rats in Mojave Desert offered an opportunity in that they had been extensively collected by zoologists since the beginning of this century. When animals were again collected within a few feet of where their presumed ancestors lived some 50 to 60 kangaroo rat-generations ago, it was shown that those ancestral rats were indeed the direct ancestors of the present day populations (Thomas et al., 1990). These results were highly encouraging since the 43 museum skins, which had been dried and stored for 50 to 80 years in the collection, all allowed the amplification of 225-bp-long mitochondrial sequences. Thus, millions of specimens curated in museums may allow us to follow genetic change over time.

Some less enlightened administrators and consultants have lately tended to condemn natural history collections as outdated storage houses of dusty skins that could be either closed down or transformed into amusement parks for a public deemed ignorant and uninterested in obtaining insights and information during museum visits. However, through the advent of the PCR, museums have obtained an additional and important role as molecular genetic data banks. It is of uttermost importance not only that the existing collections are well curated, but that collections are continuously enlarged to allow future investigators to follow the genetic impact of, for example, habitat change. Several major museums such as the Natural History Museum in London, the American Museum in New York, the Smithsonian Institution in Washington, D.C. and others have already taken up this challenge and set up molecular laboratories that not only concern themselves with extant populations, but also exploit the possibilities that their collections provide.

As with all advances, there are also risks with this development. One risk is that museum collections will be rapidly consumed by eager molecular evolutionists and ecologists, leaving little or nothing for future generations. Particularly severe is the risk that collections of rare but well known species groups such as Galapagos finches or Hawaiian honey creepers will be eroded. The resolution of the conflict between the interest of performing experiments and the need to preserve collections for the future is a new and difficult responsibility with which the curators increasingly find themselves confronted (Pääbo et al., 1992).

Controls, Controls, and More Controls

The early pioneer days of ancient DNA studies were rather quickly replaced by a period of self doubts. This was induced by the realization that the very strength of the PCR—its ability of the PCR to amplify a few intact molecules from a mixture of damaged one—could also be its Achilles' heel. For example, when primers that are able to amplify mitochondrial sequences from essentially any vertebrate (Kocher et al., 1989) were used to perform PCR from some marsupial wolf extracts, amplification products of human sequence were produced. When shorter primers were used, the same extracts yielded marsupial sequences. Thus, a few human molecules, which contaminate the extract of a museum skin, can outcompete the old molecules when longer amplifications are performed, whereas for shorter fragments, the old DNA will outcompete the contaminant. Furthermore, when working on the moa sequences, it was observed that a segment of one sequence fell out of the realm of variation among flightless birds. This sequence turned out to be of chicken rather than of moa origin and to stem from one of the primers that had become contaminated by trace amounts of a chicken DNA amplified previously in the laboratory.

This and other similar experiences demonstrated that extreme precaution was not only desirable but necessary in order that a young and attractive field of research would not be tainted by too many questionable or false results. Extensive soul-searching led to the establishment of a number of "criteria of authenticity" that we find necessary to adhere to in any ancient work (Table 22.1). Control extracts prepared with the ancient tissue extracts are needed for detecting contamination introduced from reagents and handling. Similarly, reproduction of the results from a minimum of two extracts from independent samples from the same individual will eliminate the risk of contamination from handling of one particular

TABLE 22.1. Criteria of authenticity for ancient DNA sequences.

Control extract amplification(s)
No-template amplification(s)
Inverse relationship between amplification length
  and efficiency
Unambiguous direct sequencing reactions
  (for mt and cpDNA)
Multiple extracts from independent tissue samples
Phylogenetic inference

sample or extract. In the case of mitochondrial and chloroplast DNA sequences, one expects unambiguous direct sequencing reactions since most organisms carry only one type of organellar genomes.

All these controls are necessary and will turn positive from time to time. This will result in a tedious search for the source of the contaminant that can often not be eliminated with less than the replacement of all reagents. Furthermore, a strict spacial separation of extraction and setting up of the PCR from the analysis of the amplification reactions is necessary to reduce the risk of carryover of amplification products to extracts and reagents (Kwok, 1990).

It is painfully obvious that not even these controls and protective measures will help if the specimen itself is contaminated by handling, be it by an archaeologist, a museum curator, or the experimentor. And to make things even worse, it is sometimes observed that an amplification product from a tissue extract, where all the controls look perfect, still represents a contamination and, worse still, that this result is reproducible when other extracts are performed. This is explained by a carrier effect whereby some ancient extracts can enhance the amplification efficiency so that a contamination of only a few molecules produces a visible band in the amplification where the extract is included but not in the controls. This carrier effect is the (until now) most insidious form of contamination that we have come across and is a serious concern whenever a sequence that has previous been determined in the laboratory is detected in an extract.

These tribulation has led to the sixth criterion indicated in Table 22.1, namely, that se-

quences should make phylogenetic sense. When you sequence a marsupial wolf, the sequences you come up with should look like marsupial sequences. Most projects can be designed so that they fulfill the phylogenetic criterion to some extent. For example, when an extinct species falls in an unexpected place in a phylogeny, as was the case with the moas (Cooper et al., 1992), remains of closely related species can often be found and studied. Obviously, human remains represent the worst problem in terms of the identification of contamination. This is because humans are the most likely source of contamination of the specimens themselves as well as of laboratory reagents and instruments. To some extent, one can alleviate this problem by studying the present variation in the geographic region of interest. The ancient sequences can then be compared to the modern variation and a contaminating sequence identified as not fitting into the expected variation. This approach is thus necessary not only to infer new knowledge from the ancient sequences but also to identify possible contaminations. Future work will have to show whether further criteria and procedures will have to be designed to make work on ancient human remains reliable.

It is our firm belief that only by adhering to all of the above criteria of authenticity with a quasireligious fervour can we avoid slipping into wishful thinking and minimize the risk of arriving at false conclusions.

A Challenging Future

The polymerase chain reaction has made it possible to directly study ancient DNA sequences and sequences that are the ancestors of present ones and thus, in a sense, to catch evolution red handed. This allows studies of recently extinct animals and of the population genetics of organisms that have been collected during the past few hundred years. Eventually, it will undoubtedly allow us to go back much further in time since scientists will continue to try to amplify older and older sequences from ever smaller and more exotic samples. What will there be after sequences from bones, amber, and coprolites?

However, this endeavor is threatened by the fact that the normal scientific criterion of reproducibility often cannot be implemented in ancient DNA work. If someone claims to have amplified a kilobase of DNA from a dinosaur bone and thus to have opened the way for a Jurassic Park (Crichton, 1990), one may have one's doubts about it. But no matter how many other Tyranosaurus bones that fail to yield any amplifiable DNA, it can always be claimed that the one original bone was special. Thus, the entire field runs the risk of going down the slippery slope of reliance on authoritative and irreproducible statements. The end result could be a subdiscipline that, at the most, may serve as a source of ridicule for mainstream scientists.

Indeed, one is sometimes overcome by a sense of helplessness when one observes the current deluge of work where enthusiastic scientists are describing their results that are only rarely verified by criteria such as those outlined in Table 22.1. If several published results turn out to be due to various forms of contamination, then the current enthusiasm might change into its opposite—deep depression. Such a feeling will then quickly spread to granting bodies, appointment and tenure committees, and other gatherings sensitive to scientific mood changes. This is the greatest risk for the field in the next few years.

One can only hope that scientists will do their utmost to stay scientific—which entails not only scrupulous testing of results but willingness to share extracts and reagents and have results tested by others. In this realm we all have to try to overcome our fears of being proved wrong. The future for molecular archaeologists is thus not only challenging on a technical level but on a personal level as well.

Acknowledgments. We apologize to those investigators whose work we have failed to cite due to space limitation or oversight and acknowledge comments on the manuscript from Dr. John Davison and the financial support of the DFG.

References

Ascenzi A, Brunori M, Citro G, Zito R (1985): Immunological detection of hemoglobin in bones of ancient Roman times and of Iron and Eneolithic ages. *Proc Natl Acad Sci USA* 82:7170–7172.

Cano RJ, Poinar H, Poinar GO, Jr (1992): Isolation and partial characterization of DNA from the bee Proplebeia dominicana (Apidae: Hymenoptera) in 25–40 million year old amber. *Med Sci Res* 20:249–251.

Crichton M (1990): *Jurassic Park.* New York: Knopf.

Cooper A, Mourer-Chauviré C, Chambers GK, von Haeseler A, Wilson AC, Pääbo S (1992): Independent origins of New Zealand moas and kiwis. *Proc Natl Acad Sci USA* 89:8741–8744.

Flaherty T, Haigh TJ (1986): Blood groups in mummies. In: *Science in Egyptology.* David AR, ed. Manchester: Manchester University Press.

Golenberg EM, Giannasi DE, Clegg MT, Smiley CJ, Durbin M, Henderson D, Zurawski G (1990): Chloroplast DNA sequence from a Miocene Magnolia species. *Nature (London)* 344:656–658.

Gillespie JM (1970): Mammoth hair: Stability of keratin structure and constituent proteins. *Science* 170:1100–1102.

Goloubinoff P, Pääbo S, Wilson AC (1992): The evolution of maize according to nuclear DNA sequences from archaeological specimens. *Proc Natl Acad Sci USA* 90:1997–2001.

Hagelberg E, Sykes B, Hedges R (1989): Ancient bone DNA amplified. *Nature (London)* 342:485.

Hänni C, Laudet V, Sakka M, Bègue A, Stéhelin D (1990): Amplification de fragments dÂDN mitochondrial à partir de dents et d^ós humains anciens. *CR Acad Sci Paris 310, Sér* III:365–370.

Harrison RG, Connolly RC, Abdalla A (1969): Kinship of Smenkhkare and Tutankhamen demonstrated serologically. *Nature (London)* 224:325–326.

Helentjaris T (1989): *Maize Genet Cooperation News Lett* 62:104–105.

Higuchi R, Bowman B, Freiberger M, Ryder OA, Wilson AC (1984): DNA sequences from the quagga, an extinct member of the horse family. *Nature (London)* 312:282–284.

Horai S, Hayasaka K, Murayama K, Wate N, Koike H, Nakai N (1989): DNA amplification from ancient human skeletal remains and their sequence analysis. *Proc Jpn Acad* 65 B:229–233.

Houde P (1988): Paleognateous birds from the Early Tertiary of the Northern Hemisphere. *Publ Nuttall Ornitol Club No* 22:133.

Kocher TD, Thomas WK, Meyer A, Edwards SV, Pääbo S, Wilson AC (1989): Direct sequencing of animal mitochondrial DNA via conserved primer sequences and the polymerase chain reaction. *Proc Natl Acad Sci USA* 86:6196–6200.

Krajewski C, Driskell AC, Baverstock PR, Brown MJ (1992): Phylogenetic relationships of the thylacine (Mammalia: Thylacinidae) among dasyuroid marsupials: evidence from cytochrome b DNA sequences. *Proc R Soc London B* 250:19–27.

Kwok S (1990): Procedures to minimize PCR-product carry-over. In: *PCR-Protocols and Applications—A Laboratory Manual.*

Innis MA, Gelfand DH, Sninsky JJ, White TJ, eds. San Diego: Academic Press.

Lawlor DA, Dickel CD, Hauswirth WW, Parham P (1991a): Ancient HLA genes from 7,500-year-old archaeological remains. *Nature (London)* 349:785–788.

Lindahl T, Nyberg B (1972): Rate of depurination of native deoxyribonucleic acid. *Biochemistry* 11:3610–3618.

Lowenstein JM, Sarich VM, Richardson BJ (1981): Albumin systematics of the extinct mammoth and Tasmanian wolf. *Nature (London)* 291:409–411.

Mullis KB, Faloona F (1987): Specific synthesis of DNA in vitro via a polymerase-catalyzed chain reaction. *Methods Enzymol* 155:335–350.

Niklas KJ, Brown RM, Jr (1981): Ultrastructural and paleobiochemical correlations among fossil leaf tissues from the St. Maries River (Clarkia) area, Northern Idaho, USA. *Am J Bot* 68(3):332–341.

Pääbo S (1985): Cloning of ancient Egyptian mummy DNA. *Nature (London)* 314:644–645.

Pääbo S (1989): Ancient DNA; extraction, characterization, molecular cloning and enzymatic amplification. *Proc Natl Acad Sci USA* 86:1939–1943.

Pääbo S (1990): Amplifying ancient DNA. In: *PCR-Protocols and Applications—A Laboratory Manual.* Innis MA, Gelfand DH, Sninsky JJ, White TJ, eds. San Diego: Academic Press.

Pääbo S (1993): Ancient DNA. *Sci Am* 269:86–92.

Pääbo S, Wilson AC (1988): Polymerase chain reaction reveals cloning artefacts. *Nature (London)* 334:387–388.

Pääbo S, Wilson AC (1991): Miocene DNA sequences—A dream come true? *Current Biol* 1:45–46.

Pääbo S, Gifford JA, Wilson AC (1988): Mitochondrial DNA sequences from a 7000-year-old brain. *Nucl Acids Res* 16(20):9775–9787.

Pääbo S, Higuchi RG, Wilson AC (1989): Ancient DNA and the polymerase chain reaction: The emerging field of molecular archaeology. *J Biol Chem* 264:9709–9712.

Pääbo S, Irwin DM, Wilson AC (1990): DNA damage promotes jumping between templates during enzymatic amplification. *J Biol Chem* 265:4718–4721.

Pääbo S, Wayne R, Thomas R (1992): On the use of museum collections for molecular genetic studies. *Ancient DNA Newslett* 1:4–5.

Poinar GO, Jr, Hess R (1982): Ultrastructure of 40-million-year-old insect tissue. *Science* 215:1241–1242.

Prager EM, Lowenstein JM, Sarich VM (1980): Mammoth albumin. *Science* 209:287–289.

Rollo F (1991): Nucleic acids in mummified plant seeds: Biochemistry and molecular genetics of pre-Columbian maize. *Genet Res* 58:193–201.

Sidow A, Wilson AC, Pääbo S (1991): Bacterial DNA from Clarkia fossils. *Phil Trans R Soc B* 333:429–433.

Soltis PS, Soltis DE, Smiley CJ (1992): An rbcL sequence from a Miocene Taxodium (bald cypress). *Proc Natl Acad Sci USA* 89:449–451.

Thomas RH, Schaffner W, Wilson AC, Pääbo S (1989): DNA phylogeny of the extinct marsupial wolf. *Nature (London)* 340:465–467.

Thomas WK, Pääbo S, Villablanca FX, Wilson AC (1990): Spatial and temporal continuity of kangaroo rat populations shown by sequencing mitochondrial DNA from museum specimens. *J Mol Evol* 31:101–112.

Wrischnik LA, Higuchi RG, Stoneking M, Erlich HA, Arnheim N, Wilson AC (1987): Length mutations in human mitochondrial DNA: Direct sequencing of enzymatically amplified DNA. *Nucl Acids Res* 15:529–542.

Wyckoff RWG (1972): *The Biochemistry of Animal Fossils.* Bristol, UK: Scientechnica.

23

Nonbiological Applications

Gavin Dollinger

Introduction

PCR can be only as useful in industry as DNA is, it being merely the tool that makes DNA accessible. This section accordingly first discusses the characteristics that make this biopolymer applicable to industry. Unlike statistical copolymers, which it might at first glance seem to resemble, the DNA biopolymer has impressive information storage potential in its primary structure. The industrial possibilities for DNA as a repository of information, using PCR in the elucidation of that information, are detailed. In particular, the case is argued that DNA could be used as a submicroscopic tag—a "taggant"—on commercial products to help in their identification or control their distribution, using PCR. On another tack, the secondary and higher order structural characteristics of the DNA biopolymer are shown to have potential in the new field of nanotechnology. The use of PCR in the building of DNA-based microstructures is explained.

DNA Primary Structure and Information Capacity

The primary structure of DNA, the linear sequence of nucleotides in the molecule, can be seen as a counterpart of contemporary electronic information storage and retrieval. Modern digital electronic devices such as computers use information that is encoded in a simple two-state or binary code. The two states are zero and one, and it is the linear sequence of zeroes and ones that encodes the information. The smallest piece of information (a bit) thus consists of either 0 or 1, and a typical device operates on a grouping of eight of these bits (a byte). To elaborate on the analogy, DNA uses a four-state bit, encoded by the sequence of the bases adenine (A), guanine (G), thymine (T), and cytosine (C). Although in biological systems a particular amino acid is encoded using a three-nucleotide sequence, there is no compelling physical or chemical reason for DNA technology to limit itself to this byte size. A digital eight-bit byte, in binary code, has 2^8 (= 256) possible permutations. Just as much information can be encoded in a DNA four-bit byte in quaternary code, i.e., 4^4 (= 256).

The Polymerase Chain Reaction
K.B. Mullis, F. Ferré, R.A. Gibbs, editors
© 1994 Birkhäuser Boston

Like digital electronics, DNA has well-developed operating systems for overseeing information storage, retrieval, copying, partitioning, implementation, and transfer. For example, both systems have mechanisms by which the fidelity of stored, copied, or transferred information is ensured. Watson (1977) gives a detailed and useful discussion of this subject, and is accessible to readers who might be unfamiliar with the field.

In any information system, the density and the retrieval time of stored information are important parameters of functionality. In contemporary digital systems, a 16 MB RAM chip occupies ~ 0.75 cm^3, which translates into a storage density of $\sim 10^{-15}$ bit/Å^3. In contrast, a nucleotide occupies approximately 1000 Å^3, as estimated using the known structure of its constituent chemical moieties. Thus its information storage density is theoretically 1×10^{-3} bit/Å^3. And in fact, this density is routinely achieved both synthetically and in living systems for transfer of information ("messages") of up to several thousand bits (i.e., bases) in length. Mechanical effects such as shear, which will break longer strings of bits, and entanglement, which will limit retrieval, will interfere with information transfer in long messages using current technology. In living systems, longer messages are packaged, or organized, in the highly specialized structures, cell nuclei. Using 10 μm for the size of a typical nucleus and a genome consisting of 3×10^9 bases, the information storage density here is $\sim 1 \times 10^{-5}$ Å^3 per bit—approximately 100 times less than the theoretical maximum. In either case, information storage density is many orders of magnitude greater in DNA than in state-of-the-art electronics.

The 16 MB of information on a RAM chip can be copied to another chip at a rate greater than 1×10^8 bit/sec. Decoding, or translating the information into a form decipherable by a human (e.g., output to a video monitor) takes only a second or two longer. Retrieval of the DNA message is considerably slower. It takes one second to copy a small DNA message of 1000 bases, which means information is transmitted at a rate of 1×10^3 bit/sec. With present technology, fully deciphering the message

takes on the order of hours. The DNA message usually must first be copied or amplified and then sequenced. For this reason, DNA based information storage systems will be competitive only in applications where the advantages provided by its high storage density more than compensate for the slow retrieval times. One such application, or perhaps set of applications, is the use of short ($<1 \times 10^3$ base) DNA segments as identity tags.

Industrial Need for Submicroscopic Information

There are at least three reasons for wanting to tag a commercial object with a submicroscopic label: (1) to determine its source, (2) to trace its distribution, and (3) to aid in its ultimate detection. A familiar example of this last category is the addition of putricine, which has a strong odor, to natural gas, which is odorless, so that leaks can be detected before the gas reaches explosive density in air.

The word "taggant" has been coined to name substances that tag commercial objects in this way. Essentially a taggant is any object added or attached to a substance in order to label it, or to allow subsequent identification. Table 23.1 lists some characteristics of a good taggant. Most of the terms are self-explanatory; three are discussed in more detail here.

TABLE 23.1. Some characteristics of a good taggant.

1. Traceable	Detectable in small amounts
	Suitable to the tagged object or substance
2. Identifiable	Relatively high information content
	Unique characteristics
3. Recordable	Storing and recording information is easy
4. Inert	Not chemically reactive with other substances
	Physically and chemically stable
5. Secure	Not easily removed from the tagged object or substance
	Not easily counterfeited
6. Environmentally harmless	Not dangerous to earth's atmosphere or inhabitants
7. Inexpensive	Easy to procure or manufacture

The term "traceable" refers to the necessity of being able to find the tag on or in the object of interest. Having to homogenize a piece of art to locate the taggant would obviously be unacceptable. On the other hand, if the taggant were too obvious, not only would it invite counterfeiting, it might also have the effect of defacing the object. Large taggants, visible to the consumer, are usually avoided, especially in the cosmetic or "romance" product business. Another aspect of traceability is that a taggant needs to be detectable at low concentration or copy number. "Identifiable" means that the taggant needs to provide a unique identification of the source of the object. Further, the taggant should contain enough information to relate other information on the product besides source, such as lot number, date manufactured, and intended recipient. "Recordable" refers to the ability to record and transfer the encoded information in a concise manner.

Table 23.2 is a partial list of taggants that have been used as suggested. While all of these have utility and drawbacks, some of the drawbacks will be used to motivate the selection of DNA, whose potential characteristics as a taggant are shown at the bottom of the table. Radioactive isotopes are traceable and recordable, but they have poor identifiability and are not inert or environmentally harmless. Magnetic particles have a low information content and can easily be removed from the object, making them not very secure. *Lycopodium* spores are harvested from a club moss and then dyed with one of several colors. Differently colored spores are mixed, and the presence of a certain mixture, such as a blue and green combination, identifies the tagged object. This system relies on the detection of spores bearing each of the colors added to an object. Failure to find one of the colors could cause mistaken identification of the object. Furthermore, since the colors are unordered, they cannot contain information, and the system is thereby limited in utility.

Microtaggants® are melamide alkyl chips that have been painted or dyed in layers of different colors. Since the order of the colors can be fixed and recorded, their order can convey information. Further, a magnetic or a fluores-

cence layer can also be introduced, which increases the ease of recoverability and traceability. Each chip is roughly the size of a grain of salt (~ 250 μm on a side). This simple and rather useful system was used to trace explosives for about 2 years. Close to 5 billion lb of explosives is manufactured each year for nonmilitary uses (*Chemical Marketing Reporter*, 1990). Some inducements to the tracking of explosives are (1) there is usually some detectable explosive residue at the site of a bombing; (2) only 10% of bombing investigations result in a suspect being forwarded to the criminal justice system (Peterson, 1981); and (3) most victims and perpetrators of firearm mediated crimes have detectable, residual unburnt gunpowder on their persons. It was hoped that the tagging of explosives would aid in police investigation. However, the pilot taggant program failed for two main reasons: (1) the Institute of Makers of Explosives claimed it cost $2/lb to tag one explosive [The manufacturers claimed $0.007/lb (Office of Technology Assessment, 1980), more than the cost of some explosives.]; and (2) a typical bullet with ~ 2 g of gunpowder would contain only an average of about three chips; owing to constraints on the amount of taggant one could add to the explosive without altering its explosive properties. Thus, the probability of recovering a chip from either the victim or the perpetrator proved small.

Peptides have an extremely high information content, and are inexpensive, environmentally harmless, and recordable. However, they are difficult to detect in low concentrations and are only relatively inert. They are, for example, subject to degradation by proteases and by ultraviolet radiation. Proteins store information at a density of approximately 1×10^{-2} to 1×10^{-3} bit/Å^3. However, since there are 21 amino acids, each bit has approximately 20 possible states, resulting in a much greater density than is achievable with DNA. Unfortunately, it is not at present possible to use this density, since there is no current technology capable of copying the information in any but the most tedious ways. Unless the protein or peptide is present in a large number of copies,

TABLE 23.2. Some taggants and their properties.

Taggant	Traceable	Identifiable	Recordable	Inert	Secure	Harmless	Inexpensive
Radioactive isotopes	Yes	Poorly	Yes	No	No	No	No
Magnetic particles	Yes	Poorly	Yes	Yes	No	Yes	Yes
Lycopodium spores	Poorly	Poorly	Yes	Yes	No	Yes	Yes
Microtaggants®	Poorly	Yes	Yes	Yes	No	Yes	Yes
Polypeptides	Poorly	Yes	Yes	Relatively	Yes	Yes	No
DNA (potential)	Yes[a]	Yes	Yes	Relatively	Yes	Yes	Yes

[a]Using PCR.

it is not possible to read or decipher the information, i.e., it does not have good traceability.

In some regards, DNA is similar to protein. Page et al. (1987), in a patent application, suggested its use as a taggant with the curious caveat that only long (>1000 bp) pieces be used. The advent of PCR, and the realization that short pieces (<200 bp) are sufficient, has made the use of DNA as a taggant eminently feasible. In fact, current research has addressed the poor traceability of peptides mentioned above using DNA as a taggant and PCR for amplification. One modern method of drug discovery involves the making of peptide libraries, with subsequent identification of certain peptides for particular purposes. The amino acid sequence of a synthetic peptide or peptide-like molecule is encoded by a corresponding nucleotide sequence on a chemically linked DNA taggant, as described in the musings of Brenner and Lerner (1992). The DNA taggant allows investigators to index a peptide library, and PCR amplification makes the detection and selection of desirable molecules a simple task.

Potential of DNA to Be a Taggant

Using PCR, DNA is detectable in trace amounts, and its unique characteristics are accommodated because PCR primers are sequence specific. Target DNA—a taggant, for instance—can be detected against background or environmental DNA. Because DNA is harmless to the environment and relatively inert, it is suitable for use with many different kinds of tagged objects or substances. As discussed above, DNA has a relatively high and recordable information content. Storing and recording information are easy yet secure. Finally, DNA is inexpensive to procure and to manipulate.

Potential Role of PCR in the Taggant Industry

The properties that make DNA a good taggant—its size, inertness, and so on—have, until now, made it also difficult to recover. The advent of PCR as a tool for DNA amplification and recovery diminishes this difficulty. The DNA taggant will be of a specific nucleic acid sequence, known to the manufacturer or to some other agency. Testing for the presence of that taggant requires only a PCR kit and the appropriate primer.

The use of DNA and PCR in taggant systems is categorically different from both the biological functioning of DNA and the diagnostic uses of PCR because of the possibility of designing and making a particular sequence of nucleotides for the taggant. This kind of control means that synthetic DNA targets and their PCR primers can be optimized for length, composition, and nucleotide sequence. Optimization can accommodate requirements imposed by the tagged substance, by the manufacturer of the substance, by the storage and shipping conditions of the substance, and by the PCR detection system. Carrier DNA can be added to taggants to lower the probability of nonspecific adsorption. In contrast to other taggants, which might be rendered useless by the addition of a similar substance, the presence of carrier DNA does not compromise, but actually enhances recovery and security of the taggant DNA because of the specificity of the PCR reaction.

The optimal length of a DNA taggant will vary according to the purpose for its use. Because of the high information density of the nucleotide sequence, optimal length is apparently quite short; conceivably less than 30 bases, or simply a PCR primer. The efficiency of the PCR reaction is lowered if the target DNA is too long. On the other hand, too short a taggant molecule will compromise specificity. When an appropriate balance is found, the result is high efficiency and specificity.

Optimizing the composition of the taggant means it can be made to suit its purpose. For example, it can be constructed so as not to be confused with naturally occurring DNA, ubiquitous in the environment. Another example is that the hydrophobicity of the molecule can be manipulated by modifying the phosphodiester backbone. The desired hydrophobicity can be changed according to whether the tagged substance is miscible with water. A phosphothioate linkage can be used to confer nuclease resistance to the taggant. The composition of the taggant and primer can at the same time be optimized with respect to the PCR reaction. The melting and annealing temperatures of the reaction can be controlled; the polymerase error rate can be reduced by ensuring, for example, that there are no self-complementary regions on the taggant molecule, and cross-contamination in the PCR reaction can be eliminated. The taggant can be optimized so that the same rate of DNA amplification is achieved on each PCR cycle, both within and between reactions. Detection in this case will be reliable and quantitative.

The possibility of optimizing the nucleotide sequence provides a significant technological advantage. For example, it is possible to construct a taggant to accommodate nested primers (see Fig. 23.1 for a graphic representation). The ends of the taggant have a common sequence, allowing recovery and amplification of all taggants using common primers and procedures. The section next to these consists of a

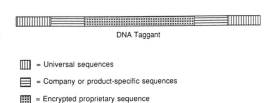

FIGURE 23.1. Example of the construction of a DNA-based, PCR-amplifiable general purpose or universal taggant.

product- or company-specific sequence, and the middle section consists of an encrypted sequence that might code for product lot number, shipment number, distributor identity, and so on.

By changing the nucleotide sequence, the environmental stability of the taggant can be strengthened. For instance, neighboring thymidine residues dimerize on exposure to ultraviolet radiation, causing a glitch in the PCR reaction because the polymerase does not process the dimer. This problem is averted if the thymidine residues are spaced far enough apart so as not to dimerize or are used only for parity checking, as explained in the paragraph below. The nucleotide sequence can also be designed so as to avoid dimerization of the PCR primer.

Error detection can be incorporated into the DNA taggant system in much the same way as parity checking is incorporated into electronic information processing, one bit per byte being dedicated to internal rules of composition. As in computers, this lowers information density, but raises the quality of communication. Similarly also, error correction can be achieved by repetition of bytes or interleaving of informational units.

Potential Industrial Applications for DNA Taggants

Drugs

The use of illegal drugs and the illegal distribution of prescription drugs present complex problems for any agency invested in control and/or prosecution. For example, although the U.S. Government has no real control over the cultivation of coca, the processing of coca leaf into cocaine and crack, whether carried out in South America or the United States, requires the use of solvents for which the primary source is U.S. manufacturers. This fact resulted in Congress passing the Chemical Diversion and Drug Trafficking Act of 1989. The act attempted to restrict the sales of these particular solvents by requiring companies to verify the legitimacy of their clients. Compliance with the act is voluntary.

An alternative to the legislative approach is possible using taggants. The solvents could be tagged at their source, imperceptibly. These tags, if later found in illegal processing labs or in illicit compounds, could be traced to the manufacturers, who might then be required to stop shipments to that particular client. The tag would have to be informative, containing enough information to allow the solvent to be traced to a manufacturer and lot number, inexpensive, not adding significantly to the cost of the solvents, and be added in such small quantities that the physical and chemical characteristics of the solvent would not be altered.

Contrary to most public perception, the substances responsible for the majority of drug-related emergencies are not illicit drugs such as cocaine, but legally manufactured prescription drugs such as valium, barbiturates, and amphetamines. In 1987, the National Institute on Drug Abuse reported that 60% of drug-related emergency room visits and 70% of drug-related deaths were due to abuse of prescription drugs. Pharmaceutical companies risk liability for emergency care and deaths that their drugs may cause. They can also be sued for proven adverse effects of counterfeit versions of their drug—unless they are able to establish that the substance was in fact counterfeit. It is therefore within the interests of pharmaceutical companies to tag their products and thereby establish authenticity, and identify any point of diversion.

In cases where manufacturers can prove they are not culpable, the parties responsible for irregularities of distribution are often pharmacists, nonprofit hospitals, and import–export firms that buy drugs for export and illegally reimport them (Le Page and Slater, 1987; *Drug*

Topics, 1985). In such cases of diversion, pharmacists, distributors, or import–export companies simply remove the lot markings from the product. The California Boards of Equalization and of Pharmacy in 1988 put the estimated street value of diverted drug products in excess of $1 billion in California alone.

The need for tracing the distribution and resale of controlled prescription drugs is obvious. In such an application, the taggant needs to be biologically inactive. The small size of DNA and the minuscule amount added make it impossible to remove. Yet, with PCR, the lot information is easily recovered. The end user, or abuser, of the drug would incur no added liability by consuming a tagged, as opposed to an untagged substance. Tagging would simply give authorities more control of the pharmaceutical distribution system. This kind of incorporation of DNA into ingestible or injectable substances would of course be subject to Food and Drug Administration (FDA) scrutiny. Approval of the substances so labeled would no doubt be considered, and concerns addressed, on a case-by-case or class-by-class basis.

Gray Market Diversion

Gray market diversion is said to occur whenever a commodity is diverted from the distribution channels intended for it by the commodity's producer. Such practices do not violate the law but only a contractual agreement between producer and distributor. The process is similar to that described above for prescription drugs. However, the social impact of gray market diversion is limited to fiscal considerations, and does not concern public health.

There may be many reasons why the maker of a product wishes to control its distribution; two commonly cited are to limit liability by keeping a product away from unqualified consumers and to maintain the exclusivity and hence the relative value of a "romance" product. As an example of the latter, the appearance of an expensive product in a discount store chain is considered to so cheapen the product's image that more exclusive department stores and boutiques might no longer carry it. Manufacturers need a method by which they can identify which one of their distributors is diverting their product. Many methods are currently being used in an attempt to limit this type of diversion, including various taggants; but it remains a growing commercial problem. The practice is apparently so lucrative that diverters are willing to spend a considerable amount of time and money to detect and neutralize the taggants used. The ideal taggant must not only be difficult for the distributor to detect, it must also be invisible to the consumer for reasons of market appeal. Many producers of (especially) cosmetics feel that any taggant that is visible will detract from the appearance of their packaging, which is often costly. DNA/PCR is applicable for several reasons. The nucleotide sequence is both easy for the manufacturer to change and virtually impossible for the distributor to counterfeit, as discussed in the next section. The very small amount of DNA necessary for tagging would not alter the appearance or properties of the product or its container. Finally, although with the appropriate PCR reaction the DNA taggant can be easily located and identified, it could be attached or admixed so as to be impossible to remove without destroying the product.

Counterfeiting

One method of trying to prevent counterfeiting is to include or attach to the authentic object a tag that itself cannot be forged or removed. Taggants of this type are already widely used. The makers of holograms, for example, rely on the technical difficulty of reproduction to resist the copying of their taggant and thus the counterfeiting of the tagged object. Such tags are readily located on the object. A different approach would be a tag resistant to reproduction by virtue of its being undetectable to would-be counterfeiters. Using DNA as the taggant, and PCR as the recovery tool, counterfeiting would be made extremely difficult. Even if the would-be counterfeiter knew the item was tagged, knowledge of the primer sequence would be necessary to effect recovery of the taggant. It could be demonstrated only against the background of environmental DNA using PCR with the taggant-specific primer.

Pollution

Current awareness of the problems of local, global, and atmospheric pollution has yet not given rise to significant restriction on the use of the internal combustion engine, one of the major polluters. However, a great deal of polluting activity has been outlawed. Illegal or accidental emission from radioactive substances and illegal disposal of hazardous or toxic waste are causing increasing public concern. The Exxon Valdez and Chernobyl incidents are but two of the more notorious and transparent incidents; in a dismaying percentage of cases of pollution, the source is unknown. Table 23.3 contains a page from a U.S. Coast Guard report on polluting incidents in and around U.S. navigable waters, categorized as "oil," "hazardous," and "other." The third category includes spills of, for example, garbage or acids. These, while noxious and often destructive of the environment, do not represent a substantial threat to people or property; acids, for example, dissipate rapidly. The last row of the table shows that the number of incidents for which the source is unknown is highly significant. In such cases, because no responsible party can be found, no pressure can be brought to bear to induce people to adopt acceptable methods for the transport, transfer, and/or disposal of their material. For example, the practice of illegal emptying of ships' bilges is thought to be a large source of pollution by oil tankers in the Mediterranean. A technique by which oil, hazardous waste, and other noxious compounds could be labeled on an either random or targeted manner would be of great use in stopping such illegal practices. Ships' captains would be less prone to illegally pumping out their bilges if they knew that the material contained a tag that could ultimately identify them.

The cost of the label and the amount needed to label the entire cargo of, for example, an oil tanker would be prohibitive. Because of the large volume of oil, an inexpensive, but highly traceable (amplifiable) taggant is needed. The possibility of using DNA and PCR as a taggant system for hazardous substances is strong and viable, for similar reasons to those given for

TABLE 23.3. Polluting incidents in and around U.S. waters (1986).[a]

Source	Oil		Hazardous		Other		Total	
	% of events	% of amount	% of events	% of amount	% of events	% of amount	% of events	% of amount
Vessels	48.9	76.5	19.7	48.6	37.9	38.0	45.5	63.5
Land vehicles	4.5	0.8	10.8	0.8	2.3	0.5	4.4	0.8
Nontransportation	10.4	14.7	19.7	5.5	8.7	59.2	10.5	20.7
Pipelines	0.7	3.9	0.5	0.0	0.1	0.0	0.6	3.0
Marine facilities	5.5	1.9	4.9	5.6	1.6	1.9	4.8	2.1
Land facilities	4.4	0.5	11.1	14.5	1.6	1.9	4.7	1.7
Unknown	26.7	6.7	34.5	25.1	46.0	34.0	30.6	12.2

[a]Source: U.S. Coast Guard (1989).

drug trafficking, the gray market, and counterfeiting. DNA provides a secure, harmless, and inexpensive informational tag that is easy to recover and identify using PCR.

Higher Order Structure and Nanotechnology

Besides the informational potential provided by the primary structure of DNA, there is non-biological engineering potential in its tertiary and higher order structures: that is, in the three-dimensional configuration of DNA molecules. The most regular and useful secondary structure of DNA is the double helix described by Watson and Crick. The potential for exploiting this secondary structure to make artificial higher order structures is also most efficiently realized using PCR.

Recent work in nanotechnology has focused on the use of DNA segments as building blocks in the construction of extremely small but carefully engineered shapes. Chen et al. (1989) found that they could design and construct DNA branched junctions—analogs of intermediate structures that occur during DNA recombination and replication. Branched junctions are composed of three or four single strands of DNA. These strands, however, are aligned heterotaxially so that their two ends form double helices with different, other strands. These double helical ends are the "branches." The "junction" consists of a central arrangement of the nonaligned middle portions of the strands.

Chen and Seeman (1991) describe their use of the three-way junction to design a three-dimensional structure consisting of DNA segments. They were able to insert single-stranded DNA between different branched junctions, connecting two branches of each to form a cyclic structure. Hybridization of the single-stranded DNA produced a stable double-helical arrangement that they called a "square." Repeating this procedure and building on the remaining free branches, they were able to make a four-rung "ladder" of squares, the ends of which were finally ligated together to make a "cube" of DNA. The DNA segments used to construct the first cyclic structure and those used in hybridization were carefully designed and synthesized so that the reactions could be controlled and monitored at every step.

This work, while not being developed for a specific industrial application, is coincident with other reports about biological molecules and the operations they can carry out *in vitro* (*Science*, 1991). Ferritin, a mammalian protein, forms a "cage" that can trap some compounds containing iron and manganese. Researchers are using nanoengineering techniques to give it specificity for other metallic compounds as well. Bacteriorhodopsin, a bacterial protein, has been found to function as a detector of acid or of chloride concentration under stimulus from light of different frequencies. The same protein, again because of its complex reactions to light, has been used to build an optical computer memory. Another bacterial protein releases electrons when exposed to light, giving it the potential of being used as a transistor. Still more possibilities for using DNA structures are control of chemical reactions by enclosing them in a nanostructure, or by positioning the reactants, orientation of another molecule on the immobilized DNA (Robinson and Seeman, 1987), and filtering of radiation, similar to a function performed by "photonic" crystals (*Science*, 1992).

Role of PCR in Nanotechnology

It has been recognized for some time that one of the attractive features of using biological molecules is their inbuilt knowledge of how to self-assemble. PCR puts the inbuilt knowledge of DNA into human hands as a tool in the automatic assembly process. The DNA cubes constructed by Chen and Seeman could be built from single-stranded DNA by using PCR to assemble complementary strands. Conceivable, extending a primer with a polymerase to assemble the complementary strand could yield different and more highly constrained structures than are possible through simply annealing the complementary strand to that already in place. Further, the annealing and melting of DNA complexes that are necessary to assemble them into the most stable configuration are intrinsic to PCR. Therefore, the use of the PCR reaction would be an advantage in the assembling of the structures described. Polymerase in the PCR reaction would substitute for many of the functions of the ligases used in the method of Chen and Seeman (1991).

In recent, unpublished work, Dollinger and Higuchi used PCR to construct a biotin-streptavidin DNA mesh. PCR primer is attached to biotin, which is in turn bound to streptavidin at a ratio of 2–4 binding sites per streptavidin molecule. Target DNA of a specific length is added with polymerase and DNTPs in a typical PCR buffer. The extension of the PCR primers during PCR results in a DNA mesh, the pore size of which depends on the length of the target DNA.

Conclusion

PCR is the product of biotechnology, and has become a standard technique in diagnostics and some areas of biological research. However, it also has potential uses in nonbiological arenas. The primary structure of DNA, the sequence of nucleotides, has impressive information-carrying possibilities, as yet untapped except in biological systems. Using PCR amplification, information can easily be retrieved from very small starting amounts of DNA, making it useful as a submicroscopic tag, or taggant, in commercial products. The secondary structure of DNA, the spatial arrangement of the double helix, has recently been used in the construction of novel, nanometrically small squares, cubes, cages, and nets. PCR can be used for implementation of these constructions, making them easier to build. In an age when nonbiological products are so heavily impinging on human existence, it is gratifying to see a biological system that has potential for use in some of the artifacts of industry and commerce.

Acknowledgments. The author is indebted to Heatherbell Fong, without whose assistance this chapter would never have materialized; and to Russell Higuchi, who made it technically possible to demonstrate the taggant concept using DNA.

References

Amato I (1992): Designing crystals that say no to photons. *Science* 255:1512.
Brenner S, Lerner RA (1992): Encoded combinatorial chemistry. *Proc Natl Acad Sci USA* 89:5381–5383.
Chemical Marketing Reporter (1990): September 10, p. 32.
Chen J, Seeman NC (1991): Synthesis from DNA of a molecule with the connectivity of a cube. *Nature (London)* 350:631–633.
Chen J-H, Kallenbach NR, Seeman NC (1989): A specific quadrilateral synthesized from DNA branched junctions. *J Am Chem Soc* 111:6402–6407.

Drug Topics (1985): August 5, pp. 24–26.

Freedman DM (1991): Exploiting the nanotechnology of life. *Science* 254:1308–1310.

Le Page RWF, Slater (1987): J. H. Patent WO 87/06383.

Office of Technology Assessment report (1980): OTA ISC 116.

Peterson AA (1981): A report on the detection and identification of explosives by tagging. *J Forens Sci JFSCA* 26(2):313–318.

Robinson BH, Seeman NC (1987): The design of a biochip: A self-assembling molecular-scale memory device. *Protein Engineer* 1(4):295–300.

Watson JD (1977): *Molecular Biology of the Gene.* Menlo Park: W. A. Benjamin.

PART TWO
Applications

SECTION II
Genetic Analysis

24

RT-PCR and Gene Expression

Didier Montarras, Christian Pinset, Jamel Chelly, and Axel Kahn

The application of the polymerase chain reaction technique (PCR) to the study of gene expression, variously referred in the literature to as cDNA-PCR reverse transcription-PCR (RT-PCR) (Chelly et al., 1988; Rappolee et al., 1988a) and sometimes as Patty (PCR aided transcript titration assay, Becker-Andre and Hahlbrock, 1989), represents a dramatic technical innovation. The RT-PCR procedure has proven more sensitive and discriminating than Northern blot analysis, nuclease protection assay, and *in situ* hybridization. It is rapid and easy to handle, allows simultaneous analysis of several transcripts from total RNA, and can be used for relative or absolute quantification of mRNAs (Chelly et al., 1990a; Rappolee et al., 1989; Becker-Andre and Hahlbrock, 1989; Wang et al., 1989; Singer-Sam et al., 1990; Gilliland et al., 1990). This technique is very powerful in detecting transcripts that have a low copy number because of their short half-life or low rate of transcription and in detecting transcripts from a small number of cells (even from a single cell) or a small amount of tissue (even from a tissue section). It is also suitable for distinguishing between closely related transcripts independently of their abundance. The aim of this chapter, which is not exhaustive, is

to illustrate how RT-PCR has improved our knowledge of biological systems with examples related to development, differentiation, tissue specificity, and pathology.

Early Development

RT-PCR has allowed studies of gene expression in the early stages of vertebrate embryogenesis (from the unfertilized egg to the postimplantation embryo). This technique has been applied to the study of genes coding for growth factors and their receptors (Rappolee et al., 1988b; Serrano et al., 1990; Telford et al., 1990) cytokines (Murray et al., 1990), and intracisternal A particles (Poznanski and Calarco, 1991). Expression of the genes coding for platelet-derived growth factor (PDGF) A chain and transforming growth factors (TGF)-α and -β was detected in preimplantation mouse embryos while no trace of mRNAs coding for epidermal growth factor (EGF), basic fibroblast growth factor (FGF), nerve growth factor (NGF)-β, and granulocyte-colony-stimulating factor (G-CSF) was found. Detection of variations in the accumulation of the transcripts have indicated that both PDGF-A and

The Polymerase Chain Reaction
K.B. Mullis, F. Ferré, R.A. Gibbs, editors
© 1994 Birkhäuser Boston

TGF-α mRNAs are initially transcribed from the maternal genome (these transcripts are present in the unfertilized egg) while TGF-β transcripts that appear after fertilization are contributed by the zygote. The presence of the corresponding proteins in mouse blastocysts further supports the notion that PDGF-A, TGF-α, and TGF-β participate in very early stages of embryogenesis (Rappolee et al., 1988b).

Further evidence has also been obtained that the insulin family of growth factors is mobilized early in mouse embryogenesis. Expression of the genes coding for insulin-like growth factors I and II (IGF I and IGF II) and their receptors has been demonstrated in early postimplantation embryos. Although expression of the insulin receptor gene has also been detected at this stage (Telford et al., 1990), the transcripts for insulin remain absent, suggesting that the early postimplantation embryo as well as the preimplantation embryo can respond to insulin of maternal origin (Heyner et al., 1989). IGF II, but neither IGF I nor insulin transcripts, has been found in preimplantation mouse embryos (Rappolee et al., 1989, cited in Telford et al., 1990). Analysis of the IGF I gene expression in the course of chicken embryogenesis using the RT-PCR procedure has revealed that IGF I transcripts are present in the embryo prior to gastrulation (Serrano et al., 1990).

Evidence has also been obtained for the early expression of cytokine genes during mouse embryogenesis (Murray et al., 1990). These authors have studied the expression of four genes encoding cytokines (interleukin 6 and 3, IL-6 and IL-3, the leukemia inhibitory factor, LIF, and the granulocyte–macrophage colony-stimulating factor, GM-CSF) in preimplantation mouse embryos. Transcripts coding for IL-6 and LIF, but not for IL-3 and GM-CSF, were found in blastocysts. Further evidence was also obtained that blastocysts produce active IL-6 and LIF. The presence of these two cytokines early in embryogenesis, particularly prior to hematopoiesis, broadens their potential role in proliferation of embryonic stem cells. Expression of intracisternal A particle genes has also been shown to occur in preimplantation mouse embryos (Poznanski and Calarco, 1991). Although difficult to relate to development, this phenomenon might contribute to a better understanding of the control of gene expression in early embryos.

Altogether these results show that the involvement of growth factors and cytokines in early vertebrate embryogenesis, hypothesized from investigation of cell systems (embryonic stem cells and teratocarcinoma), is now accessible to further studies.

Microdissected Samples

Gene expression studies by RT-PCR in very early embryos provide a dramatic illustration of how useful this procedure can be where the tissue sources are limited. In this section we wish to illustrate the use of RT-PCR coupled with microdissection procedures to investigate the distribution of specific mRNAs. Talian and Zelenka (1991) studied the spatial distribution of calpactin I mRNA and protein in differentiating embryonic chicken lens. They observed that predominant expression of the calpactin I gene occurs in the equatorial epithelium of the lens where differentiation of fibers starts. Correlation between transcripts and protein distribution suggests a role for calpactin I in fiber cell elongation during lens differentiation.

Phenotypic heterogeneity within rat nephrons was studied by RT-PCR performed on single renal nephron segments (Moriyama et al., 1990). These authors analyzed the distribution of aldose reductase transcripts in single nephron segments (glomeruli, inner medullary collecting ducts, and proximal tubule). Results of RT-PCR performed on 1-mm-long tissue fragments revealed that aldose reductase transcripts are absent from the proximal tubule and present in much lower amounts in the glomeruli than in the inner medullary collecting ducts.

The amount of tissue used in such studies can even be reduced to the amount of material present on a tissue section (Neve et al., 1990). This procedure, where *in situ* hybridization and RT-PCR are performed on adjacent sections, has been used to determine the distribution of the transcripts coding for the amyloid precursor protein and to identify new transcripts in the brain in Alzheimer's disease (Neve et al., 1990; Golde et al., 1990). This method should contribute to a better understanding of the role of the amyloid precursor protein in this disease (de la Monte et al., 1990). More generally, RT-PCR performed on tissue sections could complement histological diagnosis at the level of gene expression (Weiszacker et al., 1991). Recently, evidence has been obtained that *in situ* PCR is feasible (Haase et al., 1990). Proviral DNA has been successfully amplified and subsequently detected by classical *in situ* hybridization within cells harboring a dormant lentivirus. Despite the outrageous treatment imposed by PCR, cells are still recognizable. It would be useful to adapt this technique to the RT-PCR approach. Another variation on the theme is illustrated by the work of Rappolee (1988a) who applied their microprocedure for RNA purification from a small number of cells (a few hundred in this case) to glass adherent cells on wound cylinders. Wounds were provoked by subepidermal implantation of glass cylinders. Adherent cells were isolated 6 days after implantation of the cylinders. This approach was undertaken to study the role of macrophages in wound healing and, particularly, to determine which types of growth factors are produced by macrophages recruited at the wound site *in vivo*. The results obtained indicate that macrophages from wounds express and secrete TGF-α. The RT-PCR procedure was also used to reinvestigate expression of the estrogen receptor in the course of fracture healing (Boden et al., 1989). Although previous attempts at detecting estrogen receptor mRNAs in fracture callus total RNA using Northern blot analysis had failed, RT-PCR revealed that accumulation of the estrogen-receptor mRNA is specifically and transiently stimulated in callus to a level that represents 70% of the level found in uterus (Fig. 24.1). This observation further suggests that estrogens exert their protective effect on bone resorption directly.

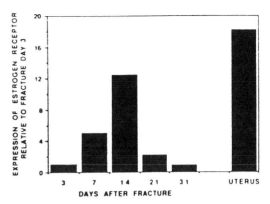

FIGURE 24.1. Quantification of the expression of the estrogen receptor by RT-PCR during rat fracture healing. Reproduced from Boden et al. (1989), *Calcified Tissue International*, 45:324-325 by copyright permission of Springer-Verlag.

Differentiation

The discovery of muscle specific regulatory genes has represented a key step in understanding commitment to cell fate and cellular differentiation processes in the context of myogenesis. Four factors, Myf5, MyoD, myogenin, and MRF4, have been characterized in vertebrates (see for review Chen and Jones, 1989; Olson, 1990; Emerson, 1990). Structural and functional studies support the notion that these factors belong to the family of basic helix–loop–helix factors and are sequence-specific DNA binding proteins that can act as transactivators of muscle genes. Although it seems clear that we are confronted with muscle specific regulatory factors—their expression is restricted to skeletal muscle—their respective roles in myogenic processes remain to be determined. It is essential to study the expression of these factors using the most sensitive techniques to unambiguously establish whether they are present in or absent from myogenic cells at a given stage of differentiation, and to determine when they are induced during the progression of myogenic cells from the determined stage to the onset of differentiation and, ultimately, to the formation of mature myotubes. Unexpectedly, RT-PCR analysis of MyoD during early embryonic development of *Xenopus laevis* has revealed ubiquitous expression throughout the embryo (although at a low level), prior to mesodermal induction (Rupp and Weintraub, 1991). This observation raises the possibility that the subsequent expression of MyoD, which is restricted to presumptive mesoderm, results from a selection process rather than from a direct activation event.

RT-PCR-based studies performed in cultured mouse muscle cells revealed striking temporal differences in the expression patterns of the genes for the four myogenic factors (Montarras et al., 1989, 1991). Myf5 expression precedes terminal differentiation. MyoD is optional at the myoblast stage and, subsequently, accompanies terminal differentiation. As shown in Figure 24.2, expression of MyoD does not occur in inducible C2 cells at the myoblast stage indicating the MyoD may not be required for the maintenance of the determined state. Expression of myogenin also accompanies differentiation, while expression of MRF4 follows expression of the other three

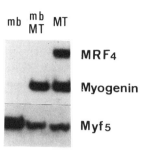

FIGURE 24.3. RT-PCR analysis of Myf5, myogenin, and MRF4 transcripts during a time course of differentiation of permissive C2 myoblasts. Constitutive expression of Myf5 occurs in myoblasts (mb), myogenin expression is induced at the onset of differentiation (mb/MT), and MRF4 expression occurs when myotubes (MT) are formed. Reproduced from Montarras et al. (1991), *The New Biologist*, 3:592–600 by copyright permission of W.B. Saunders Company.

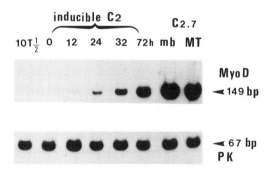

FIGURE 24.2. RT-PCR analysis of the MyoD1 transcripts during a time course of differentiation of inducible C2 myoblasts. MyoD transcripts become detectable 12 hr after addition of differentiation medium to inducible C2 myoblasts and accumulate at higher level during the next 2 days as differentiation occurs. In contrast, constitutive expression of MyoD occurs in permissive C2 myoblast (mb) and myotubes (MT). PK, rat liver pyruvate kinase used as an internal control of reverse transcription and amplification. Reproduced from Montarras et al. (1989), *EMBO Journal*, 8:2203–2207 by copyright permission of the IRL Press.

factors and occurs after the onset of terminal differentiation as illustrated in Figure 24.3. It was also observed that Myf5 is the first transcript for a myogenic regulatory gene to be detected in 8-day-old mouse embryos. *In situ* hybridization has led to the same conclusion and, further, indicates that Myf5 expression is restricted to somites (Ott et al., 1991) and, unlike myogenin and MyoD expression (Sassoon et al., 1989), occurs prior to activation of genes for muscle contractile proteins.

In contrast, expression of the gene for MRF4 appears to be a late event with respect to the onset of differentiation both in cultured myogenic cells derived from limb muscles and in developing limbs. It was further observed that in cultured myogenic cells, expression of MRF4 is temporally correlated with expression of genes coding for adult muscle proteins such as the acetylcholine receptor ϵ subunit gene (Pinset et al., 1991).

The results discussed here have strengthened the working hypothesis that the four myogenic regulatory factors, Myf5, MyoD, myogenin, and MRF4, fulfill distinct roles and do not simply serve redundant functions as transcriptional activators of muscle genes.

Repertoire of Cytokines Expressed by Immune Cells

The study of the repertoire of cytokines expressed by immune cells in the course of immune responses has also benefited from RT-PCR.

The influence of primary sensitization provoked by exposing the skin of adult mice to picrylchloride was analyzed (Mohler and Butler, 1990). Draining of the cells from the neighboring lymph nodes at various times after treatment has revealed that these cells sequentially express interleukin 2 and 4 genes (IL-2 and IL-4). The maximum level of accumulation was reached after 48 hr for IL-2 transcripts and 4 days for IL-4 transcripts. These differential time courses of expression during the primary immune response may reflect the need for early IL-2 synthesis to increase clonal expansion and late IL-4 expression to induce differentiation.

Yamamura et al. (1991) analyzed by RT-PCR the cytokine profiles in leprosy lesions and found that in paucibacillary tuberculoid lesions, IL-2 and interferon-γ predominate, while IL-4, IL-5, and IL-10 were more evident in multibacillary, lepromatous lesions. Salgame et al. (1991), analyzed the same patients and reported that the cytokine profile is different in CD4 and CD8 T cell clones from patients with a tuberculoid immunologically responsive leprosy (production of interferon by CD4 clones and CD8 cytotoxic clones and of IL-4 by CD4 B cell helper lymphocytes) and from patients with a lepromatous immunologically unresponsive form of the disease (production of IL-4 by CD8 T suppressor clones).

The signaling mechanism involved in the control of IL-2 gene expression has been analyzed in human T cells (Weider et al., 1990). While treatment of the cells by calcium ionophore results in the transient accumulation of IL-2 mRNAs, direct activation of protein kinase C by dioctanoylglycerol (diC8) has no effect. Interestingly, treatment with both compounds extends the level and the time during which IL-2 mRNA is present. These results suggest that an increase in Ca^{2+} concentration

is an initial event in the activation of IL-2 gene transcription and that PKC may be involved in the maintenance of this process.

RT-PCR is a powerful technique for studying induction events and for performing simultaneous analysis of several transcripts. The work of Ehlers and Smith (1990) further illustrates these features. These authors performed a comparative study of neonatal (unprimed or naive) and adult (primed or memory) human T cells with respect to the repertoire of lymphokine genes expressed by these cells following stimulation with anti-CD3 monoclonal antibody. Prior to stimulation, neonatal and adult T cells express none of the lymphokines studied. Three hours after stimulation (Fig. 24.4), neonatal T cells express IL-2 and IL-2 receptor p55. Later on, 24 to 48 hr after stimulation, these cells also express GM-CSF. Adult T cells stimulated under the same conditions readily express (3 hr after stimulation) (Fig. 24.4) a much broader spectrum of lymphokine genes (IL-2, IL-3, IL-4, IL-5, GM-CSF, and interferon-γ). Expression of IL-6 in these cells occurs later and at a lower level. Interestingly, the authors show that cultured neonatal T cells can acquire the adult phenotype after a secondary stimulation. This approach may contribute to a better understanding of the mechanisms involved in the acquisition of T cell memory.

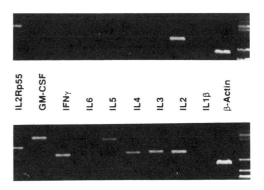

FIGURE 24.4. PCR-assisted mRNA amplification of adult (bottom) and neonatal (top) T cells 3 hr after primary activation via α-CD3. Reproduced from Ehlers and Smith (1991), the *Journal of Experimental Medicine,* 173:25–36 by copyright permission of the Rockefeller University Press.

Immune phenotyping of follicular dendritic cells (FDC), which trap and retain antigen–antibody complexes to present them to B cells, was performed on single FDC (Schriever et al., 1991). FDC can be obtained only in small number and are always contaminated by other cell types that complicate their characterization. Therefore, these authors have purified FDC by flow cytometry using a monoclonal antibody against the CD14 antigen and performed RT-PCR on single FDC. Results obtained indicate that FDC express a unique gene repertoire characterized by a high level of CD21 transcripts and, in contrast to B cells, a lack of mRNAs coding for CD20 and CD45. Furthermore, FDC do not contain transcripts for fibronectin, PDGF, or the CD4 T cell marker. This unique phenotype raises the question of the lineage from which FDC originate.

The pattern of expression of several cytokines has been studied in cultured astrocytes (Wesselingh et al., 1990). These cells are known to participate in the intracerebral immune response both by acting as antigen-presenting cells and by producing cytokines. The authors have observed that infection by cytomegalovirus leads to increased accumulation of the transcripts coding for tumor necrosis factor-α (TNF-α), GM-CSF, G-CSF, and LIF. These observations raise the question of the involvement of these cytokines in the intracerebral response and in generation of neuropathological lesions associated with viral diseases.

Tissue Specificity

The sensitivity of RT-PCR has allowed the study of tissue-specific gene expression in great detail. This technique has been used either to firmly establish the absence of expression of a given gene in a given tissue, or to confirm or reevaluate the tissue-specific expression of several genes, as illustrated by the following examples:

1. It has been confirmed by this means that fibrinogen is not synthesized by megakaryocytes (Louache et al., 1991), implying that the fibrinogen found in platelets arises from endocytosis of fibrinogen present in plasma. In contrast, the low level of activity corresponding to the enzyme 3β-hydroxy-5-ene steroid dehydrogenase, which converts progesterone into cortisol in fetal adrenals, correlates with a low level of transcripts, indicating that this activity corresponds, as expected, to an endogenous synthesis and is mainly controlled at the transcriptional level (Voutilainen et al., 1991).

2. The cytochrome P-450 gene superfamily encodes enzymes mainly detected in the liver and that are involved in xenobiotic metabolism. Within a subfamily these genes show extensive sequence homology and their products exhibit overlapping substrate specificity. For these reasons, studying the expression of a given gene is not always straightforward. RT-PCR analysis of two related genes coding for cytochrome P-450 IIB1 and IIB2 (Traber et al., 1990) established that constitutive and induced expression of the P-450 IIB1 gene occurs not only in the liver but also in the small intestine. Similarly, another study (Omiecinski et al., 1990) revealed extrahepatic expression of the P-450 IA1 gene. Corresponding mRNAs were detected in kidney, lung, and pulmonary alveolar macrophages. These results further establish that a subset of P-450 genes is mobilized in extrahepatic tissues also exposed to xenobiotics.

3. Previous observations suggested the presence of atrial natriuretic factor (ANF) in the adrenal medulla. However, local synthesis of this factor in this gland had not been established. The use of RT-PCR has led to the detection of ANF mRNAs in the adrenal medulla while Northern blot analysis revealed the presence of ANF transcripts only in the atrium (Nunez et al., 1990). This observation strengthens the results of *in situ* hybridization that, although the signal was weak, suggested the presence of ANF transcripts in the adrenal gland, and raises the question of the role of this local synthesis in adrenal steroid secretion.

4. Despite the presence of the protein, mRNA coding for the β-subunit of nerve growth factor (NGF-β) could not be detected by Northern blot analysis in the developing rat central nervous system prior to birth. However, the presence of NGF-β transcripts has

been demonstrated by RT-PCR in the developing brain (Pizzuti et al., 1990).

5. It was shown by the same approach that the expression of the pituitary-specific transcription factor gene (GHF1 or Pit 1) clearly precedes expression of the growth hormone gene and is restricted to the forming pituitary in the developing mouse embryo (Dolle et al., 1990).

6. Expression of the α_2-nicotinic acetylcholine receptor gene (α_2 n-Ach-R) was studied in the developing chicken brain (Daubas et al., 1990). *In situ* hybridization revealed that expression of the α_2 n-Ach-R gene is primarily restricted to a limited number of cells that compose the lateral spiriform nucleus of the diencephalon. Despite the scarcity of the α_2 n-Ach-R transcripts in total brain RNA, the use of the RT-PCR procedure allowed these authors to determine the relative increase of this transcript in the course of development.

7. RT-PCR was particularly useful for studying expression of the dystrophin gene in muscle and brain cells (Chelly et al., 1990a) and for investigating the specificity of expression from two distinct promoters (Chelly et al., 1990b; Barnea et al., 1990). These authors established that the dystrophin gene is transcribed from the same promoter (the muscle promoter) in muscle and glial cells and from the brain promoter in neuronal cells (Fig. 24.5).

8. Other examples of the application of RT-PCR include demonstrations

1. that the corpus luteum contains mRNA for the neurohypophyseal hormone oxytocin (Ivell et al., 1990);
2. that the two relaxin genes H1 and H2 are differentially expressed in distinct tissues (Hansell et al., 1990); both genes are expressed in decidua, trophoblast, and prostate while only the H2 gene is expressed in the corpus luteum;
3. and that basic FGF transcripts are present in the ovary during follicular development, suggesting that this growth factor participates in the angiogenic process associated with follicular maturation (Koos and Olson, 1989).

RT-PCR has also been applied to the search for sex-determining genes in males [known as testis determination factor (TDF) in human and Tdy in mouse]. Genes have been identified that map to the minimum sex determining region of the Y chromosome. One of these candidate genes, the *sry* gene, has been shown to be expressed early and transiently (between 10.5 and 11.5 days postcoitum) in the course of testis development in mice (Koopman et al., 1990) (Fig. 24.6). This observation together with genetic evidence (Jager et al., 1990) strongly suggests that *sry* plays a primary role in mouse sex determination.

RT-PCR has, in some cases, been used to reevaluate the scientific basis of therapeutic strategies. Attempts to purge leukemic cells by hyperthermia are conditioned by the possibility of predicting the thermal resistance of both tumor and normal cells. Along these lines, expression of two heat shock genes, HSP70 A and B, was reinvestigated in leukemic cells and normal and tumoral tissues (Mivechi and Rossi, 1990) to determine whether the levels of the corresponding mRNAs (basal levels as well as induced levels) could be correlated with thermal resistance.

With a similar aim in mind (Noonan et al., 1990), expression of the multidrug resistance gene, MDR1, was studied in normal and tumoral tissues and cell lines derived from these tumors to determine whether the level of expression of the MDR1 gene could be predictive for clinical resistance.

Distinction between Closely Related Transcripts

RT-PCR is not only sensitive but also discriminating and can be used to distinguish between closely related transcripts, either generated by alternative splicing or synthesized from alternative start sites of transcription. In the first category we can find very numerous examples, only some of them being presented in this review.

The neural cell adhesion (N-cam) gene can be transcribed into at least 27 alternatively

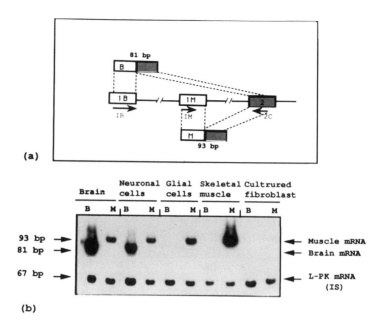

(a)

(b)

FIGURE 24.5. Promotion of the dystrophin gene in brain tissue. **(a)** Position of the different oligonucleotide primers of mouse dystrophin exons and size of amplified fragments. The brain-type transcript was amplified using primers 1B and 2C (Table 24.1) and the muscle-type transcript was amplified using primers 1M and 2C. **(b)** Promotion of the dystrophin gene in muscle and cultured neuronal and glial cells: autoradiographs of Southern blots of PCR products (15 cycles) of mouse brain and skeletal muscle dystrophin mRNA that had been co-amplified with L-PK transcipts as an internal standard. Reproduced from Chelly et al. (1990b), *Nature*, 344:64–65 by copyright permission of the Macmillan Magazines Ltd.

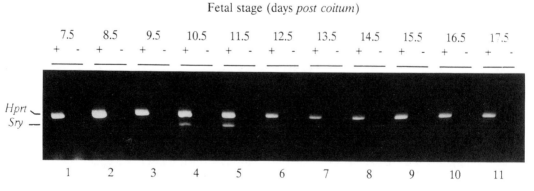

FIGURE 24.6. Time course of fetal Sry expression. dpc, day postcoitum; Hprt, hypoxanthine phosphoribosyltransferase used as an internal control of RT-PCR. Reactions were performed in the presence (+) or absence (−) of reverse transcriptase. Reproduced from Koopman et al. (1990), *Nature* 348: 450–452 by copyright permission of the Macmillan Magazines Ltd.

FIGURE 24.7. Alternative splicing at the exon 12–exon 13 function of the N-CAM mRNA1 during rat heart development. Reproduced from Reyes et al. (1991), *Molecular and Cellular Biology*, 11:1654–1661 by copyright permission of the American Society for Microbiology.

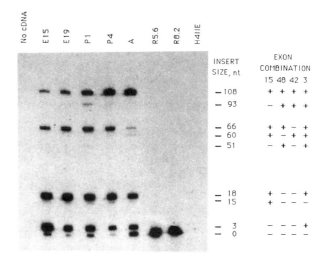

spliced mRNAs in muscle tissues (Reyes et al., 1991) (Fig. 24.7). This puzzling diversity resides in the differential usage of 4 small exons located between exons 12 and 13.

The human gene for ceruloplasmin, a plasma glycoprotein involved in the transport of copper, is transcribed into 2 mRNAs, CP1 and CP2, resulting from tissue-specific alternative splicing of 12 nucleotides (Yang et al., 1990).

The type II procallagen gene is transcribed into two distinct mRNAs generated by alternative splicing of exon 2 (Ryan and Sandell, 1990). Interestingly, it was shown subsequently that these two transcripts occur in different cell populations during vertebral development (Sandell et al., 1991).

To evaluate the relative proportion of "naive" and memory T cells in the lung, Saltini et al. (1990) studied the transcripts generated from the CD45 gene by alternative splicing. They have observed an equal proportion of "naive" cells expressing the transcripts for the 220- and 205-kDa proteins and memory cells expressing the transcripts for the 180-kDa protein in the circulating blood. In contrast, in the lung, 86 ±2% of the T cells express the 180-kDa protein. This differential distribution of T cells, which is also observed by flow cytometric analysis performed with antibodies directed against the 220–205 kDa and the 180 kDa products, may reflect the chronic exposure to diverse antigens in the lung.

It is also through the use of RT-PCR that several groups have been able to demonstrate that the huge dystrophin primary transcript could generate many different species by alternative splicing (Feener et al., 1989; Chelly et al., 1990b). This phenomenon has been proposed as the mechanism explaining the rescue of a partially functional dystrophin protein in patients with gene deletions resulting, theoretically, in out-of-frame transcripts: the frame can be restored by the splicing out of additional exons (Chelly et al., 1990c) (Fig. 24.8).

Another example where a pathological transcript is directly distinguished from its normal counterpart by RT-PCR amplification is provided by the development of Wilm's tumors that is associated with a 25-bp deletion in the 11p13 zinc finger gene, which results in the formation of an aberrant transcript missing one of the zinc finger domains (Haber et al., 1990).

One must keep in mind that RT-PCR, when used to distinguish between closely related transcripts, may also generate artifacts (appearance of additional bands on nondenaturing gels) through the formation of heteroduplexes between closely related sequences. Fractionation of the amplified products on denaturing gels allows artifactual and correct RT-PCR

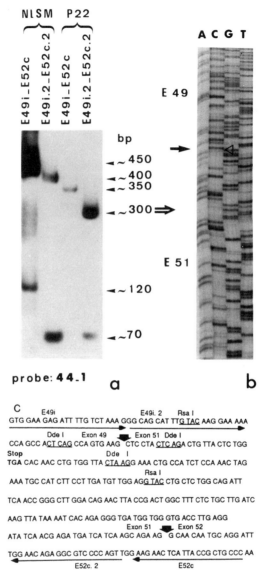

FIGURE 24.8. Analysis of truncated dystrophin transcripts in fibroblasts from a Becker patient with out-of-frame deletion of exon 50. (a) Autoradiograms of Southern blots performed on cDNA-PCR coamplified products (40 cycles) of dystrophin transcripts hybridized with a dystrophin cDNA probes. The dystrophin transcript was analyzed in normal muscle biopsy (NI SM) and in patient's fibroblasts (P22) using primer couple E49i-E52c for cDNA-PCR and nested primer couple E49i2-E52c.2 for the second run of PCR. In normal muscle the expected fragment comprising exons 49–52 is the 450-bp species (400 bp with nested primers). The additional 120-bp fragment (70 bp with nested primers) corresponds to alternative splicing of exons 50 and 5. In the patient's fibroblasts, the 350- and 300-bp fragments correspond to the expected truncated transcript (exons 49–51–52). The in-frame spliced species (exons 49–52) is seen only after reamplification between nested primers (70-bp fragment). (b) Sequencing gel of the abnormal 300-bp cDNA segment obtained after amplification using nested primers. The triangle indicates the junction point. The sequence of the abnormal 300 bp cDNA. (c) Complete nucleotide sequence of the abnormal 300-bp cDNA fragment with position of primers used for PCR and sites of restriction enzymes used to characterize the abnormal fragment. Nucleotide sequence of the fragment corresponding to the alternatively splice species was already published. Reproduced from *The Journal of Clinical Investigation*, 1991, 88:1161–1197 by copyright permission of the American Society for Clinical Investigation.

products to be readily distinguished (Zorn and Kreig, 1991).

When a gene is transcribed from alternative promoters, generating mRNAs with different 5'-ends, the use of couples of primers consisting of a common 3' primer and alternative 5' primers is the most sensitive way to analyze the activity of these different promoters in different cells and as a function of development. A good example is the dystrophin gene, which possesses at least three promoters, one specific to neurons, the second to muscle (smooth and skeletal muscle as well as heart), and the third being nonspecific (Hugnot et al., 1991; Bar et al., 1990). A similar strategy has been used to investigate several other genes with alternative promoters, for instance the glucokinase gene (Magnuson and Shelton, 1989).

The method aimed at analyzing the transcripts from genes with alternative promoters discussed above (i.e., using 5' primers specific to the different alternative 5'-ends) can be applied only to the cases where these alternative 5' sequences are known. Probably the most powerful method in determining such heterogeneity in the 5'-ends of transcripts and to demonstrate that a gene possesses several promoters (or several start sites directed by a same promoter) is by "anchored-PCR," also termed "single-sided PCR" (Frohman et al., 1988; Loh et al., 1989; Ohara et al., 1989).

The principle of this method is to tail the cDNA copies of the investigated mRNAs with terminal transferase, then to amplify cDNA fragments using a primer specific to the known mRNA sequence, supposed to be common to all transcript species, and a primer recognizing the homopolymeric tail. This second primer can be composed of a homopolymeric sequence preceded by a unique sequence that will be used for further, more specific amplification (Frohman et al., 1988; Loh et al., 1989). This approach has allowed investigators to characterize the multiple 5' extremities of transcripts for α- and β-retinoic acid receptors (Leroy et al., 1991; Zelent et al., 1991) and to analyze the repertoire of expressed T-cell receptor V_β genes in rat (Smith et al., 1991). Anchored PCR has also been used to determine the sequence of the alternative 5' exon of

the ubiquitous dystrophin transcript, corresponding to the use of an alternative, ubiquitous promoter located between the 61st and 62nd exon of the dystrophin gene as numbered from the species expressed in the muscle (Hugnot et al., 1991).

Recently, we used this approach to analyze the extremities of mRNAs for NADH-cytochrome b_5 reductase. This enzyme is deficient in patients with hereditary methemoglobinemia, a relatively mild disease, but also in patients with very severe encephalopathy resulting in death before 2 years (Leroux et al., 1975). In nucleated cells, for instance in brain and liver, NADH cytochrome b_5 reductase is a membrane-bound microsomal enzyme whereas it is soluble in red blood cells. The membrane-bound NADH-cytochrome b_5 reductase possesses, in contrast to the soluble protein, a hydrophobic N-terminal peptide (Ozols et al., 1985; Yubisui et al., 1986). It was unknown until very recently whether these proteins derived from one another by partial proteolysis or were synthesized from distinct mRNA species. Anchored PCR starting from a primer corresponding to the common protein sequence has allowed us to detect three mRNA species with 5'-ends generated by alternative first exons. Two of these forms are especially abundant in reticulocytes, the third one being ubiquitous and coding for the membrane-bound enzyme (Leroux and Motta-Vierra, in preparation).

Finally, Schaefer et al. (1991) discovered a third promoter of the Epstein–Barr nuclear antigen 1 (EBNA1) gene in some Burkitt lymphoma cell lines by using anchored PCR.

Illegitimate (or Ectopic) Transcription

The current view is that housekeeping genes are expressed in essentially all cells while tissue-specific genes are exclusively expressed at a certain stage of development of certain tissues. However, the biological controls are rarely or never absolute so that the concept that tissue-specific genes are not expressed in nonspecific cells should be interpreted as "are not expressed at a detectable level." This "detectable level," however, is clearly related to the available techniques and PCR is obviously a revolutionary technique from the point of view of sensitivity. Chelly et al. demonstrated in 1988 that dystrophin transcripts could be detected not only in muscle and brain, as expected, but also, at a very low level (about 1 copy for 500–1000 cells), in cultured fibroblasts, lymphoblasts, and HepG2 hepatoma cell lines. These transcripts were correctly spliced and seemed, therefore, to be bona fide copies of the functional dystrophin mRNA.

This approach was then extended in our laboratory to other tissue-specific genes: L-type pyruvate kinase, anti-Müllerian hormone, antihemophilic factor VIII, and β-globin genes and we proposed to term such a low-level, ubiquitous transcription of tissue-specific genes "illegitimate transcription" (Chelly et al., 1989). Sarkar and Sommer (1989) reported the same phenomenon with four tissue-specific human messenger RNAs (for blue pigment, phenylalanine hydroxylase, anti-hemophilic factor IX, and tyrosine hydroxylase and described it as "ectopic transcription." Since then the phenomenon has been confirmed and generalized in several laboratories that have been able to detect and analyze a variety of tissue-specific transcripts in any type of nonspecific cells: vitamin D-binding protein, α-fetoprotein, and albumin mRNAs (McLeod and Cooke, 1989), cystic fibrosis transmembrane regulator (CFTR) mRNA (Fonknechten et al., 1991), spermatid-specific proacrosin and protamine 2 (Slomski et al., 1991), and tissue-specific collagens (Chan and Cole, 1991). Berg et al. (1990), Fonknechten et al. (1991), Knebelman et al. (1991), Chelly et al. (1991a) (Fig. 24.8), Roberts et al. (1990, 1991), Schloesser et al. (1990), and Chan and Cole (1991) used this approach to characterize the molecular anomalies of tissue-specific mRNAs (for anti-hemophilic factor VIII, CFTR, anti-Müllerian hormone, dystrophin, and collagens) in easily accessible nonspecific cells from patients.

The very low abundance of "illegitimate transcripts" often make it necessary to use "nested PCR" and increases the risk of contamination. However, we recently found that it was also possible to increase about 10-fold the amount of such transcripts by treating cultured fibroblasts with cycloheximide, a protein synthesis inhibitor (Fig. 24.9) (Chelly et al., 1991a).

One important question concerning the mechanism of illegitimate transcription was whether illegitimate transcripts correspond to a very low level activity of the usual promoters, or to the existence of multiple, nonspecific, and very rare start sites of transcription scattered throughout the genome and used independently of cell differentiation. In fact, we have found that the ratio of transcripts initiated at the "normal" start site to transcripts initiated at any aberrant 5′ cryptic site was the same in specific and nonspecific cells, which signifies that illegitimate transcription results from a very low level activity of tissue-specific promoters outside their cognate cells (Fig. 24.10). The exact mechanism of this leaky

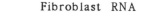

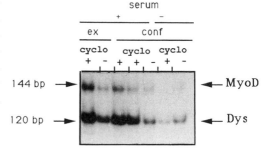

FIGURE 24.9. Effect of cycloheximide treatment on illegitimate transcript levels. Autoradiograph of Southern blot of cDNA-PCR products (obtained after 30 cycles) corresponding to the coamplification of mouse dystrophin and MyoD transcripts starting from cultured fibroblasts. RNAs were prepared from exponential (ex) or confluent (conf) cultured fibroblasts grown in the following conditions: cyclo +, cyclo −, cultures were treated or not with 1 mg/ml of cycloheximide for 7 hr; serum +, serum −, cultures were performed in the presence or absence of serum in the medium. Reproduced from Chelly et al. (1991a), *Biochemical and Biophysical Research Communications,* 178:553–557 by copyright permission of Academic Press Inc.

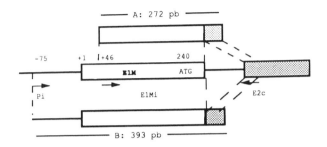

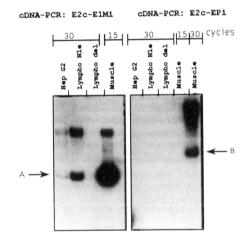

Figure 24.10. Initiation of the muscle-type dystrophin transcripts in muscle and in cultured non-specific cells. Upper part: position of the different oligonucleotide primers of the human dystrophin gene and size of amplified transcripts fragments. E1Mi and E2c were used to amplify transcripts initiated upstream of the E1Mi primer. E1Mi, a primer identical to a sequence of the first exon, is located 46 nucleotides downstream of the start site of the muscle-type dystrophin transcript. E2c is a primer complementary to a sequence of the second exon. Pi and E2c primers were used to amplify transcripts initiated 75 nucleotides upstream of the start site of initiation or further upstream. Lower part: autoradiographs of Southern blots of cDNA-PCR products (after a number of cycles as indicated) corresponding to the amplification of fragments A and B starting from skeletal muscle, HepG2 cells, normal lymphoblasts (Lympho Nle), and lymphoblasts from a patient who had a deletion encompassing the whole dystrophin gene (Lympho del, 14). The blots were hybridized with an internal specific oligonucleotide labeled by kinations. Reproduced from Chelly et al. (1991a), *Biochemical and Biophysical Research Communications,* 178:553–557 by copyright permission of Academic Press Inc.

control of tissue-specific promoters and regulatory regions remains the object of speculation. One hypothesis could be that ubiquitous transcriptional factors that cooperate with tissue-specific factors in activating transcription of tissue-specific genes are sufficient to promote transcription initiations at a very low frequency, which would explain why illegitimate transcripts are initiated at the usual cap site. It is also possible, although not proved by examination of cells sorted according to their DNA content (our unpublished data), that such transcription initiations are facilitated by chromatin disruption associated with DNA replication, making easier the binding of ubiquitous transcription factors to their cognate DNA elements.

Whatever the mechanism of illegitimate transcription, illegitimate transcripts are correctly initiated and processed and thus, by all criteria examined so far, represent faithful copies of the mRNAs accumulated in the normally expressing tissues. Therefore this phenomenon provides a powerful tool for investigating pathological transcripts by using any easily accessible cells. In addition, the use of the normal promoter outside the cells where it is physiologically activated implies that only authentic genes are expected to give rise to illegitimate transcripts, not pseudogenes or intergenic sequences. Consequently, the search for illegitimate transcripts corresponding to candidate genes isolated by any method of genome analysis should prove to be a powerful method to confirm or not confirm that they are active genes, regardless of their (unknown) tissue specificity.

Although being in principle translatable in functional proteins, it is doubtful whether these "illegitimate transcripts" play any role in most tissues, due to their very low abundance (much less than one copy per cell). In one case, however, it can be speculated that hypothetical "illegitimate proteins" may have an important function: during thymus ontogenesis, tolerance to self-antigens is most likely mediated by specific deletion of T cell clones in the thymus requiring a contact between these antigens presented by MHC molecules and thymocytes. However, most of the tissue-specific proteins are not expressed in fetal thymus and sometimes are not expressed at all in the fetus at this stage of development. It could be, in fact, that fetal thymocytes can contact the majority of proteins encoded in the genome through the phenomenon of illegitimate transcription (Linsk et al., 1989).

If this hypothesis were confirmed, illegitimate transcription would not only be a convenient means for analyzing tissue-specific mRNAs in any tissue, but also a fundamental process enabling the immune system to be informed of all (or almost all) the coding capacity of the genome.

Acknowledgments. This work was supported by the "Association Française de Lutte contre les Myopathies," the Centre National de la Recherche Scientifique, and the Institut Pasteur. We are grateful to Ms. Virginie Tourte for typing this manuscript and to Allan Strickland for his careful linguistic revision.

References

Bar S, Barnea E, Levy Z, Neuman S, Yaffe D, Nudel U (1990): A novel product of the Duchenne muscular dystrophy gene which greatly differs from the known isoforms in its structure and tissue distribution. *Biochem J* 272:557–560.

Barnea E, Zuk D, Simantov R, Nudel U, Yaffe D (1990): Specificity of expression of the muscle and brain dystrophin gene promoters in muscle and brain cells. *Neuron* 5:881–888.

Becker-André M, Hahlbrock K (1989): Absolute mRNA quantification using the polymerase chain reaction (PCR). A novel approach by a PCR aided transcript titration assay (PATTY). *Nucl Acids Res* 17:9437–9446.

Berg LP, Wieland K, Millar DS, Schlösser M, Wagner M, Kakkar VV, Reiss J, Cooper DN (1990): Detection of a novel point mutation causing haemophilia A by PCR/direct sequencing of ectopically-transcribed factor VIII mRNA. *Hum Genet* 85:655–658.

Boden SD, Joyce ME, Oliver B, Heydemann A, Bolander ME (1989): Estrogen receptor mRNA expression in callus during fracture healing in the rat. *Calcif Tissue Int* 45:324–325.

Chan D, Cole WG (1991): Low basal transcription of genes for tissue-specific collagens by fibroblasts and lymphoblastoid cells. *J Biol Chem* 266:12487–12494.

Chelly J, Kaplan JC, Maire P, Gautron S, Kahn A (1988): Transcription of the dystrophin gene in human muscle and non-muscle tissues. *Nature (London)* 333:858–860.

Chelly J, Concordet JP, Kaplan JC, Kahn A (1989): Illegitimate transcription: transcription of any gene in any cell type. *Proc Natl Acad Sci USA* 86: 2617–2621.

Chelly J, Montarras D, Pinset C, Berwald-Netter Y, Kaplan JC, Kahn A (1990a): Quantitative estimation of minor mRNAs by cDNA-polymerase chain reaction. Application to dystrophin mRNA in cultured myogenic and brain cells. *Eur J Biochem* 187:691–658.

Chelly J, Hamard G, Koulakoff A, Kaplan JC, Kahn A, Berward-Netter Y (1990b): Dystrophin gene transcribed from different promoters in neuronal and glial cells. *Nature (London)* 344:64–65.

Chelly J, Gilgenkrantz H, Lambert M, Hamard G, Chafey P, Recan D, Katz P, de la Chapelle A, Koenig M, Ginjaar IB, Fardeau M, Tome F, Kahn A, Kaplan JC (1990c): Effect of dystrophin gene deletions on mRNA levels and processing in Duchenne and Becker muscular dystrophies. *Cell* 63:1239–1248.

Chelly J, Hugnot JP, Concordet JP, Kaplan JC, Kahn A (1991a): Illegitimate (or ectopic) transcription proceeds through the usual promoters. *Biochem Biophys Res Commun* 178:553–557.

Chelly J, Gilgenkrantz H, Hugnot JP, Hamard G, Lambert M, Recan D, Akli S, Cometto M, Kahn A, Kaplan JC (1991b): Illegitimate transcription: Application to the analysis of truncated transcripts of the dystrophin gene in non-muscle cultured cells from Duchenne and Becker patients. *J Clin Invest* 88:1161–1197.

Chen J, Jones P (1989): Determination genes. *Curr Opinion Cell Biol* 1:1075–1080.

Daubas P, Devillers-Thiery A, Geoffroy B, Martinez S, Bessis A, Changeux JP (1990): Differential expression of the neuronal acetylcholine receptor $\alpha 2$ subunit gene during chick brain development. *Neuron* 5:49–60.

de la Monte SM, Ozturk M, Wands JR (1990): Enhanced expression of an exocrine pancreatic protein in Alzheimer's disease and the developing human brain. *J Clin Invest* 86:1004–1013.

Dolle P, Castrillo JL, Theill LE, Deerinck T, Ellismaen M, Karin M (1990): Expression of GHF-1 protein in mouse pituitaries correlates both temporally and spatially with the onset of growth hormone gene activity. *Cell* 60:809–820.

Ehlers S, Smith KA (1991): Differentiation of T cell lymphokine gene expression. The in vitro acquisition of T cell memory. *J Exp Med* 173:25–36.

Emerson CP (1990): Myogenesis and developmental control genes. *Curr Opinion Cell Biol* 2:1065–1075.

Feener CA, Koenig M, Kunkel LM (1989): Alternative splicing of human dystrophin mRNA generates isoforms at the carboxy terminus. *Nature (London)* 338:509–511.

Fonknechten N, Chelly J, Lepercq J, Kahn A, Kaplan JC, Kitzis A, Chomel JC (1992): CFTR illegitimate transcription in lymphoid cells: Quantification and applications to the investigation of pathological transcripts. *Hum Genet* 88:508–512.

Frohman MA, Dush MK, Martin GR (1988): Rapid production of full-length cDNAs from rare transcripts: Amplification using a single gene-specific oligonucleotide primer. *Proc Natl Acad Sci USA* 85:8998–9002.

Gilliland G, Perrin S, Blanchard K, Bunn FF (1990): Analysis of cytokine mRNA and DNA: Detection and quantitation by competitive polymerase chain reaction. *Proc Natl Acad Sci USA* 87:2725–2729.

Golde TE, Estus S, Usiak M, Younkin LH, Younkin SG (1990): Expression of β amyloid protein precursor mRNAs: Recognition of a novel alternatively spliced form and quantitation in Alzheimer's disease using PCR. *Neuron* 4:253–267.

Haase T, Retzel EF, Staskus KA (1990): Amplification and detection of lentiviral DNA inside cells. *Proc Natl Acad Sci USA* 87:4971–4975.

Haber DA, Buckler AJ, Glaser T, Call KM, Pelletier J, Sohn RL, Douglass EC, Housman DE (1990): An internal deletion within an 11p13 zinc finger gene contributes to the development of Wilms' tumor. *Cell* 61:1257–1269.

Hansell DJ, Bryant-Greenwood GD, Greenwood FC (1991): Expression of the human relaxin H1 gene in the decidua, trophoblast, and prostaste. *J Clin End Met* 72:899–904.

Heyner S, Rao LV, Jarett L, Smith RM (1989): Preimplantation mouse embryos internalize maternal insulin via receptor-mediated encodytosis: Pattern of uptake and functional correlations. *Dev Biol* 134:48–58.

Hugnot JP, Gilgenkrantz H, Vincent N, Chaffey P, Morrist G, Monaco T, Koulakoff A, Berwald-Netter Y, Kaplan JC, Kahn A, Chelly J (1992): Characterization of the products generated by the distal part of the dystrophin gene: mRNAs and protein. *Proc Natl Acad Sci USA* 89:7506–7510.

Ivell R, Furuya K, Brackmann B, Dawood Y, Khan-Dawood F (1990): Expression of the oxytocin and vasopressin genes in human and baboon gonadal tissues. *Endocrinology* 127:2990–2996.

Jager RJ, Anvret M, Hall K, Scherer G (1990): A human XY female with a frame shift mutation in the candidate testis-determining gene SRY. *Nature (London)* 348:452–453.

Knebelmann B, Boussin L, Guerrier D, Legeai L, Kahn A, Josso N, Picard JY (1991): Anti-Müllerian hormone Bruxelles: A nonsense mutation associated with the persistent Müllerian duct syndrome. *Proc Natl Acad Sci USA* 88:3767–3371.

Koopman P, Münsterberg A, Capel B, Vivian N, Lovell-Badge R (1990): Expression of a candidate sex-determining gene during mouse testis differentiation. *Nature (London)* 348:450–452.

Koos RD, Olson CE (1989): Expression of basic fibroblast growth factor in the rat ovary: Detection of mRNA using reverse transcription-polymerase chain reaction amplification. *Mol Endocrinol* 3:2041–2048.

Leroux A, Junien C, Kaplan JC, Bamberger J (1975): Generalized deficiency of cytochrome b5 reductase in congenital methemoglobinemia with mental retardation. *Nature (London)* 258:619–620.

Leroy P, Krust A, Zelent A, Mendolsohn C, Garnier JM, Kastner P, Dierich A, Chambon P (1991): Multiple isoforms of the mouse retinoic acid receptor α are generated by alternative splicing and differential induction by retinoic acid. EMBO J 10:59–69.

Linsk R, Gottesman M, Pernis B (1989): Are tissues a patch quilt of ectopic gene expression? *Science* 246:261.

Loh EY, Elliott JF, Cwirla S, Lanier LL, Davis MM (1989): Polymerase chain reaction with single-sided specificity: Analysis of T cell receptor δ chain. *Science* 243:217–220.

Louache F, Debili N, Cramer E, Breton-Gorius J, Vainchenker W (1991): Fibrinogen is not synthesized by human megakaryocytes. *Blood* 77:311–316.

Magnuson MA, Shelton KD (1989): An alternate promoter in the glucokinase gene is active in the pancreatic β cell. *J Biol Chem* 264:15936–15942.

McLeod JF, Cooke NE (1989): The vitamin D-binding protein, α-fetoprotein, albumin multi-

gene family: Detection of transcripts in multiple tissues. *J Biol Chem* 264:21760–21769.

Mivechi NF, Rossi JJ (1990): Use of polymerase chain reaction to detect the expression of the M_r 70,000 heat shock genes in control or heat shock leukemia cells as correlated to their heat response. *Cancer Res* 50:2877–2884.

Mohler KM, Butler LD (1990): Differential production of IL-2 and IL-4 mRNA *in vivo* after primary sensitization. *J Immunol* 145:1734–1739.

Montarras D, Pinset C, Chelly J, Kahn A, Gros F (1989): Expression of *MyoD1* coincides with terminal differentiation in determined but inducible muscle cells. *EMBO J* 8:2203–2207.

Montarras D, Chelly J, Bober E, Arnold H, Ott MO, Gros F, Pinset C (1991): Developmental patterns in the expression of *Myf5, MyoD, myogenin,* and *MRF4* during myogenesis. *New Biol* 3:592–600.

Moriyama T, Murphy HR, Martin BM, Garcia-Perez A (1990): Detection of specific mRNAs in single nephron segments by use of the polymerase chain reaction. *Am J Physiol* 258:F.1470–1474.

Murray R, Lee F, Chiu CP (1990): The genes for leukemia inhibitory factor and interleukin-6 are expressed in mouse blastocysts prior to the onset of hemopoiesis. *Mol Cell Biol* 10:4953–4956.

Neve RL, Rogers J, Higgins GA (1990): The Alzheimer amyloid precursor-related transcript lacking the β/A4 sequence is specially increased in Alzheimer's disease brain. *Neuron* 5:329–338.

Noonan KE, Beck C, Holzmayer TA, Chin JE, Wunder JS, Andrulis IL, Gazdar AF, Willman CL, Griffith B, Von Hoff DD, Roninson IB (1990): Quantitative analysis of *MDR1* (multidrug resistance) gene expression in human tumors by polymerase chain reaction. *Proc Natl Acad Sci USA* 87:7160–7164.

Nunez DJR, Davenport AP, Brown MJ (1990): Atrial natriuretic factor mRNA and binding sites in the adrenal gland. *Biochem J* 271:555–558.

Ohara O, Dorit RL, Gilbert W (1989): One-sided polymerase chain reaction: The amplification of cDNA. *Proc Natl Acad Sci USA* 86:5673–5677.

Olson EN (1990): MyoD family: A paradigm for development. *Genes Dev* 4:1454–1461.

Omiecinski CJ, Redlich CA, Costa P (1990): Induction and developmental expression of cytochrome P450IA1 messenger RNA in rat and human tissues: Detection by the polymerase chain reaction. *Cancer Res* 50:4315–4321.

Ott MO, Bober E, Lyons G, Arnold H, Buckingham M (1991): Early expression of the myogenic regulatory gene, *myf-5,* in precursor cells of skeletal muscle in the mouse embryo. *Development* 111: 1097–1107.

Ozols J, Korza G, Heinemann FS, Hediger MA, Strittmatter P (1985): Complete amino acid sequence of steer liver microsomed NADH-cytochrome *b5* reductase. *J Biol Chem* 260:11953–11961.

Pinset C, Mulle C, Benoit P, Changeux JP, Chelly J, Gros F, Montarras D (1991): Functional adult acetylcholine receptor develops independently of motor innervation in Sol 8 mouse muscle cell line. *Embo J* 10:2411–2418.

Pizzuti A, Borsani G, Falini A, Rugarli EI, Sidoli A, Baralle FE, Scarlato G, Silani V (1990): Detection of β-nerve growth factor mRNA in the human fetal brain. *Brain Res* 518:337–341.

Poznanski AA, Calarco PG (1991): The expression of intracisternal A particle genes in the preimplantation mouse embryo. *Dev Biol* 143:271–281.

Rappolee DA, Mark D, Banda MJ, Werb Z (1988a): Wound macrophages express TGF-α and other growth factors in vivo: Analysis by mRNA phenotyping. *Science* 241:708–712.

Rappolee DA, Brenner CA, Schultz R, Mark D, Werb Z (1988b): Developmental expression of PDGF, TGF-α, and TGF-β genes in preimplantation mouse embryos. *Science* 241:1823–1825.

Rappolee DA, Wang A, Mark D, Werb Z (1989): Novel method for studying mRNA phenotypes in single or small numbers of cells. *J Cell Biochem* 39:1–11.

Reyes AA, Small SJ, Akeson R (1991): At least 27 alternatively spliced forms of the neural cell adhesion molecule mRNA are expressed during rat heart development. *Mol Cell Biol* 11:1654–1661.

Roberts RG, Bentley DR, Barby TFM, Manners E, Bobrow M (1990): Direct diagnostic of carriers of Duchenne and Becker muscular dystrophy by amplification of lymphocyte RNA. *Lancet* 336: 1523–1526.

Roberts RG, Barby TFM, Manners E, Bobrow M, Bentley DR (1991): Direct detection of dystrophin gene rearrangements by analysis of dystrophin mRNA in peripheral blood lymphocytes. *Am J Hum Genet* 49:298–310.

Rupp RAW, Weintraub H (1991): Ubiquitous MyoD transcription at the midblastula transition precedes induction-dependent MyoD expression in presumptive mesoderm of X. laevis. *Cell* 65:927–937.

Ryan MC, Sandell LJ (1990): Differential expression of a cysteine-rich domain in the amino-terminal propeptide of type II (cartilage) procollagen by alternative splicing of mRNA. *J Biol Chem* 265:10334–10339.

Salgame P, Abrams JS, Clayberger C, Goldstein H, Convit J, Modlin RL, Bloom BR (1991): Differing lymphokine profiles of functional subsets of human CD4 and CD8 T cell clones. *Science* 277:279–282.

Saltini C, Kirby M, Trapnell BC, Tamura N, Crystal RG (1990): Biased accumulation of T lymphocytes with "memory" type CD45 leukocyte common antigen gene expression on the epithelial surface of the human lung. *J Exp Med* 171:1123–1140.

Sandell LJ, Morris N, Robbins JR, Goldring MB (1991): Alternatively spliced type II procollagen mRNAs define distinct populations of cells during vertebral development: Differential expression of the amino-propeptide. *J Cell Biol* 114: 1307–1319.

Sarkar G, Sommer SS (1989): Access to a messenger RNA sequence or its protein product is not limited by tissue or species specificity. *Science* 244:331–334.

Sassoon D, Lyons G, Wright WE, Lin V, Lassar A, Weintraub H, Buckingham M (1989): Expression of two myogenic regulatory factors myogenin and MyoD1 during mouse embryogenesis. *Nature (London)* 341:303–307.

Schaefer BC, Woisetschlaeger M, Strominger JL, Speck SH (1991): Exclusive expression of Epstein-Barr virus nuclear antigen 1 in Burkitt lymphoma arises from a third promoter, distinct from the promoters used in latently infected lymphocytes. *Proc Natl Acad Sci USA* 88:6550–6554.

Schloesser M, Slomski R, Wagner M, Reiss J, Berg LP, Kakkar VV, Cooper DN (1990): Characterization of pathological dystrophin transcripts from the lymphocytes of a muscular dystrophy carrier. *Mol Biol Med* 7:519–523.

Schriever F, Freeman G, Nadler LM (1991): Follicular dendritic cells contain a unique gene repertoire demonstrated by single-cell polymerase chain reaction. *Blood* 77:787–791.

Serrano J, Shuldiner AR, Roberts CT, LeRoith D, de Pablo F (1990): The insulin-like growth factor I (IGF-I) gene is expressed in chick embryos during early organogenesis. *Endocrinology* 127: 1547–1549.

Singer-Sam J, Robinson MO, Bellvé AR, Simon MI, Riggs AD (1990): Measurement by quantitative PCR of changes in HPRT, PGK-1, PGK-2,

APRT, MTase, and Zfy gene transcripts during mouse spermatogenesis. *Nucl Acids Res* 18: 1255–1259.

Slomski R, Schloesser M, Chlebowska H, Reiss J, Engel W (1991): Detection of human spermatid-specific transcripts in peripheral blood lymphocytes of males and females. *Hum Genet* 87:307–310.

Smith LR, Kono DH, Theofilopoulos AN (1991): Complexity and sequence identification of 24 rat Vβ genes. *J Immunol* 147:375–379.

Talian JC, Zelenka PS (1991): Calpactin I in the differentiating embryonic chicken lens: mRNA levels and protein distribution. *Dev Biol* 143:68–77.

Telford NA, Hogan A, Franz CR, Schultz GA (1990): Expression of genes for insulin and insulin-like growth factors and receptors in early postimplantation mouse embryos and embryonal carcinoma cells. *Mol Repro Dev* 27:81–92.

Traber PG, Wang W, McDonnell M, Gumucio JJ (1990): P450IIB gene expression in rat small intestine: Cloning of intestinal P450IIB1 mRNA using the polymerase chain reaction and transcriptional regulation of induction. *Mol Pharmacol* 37:810–819.

Voutilainen R, Ilvesmäki V, Miettinen PJ (1991): Low expression of 3β-hydroxy-5-ene steroid dehydrogenase gene in human fetal adrenals in vivo; adrenocorticotropin and protein kinase C-dependent regulation in adrenocortical cultures. *J Clin End Met* 72:761–767.

Wang AM, Doyle MV, Mark DF (1989): Quantitation of mRNA by the polymerase chain reaction. *Proc Natl Acad Sci USA* 86:9717–9721.

Weider KJ, Walz G, Zanker B, Sehajpal P, Sharma VK, Skolnik E, Strom TB, Suthanthiran M (1990): Physiologic signaling in normal human T-cells: mRNA phenotyping by Northern blot analysis and reverse transcription-polymerase chain reaction. *Cell Immunol* 128:41–51.

Weizsächer FV, Labeit S, Koch HK, Oehlert W, Gerok W, Blum HE (1991): A simple and rapid method for the detection of RNA in formalin-fixed, paraffin-embedded tissues by PCR amplification. *Biochem Biophys Res Commun* 174:176–180.

Wesselingh SL, Gough NM, Finlay-Jones JJ, McDonald PJ (1990): Detection of cytokine mRNA in astrocyte cultures using the polymerase chain reaction. *Lymphokine Res* 9:177–185.

Yamamura M, Uyemura K, Deans RJ, Weinberg K, Rea TH, Bloom BR, Moddlin RL (1991): Defining protective responses to pathogens: Cytokine profiles in leprosy lesions. *Science* 277:277–279.

Yang F, Friedrichs WE, Cupples RL, Bonifacio MJ, Sanford JA, Horton WA, Bowman BH (1990): Human ceruloplasmin tissue-specific expression of transcripts produced by alternative splicing. *J Biol Chem* 265:10780–10785.

Yubisui T, Miyata T, Iwanaga S, Tamura M, Yoshida S, Takeshita M, Nakajima H (1984): Amino acid sequence of NADH-cytochrome *b5* reductase of human erythrocytes. J Biochem 96:579–582.

Zelent A, Mendelsohn C, Kastner P, Krust A, Garnier JM, Ruffenach F, Leroy P, Chambon P (1991): Differentially expressed isoforms of the mouse retinoic acid receptor β are generated by usage of two promoters and alternative splicing. *EMBO J* 10:71–81.

Zorn AM, Krieg PA (1991): PCR analysis of alternative splicing pathways: Identification of artifacts generated by heteroduplex formation. *Biotechniques* 11:181–183.

25

Fingerprinting Using Arbitrarily Primed PCR: Application to Genetic Mapping, Population Biology, Epidemiology, and Detection of Differentially Expressed RNAs

John Welsh and Michael McClelland

Introduction

Arbitrarily Primed PCR for Genetic Mapping and Phylogeny

Several approaches to genetic mapping and phylogenetic analysis using PCR have been developed over the past few years. The ability to examine specific sequences of DNA from many organisms simultaneously and without the need of standard cloning has streamlined several types of analysis that were already commonly used but rather labor intensive and has also made possible several types of analysis that were previously not possible. For example, RFLP analysis using Southern blotting has been the principal tool for chromosomal mapping in mammals and plants and, in some situations, has been replaced by PCR-based methods (e.g., Litt and Luty, 1989; Nelson et al., 1989; Orita et al., 1990; Sinnet et al., 1990; Ledbetter et al., 1990). Methods based on PCR have also been developed for studies in phylogenetics and population biology. Specific sequences of phylogenetic significance, such as ribosomal DNA or DNA from surface antigen genes, can be amplified and sequenced to derive phylogenetic and population genetics information (e.g., see Woese, 1987). Prior to the invention of PCR, these analyses required cloning and were correspondingly labor intensive. PCR allows for the direct amplification and sequencing of interesting sequences without the need for cloning (e.g., Medlin et al., 1988).

In addition to these obvious extensions of PCR, novel applications of PCR have also evolved. For example, we have developed a method for genomic fingerprinting based on PCR, termed arbitrarily primed PCR, which relies on chance homologies between an oligonucleotide primer and genomic DNA or, more recently, RNA. Such interactions can be extended by polymerase under low stringency annealing conditions. Arbitrarily primed PCR-based genomic fingerprinting reveals sequence polymorphisms that can be used similarly to RFLPs in genetic mapping, and differences between fingerprints for closely related organisms can be used to determine their relatedness in phylogenetic and population biology experiments. The purpose of this brief review is to explore these new possibilities that are facilitated by PCR with an emphasis on our own research in this area.

The Polymerase Chain Reaction
K.B. Mullis, F. Ferré, R.A. Gibbs, editors
© 1994 Birkhäuser Boston

Mapping Genetic Polymorphisms in Sexual Species

There are two high throughput methods based on PCR for mapping sequence polymorphisms. Jeffreys et al. (1985) recognized that the level of polymorphism in variable number tandem repeats (VNTRs) between different members of a population make them particularly suited as polymorphic markers in genetic analysis. Rapid variation in the length of a VNTR results from the instability of simple repeats. By following the segregation of VNTRs in families or in a breeding population, recombination frequencies, and therefore genetic distances, can be determined. These experiments first used Southern analysis, and in some situations, this is still the method of choice. However, as the sequence database for important experimental organisms such as human and mouse expands, sequences flanking potential VNTRs are being identified. This allows primers that bracket VNTRs to be constructed and used to detect VNTR length polymorphisms in the mapping population. Because there are over 13,000 potential VNTRs in each mammalian genome, the possible resolution of a genetic map based on this approach is restricted only by the nature of the mapping population. An advantage of this approach is that once a polymorphism is mapped, the primers used for each polymorphism are immediately available for further experiments. This method does, however, have some practical limitations. First, oligonucleotide primers are expensive, so each polymorphism is obtained at a cost of several hundred dollars in reagents. Second, these primers are designed for the genetic mapping of polymorphisms in a *particular* organism or set of closely related species and often cannot be used to map other organisms. Also, there is some concern that the nonrandom distribution of VNTRs in the genome may lead to the incompleteness of maps generated by this method (Moyzis et al., 1989).

Another approach to genetic mapping uses the often observed but seldom appreciated property of PCR that, if the stringency of the annealing step is not properly adjusted, products other than the desired sequence result. By intentionally reducing the stringency of the annealing step and choosing a single primer that is unlikely to match *anything* is the genome very well, an information-rich genomic fingerprint can be obtained reproducibly (Welsh and McClelland, 1990; Williams et al., 1990; Welsh et al., 1991a,b,c; Welsh and McClelland, 1991a,b; Martin et al., 1991; Michelmore et al., 1991). In Figure 25.1, the strategy for arbitrarily primed PCR is outlined. Two or more cycles are performed at low stringency during the annealing step (at which time some synthesis occurs, thereby stabilizing the template–primer interaction). Following these two low stringency steps, subsequent cycles are performed under standard, high stringency PCR conditions. This procedure is sensitive to sequence polymorphisms in the target genome. Thus, the segregation of arbitrarily primed PCR polymorphisms in a recombinant inbred or other mapping population can be used to place the polymorphisms on the genetic map. In Figure 25.2, the results of arbitrarily primed PCR applied to genomic DNAs from a collection of recombinant inbred mice are shown. As can be seen, the patterns are nonidentical. In this rather unusual case, there appear four independent length polymorphisms. In general, four to seven polymorphisms can be mapped with each primer in this particular cross with about 80% being the presence or absence of a band and 20% being length polymorphisms.

New arbitrarily primed PCR patterns can be generated by the application of primers in pairwise combinations as long as the primers are designed so as to minimize the primer artifacts that can occur with low stringency annealing. The experiment in Figure 25.2 uses two primers in pairwise combination. When primers are used in pairwise combinations, the patterns generated are very different from the simple sum of the patterns generated by the same primers used independently. Thus, 50 primers can be used to generate $(50)^2/2 = 1250$ different fingerprints (Welsh and McClelland, 1991b). Due to the complex kinetics of arbitrarily primed PCR, less than 50% of the bands are shared in a band-by-band com-

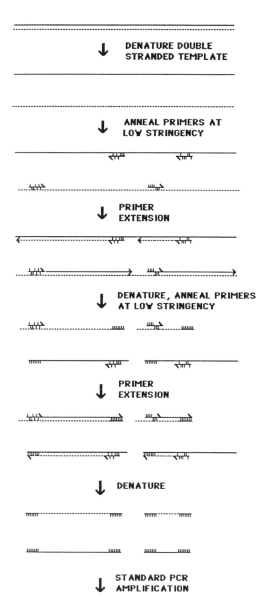

FIGURE 25.1. Arbitrarily primed PCR can be used to generate polymorphic fingerprints for genetic mapping. Oligonucleotide primers are annealed at low stringency to the template. This reaction depends on the sequence of the template and the details of the interaction are influenced by sequence polymorphisms. Two low stringency cycles are performed, followed by 40 high stringency cycles. Those sequences that lie between two sites where primer extension occurs during the first two low stringency cycles can be amplified in subsequent high stringency cycles.

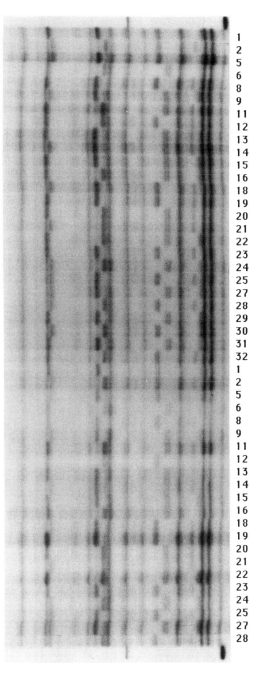

FIGURE 25.2. Arbitrarily primed PCR applied to mouse recombinant inbreds: lanes 1–32 are the result of arbitrarily primed PCR on genomic DNA from 26 recombinant inbreds. The parentals of this population are C57BL/6J and DBA/2J. Polymorphisms segregating between these two strains are clearly visible. The experiment was performed at two concentration of genomic DNAs. DNA from recombinant inbreds was kindly supplied by Benjamin Taylor, Jackson Labs.

parison with the patterns produced by either primer alone. Given that about four polymorphisms can be detected in genomes of the quite closely related mouse strains C57BL/6 and DBA with each new primer or primer pair, the cost of mapping is correspondingly low. A disadvantage of arbitrarily primed PCR is that each new polymorphism must be purified to be of further use, but this procedure is very straightforward. Also, only length polymorphisms can be scored in heterozygotes using this method.

Arbitrarily primed PCR requires no prior knowledge of sequence and probably samples the genome randomly. Since primers can be chosen arbitrarily, any organism can be mapped with the same set of primers. However, if desired, a sequence bias can be engineered into the primer. Primers can be directed against repeated or motif sequences (Welsh and McClelland, 1992). In principle, GC-rich regions can be mapped preferentially by constructing a GC-rich primer. Similarly, primers that contain octamers at their 3'-end that are very common in a particular genome will give complex patterns, whereas primers that contain rare octamers give few or no bands (Griffais et al., 1991).

Another advantage of arbitrarily primed PCR is that it can be used to detect polymorphisms in near isogenic strains (or congenics). Thus, if a phenotype is followed as it is introgressed any polymorphisms that are detected are likely to map to the gene(s) responsible for the phenotype (Martin et al., 1991). Alternatively, one can perform bulk segregant analysis. In this method a phenotype is scored in an F_2 population and five individuals from one extreme phenotype are placed in a pool and five individuals from the opposite phenotype are placed in another pool. If arbitrarily primed PCR is performed on each pool, any polymorphisms detected between pools have a reasonable chance of being linked to the gene(s) responsible for the phenotype since nonlinked polymorphisms have only a 1/32 of being absent in one pool (Michelmore et al., 1991). The likelihood of linkage in both these strategies is a function of the level of inbreed-

ing, in the former case, and a function of the number of individuals examined in the latter case.

The Use of Arbitrarily Primed PCR Fingerprinting to Characterize Individuals

Polymorphisms in fingerprint patterns generated by arbitrarily primed PCR can be used to distinguish between even very closely related individuals. Arbitrarily primed PCR fingerprints are quite complex or "information rich," and because this information is easily and inexpensively obtainable, the resolution of arbitrarily primed PCR for taxonomic comparison is very high. Thus, for example, we have been able to distinguish between isolates of the same species of bacteria including *Staphylococcus haemolyticus* (Welsh and McClelland, 1990; Fang et al., 1973), *Streptococcus pyogenes*, and *Borrelia burgdorferi* (Welsh et al., 1991c).

Polymorphisms in fingerprints generated by arbitrarily primed PCR can be treated as apomorphic characters in phylogenetic analysis and population biology. Using this approach, *Streptococcus pyogenes* strains can be resolved by arbitrarily primed PCR into groups that correspond to their surface antigen types. In Figure 25.3, a sample of fingerprinting data for a collection of *Streptococcus pyogenes* is presented, along with the resultant unrooted tree. The numbers refer to the surface antigen types of the strains. In this analysis, strains having the surface antigen type 49 appear to be ancestral to those having types 4, 18, and 55 (Welsh et al., in preparation).

In principle, genotypes characterized by fingerprinting can be used to study a number of problems in population biology. For example, linkage disequilibrium of various sorts, such as fixed heterozygosity in diploids, can shed light on such problems as clonality. By reconstructing the phylogeny of a bacterial pathogen and identifying polymorphisms for individual phylogenetic groups, genetic and ecological interactions between populations can be studied.

When we applied arbitrarily primed PCR to a collection of *Borrelia burgdorferi*, the etio-

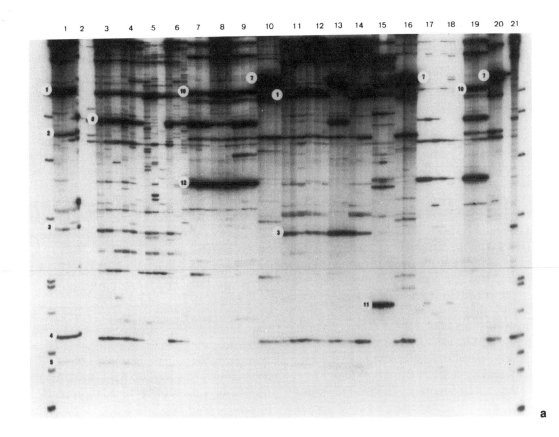

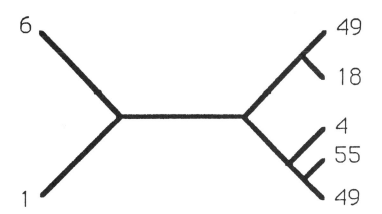

FIGURE 25.3. (a) All lanes contain fingerprints of S. pyogenes except lanes 10 and 20, which contain fingerprints from E. faecalis. Each strain has a characteristic antigenic type. Genomic fingerprinting was performed as described in the text. Polymorphic bands, indicated by small numbered circles, were scores as either present (1) or absent (0). This gel represents one of three experiments from which polymorphisms were scored. (b) The most parsimonious trees generated from this and other data, placing antigenic types 1, 6, 49, 55, 18, and 4 in their positions relative to one another. Outgroup analysis suggests that antigen type 49 is ancestral to types 4, 18, and 55.

logical agent of Lyme disease we discovered that this species is actually comprised of three distinct phyletic groups that, by DNA homology criteria, differ from one another around the level of species (Welsh et al., 1992). This may eventually be important in understanding various clinical manifestations of the disease. Like most bacteria (with the exception of *E. coli*) the population biology of *Borrelia burgdorferi* and other spirochetes is in its infancy.

In another set of experiments a set of nosocomial (hospital derived) infections with Methicilin-resistant *Staphylococcus aureus* (MRSA) was compared to determine how many different strains were responsible for an outbreak of this problem. In this study, arbitrarily primed PCR was used to resolve an ambiguity that remained after plasmid profile analysis (Fang et al., 1993). Thus, arbitrarily primed PCR can distinguish between very closely related strains for which other convenient markers may not exist.

In general, arbitrarily primed PCR can be used to survey for polymorphisms between any two sufficiently divergent DNAs. The fraction of arbitrarily primed PCR bands that will be polymorphic given two divergent templates is roughly equal to their genetic distance (Welsh et al., 1992). In humans losses of heterozygosity associated with cancer have been detected (Ionov et al., 1993).

Arbitrarily Primed PCR Fingerprinting of RNA

Recently, fingerprinting of RNA populations was achieved (Welsh et al., 1992b; Liang and Pardee, 1992) using an arbitrarily selected primer at low stringency for first and second strand cDNA synthesis. PCR amplification is then used to amplify the products. The method requires only a few nanograms of total RNA and is unaffected by low levels of genomic double-stranded DNA contamination. A reproducible pattern of 10 to 20 clearly visible PCR products is obtained from any one tissue. Differences in PCR fingerprints are detected for RNAs from the same tissue isolated from dif-

ferent mouse strains and for RNAs from different tissues from the same mouse. The *strain-specific* differences revealed are probably due to sequence polymorphisms and are useful for genetic mapping of genes. The *tissue-specific* differences revealed are useful for studying differential gene expression. Examples of tissue-specific differences have been cloned. Differential expression was confirmed for these products by Northern analysis and DNA sequencing uncovered two new tissue-specific messages. The method should be applicable to the detection of differences between RNA populations in a wide variety of situations (Ralph et al., 1993).

PCR between tRNA Gene Repeats

PCR primers can be designed to recognize specific sequences that are interspersed throughout the genome. Amplification of sequences between interspersed sequence elements results in a genomic fingerprint. Amplification of sequences between *Alu* repeats in somatic cell hybrids containing fragments of human chromosomes in rodent backgrounds was one of the first demonstrations of this principle (Nelson et al., 1989; Ledbetter et al., 1990). Some of our work has focused on the amplification of sequences between tRNA genes in bacteria (Welsh et al., 1991a). In bacterial genomes there are about 100 tRNA genes, generally clustered head to tail with short intergenic spacers (Jinks-Robertson and Nomura, 1987; Vold, 1985). Because tDNA sequences evolve slowly, distinctions between genera of bacteria on the basis of intergenic sequence length polymorphism and tDNA cluster rearrangement can be achieved. The method works as follows: first, consensus tDNA primers are constructed that amplify tDNA spacer regions for any eubacteria. These primers point out of the consensus gene and are slightly recessed from the ends of the tDNA sequence, for reasons that will become clear later. PCR amplification is performed at moderate rather than high stringency and a pattern of bands is obtained. The primers anneal to the best matches available and some pairs of matches are close enough on opposite strands

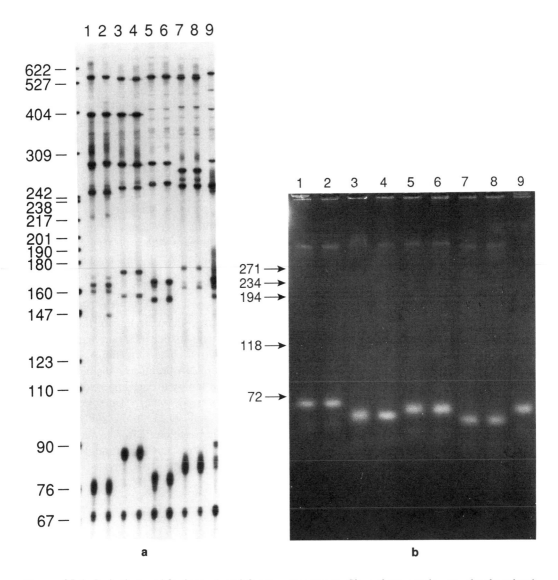

FIGURE 25.4. In both **a** and **b**, lanes 1 and 2 are *Staphylococcus hominis*, lanes 3 and 4 are *S. warneri*, lanes 5 and 6 are *S. aureus*, lanes 7 and 8 are *S. haemolyticus*, and lane 9 is *S. cohnii*. (**a**) tDNA-PCR using consensus primers was performed as described in the text. Polymorphisms can result from three sources: (1) polymorphic inter-tDNA spacer lengths, (2) selection of different tDNA sequences by the primer, and (3) tDNA cluster rear- rangement. Since these species are closely related and since tDNA sequences and clusters evolve only very slowly, most of the polymorphisms here reflect spacer length differences. (**b**) tRNA intergenic length polymorphisms (tRNA-ILPs). Primer se- quences based on the results shown in **a** were used to amplify specific polymorphisms the lengths of which are generally characteristic of each species.

to allow PCR. The resulting pattern displays differences in spacer length and tDNA cluster organization between genera and species that are phylogenetically useful (see Fig. 25.4).

While the consensus primers we have derived are suitable for eubacteria, others could equally easily be designed for other groups of organisms, for example, insect nuclear tRNA genes or vertebrate mitochondrial tRNA genes.

The tDNA-PCR experiment described above used weak consensus primers at moderate stringency. Such primers will not amplify the desired tDNA spacer regions if the bacterial DNA is heavily contaminated with DNA from another source, as is the case with medical specimens, for example. However, because the primers are slightly recessed from the ends of the tDNA sequences, primers that can be used at *high* stringency can now be derived from the tDNA-PCR fingerprint. The tDNA-PCR length polymorphism that most clearly distinguishes between the set of related test species is chosen, reamplified, and sequenced from both ends. The sequences immediately 3′ to the original primers are still within conserved tRNA genes and can be used to design perfectly homologous primers. These new primers can be used in PCR identify *intergenic length polymorphisms* (tRNA-ILPs) that classify members of the genus into species or subspecies. These primers can be used for medical diagnostics by high stringency PCR where samples are contaminated with human DNA and in epidemiology where culturing various organisms of interest may be cumbersome. In Figure 25.4b, we show how primers derived in this way can be used to generate products (tRNA-ILPs) whose lengths are characteristic of different clonal groups (e.g., species) of bacteria. In this particular experiment, the primers were derived from tDNA sequence from products around 160 bp (Fig. 25.4a). DNA gene sequences and the order of the genes in the clusters evolve rather slowly, so PCR primers homologous to two particular adjacent tRNA genes give a positive signal for almost any species within the same genus.

Using this approach, we have developed a pair of primers for high stringency tRNA-ILP

PCR that identify most, if not all, *Staphylococci* and define species based on the lengths of the products (Welsh and McClelland, 1991c, 1992). Similarly, we have developed a pair of primers for tRNA-ILP PCR that identify and distinguish between members of the *Streptococcus pyogenes* cluster of species (McClelland et al., 1992).

Summary

The versatility of PCR as an analytical tool seems to increase with each new twist on the basic methodology. Taking advantage of the ability of oligonucleotide primers to prime DNA synthesis at imperfect matches, we and others have extended PCR to genomic fingerprinting. Genomic fingerprinting is useful in genetic mapping, strain identification, and population characterization. Now the application to RNA promises a distinct improvement in our ability to detect and clone differentially expressed genes. Due to relatively simplicity and speed, molecular methods of comparison based on PCR have made possible a number of experiments that might otherwise be impractical.

References

Fang FC, McClelland M, Guiney DG, Jackson MM, Hartstein AI, Morthland VH, Davis CE, McPherson DC, Welsh J (1993): Value of molecular epidemiologic analysis in a nosocomial methicillin-resistant *Staphylococcus aureus* outbreak. *J Am Med Assoc* 270:1323–1328.

Griffais R, Andre PM, Thibon M (1991): K-tuple frequency in the human genome and polymerase chain reaction. *Nucl Acids Res* 19:3887–3891.

Ionov Y, Peinado MA, Malkhosyan S, Shibata D, Perucho M (1993): Ubiquitous somatic mutations in simple repeated sequences reveal a new mechanism for colonic carcinogenesis. *Nature* 363: 558–561.

Jeffreys AJ, Wilson V, Thein SL (1985): Individual-specific "fingerprints" of human DNA. *Nature (London)* 316:76–79.

Jinks-Robertson, Nomura M (1987): Ribosomes and tRNA, In *E. coli and S. typhimurium.*

Neidhardt FC, ed. Washington: ASM Press, pp. 1358–1385.

Ledbetter SA, Nelson DL, Warren ST, Ledbetter DH (1990): Rapid isolation of DNA probes within specific chromosome regions by interspersed repetitive sequence polymerase chain reaction. *Genomics* 6:475–481.

Liang P, Pardee A (1992): Differential display of eukaryotic messenger RNA by means of the polymerase chain reaction. *Science* 257:967–971.

Litt M, Luty JA (1989): A hypervariable microsatellite revealed by in vitro amplification of a dinucleotide repeat within the cardiac muscle actin gene. *Am J Hum Genet* 44:397–401.

Martin GB, Williams, JG, Tanksley SD (1991): Rapid identification of markers linked to a Pseudomonas resistance gene in tomato by using random primers and near-isogenic lines. *Proc Natl Acad Sci USA* 88:2336–2340.

McClelland M, Ivarie R (1982): Asymmetrical distribution of CpG in an "average" mammalian gene. *Nucl Acids Res* 10:7865–7877.

McClelland M, Peterson C, Welsh J (1992): Length polymorphisms in tRNA intergenic spacers detected using the polymerase chain reaction can distinguish streptococcal strains and species. *J Clin Microbiol* 30:1499–1504.

Medlin L, Elwood HJ, Stickel S, Sogin M (1988): The characterization of enzymatically amplified eukaryotic 16S-like rRNA-coding regions. *Gene* 71:491–499.

Michelmore RW, Paran I, Kesseli RV (1991): Identification of markers linked to disease resistance genes by bulked segregant analysis: A rapid method to detect markers in specific genomic regions using segregating populations. *Proc Natl Acad Sci USA* 88:9828–9832.

Moyzis RK, Torney DC, Meyne J, Buckingham JM, Wu J-R, Burks C, Sirotkin KM, Goad WB (1989): The distribution of interspersed repetitive DNA sequences in the human genome. *Genomics* 4:273–289.

Nelson DL, Ledbetter SA, Corbo L, Victoria MF, Ramirez-Solis R, Webster TD, Ledbetter DH, Caskey CT (1989): *Alu* polymerase chain reaction: a method for rapid isolation of human-specific sequences from complex DNA sources. *Proc Natl Acad Sci USA* 86:6686–6690.

Orita M, Sekiya T, Hayashi K (1990): DNA sequence polymorphisms in Alu repeats. *Genomics* 8:271–278.

Ralph D, Welsh J, McClelland M (1993): RNA fingerprinting using arbitrarily primed PCR identifies differentially regulated RNAs in Mink lung (MvlLu) cells growth arrested by TGF-β. *Proc Natl Acad Sci USA* 90:10710–10714.

Sinnet D, Deragon J-M, Simard LR, Labuda D (1990): Alumorphs-human DNA polymorphisms detected by PCR using *Alu*-specific primers. *Genomics* 7:331–334.

Vold B (1985): Structure and organization of genes for transfer ribonucleic acid in *Bacillus subtilis*. *Microbiol Rev* 49:71–80.

Welsh J, McClelland M (1990): Fingerprinting genomes using PCR with arbitrary primers. *Nucl Acids Res* 18:7213–7218.

Welsh J, McClelland M (1991a): Species-specific genomic fingerprints produced by PCR with consensus tRNA gene primers. *Nucl Acids Res* 19:861–866.

Welsh J, McClelland M (1991b): Genomic fingerprinting using arbitrarily primed PCR and a matrix of pairwise combinations of primers. *Nucl Acids Res* 19:5275–5279.

Welsh J, McClelland M (1992): PCR-amplified length polymorphisms in tRNA intergenic spacers for categorizing staphylococci. *Mol Microbiol* 6:1673–1680.

Welsh J, Petersen C, McClelland M (1991a): Polymorphisms generated by arbitrarily primed PCR in the mouse: Application to strain identification and genetic mapping. *Nucl Acids Res* 19:303–306.

Welsh J, McClelland M, Honeycutt RJ, Sobral BWS (1991b): Parentage determination in maize hybrids using arbitrarily primed PCR. *Theoret Appl Genet* 82:473–476.

Welsh J, Pretzman C, Postic D, Saint Girons I, Baranton G, McClelland M (1991c): Genomic fingerprinting by arbitrarily primed PCR resolves *Borrelia burgdorferi* into three distinct phyletic groups. *Int J System Bacteriol* 42:370–377.

Welsh J, Chada K, Dalal SS, Ralph D, Chang R, McClelland M (1992): Arbitrarily primed PCR fingerprinting of RNA. *Nucl Acids Res* 20:4965–4970.

Williams JG, Kubelik AR, Livak KJ, Rafalski JA, Tingey SV (1990): DNA polymorphisms amplified by arbitrary primers are useful as genetic markers. *Nucl Acids Res* 18:6531–6535.

Woese CR (1987): Bacterial evolution. *Microbiol Rev* 51:221–271.

26

Genetics, Plants, and the Polymerase Chain Reaction

Bruno W.S. Sobral and Rhonda J. Honeycutt

Introduction

The polymerase chain reaction (PCR) has given plant geneticists, ecologists, evolutionary, and population biologists a powerful new tool for studying their favorite organisms. In this chapter, we will use specific PCR to mean a standard, two-primer amplification that has as a target a specific genomic region, or gene, and therefore requires specific primers to be designed based on knowledge of DNA sequence. We differentiate this from PCR that uses primers of arbitrary sequence to specifically amplify a set of arbitrary loci in any genome, without the requirement for prior sequence knowledge. This is usually referred to as arbitrarily primed PCR or random amplified polymorphic DNA (RAPD) markers; herein, we will use the term arbitrarily primed PCR.

The first part of this chapter will discuss the applications that specific PCR has had in the plant sciences. The second part will discuss applications of arbitrarily primed PCR. In both sections we will attempt to exemplify existing applications and identify potential areas of improvement and research. We also note that although a fairly recent introduction, the

amount of published work using PCR in its various forms has exploded and therefore we will obviously be required to omit a variety of good work from various authors, because of space constraints. Our tendency will be to focus on areas of research that are similar to our own. Finally, we shall end by summarizing and commenting on future directions.

Specific PCR

Applications of specific PCR (Saiki et al., 1985) to plant sciences have been of two major types: (1) to amplify and directly sequence or otherwise characterize specific DNA sequences for phylogenetic or parentage analyses, strain, or cultivar identification, and (2) to identify pathogens or soil microbes in mixtures of complex biological samples with minimal purification.

Phylogenetic analysis of a variety of loci has become easier because of PCR. A general strategy that can be used is to apply a set of nested primers to amplify then sequence the region of interest directly, using *Taq* polymerase (Ruanto and Kidd, 1991). Usually the primers flank a hypervariable region and hy-

The Polymerase Chain Reaction
K.B. Mullis, F. Ferré, R.A. Gibbs, editors
© 1994 Birkhäuser Boston

bridize to conserved flanking regions such that comparisons can be made against a wide variation of genotypes. Introns are particularly good candidates to be amplified for this approach because they generally evolve more rapidly than exons (Wolfe et al., 1989) and tend to be short in plants (Hanley and Schuler, 1988; Hawkins, 1988). An internal pair of nested primers gives a secondary step of purification, during the sequencing reaction itself, and typically yield cleaner sequences. Longer sequences still require cloning before sequencing. Direct sequencing of templates, without prior amplification, has been shown on chloroplast DNA (To et al., 1992), suggesting that a variety of phylogenetic studies on chloroplast-encoded genes should be forthcoming.

The approach of amplifying and sequencing or digesting with restriction enzymes, not always using nested primers, has been successfully used on wild rice species (Barbier and Ishihama, 1990; Barbier et al., 1991) and sugarcane (Sobral et al., 1991; Al-Janabi and Sobral, unpublished data). Waugh et al. (1991) applied a similar strategy by using primers directed against the intergenic nucleotide sequences of the *U2snRNA* multigene family in potato, allowing identification of six new variant forms and determination of their genetic linkage. PCR amplification of the first intron in maize α-tubulin has been used to estimate the number of different genes present in this multigene family, which was found to be higher than revealed by RFLP approaches (Montoliu et al., 1989, 1992).

Another approach based on the high specificity of the PCR reaction is known as PCR amplification of specific alleles (PASA, Sarkar et al., 1990; Sommer et al., 1992), allele-specific PCR (ASPCR or ASP, Nichols et al., 1989; Okayama et al., 1989), and amplification-refractory mutation system (ARMS, Newton et al., 1989). No matter what the acronym, the idea is to selectively amplify specific alleles by using primers that match the nucleotide sequence of one allele, but mismatch the sequence of a dissimilar allele. This method has been applied to analysis of the *waxy* locus in maize inbred lines (Shattuck-Eidens et al., 1991). Development of allele-specific primers

requires substantial time and effort, but once the primers have been developed, large numbers of individuals can be quickly screened. Perhaps the PASA approach is a small glimpse of applications that will rely on specific PCR to identify superior genotypes in plant breeding. In this regard, a genetic linkage map of the mouse has been generated by Dietrich et al. (1992) that allows the specific PCR typing of intraspecific cross-progeny and contains 317 simple sequence length polymorphisms (SSLPs) based on primers that flank simple sequence repeats (SSRs, also known as microsatellites). SSRs are found in most eukaryotic genomes (Hamada et al., 1982), suggesting that a similar approach could be taken in plant species. The main advantage of specific PCR polymorphisms is that they can be codominant (as SSLPs are) and, in some cases, multiallelic, thereby having the potential for more information per marker.

Because of phylogenetic conservation of some regulatory motifs across kingdoms, specific PCR approaches can also be used to determine whether specific types of regulators exist in other kingdoms, thereby allowing knowledge to be generated almost in parallel. For example, Singh et al. (1991) designed a pair of primers that hybridized to a cDNA clone of *Drosophila melanogaster* known to encode a modifier that suppresses variegation. Those primers amplified a 111-bp DNA fragment that was used as a heterologous probe to screen and clone full length murine cDNAs containing conserved chromo box motifs, now suggested to be a major regulatory motif (Singh et al., 1991). Similar sequences were detected in plants (Singh et al., 1991). These results should allow isolation and genetic studies on putative modifier genes in plant species where chromosomal imprinting has been described, and propel PCR applications into the study of epigenetic factors. Phylogenetic conservation of important motifs has also allowed specific PCR to aid in systematic studies of plant retrotransposons, as well as permitting identification of elements in new species (Hirochika et al., 1992). Perhaps more surprising, data accumulated from a variety of retrotransposons lead to the suggestion that horizontal transmission between different species has played a role in the evolution of these elements (Flavell and Smith, 1992; Flavell et al., 1992). Homologues of the cdc2 protein kinase of *Saccharomyces cerevisiae,* which plays a central role in the regulation of cell division of eukaryotes (reviewed in Nurse, 1990), have been isolated from rice using PCR amplification of probes (Hashimoto et al., 1992). PCR-based approaches can be used to study phylogeny of plant viral genomes as well. Asymmetric PCR amplification, followed by DNA sequencing, has been used to study variability within the bipartite genome of bean golden mosaic geminivirus (Gilbertson et al., 1991).

Pathogen identification is a major concern to those working with exchange and conservation of plant germplasm. A large number of plant pathogens can be found in a variety of plant tissues and locations, intracellularly, extracellularly, and superficially. In best-case scenarios, detection of plant pathogens has usually been at the level of antigen–antibody interactions, using antibodies tagged with some type of fluorescent or other type of label. More often, detection has been based on inoculation of susceptible (tester) genotypes and subsequent detection of specific symptoms, which is slow and laborious. Sophisticated approaches such as antibody detection can require relatively pure materials on which binding assays are performed. Such assays also require monoclonal or cross-adsorbed antibodies resulting in high cost and technical difficulty for many laboratories and quarantine facilities. Furthermore, detection of phloem pathogens, such as mycoplasma-like organisms (MLOs), has been a persistent problem because they resist laboratory culture, as do obligate parasites, such as some rusts and smuts.

Specific PCR approaches to pathogen identification in complex biological samples has been achieved by targeting conserved regions of their genomes, such as rDNA (Wilson et al., 1989) and tDNA (McClelland et al., 1992; Welsh and McClelland, 1992) genes. In general terms, the strategy involves aligning se-

quences from the organism under study and comparing those with homologous sequences from plants. The goal is to find regions that are specific to the pathogen in question (usually at the genus level) and yet not found in plants or other potential sources of contaminating DNA (such as human DNA from the operator or a variety of saprophytes that colonize plant surfaces or tissues) that may be in the PCR mixture. Variability of the amplified region is a plus, in that it allows strains or species to be separated, which in turn is useful for studies in epidemiology and population genetics. Primers are designed to hybridize and allow amplification *when and only when* genomic DNA from the pathogen is encountered. DNA sequence analysis of the amplified region, either using direct cycle-sequencing with *Taq* polymerase (circumventing cloning; Ruanto and Kidd, 1991) or traditional cloning and sequencing, allows identification of polymorphic restriction enzyme sites. Once a restriction map is made, then restriction enzyme analysis of the amplified region can be used to generate mapped restriction site polymorphism (MRSP) data for phylogenetic analysis (Ralph et al., 1992). Using primers directed to 16 S rDNA, Ahrens and Seemuller (1992) have designed a set of primers to detect MLOs in complex mixtures of field grown woody species. This required as little as 170 pg of DNA from infected woody plants. A similar approach for detecting plant MLOs, targeting different regions, was reported by Deng and Hiruki (1991). These approaches have not only aided pathologists to quickly identify MLOs, they also are supplying information that is useful for systematic purposes. Viruses, both RNA and DNA, can also be quickly identified in complex mixtures using specific PCR or reverse-transcription PCR (RT-PCR). RT-PCR has been used to detect RNA viruses in apple, citrus, plum, peach, and grape (Yang et al., 1992; Hadidi and Yang, 1990).

Identification of plant symbionts has also been a difficult area of research that has benefited by application of specific PCR. For example, identification of symbiotic nitrogen-fixing bacteria, such as *Rhizobium* or *Frankia,* from large numbers of plant-derived nodules has been a difficult task that has also relied mainly on antibodies. Recent work in *Frankia* has made use of specific primers that amplify a portion of the *nifH* gene, one of the structural genes for nitrogenase (Simonet et al., 1990). Because nitrogenase is not present in plants, nodules can be crushed directly in microtiter plates and the crude extract subjected to PCR. Strain-specific primer pairs could be developed such that PCR could be used to study important questions of competition for nodule occupancy and survival in the soil. Similar work, using primers targeted against the T-DNA, has been reported for *Agrobacterium tumefaciens,* another difficult-to-detect plant pathogen (Dong et al., 1992).

Following the fate of genetically engineered, introduced bacteria in complex environments, such as the soil, has also been an elusive goal that has become closer to reality by application of PCR strategies. For example, Van Elsas et al. (1991) used specific primers against a non-selected segment of a patatin cDNA, introduced to *Pseudomonas florescens,* to follow the fate of the strain and its plasmid (RP4) in the soil. This represents a large improvement over previous methods of detection of engineered organisms, such as antibiotic resistance, particularly because transfer of genes to nonculturable soil microbes can also be determined. RP4 is a broad host range, self-transmissible plasmid, and its lateral transfer is expected, even though the range of transfer may not be known. It would be interesting to insert similar genes into chromosomal loci to determine the amount of lateral transfer of chromosomal markers within a species or genus, as little is known about the population structure in most bacteria.

Because PCR is a highly automatable technique (Sobral and Honeycutt, 1993; Nelson et al., 1992; Dietrich et al., 1992), and because scoring of specific PCR amplifications can be of the DNA present or DNA absent type, we expect it will soon be possible to quickly type very large numbers (thousands) of nodules or soil samples for the presence of specific strains

of symbiotic bacteria or engineered, introduced bacteria. This type of high output will require development of nonelectrophoretic detection of amplified products, such as ethidium bromide (EtBr) staining, followed by direct data acquisition via computer reading of stained microtiter plates. Quantitative methods for typing via PCR would be important for such applications.

Fungi are major pathogens of crops. Cereal rusts are among the major biotic pathogens limiting cereal production. Classification of many obligate parasites has been based on genetics of the interaction between host and pathogen, meaning that many of the pathogens have been classified primarily (if not only) by their avirulence gene content, as determined by inoculation on tester plants. Although such classifications have been useful for breeding, little is known about the genetic diversity, epidemiology, population structure, and phylogenetic relations of most phytopathologically important fungal species. This is mainly caused by the inability of avirulence gene phenotype to characterize the genetic variability within the pathogen, just as seen above for major epitopes against which antibodies are prepared. Approaches relying on protein differences have generally not yielded sufficiently discriminatory patterns to be a significant improvement, besides being costly, time-consuming, and technically difficult (Kim et al., 1992). Specific PCR of an intergenic region between the 26 S and 5 S rDNA genes of *Puccinia graminis* (cereal stem rust) allowed development of a rapid method for identification of races of *P. graminis* and opened the door for the study of genetic relations within this important species of fungal pathogen (Kim et al., 1992). Liu and Sinclair (1992) used a series of six primers directed against the nuclear rDNA loci of *Rhizoctonia solani,* a very important soil pathogen of many crop species, to investigate MSRPs within anastomosis group 2. Five groups were obtained, either through analysis of isozyme alleles or PCR amplification followed by restriction enzyme digestion, demonstrating that genetically independent groups can be established and monitored using this approach.

Arbitrarily Primed PCR

The discovery that the use of PCR with an arbitrarily selected primer to amplify a specific set of arbitrarily distributed loci in any genome laid the foundation for high output of genetic markers that can be used for a variety of purposes (Welsh and McClelland, 1990; Williams et al., 1990). The impact of arbitrarily primed PCR on plant genetics has been great. Less than one year after publication of the protocol (Welsh and McClelland, 1990; Williams et al., 1990), there were more than 30 posters describing work in progress at the biennial meeting of the International Society for Plant Molecular Biology (Tucson AZ, October 1991); one year after that, the Plant Genome I conference (San Diego CA, November 1992) was filled almost exclusively with posters that reported progress on genetic and systematic studies of various plant species and their pathogens, mostly using arbitrarily primed PCR.

Perhaps the main reason for the immediate success of arbitrarily primed PCR among plant scientists was the need for a high output marker acquisition method that was also low technology and immediately accessible to a variety of research or end-user environments. Because arbitrarily primed PCR is easily done with small amounts of DNA and without the requirement for clone banks or other forms of molecular characterization of the species in question, many crop species that were orphans because they lacked sufficient research investments became amenable to genetic studies. In addition, arbitrarily primed PCR does not normally require radioactively labeled nucleotides, a limiting factor in most non-first-world countries. Finally, because any PCR method is inherently automatable, there is the prospect for fulfilling the promise of routine use of molecular markers by breeding programs *in loco,* something that has not been possible with RFLP technology.

The main applications of arbitrarily primed PCR in plant sciences have been (1) genetic mapping, (2) systematic studies with various goals, and (3) identification of controlling regions for traits of agronomic importance, though this area is still embryonic. Development of plant genetic maps using arbitrarily primed PCR has progressed impressively. Some plant species that have been mapped by this approach include *Arabidopsis thaliana* (Reiter et al., 1992), *Saccharum spontaneum,* a wild relative of sugarcane (Al-Janabi et al., 1992, 1993), species of pines (Carlson et al., 1991; Chaparro et al., 1992), alfalfa (Echt et al., 1992), soybeans (Williams et al., 1990), peach (Chaparro et al., 1992b), citrus (Cai et al., 1992), flax (Gorman and Parojcic, 1992), grapes (Lodhi et al., 1992), tomato (Klein-Lankhorst et al., 1991), and *Eucalyptus* trees (Grattapagalia et al., 1992; Grattapagalia and Sederoff, 1992).

Arbitrarily primed PCR polymorphisms presumably are based on mismatches in primer binding sites or insertion/deletion events, and therefore usually result in the presence or absence of an amplified product from a single locus (Welsh et al., 1992; Williams et al., 1990). This means the arbitrarily primed PCR markers are usually dominant because individuals containing two copies of an allele (homozygous with presence phenotype) cannot be distinguished from individuals with one copy of the allele (heterozygous with presence phenotype). Mapping with dominant markers usually means that information is less per marker in F_2 populations because dominant markers in repulsion provide little information for genetic distance estimation, although selection of markers in coupling phase or from a single parent can increase the per-gamete informativeness of the marker to levels similar to those of codominant markers (Tingey et al., 1992).

Although the dominant nature of arbitrarily primed PCR polymorphisms can be seen as a hindrance to their informativeness for genetic mapping, there are specific situations in the plant sciences that cannot use but dominant markers. In particular, genetic mapping of polyploid species and tree species that have high amounts of DNA and long generation times have been brought out of a near standstill by application of arbitrarily primed PCR technology. In polyploids of unknown genomic constitution, Al-Janabi et al. (1992, 1993) adopted an approach based on selection of single-dose polymorphisms and subsequent determination of their linkages by analysis of what has been called the pseudo-testcross strategy by Grattapagalia and Sederoff (1992), which the latter authors have applied to mapping in tree species using existing crosses. This strategy has been proposed with various levels of detail by Bonierbale et al. (1988), Ritter et al. (1990), and Wu et al. (1992). In this approach, markers are selected from any cross between any two species from which an F_1 can be produced. Markers selected for mapping must fit two criteria: (1) they must be present in one parent and absent in the other and (2) they must segregate 1 : 1 in the progeny. In the case of polyploid species, no matter what the genomic constitution (allopolyploid vs. autopolyploid) or ploidy level of the material, single-dose markers correspond to simplex alleles (autopolyploids) or heterozygous alleles in diploid loci (allopolyploids) (Wu et al., 1992; Al-Janabi et al., 1992, 1993). In tree species, crosses normally cannot be made and analyzed on short notice, so the method allows mapping of existing crosses. In addition, in pine species there is haploid, maternally inherited tissue in the megagametophyte, meaning that all single-dose markers can be mapped and single-tree maps can be readily made (Chaparro et al., 1992a). Not only are these maps readily made, they typically require approximately four to six person-months per 200 mapped markers (Reiter et al., 1992; Al-Janabi et al., 1993), which is significantly less than required to make similar RFLP maps. Of course, single-dose RFLP maps could be made in polyploid species as well, but single-copy RFLP probes tend to hybridize to many fragments in polyploids and the resulting complex fingerprint may cause difficulties in interpreting alternate alleles. In addition, in some tree species, DNA content is so high that single-copy Southern hybridization may be impractical, or at least very lengthy exposures are required. Therefore, one large impact of arbitrarily primed PCR has been to increase the species amenable to mapping activities. Furthermore, automation of PCR has progressed to the point that data generation for a 200 marker map can be done in 1 or 2 weeks by a robotic liquid handling station (Sobral and Honeycutt, 1993; Sobral et al., 1993; Crawford et al., 1992). Robotic liquid handling stations can be programmed to handle 384-well (24 × 16) microtiter plates, and should be able to handle even larger numbers of wells/plate. So, arbitrarily primed PCR also has increased the speed of mapmaking.

Fingerprinting of plant genomes using arbitrarily primed PCR polymorphisms has been done for a variety of systematic and population genetic studies. Although discussions abound as to the appropriate manner to analyze the data, this is due less to methodological constraints than to different perceptions of how systematics, population genetics, and phylogenetic inference are related and what are the appropriate ways to analyze data (for a brief review, see Moritz and Hillis, 1991). Once again, adjustments need to be made because of the dominant nature of the polymorphisms detected by arbitrarily primed PCR, which lowers their polymorphism information content (PIC, Botstein et al., 1980) but does not invalidate phylogenetic analysis of appropriate biological situations. In particular, phylogenetic approaches can be taken if the genome in question fits the assumptions made by all methods of inference, that is, that organisms evolve mainly by drift and mutation under a bifurcating tree assumption (Swofford and Olsen, 1991). Most plant nuclear genomes are at least diploid and sexual, and presumably have reticulating trees that trace their evolutionary history, rather than bifurcating trees (Swofford and Olsen, 1991), so such analyses invalidate assumptions no matter what type of method is used to generate the data. If the biology of your organism fits the assumptions of the algorithms, then you can use PAUP (Swofford, 1991), with appropriate weighting of character state transformations (Albert et al., 1992). Chloroplast, mitochondria, and some bacterial and fungal pathogens are generally believed to fit assumptions of bifurcating trees. If modest reticulation is expected, cladistic parsimony can be applied and resulting hypotheses can be tested within a framework of maximum likelihood (Felsenstein, 1973; Lathrop, 1982; Thompson, 1973, 1975).

Even when phylogenetic analyses should not be conducted, fingerprinting data can be used for systematic or classification purposes (Honeycutt et al., 1992), parentage determination (Welsh et al., 1991), estimation of gene flow (Arnold et al., 1991), and detection of genetic variation in natural populations (Chalmers et al., 1992; Chapco et al., 1992). These areas of research have not progressed greatly with development of molecular markers because thus far they have been either too costly and laborious to be used on large numbers of individuals (as is the case for RFLPs) or too limited in their genomic distribution and the level of diversity they can reveal (as is the case for isozymes). Arbitrarily primed PCR has largely resolved these problems and we expect that large amounts of fingerprinting data from various plant species will be analyzed in the near future. These data will certainly have an impact on management, conservation, and improvement of plant genetic resources worldwide.

Analysis of arbitrarily primed PCR fingerprints for systematic or classification purposes can be done using similarity coefficients, as the general objective is to group similar germplasm. Choices of coefficients and their implications on subsequent analyses should be carefully considered (Jackson et al., 1989; Swofford and Olsen, 1991; Weir, 1991), as should earlier choices regarding sampling (Baverstock and Moritz, 1991). For population studies, gene flow and mating system are known to be important determinants of genetic structure of plant populations and require the ability to detect heterozygotes (Clegg, 1980), which means that uses of arbitrarily primed PCR are limited. However, Chalmers et al. (1992) and Baird et al. (1992) noted that arbitrarily primed PCR polymorphisms may be used to detect heterozygous individuals when a single primer generates at least one complementary polymorphism from each parent. In most studies of this type, each primer detects a variety of polymorphisms so this should not be difficult to achieve. Population-specific or species-specific markers can be generated in this way (Crowhurst et al., 1991; Hadrys et al., 1992; Sellstedt et al., 1992; Smith et al.,

1992) and used to further characterize differences among populations or species, especially when genetic maps are available for the species being studied. For genealogical studies, polymorphisms can be used to infer parentage (Welsh et al., 1991; Honeycutt et al., 1992). Preliminary data for our work with elite maize inbred lines, using 15 arbitrarily selected primers on 22 genotypes, showed a high correlation between genetic distances measured by 99 mapped RFLP probes (Smith et al., 1991) and those measured by the 15 primers (119 characters) (Fig. 26.1). The RFLP probes have a distribution that allows coverage of most of the maize genome. In addition, good correlation was shown for pedigree coefficients and distances as measured by arbitrarily primed PCR (Fig. 26.2), although the level of correlation was smaller than observed with the 99 mapped RFLP probes on a larger set of inbreds (Smith et al., 1991). In maize inbreds, the incapacity to detect heterozygotes is not important, so the dominant nature of the polymorphisms is not relevant. In parentage analysis work, we have not observed nonparental bands (Reidy et al., 1992). However, we note that we use a modified protocol of arbitrarily primed PCR (Sobral and Honeycutt, 1993), which produces a larger number of amplified products per primer, when compared to standard conditions (Welsh and McClelland, 1990; Williams et al., 1990). Perhaps we have not experienced this problem because there may be a smaller context effect on the competition for primer binding when more amplified products are produced. For plant breeders, it is important to have information on genetic diversity because such data can be used to inform them of the degree of relatedness of the materials they work with, and therefore select which new crosses should be made and which materials need to be preserved in germplasm collections. This is clearly another important application that arbitrarily primed PCR has filled, especially in crops that have been classified exclusively by morphological or geographical attributes.

The other criticism frequently mentioned when arbitrarily primed PCR polymorphisms

Comparison of arbitrarily primed PCR and RFLP distances in 22 maize inbred lines

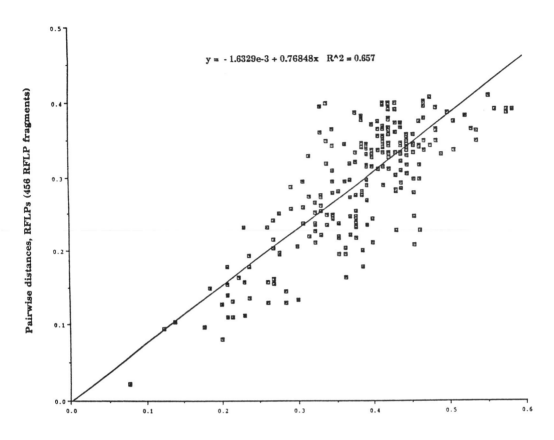

$$y = -1.6329\text{e-}3 + 0.76848x \quad R^2 = 0.657$$

Pairwise distance, arbitrarily primed PCR (130 characters)

FIGURE 26.1. Regression analysis of RFLP genetic distance × arbitrarily primed PCR genetic distance on 22 maize inbred lines (from Honeycutt et al., 1992). Data were scored as presence or absence of a DNA fragment of specified size. RFLP data are based on hybridization with 99 mapped probes that are known to be distributed throughout the maize genome (these data kindly furnished by Stephen Smith, Pioneer Hi-Bred International, Iowa). Arbitrarily primed PCR data were generated using 15 arbitrarily selected 10-mers (Operon Technologies). Genetic distances were calculated using PAUP 3.0s (Swofford, 1991). Pairwise genetic distances were then plotted for all possible combinations of the 22 inbred lines and linear regression was performed with the resulting regression coefficients shown above the line.

are used in a variety of studies is the potential comigration of amplification products that are not from the same locus. On statistical grounds this should occur rarely, but gel resolution systems and the relatedness of the genomes in question also play a large role in how often this occurs. Our work in sugarcane and its relatives has suggested that higher resolution, polyacrylamide sequencing gels are superior to agarose gels for interspecific comparisons (Fig. 26.3), whereas longer (20 cm usable running length) 2% agarose gels provided sufficient resolution for the aforementioned analysis of maize inbred lines (Fig. 26.4). In any event, dubious polymorphisms can always be excised, reamplified in the presence of a labeled nucleotide, and used in a Southern blot to show whether homology exists at the DNA sequence level (Peinado et al., 1992).

Comparison of arbitrarily primed PCR and pedigree distances in 22 maize inbred lines

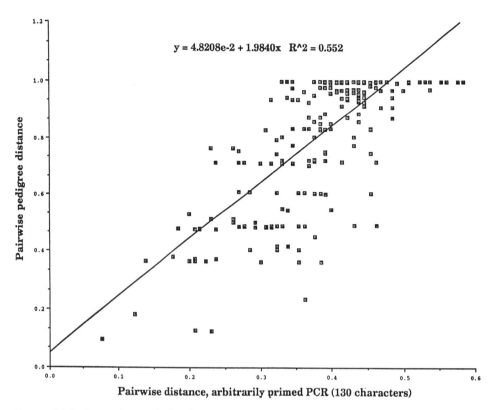

FIGURE 26.2. Regression analysis of genetic distance calculated by arbitrarily primed PCR × pedigree coefficient for 22 maize inbred lines. Pedigree coefficients were determined by Smith et al. (1991).

The third major area of application of arbitrarily primed PCR has been the targeting of markers to specific genetic regions. This area of research has been substantially forwarded by Michelmore et al. (1991), who developed an elegant method of creating "*in vitro* near-isogenic lines (NILs)" by bulking segregants from a cross between parents that contrasted for a specific trait. The process is called bulked segregant analysis (BSA) and the idea is to select from an F_2 population individuals that represent the phenotypic extremes for the trait in question and separately pool their genomic DNAs in equimolar amounts. The assumption is that the ends of the phenotyic distribution represent individuals that have opposing homozygote alleles ("good" vs. "bad") for

the trait in question. The number of individuals to be bulked can be as few as three or four and there is no need to construct near-isogenic lines, a procedure that is at best time-consuming, and virtually impossible for some species. Of course, use of traditional NILs and arbitrarily primed PCR can be done when such genotypes exist (Paran et al., 1991; Martin et al., 1991). BSA also can be used to target multiple loci of highly heritable quantitative traits that are controlled by few loci of large phenotypic effect (Michelmore et al., 1992). Not only does BSA allow for very quick screening and enrichment for markers linked to specific traits, but the procedure also generates a genetic map for the region(s) under study (Michelmore et al., 1991). This regional map can

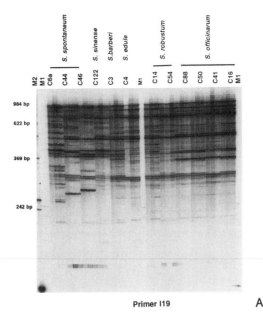

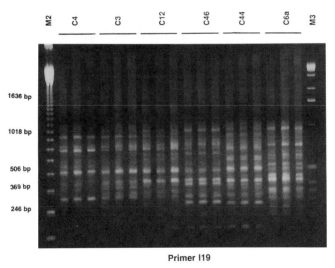

FIGURE 26.3. Comparison of gel resolution systems in study of sugarcane and its relatives. Arbitrarily primed PCR products were generated from *Saccharum* species according to Sobral and Honeycutt (1993), using AmpliTaq Stoffel fragment (Perkin-Elmer), and resolved on a 4% polyacrylamide denaturing sequencing gel (**A**) run at 50 mA for 4 hr or on a 2% agarose gel (**B**) run for 1100 V-hr. Amplifications were done in 30-μl reaction volumes in the presence of [α-^{32}P]dCTP (Welsh and McClelland, 1990). For polyacrylamide gels, 4 μl of sample was taken and mixed with 14 μl of denaturing dye, the mixture was incubated at 85°C for 5 min, put im-

mediately on ice, after which 4 μl was loaded onto the gel. For agarose gels, 20 μl of the reaction was loaded directly. Saccharum DNAs were used at three template concentrations (0.3, 1, and 1.7 ng/μl, respectively), to detect potential "sporadic" fragments that are template-concentration-dependent. Molecular weight markers were M1, pBR322 digested with *Msp*I; M2, BRL 123 bp ladder; M3, BRL 1 kb ladder. Arrows indicate the position of a fragment that potentially would be misscored on the agarose gel, especially if it were shorter than 20 cm.

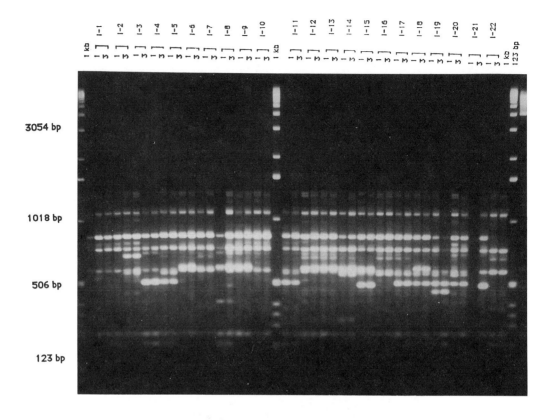

Primer B11

FIGURE 26.4. Twenty-centimeter-long 2% agarose gel (Stratagene Cloning Systems test box) used to resolve arbitrarily primed PCR products in maize inbred line study (Honeycutt et al., 1992). Electrophoresis was done at 5 V/cm for a total of 1100 V-hr. Data shown are for one 10-mer primer (Operon Technologies). Maize DNAs were analyzed using two template concentrations (1 and 3 ng/μl, loaded sequentially for each genotype) to allow detection of rare, "sporadic," template-concentration-dependent faint products, which were not scored. Amplifica-tions were done in 30-μl reaction volumes in a PTC-100 thermocycler (MJ Research) using a 96-well microtiter plate heating block. Cycling parameters were 94°C for 3 min, followed by 30 cycles of 94°C for 1 min, 35°C for 1 min, increase to 72°C at 1°C for 2 sec, 72°C for 2 min; cycling was completed by a single 72°C for 7 min, and reaction products were maintained at 12°C until loading. AmpliTaq Stoffel fragment (Perkin-Elmer) was used as the thermo-stable polymerase (Sobral and Honeycutt, 1993).

be refined by selection of appropriate progeny for further bulking and analysis as well as individual progeny testing. In addition, these regional maps can be integrated into existing genetic maps for the species being studied by using bulking to make specific, regional maps, and then cross-mapping those regions in the standard mapping population, as has been done in lettuce for disease resistance loci (Mi-chelmore et al., 1992). Cross-mapping the region of interest onto the general map is particularly important because the final product is a single, comprehensive genetic linkage map for any given species. Furthermore, regions on existing linkage maps that are poorly populated with markers can be mapped using bulks of informative individuals from existing mapping populations (Giovannoni et al., 1991).

Because of the elegant simplicity and wide applicability of BSA, we expect it to be used on a variety of important crop species.

Summary and Future Directions

In summary, there is little doubt that application of PCR in its various forms has caused a large increase in genetic knowledge of plant species and of the many species of other organisms important to plants. There is also little doubt that further advances in methodology, particularly those that relate to increased speed and increased automation, will allow further leaps in genetic knowledge of plant genomes and their evolution. Of course, the ultimate DNA marker is DNA sequence information, and when it becomes sufficiently cheap and expedient to obtain and analyze large amounts of DNA sequence data, we would expect that other methods might be superseded, at least for well-funded species.

In the meantime, it seems that with small increments in data acquisition technologies, such as nonelectrophoretic means of visualizing amplification results, and computer-assisted scoring of gel images, it may be possible to make genetic maps, screen thousands of genetic loci, or all mRNAs in a cell type (Welsh et al., 1992; Liang and Pardee, 1992) in a matter of days, rather than years. We expect this to directly benefit a large number of orphan crops that have not received much attention by funding agencies. It will also allow ecological and population genetics to address novel questions because of high marker output and the capacity to analyze large numbers of individuals through automation. Further improvements to arbitrarily primed PCR markers, such as their conversion to sequence characterized amplified regions (SCARs; Michelmore et al., 1992), which are codominant and based on specific PCR reactions, as well as novel strategies that surely will be devised, may well realize the dream of applied marker-based breeding and construction of superior genotypes, and large studies in population genetics and germplasm conservation. In addition, we expect marker-assisted introgression, marker-

aided selection, and, eventually, map-based gene cloning to progress more quickly and be attempted on a larger number of plant species because of the lowered cost per data point and lower technological requirements of arbitrarily primed PCR in relation to other molecular markers. This will be especially true when the cost of thermostable polymerases reaches the levels of cloned restriction enzymes, as the major cost component of PCR-based analyses is the polymerase.

Finally, diagnostic techniques for biotrophic plant disease agents, as well as markers for the study of pathogens, should allow large gains in knowledge to be achieved by plant pathologists and entomologists. In particular, the ability to identify and characterize pathogens in complex biological mixtures, and without the need for a capacity to culture them in the laboratory, has allowed previously impossible studies to be idealized and executed. Our general lack of understanding of fungal and bacterial pathogens most likely makes practical, energy-efficient control of these pathogens difficult if not impossible. As application of the various PCR-based strategies reaches these organisms, we may learn enough about their lives to control them more rationally in the future. Perhaps the most interesting results of the application of PCR to the plant sciences are already in the making and will soon be available from the ongoing population studies that will eventually tell us more about plants and their environment. For those, we need only to wait for their completion.

References

Ahrens U, Seemuller E (1992): Detection of DNA of plant pathogenic mycoplasmalike organisms by a polymerase chain reaction that amplifies a sequence of the 16S rRNA genes. *Phytopathology* 82:828–832.

Albert VA, Mischler BD, Chase MW (1992): Character-state weighting for restriction site data in phylogenetic reconstruction, with an example from chloroplast DNA. In *Molecular Systematics of Plants*. Soltis PS, Soltis DE, Doyle JJ, eds. New York: Chapman and Hall, pp. 369–403.

Al-Janabi SM, Honeycutt RJ, McClelland M, Sobral BWS (1992): A genetic linkage map of

Saccharum spontaneum 'SES 208'. Plant Genome I Abstracts:31, San Diego, CA.

Al-Janabi SM, Honeycutt RJ, McClelland M, Sobral BWS (1993): A genetic linkage map of *Saccharum spontaneum* (L.) 'SES 208'. *Genetics* 134:1249-1260.

Arnold ML, Buckner CM, Robinson JJ (1991): Pollen-mediated introgression and hybrid speciation in Louisiana irises. *Proc Natl Acad Sci USA* 88: 1398-1402.

Baird E, Cooper-Bland S, Waugh R, DeMaine M, Powell W (1992): Molecular characterisation of inter- and intra-specific somatic hybrids of potato using randomly amplified polymorphic DNA (RAPD) markers. *Mol Gen Genet* 233:469-475.

Barbier P, Ishihama A (1990): Variation in nucleotide sequence of a prolamine gene family in wild rice. *Plant Mol Biol* 15:191-195.

Barbier P, Morishima H, Ishihama A (1991): Phylogenetic relationships of annual and perennial wild rice: probing by direct DNA sequencing. *Theor Appl Genet* 81:693-702.

Baverstock PR, Moritz C (1991): Sampling design. In *Molecular Systematics*. Hillis DM, Moritz C, eds. Sunderland, MA: Sinauer Associates, pp. 13-24.

Bonierbale MW, Plaisted RL, Tanksley SD (1988): RFLP maps based on a common set of clones reveal modes of chromosomal evolution in potato and tomato. *Genetics* 120:1095-1103.

Botstein D, White RL, Skolnick M, Davis RW (1980): Construction of a genetic linkage map in man using restriction fragment length polymorphisms. *Am J Hum Genet* 32:314-331.

Cai Q, Guy C, Moore GA (1992): Genetic mapping of random amplified polymorphic DNA (RAPD) markers in *Citrus*. Plant Genome I Abstracts:20, San Diego, CA.

Carlson JE, Tulsieram LK, Glaubitz JC, Luk V, Kauffeldt C, Rutledge R (1991): Segregation of random amplified polymorphic DNA markers in F1 progeny of conifers. *Theor Appl Genet* 83: 194-200.

Chalmers KJ, Waugh R, Sprent JI, Simons AJ, Powell W (1992): Detection of genetic variation between and within populations of *Gliricidia sepium* and *G. maculata* using RAPD markers. *Heredity* 69:465-472.

Chaparro J, Wilcox P, Grattapaglia D, O'Malley D, McCord S, Sederoff R, McIntyre L, Whetten R (1992a): Genetic mapping of pine using RAPD markers: construction of a 191-marker map and development of half-sib genetic analysis. Advances in Gene Technology: Feeding the world in

the 21st century. Miami Winter Symposium, Miami, FL.

Chaparro J, Werner D, O'Malley D, Sederoff R (1992b): Targeted mapping and linkage analysis in peach. Plant Genome I Abstracts:21, San Diego, CA.

Chapco W, Ashton NW, Martel RKB, Antonishyn N (1992): A feasibility study of the use of random amplified polymorphic DNA in the population genetics and systematics of grasshoppers. *Genome* 35:569-574.

Clegg MT (1980): Measuring plant mating systems. *Bioscience* 30:814-818.

Crawford ML, Nance WL, Nelson CD, Doudrick RL (1992): An automated approach to genetic mapping with randomly amplified polymorphic DNA markers. Plant Genome I Abstracts:39, San Diego, CA.

Crowhurst RN, Hawthorne BT, Rikkerink EHA, Templeton MD (1991): Differentiation of *Fusarium solani* f. sp. *cucurbitae* races 1 and 2 by random amplification of polymorphic DNA. *Curr Genet* 20:391-396.

Deitrich W, Katz H, Lincoln SE, Shin H-S, Friedman J, Dracopoli NC, Lander ES (1992): A genetic map of the mouse suitable for typing intraspecific crosses. *Genetics* 131:423-447.

Deng S, Hiruki C (1991): Genetic relatedness between two nonculturable mycoplasmalike organisms revealed by nucleic acid hybridization and polymerase chain reaction. *Phytopathology* 81: 1475-1479.

Dong LC, Sun CW, Thies KL, Luthe DS, Graves CH (1992): Use of polymerase chain reaction to detect pathogenic strains of *Agrobacterium*. *Phytopathology* 82:434-439.

Echt CS, Erdahl LA, McCoy TJ (1992): Genetic segregation of random amplified polymorphic DNA in diploid cultivated alfalfa. *Genome* 35: 84-87.

Felsenstein J (1973): Maximum-likelihood estimation of evolutionary trees from continuous characters. *Am J Hum Genet* 25:471-492.

Flavell AJ, Smith DB (1992): A *Ty1-copia* group retrotransposon sequence in a vertebrate. *Mol Gen Genet* 233:322-326.

Flavell AJ, Dunbar E, Anderson R, Pearce SR, Hartley R, Kumar A (1992): *Ty1-copia* group retrotransposons are ubiquitous and heterogeneous in higher plants. *Nucl Acids Res* 20:3639-3644.

Gilbertson RL, Rojas MR, Russell DR, Maxwell DP (1991): Use of the asymmetric polymerase chain reaction and DNA sequencing to determine genetic variability of bean golden mosaic geminivirus in the Dominican Republic. *J Gen Virol* 72:2843-2848.

Giovannoni JJ, Wing RA, Ganal MW, Tanksley SD (1991): Isolation of molecular markers from specific chromosomal intervals using DNA pools from existing mapping populations. *Nucl Acids Res* 19:6553-6558.

Gorman M, Parojcic M (1992): Genome mapping in flax (*Linum usitatissimum*). Plant Genome I Abstracts:27, San Diego, CA.

Grattapagalia D, Sederoff R (1992): Pseudo-testcross mapping strategy in forest trees: single tree rapid maps of *Eucalyptus grandis* and *E. urophylla*. Plant Genome I Abstracts:27, San Diego, CA.

Grattapaglia D, Chaparro J, Wilcox P, McCord S, Werner D, Amerson H, McKeand S, Bridgewater F, Whetten R, O'Malley D, Sederoff R (1992): Mapping in woody plants with RAPD markers: applications to breeding in forestry and horticulture. In *Proceedings of the Symposium on Applications of RAPD Technology to Plant Breeding.* Crop Science Society of America, American Society of Horticultural Science, American Genetic Association, pp. 37-40.

Hadidi A, Yang X (1990): Detection of pome fruit viroids by enzymatic cDNA amplification. *J Virol Methods* 30:261-270.

Hadrys H, Balick M, Schierwater B (1992): Applications of random amplified polymorphic DNA (RAPD) in molecular ecology. *Mol Ecol* 1:55-63.

Hamada H, Petrino MG, Takunga T (1982): A novel repeated element with z-DNA-forming potential is widely found in evolutionary diverse eukaryotic genomes. *Proc Natl Acad Sci USA* 79:6465-6469.

Hanley BA, Schuler MA (1988): Plant intro sequences: evidence for distinct groups of introns. *Nucl Acids Res* 16:7159-7175.

Hashimoto J, Hirabayashi T, Hayano Y, Hata S, Ohashi Y, Suzuka I, Utsugi T, Toh-E A, Kikuchi Y (1992): Isolation and characterization of cDNA clones encoding *cdc2* homologues from *Oryza sativa*: A functional homologue and cognate variants. *Mol Gen Genet* 233:10-16.

Hawkins JD (1988): A survey on intron and exon length. *Nucl Acids Res* 16:9893-9908.

Hirochika H, Fukuchi A, Kikuchi F (1992): Retrotransposon families in rice. *Mol Gen Genet* 233:209-216.

Honeycutt RJ, Smith S, Sobral BWS (1992): Reconstructing histories of maize inbreds using molecular characters. Plant Genome I Abstracts:29, San Diego, CA.

Jackson DA, Somers KM, Harvey HH (1989): Similarity coefficients: Measures of co-occurrence, and association or simply measures of occurrence? *Am Nat* 133:436-453.

Kim WK, Zeruch T, Klassen GR (1992): A region of heterogeneity adjacent to the 5S ribosomal RNA gene of cereal rusts. *Curr Genet* 22:101-105.

Klein-Lankhorst RM, Vermut A, Weide R, Liharska T, Zabel P (1991): Isolation of molecular markers for tomato (*L. esculentum*) using random amplified polymorphic DNA (RAPD). *Theor Appl Genet* 83:108-114.

Lathrop GM (1982): Evolutionary trees and admixture: Phylogenetic inference when some populations are hybridized. *Ann Hum Genet* 46:245-255.

Liang P, Pardee AB (1992): Differential display of eukaryotic messenger RNA by means of the polymerase chain reaction. *Science* 257:967-971.

Liu ZL, Sinclair JB (1992): Genetic diversity of *Rhizoctonia solani* anastomosis group 2. *Phytopathology* 82:778-787.

Lodhi MA, Reisch BI, Weeden NF (1992): Molecular genetic mapping and genome size. Plant Genome I Abstracts:37, San Diego, CA.

Martin GB, Williams JGK, Tanskley SD (1991): Rapid identification of markers linked to a *Pseudomonas* resistance gene in tomato by using random primers and near-isogenic lines. *Proc Natl Acad Sci USA* 88:2336-2340.

McClelland M, Petersen C, Welsh J (1992): Length polymorphisms in tRNA intergenic spacers detected by using the polymerase chain reaction can distinguish *Streptococcal* strains and species. *J Clin Microbiol* 30:1499-1504.

Michelmore RW, Paran I, Kesseli RV (1991): Identification of markers linked to disease resistance genes by bulked segregant analysis: A rapid method to detect markers in specific genomic regions using segregating populations. *Proc Natl Acad Sci USA* 88:9828-9832.

Michelmore RW, Kesseli RV, Francis DM, Paran I, Fortin MG, Yang C-H (1992): Strategies for cloning plant disease resistance genes. *Molecular Plant Pathology 2. A Practical Approach.* Oxford: Oxford University Press.

Montoliu L, Rigau J, Puigdomenech P (1989): A tandom of α-tubulin genes preferentially expressed in radicular tissues of *Z. mays*. *Plant Mol Biol* 14:1-15.

Montoliu L, Rigau J, Puigdomenech P (1992):
Analysis by PCR of the number of homologous
genomic sequences to α-tubulin in maize. *Plant
Sci* 84:179–185.

Moritz C, Hillis DM (1991): Molecular systematics: context and controversies, In *Molecular
Systematics*. Hillis DM, Moritz C, eds. Sunderland, MA: Sinauer Associates, pp. 1–10.

Nelson LS, Johnson GN, Crawford ML, Nance
WL, Nelson CD, Doudrick RL (1992): An automated approach to genetic mapping with randomly amplified polymorphic DNA markers.
Plant Genome I Abstracts:39, San Diego, CA.

Newton CR, Graham A, Heptinstall IE, Powell SJ,
Summers C, Kalsheker N (1989): Analysis of any
point mutation in DNA. The amplification refractory mutation system (ARMS). *Nucl Acids Res*
17:2503–2515.

Nichols WC, Liepnicks JJ, McKusick VA, Benson
MD (1989): Direct sequencing of the gene for
Maryland/German familial amyloidotic plyneur-
opathy type II and genotyping by allele-specific
enzymatic amplification. *Genomics* 5:535–540.

Nurse P (1990): Universal control mechanism regu-
lating the onset of M-phase. *Nature (London)*
344:503–508.

Okayama H, Curiel DT, Brantly ML, Holmes MD,
Crystal RG (1989): Rapid nonradioactive detection of mutations in the human genome by allele-
specific amplification. *J Lab Clin Med* 114:105–
113.

Paran I, Kesseli R, Michelmore R (1991): Identification of restriction fragment length polymorphism and random amplified polymorphic DNA
markers linked to downy mildew resistance in
lettuce, using near-isogenic lines. *Genome* 34:
1021–1027.

Peinado MA, Malkhosyan S, Velasquez A, Perucho
M (1992): Isolation and characterization of allelic losses and gains in colorectal tumors by arbitrarily primed polymerase chain reaction. *Proc
Natl Acad Sci USA* 89:10065–10069.

Ralph D, McClelland M, Welsh J, Baranton G, Pre-
lot P (1992): Pathogenic *Leptospira* categorized
by arbitrarily primed PCR and by mapped restriction polymorphisms in PCR-amplified rDNA.
J Bacteriol 175:973–981.

Reidy MF, Hamilton III J, Aquadro CF (1992): Excess of non-parental bands in offspring from
known primate pedigrees assayed using RAPD
PCR. *Nucl Acids Res* 20:918.

Reiter RS, Williams JGK, Feldmann KA, Rafalski
JA, Tingey SV, Scolnik PA (1992): Global and
local genome mapping in *Arabidopsis thaliana* by

using recombinant inbred lines and random amplified polymorphic DNAs. *Proc Natl Acad Sci
USA* 89:1477–1481.

Ritter E, Gebhardt C, Salamini F (1990): Estimation of recombination frequencies and construction of RFLP linkage maps in plants from crosses
between heterozygous parents. *Genetics* 125:
645–654.

Ruanto G, Kidd KK (1991): Coupled amplification
and sequencing of genomic DNA. *Proc Natl Acad
Sci USA* 88:2815–2819.

Saiki RK, Scharf S, Faloona F, Mullis KB, Horn
GT, Erlich HA, Arnheim N (1985): Enzymatic
amplification of β-globin genomic sequences and
restriction site analysis for diagnosis of sickle cell
anemia. *Science* 230:1350–1354.

Sarkar G, Cassady J, Bottema CDK, Sommer SS
(1990): Characterization of polymerase chain reaction amplification of specific alleles. *Anal Biochem* 186:64–68.

Sarkar G, Yoon H-S, Sommer SS (1992): Dideoxy
fingerprinting (ddF): a rapid and efficient screen
for the presence of mutations. *Genomics* 13:441–
443.

Sellstedt A, Wullings B, Nystrom U, Gustafsson P
(1992): Identification of *Casuarina-Frankia*
strains by use of polymerase chain reaction
(PCR) with arbitrary primers. *FEMS Microbiol
Lett* 93:1–6.

Shattuck-Eidens DM, Bell RN, Mitchell JT,
McWhorter VC (1991): Rapid detection of maize
DNA sequence variation. *GATA* 8:240–245.

Simonet P, Normand P, Moiroud A, Bardin R
(1990): Identification of *Frankia* strains in nodules by hybridization of polymerase chain reaction products with strain-specific oligonucleotide
probes. *Arch Microbiol* 153:235–240.

Singh PB, Miller JR, Pearch J, Kothary R, Burton
RD, Paro R, James TC, Gaunt SJ (1991): A sequence motif found in a *Drosophila* heterochro-
matin protein is conserved in animals and plants.
Nucl Acid Res 19:789–794.

Smith JSC, Smith OS, Bowen SL, Tenborg RA,
Wall SJ (1991): The description and assessment
of distances between inbred lines of maize. III. A
revised scheme for testing of distinctiveness
between inbred lines utilizing DNA RFLPs.
Maydica 36:213–226.

Smith ML, Bruhn JN, Anderson JB (1992): The
fungus *Armillaria bulbosa* is among the largest
and oldest living organisms. *Nature (London)*
356:428–431.

Sobral BWS, Honeycutt RJ (1993): High output genetic mapping in polyploids using PCR-generated markers. *Theor Appl Genet* 86:105–112.

Sobral BWS, Honeycutt RJ, Irvine JI, McClelland M (1991): Evolution of sugarcane. III International Congress of the ISPMB:1783, Tucson, Arizona, USA.

Sobral BWS, Al-Janabi SM, McClelland M, Honeycutt RJ (1993): Novel approaches for molecular mapping and fingerprinting. In *Proceedings of the First International Scientific Meeting of the Cassava Biotechnology Network*. Roca WM, Thro AM, eds. Cali, Colombia: CIAT Press, pp. 31–46.

Sommer SS, Groszbach AR, Bottema CDK (1992): PCR amplification of specific alleles (PASA) is a general method for rapidly detecting known single-base changes. *BioTechniques* 12:82–87.

Swofford DL (1991): *PAUP: Phylogenetic Analysis Under Parsimony,* version 3.0s. Computer program distributed by the Illinois Natural History Survey, Champaign, IL.

Swofford DL, Olsen GJ (1991): Phylogeny reconstruction. In *Molecular Systematics*. Hillis DM, Moritz C, eds. Sunderland, MA: Sinauer Associates, pp. 411–510.

Thompson EA (1973): The Icelandic admixture problem. *Ann Hum Genet* 37:69–80.

Thompson EA (1975): *Human Evolutionary Trees*. Cambridge: Cambridge University Press.

Tingey SV, Rafalski JA, Williams JGK (1992): Genetic analysis with RAPD markers. *Applications of RAPD Technology to Plant Breeding*, pp. 3–8.

To K-Y, Li C-Y, Chang Y-S, Liu S-T (1992): Direct sequencing of tobacco chloroplast genome by the polymerase chain reaction. *Plant Mol Biol* 19:1073–1077.

Van Elsas JD, Van Overbeek LS, Fouchier R (1991): A specific marker, *pat*, for studying the fate of introduced bacteria and their DNA in soil using a combination of detection techniques. *Plant Soil* 138:49–60.

Waugh R, Clark G, Brown JWS (1991): Sequence variation and linkage of potato U2snRNA-encoding genes established by PCR. *Gene* 107:197–204.

Weir B (1991): Intraspecific differentiation. In *Molecular Systematics*. Hillis DM, Moritz C, eds. Sunderland, MA: Sinauer Associates, pp. 373–405.

Welsh J, McClelland M (1990): Fingerprinting genomes using PCR with arbitrary primers. *Nucl Acids Res* 18:7213–7218.

Welsh J, McClelland M (1992): PCR-amplified length polymorphisms in tRNA intergenic spacers for categorizing staphylococci. *Mol Microbiol* 6:1673–1680.

Welsh J, Honeycutt RJ, McClelland M, Sobral BWS (1991): Parentage determination in maize hybrids using the arbitrarily primed polymerase chain reaction (AP-PCR). *Theor Appl Genet* 82:473–476.

Welsh J, Chada K, Dalal SS, Cheng R, Ralph D, McClelland M (1992): Arbitrarily primed PCR fingerprinting of RNA. *Nucl Acids Res* 20:4965–4970.

Williams JGK, Kubelik AR, Livak KG, Rafalski JA, Tingey SV (1990): DNA polymorphisms amplified by arbitrary primers are useful as genetic markers. *Nucl Acids Res* 18:6531–6535.

Wilson KH, Blitchington R, Shah P, McDonald G, Gilmore RD, Mallavia LP (1989): Probe directed at a segment of *Rickettsia reckettsii* rRNA amplified with polymerase chain reaction. *J Clin Microbiol* 27:2692–2696.

Wolfe KH, Sharp PM, Li W-H (1989): Rates of synonomous substitution in plant nuclear genes. *J Mol Evol* 29:208–211.

Wu KK, Burnquist W, Sorrells ME, Tew TL, Moore PH, Tanskley SD (1992): The detection and estimation of linkage in polyploids using single-dose restriction fragments. *Theor Appl Genet* 83:294–300.

Yang X, Hadidi A, Garnsey SM (1992): Enzymatic cDNA amplification of citrus exocortis and cachexia viroids from infected citrus hosts. *Phytopathology* 82:279–285.

PART TWO
Applications

SECTION III
Assessment of Therapy Effectiveness

27

PCR Assessment of the Efficacy of Therapy in Philadelphia Chromosome-Positive Leukemias

Stephen P. Hunger and Michael L. Cleary

Introduction

As discussed in Chapter 31, the PCR has rapidly assumed an important role in the molecular diagnosis of cancer. Neoplastic transformation is accompanied by a series of somatic genetic mutations that culminate in clinical manifestation of the malignant phenotype. Molecular characterization of these neoplasia-associated genetic alterations has led to the identification of DNA (and resultant) RNA sequences that differ between normal and malignant cells. These altered nucleic acid sequences can be detected by PCR either by the use of specific primers that will amplify the mutant, but not the wild-type, sequence, or by the use of allele-specific oligonucleotide hybridization after amplification of the informative sequence. PCR amplification of these somatic mutations also allows the detection of minimal residual disease (MRD), which is defined as malignant cells that are below the standard limits of detection in a patient who has no clinical evidence of residual neoplastic cells. In this section we will discuss PCR detection of MRD by amplification of chimeric RNA sequences that result from the presence of the Philadelphia chromosome (Ph^1), the cytogenetically abnormal chromosome 22 resulting from reciprocal translocation with chromosome 9 in various human leukemias.

Molecular Features of the Ph^1

Chromosomal abnormalities are frequently observed in neoplastic cells, and careful cytogenetic analysis detects such changes in over 90% of leukemias (Pui et al., 1990). Many of these changes are nonrandom, and specific cytogenetic, and resultant molecular, abnormalities are associated with distinct clinical subtypes of leukemia. Translocations, or exchanges of genetic material between chromosomes, represent the best characterized cytogenetic abnormalities. The prototype of translocations associated with leukemia is the t(9;22)(q34;q11), which results in an abnormal chromosome 22 called the Philadelphia chromosome. The Ph^1 is detected in almost all patients with chronic myelogenous leukemia (CML) and also in a subset of patients with either acute lymphoblastic leukemia (ALL) or acute myelogenous leukemia (AML) (for a comprehensive review of the clinical and mo-

The Polymerase Chain Reaction
K.B. Mullis, F. Ferré, R.A. Gibbs, editors
© 1994 Birkhäuser Boston

lecular features of Ph^1-positive leukemias the reader is referred to Kurzrock et al., 1988).

The t(9;22) results in translocation of a portion of the *ABL* proto-oncogene from its normal location on chromosome 9 into the *BCR* gene on chromosome 22, leading to the formation of a *BCR/ABL* fusion gene, which produces fusion messenger RNA (mRNA) that codes for a chimeric protein. The Bcr-Abl fusion protein has enhanced tyrosine kinase activity compared with the wild-type Abl protein and is crucial to the pathogenesis of Ph^1-positive leukemias, as evidenced by the fact that its overexpression in murine systems results in neoplasms that mimic human malignancies (Daley et al., 1990). At the genomic DNA level, the breakpoints in the *BCR* and *ABL* genes vary widely in location; however, they always occur within introns resulting in fusion of specific *BCR* exons to specific *ABL* exons in the processed *BCR/ABL* mRNA. Because of the widely dispersed DNA breakpoint locations in the *BCR* and particularly the *ABL* genes, DNA-based PCR strategies cannot be used and one must utilize the so-called reverse PCR or RT-PCR. In this method, the fusion mRNA is reverse transcribed into cDNA and then a portion of the transcript is amplified by PCR using one primer specific for *BCR* sequences and another for *ABL* sequences flanking the site of *BCR/ABL* fusion (Kawasaki et al., 1988). In normal cells no *BCR/ABL* amplification occurs since the genes are located on different chromosomes, whereas in cells that contain the t(9;22)-associated *BCR/ABL* fusion gene and transcript, amplification products are observed.

Breakpoints in the *ABL* gene occur over a large (200-kb) region in the 5' portion of the gene usually in intron 1, whereas breakpoints in *BCR* occur either within the 5.8-kb breakpoint cluster region (Mbcr) in the central portion of the gene or more proximally between the first and second exons (mbcr). Breakpoints within the Mbcr occur either between exons 2 and 3 or 3 and 4 of the bcr region (exons 9–11 of the *BCR* gene). Thus, two types of M*BCR/ABL* transcripts may be observed (referred to as b2a2 and b3a2) that join proximal *BCR* exons with *ABL* exons 2–11. The mbcr transloca-

tions result in fusion of the first exon of the *BCR* gene with *ABL* exons 2–11, resulting in formation of a transcript referred to as e1a2. Table 27.1 shows the molecular incidence of the Ph^1 in various subtypes of leukemia and the associated *BCR/ABL* molecular variants in each disease category.

Amplification of *BCR/ABL* Fusion Transcripts

Molecular detection of *BCR/ABL* fusion transcripts involves several discrete experimental steps. The primer sequences and conditions of amplification and hybridization used in our laboratory have been previously described (Kohler et al., 1990; Suryanarayan et al., 1991) and are depicted in Figure 27.1. Total RNA is converted to cDNA by reverse transcription primed by an oligonucleotide (ABLX3) complementary to sequences in the third exon of the *ABL* gene. Alternatively, reverse transcription may be performed using random hexamer priming. The cDNA is then divided into three equal aliquots, and an amplification cocktail containing one of three upstream oligonucleotides is added to each aliquot. The ABLX2 primer is homologous to sequences in the second exon of *ABL* and in conjunction with ABLX3 will amplify a 290-bp portion of the normal *ABL* transcript. This control reaction ensures that amplifiable RNA has been isolated and that *ABL* cDNA was transcribed in the reverse transcription reaction. Since *ABL* mRNA is expressed ubiquitously, failure to amplify this product invalidates any results obtained in the parallel reactions. If the input RNA is contaminated with genomic DNA, a larger product of approximately 920 bp will be amplified due to the presence of intronic DNA between *ABL* exons 2 and 3. The CML–BCR primer, homologous to sequences in exon 2 of the bcr region, will amplify M*BCR/ABL* fusion products of 324 (b2a2) and 399 (b3a2) bp if the t(9;22) breakpoint occurs within the Mbcr. The ALLE2 primer is homologous to sequences in the first exon of *BCR*. A 506-bp e1a2 *BCR/ABL* tran-

TABLE 27.1. Molecular incidence of the Ph[1] and *BCR/ABL* transcripts in leukemia.

Disease	Incidence of Ph[1] (%)	Breakpoint location	Type of *BCR/ABL* transcript
CML	95–100	Mbcr only	b2a2, b3a2
ALL			
Adults	25–33	50% mbcr/50% Mbcr	e1a2, b2a2, b3a2
Children	5	90% mbcr/10% Mbcr	e1a2, b2a2, b3a2
AML	1–2	Mbcr or mbcr	e1a2, b2a2, b3a2

script will be amplified using ALLE2 and ABLX3 if an mbcr type translocation has occurred.

Following PCR, an aliquot of the amplification product is size fractionated by electrophoresis in agarose gel and then transferred onto nylon membranes. The identity of the products is confirmed by hybridizing the membrane with a ^{32}P-labeled oligonucleotide (nonradioactively labeled detection probes may also be used) homologous to sequences in the amplified portion of *BCR/ABL* fusion cDNAs. The detection probe may consist of either a universal detection oligonucleotide from *ABL* exon 2 downstream of the ABLX2 primer, or product-specific oligonucleotides that span

each of the *BCR/ABL* fusion sequences. In our experience, bands are visible on ethidium bromide-stained gels when the malignant cells comprise at least 1% of the population. Using radiolabeled internal oligonucleotides, it is possible to detect the *BCR/ABL* fusion mRNA from 1 to 10 Ph[1]-carrying cells diluted in 10,000 normal cells after 35 cycles of PCR amplification. Some investigators perform two-step PCR using nested primers to increase the extent of amplification and obviate the need for hybridization with an internal oligonucleotide. The time required for sample analysis from collection to determination of results is usually several days in our laboratory. We have not encountered any patient with a cytogeneti-

A. t(9;22)(q34;q11) Mbcr transcripts:

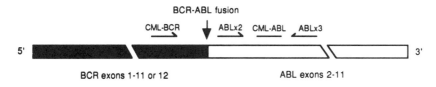

B. t(9;22)(q34;q11) mbcr transcript:

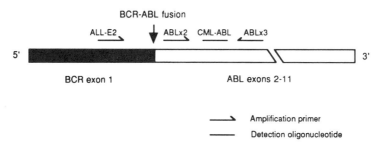

FIGURE 27.1. (**A, B**) Schematic depiction of *BCR-ABL* reverse PCR. Shaded boxes correspond to *BCR* sequences and open boxes correspond to *ABL* sequences in the *BCR–ABL* fusion RNA. Amplification and detection oligonucleotides are indicated by horizontal arrows and lines, respectively.

cally evident Ph[1] in whom *BCR/ABL* fusion transcripts could not be amplified using these primers, nor have we observed any patients with classic CML (with or without a cytogenetically detected Ph[1]) in whom *BCR/ABL* transcripts were not detected.

Two major problems are associated with PCR detection of *BCR/ABL* transcripts. One concerns false positive results that occur due to cross-contamination from other samples, cross-contamination from PCR end products, or plasmids that contain the target sequence. The other pitfall relates to the variability of results both within and between PCR reactions. As discussed elsewhere in this volume, strict precautions must be taken throughout the process from RNA extraction through amplification to avoid false positive results. This is particularly a problem in the analysis of MRD, as very faint signals may be observed in patients with a low percentage of malignant cells and one must be confident that these are not the result of contamination. Thus, stringent internal negative controls must be included in each set of amplifications. To ensure that efficient amplification has occurred, we include samples of RNA extracted from known Ph[1]-positive leukemia cells diluted in normal leukocytes in each PCR experiment when MRD is being assayed. *BCR/ABL* transcripts from a 10^{-2} dilution must give a visible signal on an ethidium bromide-stained gel, and a signal from the 10^{-3} dilution must be detected after hybridization with a radiolabeled internal oligonucleotide for us to conclude that the results are valid within the limits of sensitivity of our laboratory. If these signals are not detected, then efficient amplification has not occurred and negative results cannot be interpreted. We are also exploring the use of a synthetic internal RNA construct at low copy number within each reaction tube.

Another problem inherent in RT-PCR analysis of MRD is the difficulty associated with quantitation of the level of Ph[1]-positive cells present in the input sample based upon the amount of *BCR/ABL* product obtained after amplification. This problem is addressed elsewhere in this volume, and suggestions are given. However, it must be recalled that RT-

PCR amplifies messenger RNA, the levels of which may vary significantly between individual cells/patients or timepoints in the disease process. Furthermore, the absolute concentration of target RNA is partly dependent on its rate of synthesis or transcription. If the *BCR/ABL* fusion gene is present but not transcribed in a particular cell, RT-PCR amplification of target RNA will not occur resulting in the erroneous conclusion that no Ph[1]-containing cells are present in the specimen under analysis. Thus, even if one can accurately quantitate the number of input transcripts corresponding to a specific PCR product, extrapolation to the number of malignant cells in the input sample is troublesome. For these reasons we have elected not to attempt to quantitate the signal in RT-PCR detection of MRD at the current time.

Clinical Application of *BCR/ABL* PCR in Patients with CML

The natural history of CML classically includes three clinical phases. Patients usually present in chronic phase with greatly increased numbers of circulating mature granulocytes and splenomegaly without signs of severe marrow failure or infection. Chronic phase CML can generally be easily controlled with oral medications and patients generally lead a relatively normal life during this phase of the illness. However, chronic phase CML inevitably progresses to an accelerated phase and then blast crisis that clinically resembles acute leukemia, and is rapidly fatal without therapy. Approximately 20–25% of patients progress from chronic phase per year and the average survival is 3.5 years from the time of initial diagnosis. The duration of chronic phase does exhibit a great deal of variability, and a small minority of patients may remain in chronic phase for a much longer period of time. Standard medical therapy improves the quality of life, but does not affect the natural history of the disease. Allogeneic bone marrow transplantation (BMT) is, however, an effective therapy. When transplanted in chronic phase with unmanipulated marrow from a histocompatible sibling donor, 55–70% of patients are alive in complete remission, and presumably cured, 3 years post-BMT (McGlave, 1990).

Intriguingly, a subset of patients has been observed in whom Ph[1]-positive metaphases are detected post-BMT without clinical evidence of recurrent CML, a condition referred to as cytogenetic relapse (Thomas et al., 1986; Arthur et al., 1988; Zaccaria et al., 1988). Some of these patients will go on to experience a true hematologic and clinical relapse, yet others may have Ph[1]-positive host cells detected either transiently or persistently post-BMT without clinical relapse. The incidence of cytogenetic relapse is much higher in recipients of T-cell-depleted, compared with unmanipulated, grafts (Arthur et al., 1988). In one series, patients with high levels of Ph[1]-positive metaphases (50–100%) went on to develop clinical relapse, whereas those with lower levels remained in hematologic remission, in contrast to the experience with acute leukemia where the detection of cytogenetically abnormal metaphases is almost always followed rapidly by clinical relapse (Zaccaria et al., 1988). These observations have prompted a number of groups to further investigate the prevalence of residual Ph[1]-carrying cells using PCR to monitor patients with CML post-BMT.

There have now been a number of reports published delineating the incidence of PCR-detectable BCR/ABL fusion transcripts in patients with CML post-BMT, yet at this point in time there is no firm consensus on the clinical significance of this phenomenon. In our experience, many patients are transiently PCR positive in the first few months post-BMT and then revert to PCR-negative status; we have not found these early results to be predictive of later outcome (Kohler et al., 1990; Hunger et al., unpublished observations). Several other groups have also found that early post-BMT PCR results are not predictive of outcome (Martiat et al., 1990; Sawyers et al., 1990; Hughes et al., 1991a; Roth et al., 1989, 1992). In contrast, Delage (1991) reported that the presence of detectable BCR/ABL transcripts in the first 2–10 weeks post-BMT was associated with a high risk of later relapse.

The published results of PCR analyses outside the immediate posttransplant period are extremely variable between centers, but generally fall into three groups as is schematically represented in Figure 27.2. At one end of the spectrum are those who have found very few patients to be PCR positive (Group 1), at the other end (Group 3) are groups who report that most or all patients are positive, and in the middle are groups who find both positive and negative results (Group 2). In all the series discussed herein, adequate precautions appear to have been taken to exclude both false positive and false negative results. The level of sensitivity appears similar between studies with most centers reporting the ability to detect 1–10 BCR/ABL positive cells per 10^5–10^6 normal cells. Thus, it does not appear that technical reasons adequately account for the conflicting results.

The experience at our center has been that no patient transplanted with unmanipulated donor marrow for chronic phase (CP) CML has had BCR/ABL transcripts detected by PCR beyond 6 months post-BMT, and no patients in this group have relapsed, nor have any Ph[1]-positive metaphases been observed cytogenetically (Kohler et al., 1990; Hunger et al., unpublished observations). Thus, we have found the clinical, cytogenetic, and molecular results to be in complete concordance; however, we are not in a position to determine the predictive value of positive analyses beyond the first 6 months. Several other groups have also found that most patients transplanted with unmanipulated donor marrow for CP CML remain PCR negative after the immediate posttransplant period, and that these patients have a very low risk of relapse (Morgan et al., 1989; Martiat et al., 1990; Sawyers et al., 1990; Hughes et al., 1991a). In contrast, others have reported that most or all patients are PCR positive post-BMT, even those who are 2 or more years posttransplant and presumably at very low risk of relapse (Gabert et al., 1989; Pignon et al., 1990).

Recently, several groups have reported more intriguing results; namely, that patients can be divided into several distinct subsets on the basis of PCR and that these subsets have differing

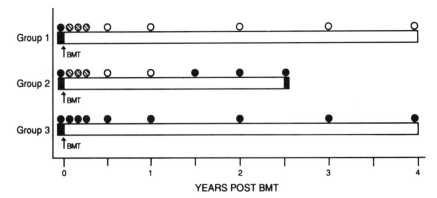

FIGURE 27.2. Schematic illustration of results obtained from longitudinal *BCR/ABL* PCR studies on CML patients following BMT. Group 1 represents the typical results obtained for a subset of patients who are PCR negative after the early posttransplant period and have a very low risk of clinical relapse. Group 2 represents the subset of patients who are PCR positive after the early posttransplant period and these patients are at increased risk for subsequent relapse. Group 3 represents a subset of patients who are PCR positive at most or all time points post-BMT but these results are not predictive of subsequent relapse. Circles indicate PCR status of patient: Open circle, negative PCR assay; closed circle, positive PCR assay; crosshatched circle, PCR results may be either positive or negative. Bars indicate clinical status of patient's leukemia: open bar, clinical and cytogenetic remission; closed bar, clinically apparent leukemia.

risks of relapse. Hughes et al. (1991a) found that all patients transplanted with unmanipulated donor marrow for CP-CML were PCR negative 8 months to 8 years post-BMT, whereas 5 of 9 patients who received T-cell-depleted BMT for CP-CML and 4 of 4 transplanted while no longer in CP were PCR positive. As patients in the latter two groups are known to be at significantly higher risk of relapse post-BMT, they suggest that the PCR results may be indicative of later outcome. Indeed, some of the PCR-positive patients did go on to experience relapse, yet others remained in remission. In another study, Delage and coworkers (1991) studied 24 patients by *BCR/ABL* PCR after T-cell-depleted BMT for CML; they observed that those patients who were persistently PCR positive had a higher risk of relapse than those who were intermittently positive. Furthermore, they used a limiting dilution titration assay to estimate the residual tumor cell burden over time in a subset of patients and found that the PCR-positive patients who relapsed had a progressive increase in tumor cell number, while the PCR-positive

patients who remained in remission had a relatively stable, low number of tumor cells.

Roth (1992) has also recently reported that PCR results were predictive of subsequent outcome. They studied 64 patients post-BMT and divided the patients into several groups on the basis of these results. Twenty-seven patients were persistently PCR negative and none of these has relapsed, whereas 37 had at least one positive PCR assay and 15 have relapsed. In the PCR-positive subgroup, 8 patients were persistently positive and only 2 of these remain in remission; 7 of 23 patients with both positive and negative results have relapsed. Thus, there were significant correlations between the PCR status and the risk of later relapse. In this study a two-step PCR amplification was performed using nested primers. Bands were visualized on ethidium bromide-stained gels after the first round of amplification in 10 patients, and 7 of 10 relapsed, suggesting that tumor cell burden (as estimated by amplification above the visualization threshold) correlated with outcome.

Thus at this time it appears that several tentative conclusions can be made concerning the predictive value of PCR detection of *BCR/ABL* fusion mRNA in patients with CML who have undergone BMT. First, many patients are PCR positive in the early posttransplant period and these results generally appear to have little or no clinical significance as most of them will later convert to PCR-negative status and will remain in clinical and cytogenetic remission. However, some groups have suggested that these early positive results are indeed predictive of later outcome (Delage et al., 1991). Second, most patients who have received an unmodified graft for CML in chronic phase are PCR negative after the initial early post-BMT phase, and have a very low risk of subsequent relapse (Fig. 27.2, Group 1 patients). Third, a subset of patients exists that is persistently or intermittently PCR positive after the early post-BMT phase, and these patients, as a group, may indeed be at higher risk of clinical relapse (Fig. 27.2, Group 2 patients). However, the clinical significance of detectable *BCR/ABL* transcripts in an individual patient in hematologic and cytogenetic remission is uncertain at the present time. It appears too early to recommend that therapeutic decisions can be made on the basis of PCR results after BMT for CML, although several recent studies certainly suggest that this may be possible in the near future.

Clinical Application of *BCR/ABL* PCR in Patients with Ph[1]-Positive Acute Leukemias

At the present time, the data on monitoring MRD by PCR in patients with Ph[1]-positive acute leukemias are much more limited than that available for patients with CML. As Ph[1]-AML is rare, we will limit our discussion in this section to cases of Ph[1]-ALL. Patients with Ph[1]-ALL have an extremely poor prognosis when treated with modern chemotherapeutic regimens, and few, if any, are successfully cured (Crist et al., 1990; Fletcher et al., 1991). In contrast, there are now a number of patients with Ph[1]-ALL who remain in complete hematologic and cytogenetic remission 2

or more years after allogeneic BMT, and who may indeed be cured by this treatment modality (Forman et al., 1987). The natural history of acute leukemia is distinctly different from that of CML, and remission patients in whom cells reappear containing the diagnostic cytogenetic abnormality (such as the Ph[1]) almost always go on to relapse within a short time unless therapeutic intervention occurs. Thus, it can be hoped that the predictive value of *BCR/ABL* PCR in patients with Ph[1]-ALL may be more apparent than is the case for patients with CML.

During standard antileukemic treatment, when complete remission is attained, the bone marrow karyotype normalizes and any cytogenetic abnormalities present at diagnosis are no longer detected. However, it is clear that low levels of leukemic cells are indeed present in remission, and can be readily detected by more sensitive PCR methods in most children with ALL during the first 18 months of therapy (Yamada et al., 1990). It is possible that methods of monitoring MRD, such as *BCR/ABL* PCR, which detect expression of mRNA for a transforming oncogene may give a better indication of imminent relapse than those that utilize amplification of nonpathogenic markers such as immunoglobin/T-cell receptor gene rearrangements.

Miyamura et al. (1992) recently reported their experience monitoring MRD by *BCR/ABL* PCR in 15 patients with Ph[1]-ALL who received either allogeneic or autologous BMT. Twelve of the patients were in hematologic and cytogenetic remission at the time of transplantation; nevertheless, *BCR/ABL* transcripts were detected in 8 of the 10 patients assayed prior to BMT. The PCR results post-BMT stand in marked contradistinction to those generally reported in patients with CML following transplantation. Each of the seven patients who had a positive PCR result post-BMT has subsequently relapsed, and the tempo of relapse has been quite rapid with recurrence developing within 3–9 weeks of positive PCR assays. Five of these seven patients had one or more negative PCR assays preceding the positive assays suggesting that the leukemic clone was transiently reduced in abundance to a level below the PCR detection threshold. Relapse also occurred in one patient without an antecedent positive PCR assay; this patient had been PCR negative at 3 months posttransplant and relapsed 4 months later. It should also be noted that all relapses occurred within the first 8 months posttransplant. Eight patients remained in CR 15–64 months post-BMT and each was PCR negative on all posttransplant assays. These results suggest several features of Ph[1]-ALL that differ significantly from the experience with CML. In this study, a positive PCR assay post-BMT was 100% predictive of relapse within the following 3–9 weeks; negative results did not exclude the possibility of subsequent relapse. The tempo of relapse was also much more rapid than the often slow evolution of recurrent disease seen in patients with CML following BMT, suggesting that frequent sampling would be necessary to identify patients prior to overt clinical relapse. Furthermore, if such patients were accurately identified, there would be a very narrow window of opportunity in which to initiate additional therapies. It should be emphasized that these patients had all undergone BMT, and thus no active therapy (excluding any graft-versus-leukemia effect) was being received after the detection of subclinical levels of MRD. It is conceivable that the rate of relapse could be more gradual or even reversed in patients receiving ongoing chemotherapy, thus expanding the "window of therapeutic opportunity."

Our experience monitoring MRD during the course of therapy (chemotherapy and/or BMT) in patients with Ph[1]-ALL by *BCR/ABL* PCR is more limited, but our results are generally in agreement with those of Miyamura (selected results are graphically displayed in Fig. 27.3). In the case of Patient 1, there were four negative *BCR/ABL* PCR assays in the first 6 months after allogeneic BMT (Kohler et al., 1990), yet relapse occurred 18 months after the last negative assay (no intervening data points are available). Patient 2 was PCR negative at 6 months post-BMT, but still relapsed 5 months later. The most instructive case is that of Patient 3 who had several negative PCR assays over a 14-month period while he was in CR and receiving maintenance chemotherapy

for ALL. However, at the time therapy was discontinued (as per the treatment protocol in which he was enrolled) he had converted to being clearly PCR positive in the bone marrow (while negative in the peripheral blood) despite a histologically and cytogenetically normal marrow. He relapsed within 2 months, again demonstrating the more rapid tempo of recurrent disease in acute leukemia. A second remission was attained, but was not as "deep" as the first as evidenced by the fact that he remained PCR positive on all assays. A second relapse occurred despite continued therapy, and the patient died of progressive disease. This case also illustrates the important point that analysis of bone marrow may be significantly more sensitive than assays of peripheral blood. Thus our results, although based on limited and uncontrolled sampling, agree that negative PCR results during therapy or after BMT are not predictive of subsequent outcome in patients with Ph[1]-ALL. Conversion from PCR-negative to positive status, however, may be predictive of impending relapse, especially in the absence of continued therapy.

Several other small series of PCR analyses of patients with Ph[1]-ALL have been published in the literature. Gehly (1991) reported limited results on four patients with Ph[1]-ALL post-BMT. One patient was PCR negative on days 21 and 75 post-BMT, yet clinically relapsed on day 115, again demonstrating the rapidity of clonal expansion in Ph[1]-ALL. Another patient was PCR negative on two occasions within the first 2 months post-BMT and died on day 123 of BMT complications. Two patients were PCR negative on two occasions within the first 3 months and remained in complete remission during 7–10 months of follow-up. In the same report 8 patients with Ph[1]-ALL were studied while in hematologic remission (although 5 of 8 had Ph[1]-positive metaphases detected cytogenetically) and *BCR/ABL* transcripts were detected by PCR in all eight. Of these eight patients, two were alive and well after allogeneic BMT (as discussed above), two died of BMT complications in remission, and 4 relapsed. Thus, none has remained in remission without BMT.

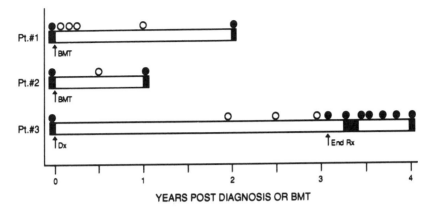

YEARS POST DIAGNOSIS OR BMT

FIGURE 27.3. Longitudinal results of *BCR/ABL* PCR in selected patients with Ph[1]-ALL during the course of chemotherapy, or following BMT. Patient 1 has been previously reported as SPN 82 in Kohler et al. (1990). Patient 3 was described in Hunger et al. (1991b). See legend for Figure 27.2 for an explanation of the symbols. For patient 3, Dx indicates the time of initial diagnosis and End Rx indicates the time at which treatment was discontinued.

At the present time, the data on the clinical utility of PCR detection of *BCR/ABL* transcripts in patients with Ph[1]-ALL are limited. It is clear that many patients have detectable malignant cells during remission, yet others are negative. Currently available chemotherapy (without BMT) cannot be considered curative (Fletcher et al., 1991), so one would expect that most, if not all, of these patients will eventually relapse. Conversion from PCR negative to positive status was rapidly followed by relapse in one of our patients and five of the patients reported by Miyamura (1992) in the absence of ongoing therapy. It is also clear that patients can relapse after previous negative PCR assays, even those performed within several months, thus the tempo of clonal expansion and clinical relapse in Ph[1]-ALL appears to be much more rapid than the more gradual process observed in patients with CML. Therefore, if such monitoring is to be clinically useful it should be performed frequently, and it appears prudent to sample the bone marrow rather than peripheral blood. Detection of patients who convert from PCR negative to positive status, or increasing levels of transcripts might allow reintensification of therapy prior to overt clinical relapse. It is generally agreed that all eligible patients with Ph[1]-ALL

should undergo allogeneic BMT if a suitable donor exists. Most patients do not have a histocompatible sibling donor, and many centers are exploring the use of transplants from matched unrelated donors and/or autologous transplants. Close monitoring of high-risk patients by PCR might allow therapy to be "tailored" prior to relapse while a search for a compatible donor continues. Clearly the role of PCR detection of MRD in this aggressive subtype of leukemia requires further investigation and such studies are ongoing in many laboratories, including our own.

Future Directions

A number of novel therapies are now, or will shortly be, available for patients with Ph[1]-positive leukemias. Interferon-α is currently being used in patients with CML who are not candidates for BMT, with encouraging preliminary results. Detection of MRD by *BCR/ABL* PCR is an important tool for assessing the efficacy of such therapies and comparing them to currently available treatments (Opalka et al., 1991). Autologous transplants, in which the patients own bone marrow is used, are also being employed with increasing frequency in patients with both CML and Ph[1]-positive acute leukemias. The marrow is often treated with chemotherapeutic agents or monoclonal antibodies to selectively remove residual tumor cells prior to reinfusion into the patient. The efficiency of such methods of "negative selection" can be assessed by PCR examination of the marrow specimen before and after purging procedures. This may allow the *in vitro* comparison of different purging techniques, or might allow one to choose which marrows are "clean" enough to be reinfused. Other groups are investigating methods of "positive selection" to separate normal Ph[1]-negative progenitor cells from Ph[1]-positive cells and then to use these cells for autologous BMT. Obviously the PCR will play an important role in evaluating such therapeutic strategies (Verfaillie et al., 1992). In the absence of any allogeneic graft-versus-leukemia effect, one might expect that the reinfusion of even one autologous Ph[1]-positive cell could ultimately lead to recurrence; thus, extremely sensitive measures of purity of the autograft are essential.

The genes involved in a number of other translocations associated with leukemia have now been identified and sequenced. Several of these translocations lead to the formation of fusion genes, and analogous modes of detection of MRD can be pursued by amplification of the resultant chimeric transcripts such as *E2A/PBX1* in the t(1;19) in pre-B ALL (Hunger et al., 1991a), the *RARα/PML* in the t(15;17) in promyelocytic leukemia (de The et al., 1990), and *DEK/CAN* in the t(6;9) in AML (von Lindern et al., 1990). As discussed elsewhere in this volume, one can also amplify unique sequences resulting from immunoglobulin or T-cell receptor gene rearrangements (which are a marker for the malignant clone) to detect MRD in ALL (Hansen-Hagge et al., 1989; Yamada et al., 1990). One would anticipate that a prominent trend of the 1990s will be the initial determination of the role that PCR detection of MRD has to play in monitoring the efficacy of various antileukemic therapies, and the rapid incorporation of methods proven beneficial into the routine clinical management of patients with leukemia. Historically, patients have been prospectively divided into risk sub-groups on the basis of clinical and biologic features present at the time of diagnosis, but no accurate means has existed to define risk subgroups on the basis of response to therapy. This powerful new tool of molecular biology has the potential to revolutionize the manner in which therapy is delivered to patients, by allowing a sensitive evaluation of the individual patient's response to treatment. This could lead to "tailored therapy," allowing treatment to be safely discontinued in patients who are cured and intensified early in the course of those who will not be cured with standard treatments. Furthermore, it potentially enables a sensitive monitoring of new therapeutic strategies, so that the clinical utility, or lack thereof, of such novel treatments could be more rapidly assessed.

References

Arthur CK, Apperley JF, Guo AP, et al. (1988): Cytogenetic events after bone marrow transplantation for chronic myeloid leukemia in chronic phase. *Blood* 71:1179–1186.

Bartram CR, Janssen JWG, Schmidberger M, et al. (1989): Minimal residual leukemia in chronic myeloid leukemia patients after T-cell depleted bone marrow transplantation. *Lancet* 1:1260 (letter).

Crist W, Carroll A, Shuster J, et al. (1990): Philadelphia chromosome positive childhood acute lymphoblastic leukemia: Clinical and cytogenetic characteristics and treatment outcome. A Pediatric Oncology Group study. *Blood* 76:489–494.

Daley GC, van Etten RA, Baltimore D (1990): Induction of chronic myelogenous leukemia in mice by the p210 bcr/abl gene of the Philadelphia chromosome. *Science* 247:824–830.

Delage R, Soiffer RJ, Dear K, Ritz J (1991): Clinical significance of bcr/abl gene rearrangement detected by polymerase chain reaction after allogeneic bone marrow transplantation in chronic myelogenous leukemia. *Blood* 78:2759–2767.

Delfau MH, Kerckaeut J-P, D'Hoeghe MS, et al. (1990): Detection of minimal residual disease in chronic myeloid leukemia patients after bone marrow transplantation by polymerase chain reaction. *Leukemia* 4:1–5.

de The H, Chomienne C, Lanotte M, et al. (1990): The t(15;17) translocation of acute promyelocytic leukemia fuses the retinoic acid α gene to a novel transcribed locus. *Nature (London)* 347: 558–561.

Fletcher JA, Lynch EA, Kimball VM, et al. (1991): Translocation (9;22) is associated with extremely poor prognosis in intensively treated children with acute lymphoblastic leukemia. *Blood* 77:435–439.

Forman SJ, O'Donnell MR, Nademanee AP, et al. (1987): Bone marrow transplantation for patients with Philadelphia chromosome-positive acute lymphoblastic leukemia. *Blood* 70:587–588.

Gabert J, Lafage M, Maraninchi D, et al. (1989): Detection of residual bcr/abl translocation by polymerase chain reaction in chronic myeloid leukemia patients after bone marrow transplantation. *Lancet* 2:1125–1128.

Gehly GB, Bryant EM, Lee AM, et al. (1991): Chimeric BCR-abl Messenger RNA as a marker for minimal residual disease in patients transplanted for Philadelphia chromosome-positive acute lymphoblastic leukemia. *Blood* 98:458–465.

Hansen-Hagge T, Yokota S, Bartram CR (1989): Detection of minimal residual disease in acute lymphoblastic leukemia by in vitro amplification of rearranged T cell receptor δ chain sequences. *Blood* 74:1762–1767.

Hughes TP, Morgan GJ, Martiat P, et al. (1991a): Detection of residual leukemia after bone marrow transplant for chronic myeloid leukemia: Role of polymerase chain reaction in predicting relapse. *Blood* 77:874–878.

Hughes TP, Ambrosetti A, Barbu V, et al. (1991b): Clinical value of PCR in diagnosis and followup of leukemia and lymphoma: Report of the third workshop of the molecular biology/BMT study group. *Leukemia* 5:448–451.

Hunger SP, Galili N, Carroll A, et al. (1991a): The t(1;19)(q23;p13) results in consistent fusion of E2A and PBX1 coding sequences in acute lymphoblastic leukemias. *Blood* 77:687–693.

Hunger SP, Amylon MD, Donlon TA, et al. (1991b): Longitudinal monitoring of minimal residual disease by PCR in a patient with Philadelphia chromosome positive ALL. *Blood* 78:443a. (abstr)

Kawasaki ES, Clark SS, Coyne MY, et al. (1988): Diagnosis of chronic myeloid and acute lymphoblastic leukemias by detection of leukemia-specific mRNA sequences amplified in vitro. *Proc Natl Acad Sci USA* 85:5698–5702.

Kohler S, Galili N, Sklar JL, et al. (1990): Expression of BCR-ABL fusion transcripts following bone marrow transplantation for Philadelphia

chromosome-positive leukemia. *Leukemia* 8: 541–547.

Kurzrock R, Gutterman JL, Talkpaz M (1988): The molecular genetics of Philadelphia chromosome-positive leukemias. *N Engl J Med* 319:990–998.

Martiat P, Maisin D, Philippe M, et al. (1990): Detection of residual bcr/abl transcripts in chronic myeloid leukemia patients in complete remission using the polymerase chain reaction and nested primers. *Br J Haematol* 75:355–358.

McGlave P (1990): Bone marrow transplants in chronic myelogenous leukemia: An overview of determinants of survival. *Sem Hematol* 27:23–30 (Suppl).

Miyamura K, Tanimoto M, Morishiwa Y, et al. (1992): Detection of Philadelphia chromosome-positive acute lymphoblastic leukemia by polymerase chain reaction: Possible eradication of minimal residual disease by marrow transplantation. *Blood* 79:1366–1370.

Morgan GJ, Janssen JWG, Guo A-P (1989): Polymerase chain reaction for detection of residual leukemia. *Lancet* 1:998–929.

Opalka B, Wandl UR, Becher R, et al. (1991): Minimal residual disease in patients with chronic myelogenous leukemia undergoing long-term treatment with recombinant interferon α-2b alone or in combination with interferon γ. *Blood* 78:2188–2193.

Pignon JM, Henni T, Amselem S, et al. (1990): Frequent detection of minimal residual disease by use of the polymerase chain reaction in long-term survivors after bone marrow transplantation for chronic myeloid leukemia. *Leukemia* 4:83–86.

Pui C-H, Crist WM, Look AT (1990): Biology and clinical significance of cytogenetic abnormalities in childhood acute lymphoblastic leukemia. *Blood* 76:1449–1463.

Roth MS, Antin JH, Bingham EL, et al. (1989): Detection of Philadelphia chromosome-positive cells by the polymerase chain reaction following bone marrow transplant for chronic myelogenous leukemia. *Blood* 74:882–885.

Roth MS, Antin JH, Ash R, et al. (1992): Prognostic significance of Philadelphia chromosome-positive cells detected by the polymerase chain reaction after allogeneic bone marrow transplant for chronic myelogenous leukemia. *Blood* 79:276–282.

Sawyers CL, Timson L, Kawasaki ES, et al. (1990): Molecular relapse in chronic myelogenous leukemia patients after bone marrow transplantation detected by polymerase chain reaction. *Proc Natl Acad Sci USA* 87:563–567.

Suryanarayan K, Hunger SP, Kohler S, et al. (1991): Consistent involvement of the BCR gene by 9;22 breakpoints in Pediatric acute leukemias. *Blood* 77:324–330.

Thomas ED, Clift RA, Fefer A, et al. (1986): Marrow transplantation for the treatment of chronic myelogenous leukemia. *Ann Int Med* 104:155–163.

Verfaillie CM, Miller WJ, Boylan K, McGlave PB (1992): Selection of benign primitive hematopoietic progenitors in chronic myelogenous leukemia on the basis of HLA-DR antigen expression. *Blood* 79:1003–1010.

von Lindern M, Poustka A, Lerach H, et al. (1990): The (6;9) chromosome translocation, associated with a specific subtype of acute nonlymphocytic leukemia, leads to aberrant transcription of a target gene on 9q34. *Mol Cell Biol* 10:4016–4026.

Yamada M, Wasserman R, Lange B, et al. (1990): Minimal residual disease in childhood B-lineage leukemia. Persistence of leukemia cells during the first 18 months of treatment. *N Engl J Med* 323:448–455.

Zaccaria A, et al. and the Cooperative study group on chromosomes in transplanted patients (1988): Cytogenetic follow-up of 100 patients submitted to bone marrow transplantation for Philadelphia chromosome-positive chronic myeloid leukemias. *Eur J Haematol* 40:50–57.

28

The Detection of Minimal Residual Disease (MRD) in Acute Lymphoblastic Leukemia Using Clone-Specific Probes Directed against V(D)J Junctional Sequences

Luc d'Auriol and François Sigaux

The monitoring of remaining malignant cells after intensive therapy is of fundamental importance in the management of leukemia (Campana and Janossy, 1990; Potter, 1992; Von Dongen et al., 1992). This is true for the study of the natural history of the disease but also for the assessment of the treatment itself. Until recently, available techniques lacked both sensitivity and specificity. The emergence of PCR-derived approaches in clinical laboratories has radically changed the detection of residual disease as they allow the detection of nucleotide sequences that are specific of the malignant clone. These studies were first restricted to chromosomal translocations that represent only a small fraction of acute leukemias. In 1989, our group (d'Auriol et al., 1989), J. Sklar's (Tycko et al., 1989), and Rovera's (Yamada et al., 1989) independently reported general strategies based on the construction of oligonucleotides targeting the random sequences generated during the V(D)J rearrangement of genes coding for antigen receptors. For reasons that will be developed later we chose to focus on genes coding for the TCR-γ and -δ chains. This strategy has been recently extended, by our group (Macintyre et al., 1990). In a second step, a number of teams have proposed modifications to that approach so as to avoid determining the nucleotide sequence of the rearrangement (Hansen-Hagge et al., 1989). Recently, reports have appeared suggesting the clinical relevance of such studies (Neale et al., 1991; Nizet et al., 1991; Wasserman et al., 1992a; Yokota et al., 1991).

In this brief review, we will show the rationale of this approach and will describe its advantages and limitations.

V(D)J Junctional Sequences Can Be Considered as Clonal Markers

Antigen recognition by lymphoid cells is mediated by clone-specific cell surface receptors. B cells recognize antigens using surface immunoglobulins (Ig). The T-cell antigen receptor (TCR) is made of an $\alpha\beta$ or $\gamma\delta$ heterodimer noncovalently associated with the CD3 multichain complex. The specificity of recognition is carried by the heterodimer and is due to somatic rearrangements of V, J, and sometimes D fragments during the early stages of lymphoid cell differentiation. These rearrangements

The Polymerase Chain Reaction
K.B. Mullis, F. Ferré, R.A. Gibbs, editors
© 1994 Birkhauser Boston

are dependent on the presence of recognition sequences (RSS) that are found in the 3' portion of V segments, in the 5' and 3' portions of D segments, and in the 5' portion of J segments. During the recombination event the genomic DNA is cut in the vicinity of the RSS and the different segments are ligated together. Before ligation takes place, nucleotide deletions frequently occur as well as additions that are due to the terminal transferase enzyme (Alt et al., 1992; Schatz, 1992). Junctional sequences are therefore quite random in essence and can be considered as specific of a given recombination event. This junction will be carried by all the cells originating from the cell in which the rearrangement occurred. We and others postulated that an oligonucleotide derived from this junctional V(D)J sequence would be able to specifically recognize a given clone (d'Auriol et al., 1989; Macintyre et al., 1990; Tycko et al., 1989; Yamada et al., 1989).

Targeting TCR$\gamma\delta$ Gene Rearrangements

TCR$\gamma\delta$ Genes Show a Limited Combinatory Diversity While Presenting a Very High Junctional Diversity

The genetic organization of the TCRγ locus has been completely established (Chen et al., 1988; Font et al., 1988; Huck et al., 1988; Huck and Lefranc, 1987; Lefranc et al., 1986a,b; Lefranc and Rabbitts, 1985). It comprises two J–C regions that have been tandemly duplicated and contain five J segments and two constant regions. The V_γ locus is located 150 kb upstream of the J–C regions and comprises, in addition to three less conserved pseudogenes ($\psi V_\gamma A$, $\psi V_\gamma B$, $\psi V_\gamma C$), four different subgroups (V_γ I, V_γ II, V_γ III, V_γ IV). Subgroup I shows a frequent repertoire polymorphism. The most frequent haplotype is composed of 9 V_γ segments, including 5 pseudogenes that never rearrange in normal T cells. In 15% of chromosomes one can find a

short haplotype that does not have $V_\gamma 4$ and $V_\gamma 5$ (Font et al., 1988). Subgroups II, III, and IV are made of only one segment ($V_\gamma 9$, $V_\gamma 10$, and $V_\gamma 11$, respectively). There is no D segment.

The genetic organization of the TCRδ locus has been more recently explored (Hata et al., 1989; Loh et al., 1988; Takiyara et al., 1988, 1989). The most peculiar of its features is that the $D_\delta - J_\delta - C_\delta$ region lies between the V_α and J_α regions. This TCRδ region is deleted by loop excision during $V_\alpha - J_\alpha$ rearrangements. Three D segments upstream of the three J segments and one C segment have been described. Rearrangements can be in the form VD, DJ, or VDJ, and D segments can be tandemly used. Six V_δ segments can be used in rearrangements. $V_\delta 1$ is preferentially used by thymocytes while $V_\delta 2$ is used by a majority of $\gamma\delta$ T cells (5% of all T cells).

TCR$\gamma\delta$ Genes Are Rearranged in Nearly all T-ALLs and in a Large Fraction of B-Lineage ALLs

The extensive use of monoclonal antibodies directed against differentiation antigens has shown that nearly all nonmyeloid acute leukemias can be considered as expansions of cells that have been blocked at early stages of lymphoid differentiation. These leukemias are called acute lymphoblastic leukemias (ALLs). About 85% of ALLs are from the B lineage while 15% are from the T lineage. TCR$\gamma\delta$ genes undergo somatic recombination during very early stages of pre-T differentiation. As would be expected, these genes are clonally rearranged in almost 95% of T lineage ALLs. In these cells, TCRγ genes are frequently rearranged on both alleles and one can demonstrate a preferential usage of the $J_\gamma 2$ segment (Chen et al., 1987). Of TCRδ rearrangements 30% are deletions due to a $V_\alpha - J_\alpha$ rearrangement while in the other cases the most commonly used segments are $V_\delta 1$ and $J_\delta 1$ (about 50% of all T ALLs) (Loiseau et al., 1989).

Although it was thought that TCRγ and TCRδ gene rearrangements are specific for T cells, it has been clearly shown that these genes undergo rearrangements in, respectively, 50 and 80% of ALLs from the B lineage (Chen et al., 1987; Loiseau et al., 1989). These rearrangements are different from those observed in the T ALLs. TCRγ genes preferentially rearrange in neoplastic B cells in a monoallelic way and in most cases the $J_\gamma 1$ segment is used (Chen et al., 1987). On the other hand, TCRδ rearrangements preferentially involve $V_\delta 2$–$D_\delta 3$ (in about 50% of B lineage ALLs) (Biondi et al., 1990; Hansen-Hagge et al., 1992; Loiseau et al., 1989).

V(D)J Junctional Sequences Are Clone Specific

The variability of junctional V(D)J sequences from TCRγδ genes has been extensively studied in normal cells by sequencing of genomic or cDNA clones and more recently through the sequencing of PCR products. The study of thymocytes at different stages of ontogenesis as well as the study of peripheral T cells has revealed that this diversity is very large, especially in adults (Lafaille et al., 1989; Loh et al., 1988; McVay et al., 1991; Takiyara et al., 1989) with the exception of the $V_\delta 1$–$J_\delta 1$ rearrangements, which present a frequent restriction of their junctional diversity (Beldjord et al., 1993). On the other hand, these studies have shown that the junctional diversity is low in γδ T cells early in ontogeny.

Similar studies were done with leukemic cells. TCRγ rearrangements on the one hand and $V_\delta 1$–$J_\delta 1$ and $V_\delta 2$–$D_\delta 3$ rearrangements on the other hand have been most extensively studied. Our group was able to show that junction regions of TCRγ genes were extremely diverse in rearrangements occurring in the T lineage ALLs as well as in those from the B lineage (Macintyre et al., 1990). This allows the construction of an oligonucleotide that is specific for the junction. It is of interest to note that junctional sequences from $V_\delta 1(DD)J_\delta 1$ are even more diverse due to the fact that D regions are frequently used and that they rearrange tandemly (Macintyre et al., 1989). On the other hand, the diversity of $V_\delta 2$–$D_\delta 3$ rearrangements seems more limited due to the

fact that the 5' part of $D_\delta 3$ is rarely deleted during the rearrangement event (Yokota et al., 1991).

All the junctional sequences have been found once with two exceptions:

1. a $V_\delta 2$–$D_\delta 3$ with no N region was found in a leukemic patient and in a normal blood sample, and
2. a canonical V_γ–J_γ junctional sequence is present in almost all individuals.

This rearrangement maintains the reading frame of the protein and corresponds only to the deletion of 3 bases in the 5' part of the J segment (Delfau et al., 1992).

Strategies for the Study of Residual Disease Using Junctional Regions Resulting from TCRγδ Genes Rearrangements

The different strategies using the specificity of TCRγδ genes junctional regions are shown in Figure 28.1. All these approaches use PCR amplification of junctional regions. They all imply that the starting material is a sufficiently pure sample of clonal tumor cells.

According to the technology used they can be divided into three groups:

1. Use of probes that allow the recognition of junctional sequences. These methods have been developed by our group for the TCRγ and for the preferential $V_\delta 1$–$J_\delta 1$ rearrangement (Macintyre et al., 1990). An elegant simplification of this approach has been proposed by C. Bartram's group for the $V_\delta 1$–$J_\delta 1$ and $V_\delta 2$–$D_\delta 3$ recombination events (Hansen-Hagge et al., 1989; Yokota et al., 1991).

The initial stage is the construction of a specific probe for the given rearrangement. In our approach this probe is an oligonucleotide that is specific for the V(D)J region that has been determined either by direct sequencing of the amplified product or after cloning. Direct sequencing can be in some cases difficult due to a high proportion of polyclonal T cells in the

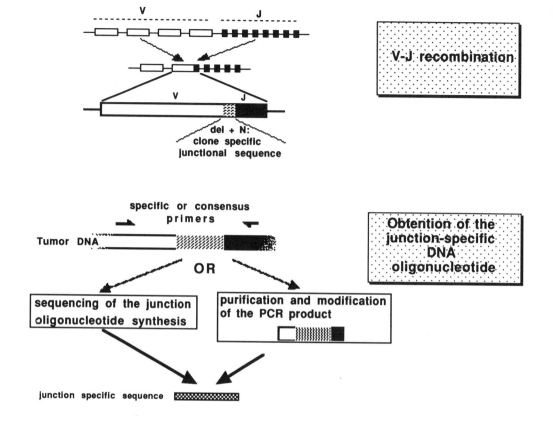

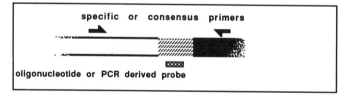

PCR using V-J amplimers

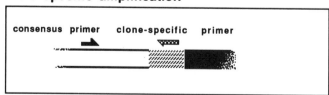

Allele specific amplification

FIGURE 28.1. Strategies using the specificity of TCRγδ genes junctional regions.

sample or when a consensus oligo for the I family is used for amplification. In Bartram's approach, a short amplified fragment is used as probe. This method does not require prior sequencing of the V(D)J junction. In the case of $V_\delta 1-J_\delta 1$ rearrangement the probe is obtained after a second round of amplification or "nested-PCR" followed by a digestion with the restriction enzyme *Fok*I. The restriction enzyme treatment allows the elimination of most $J_\gamma 1$ sequences, which renders the fragment small enough to be discriminant and therefore act as a specific probe for the amplified junction. In the case of $V_\delta 2-V_\delta 3$ rearrangements the probe is simply obtained by "nested-PCR."

Sample analysis is done either by dot-blot or by Southern blot analysis of the PCR products, the probe being an oligonucleotide encompassing the V(D)J junction or an amplified fragment of the same region.

In such approaches, the rearrangement must have been characterized beforehand so that the oligonucleotides used for amplification can be chosen for a specific V(D)J or VD combination. This can be done either through classical restriction enzyme analysis (Chen et al., 1987; Loiseau et al., 1989) or through PCR.

2. Allele-specific amplification. This method was proposed by J. Sklar's group for the detection of clones that had rearranged V_γ segments from family I and $J_\gamma 1/J_\gamma 2$ (Tycko et al., 1989). The junctional sequence is determined after amplification using a consensus oligonucleotide from the $V_\gamma I$ family. Another oligonucleotide directed against the clone-specific junctional sequence is then synthesized and used in conjunction with the consensus one to screen the remission samples.

3. RNase A analysis of *in vitro* transcribed RNA/RNA hybrids. This approach was reported by J. Sklar's group for the study of TCRγ gene rearrangements involving $V_\gamma I$ and $J_\gamma 1-2$ (Veelken et al., 1991). In this case an RNA radiolabeled probe is synthesized *in vitro* by means of a $V_\gamma I$ oligo and a J_γ oligo to which a T_7 promoter sequence has been added at the 5'-end. Similarly, the sample to be tested is amplified using a $J_\gamma 1-2$ oligo and a $V_\gamma I$ consensus oligo with a T_7 promoter at the 5'-end.

The use of T_7 polymerase allows the *in vitro* synthesis of RNAs with opposite polarities. After digestion by RNase-free DNase I, the transcripts are annealed and duplexes are treated with RNase I that creates nicks at mismatched positions. The digestion products are analyzed by polyacrylamide gels and autoradiographed. If malignant cells are present in the test sample one finds a fragment whose size corresponds to the mismatch free region.

Specificity and Sensitivity

The specificities and sensitivities of the different methods are similar. This can be roughly estimated by the inclusion of a series of tumor DNA dilutions in each experiment for a given patient. When tumor DNA (1 µg) is diluted in water or in a solution of DNA where the TCR genes are in the germline configuration, one can detect as little as one malignant cell out of 10^5 normal cells.

In our experience with the TCRγ locus, this sensitivity is lowered when the percentage of polyclonal T cells rises above 10%. We assume this to be due to a competition of targets for amplification. In any case, tumor DNA dilutions in water or in DNA with TCRγ genes in the germline configuration cannot be used for the quantitation of tumor cells in peripheral blood if polyclonal T cells have not been removed from the sample.

Besides the problem that might arise from rearrangements that generate very small N regions the specificity of this approach is almost absolute.

Limitations of the Approach

Limitations come from three different sources:

1. ALLs that do not rearrange TCRγ or TCRδ: TCRγ or TCRδ are almost always rearranged in ALLs from the T lineage but only in about 70% of ALLs from the B cell lineage. In these cases other markers can be used that are amenable to PCR and can allow the detection of residual disease: in particular, IgG

heavy chain rearrangements are present in the vast majority of ALLs from B lineage and a strategy based on the use of specific V(D)J probes has been proposed by Rovera's group (Wasserman et al., 1992a; Yamada et al., 1989, 1990). The usefulness of this approach is hampered by the very high frequency of oligoclonal rearrangements (Beishuizen et al., 1991; Bird et al., 1988). Besides this alternative, two translocations leading to the production of a hybrid mRNA can be used in RT-PCR experiments when TCRs are not rearranged. Translocation t(9;22) is present in about 30% of ALLs from the B lineage of adults (5% in children) while translocation t(1;19) is present in a number of pre-B ALLs (Kamps et al., 1990; Nourse et al., 1990). Recently, t(4;11) and t(11;19) have been cloned and fusion mRNA has been characterized (Gu et al., 1992; Tkachuk et al., 1992). These translocations are present in a small number of B-lineage ALL cases. In about 10% of T-ALLs, a Sil-Tal1 recombination is observed. This chromosomal abnormality can be PCR amplified (Bernard et al., 1991; Brown et al., 1990) and is a good target for the detection of minimal residual disease.

2. Heterogeneity of the residual disease. The strategies described above are well adapted for the study of bone marrow and blood. Bone marrow is the best place for sampling as it constitutes the preferential site of leukemic proliferation and the most frequent site of relapse. But one has to take into account the fact that the leukemic residual infiltration of the marrow can be anatomically heterogeneous. The repeated study of marrow in possibly two different areas is difficult for technical as well as ethical reasons. The study of blood is much easier but represents a compromise. In the case of relapse, malignant cells probably appear later in the blood than in the bone marrow. Moreover, in our hands, the sensitivity of the detection of residual disease drops by at least one degree of magnitude when blood cells are used instead of bone marrow for the study of TCRγ. Of course these methods need to be tested for the detection of residual disease or for relapses that occur outside the bone marrow (CNS, testis).

3. Clonal evolution. Clonal evolution and clonal heterogeneity are major causes of false negatives that can be observed with the techniques described in this chapter. All the proposed strategies rely on the hypothesis that the rearrangement that is recognized by the specific probe is present in all leukemic cells and is stable during the course of the disease. Clonal evolution of TCRγ or TCRδ is observed in about 20% of cases for a given rearrangement (unpublished results). In the case of the IgH locus, the frequency of oligoclonal rearrangements has been estimated to be 30% (Beishuizen et al., 1991; Bird et al., 1988). The frequency and the structure of novel rearrangements during relapse have been documented (Wasserman et al., 1992b). Since we have seldom seen clonal evolution of more than one allele at a given locus, we suggest using at least two clone-specific probes for each patient.

Clinical Value and Strategies for the Study of Residual Disease

There has been no prospective study demonstrating the usefulness of these approaches. Nevertheless the interest in these techniques stems from recent retrospective studies that can be summarized as follows (Neale et al., 1991; Nizet et al., 1991; Wasserman et al., 1992; Yokota et al., 1991):

1. Leukemic cells can be found in the blood or marrow of samples obtained in the year following complete remission of patients with ALLs.
2. The persistence after 1 year and moreover the increase of the number of malignant cells at successive times are very suggestive of the evolutive character of the residual disease and are signs of a relapse.
3. The presence at the end of induction therapy of a significant percentage of leukemic cells among total marrow B cells is indicative of an increased risk for relapse during therapy.

In conclusion, detection of minimal residual disease with clone-specific probes needs evaluation in large prospective clinical studies. However, the very high specificity of the strategy as well as its wide applicability position these methods among the major tools for the monitoring of therapies in malignant hematopoietic disorders.

References

Alt F, Oltz E, Young F, Gorman J, Taccioli G, Chen J (1992): VDJ recombination. *Immunol Today* 13:306–314.

Beishuizen A, Hählen K, Hagemeijer A, Verhoeven M, Hooijkaas H, Adriaansen H, Wolvers-Tettero I, Van Werin E, Van Dongen J (1991): Multiple rearranged immunoglobulin gene in childhood acute lymphoblastic leukemia of precursor B-cell origin. *Leukemia* 5:657–667.

Beldjord K, Beldjord C, Macintyre E, Even P, Sigaux F (1993): Peripheral selection of Vδ1+ cells with restricted T cell receptor δ gene junctional repertoire in the peripheral blood of healthy donors. *J Exp Med* 178:121–127.

Bernard O, Lecointe N, Jonveaux P, Souyri M, Mauchauffe M, Berger R, Larsen C, Mathieu-Mahul D (1991): Two site-specific deletions and t(1;14) translocation restricted to human T-cell acute leukemias disrupt the 5′ part of the tal1 gene. *Oncogene* 6:1477–1488.

Biondi A, Francia di Cell P, Rossi V, Casorati G, Matullo G, Giudici G, Foa R, Migone N (1990): High prevalence of T-cell receptor Vδ2-(D)-Dδ3 or Dδ1/2-Dδ3 rearrangements in B-precursor acute lymphoblastic leukemias. *Blood* 75:1834–1840.

Bird J, Gahli N, Link M, Stites D, Sklar J (1988): Continuing rearrangement but absence of somatic hypermutation in immunoglobulin genes of human B cell precursor leukemia. *J Exp Med* 168:229–245.

Brown L, Cheng J, Chen Q, Siciliano M, Crist W, Buchanan G, Baer R (1990): Site-specific recombination of the tal-1 gene is a common occurrence in human T-cell leukemia. *EMBO J* 9:3343–3351.

Campana D, Janossy G (1990): Critical analysis of detecting minimal residual leukemia. In *Acute Lymphoblastic Leukemia*. New York: Alan R. Liss.

Chen Z, Le Paslier D, Dausset J, Degos L, Flandrin G, Cohen D, Sigaux F (1987): Human T-cell re-arranging genes gamma are frequently re-arranged in B-lineage acute lymphoblastic leukemias but not in chronic B-cell proliferations. *J Exp Med* 165:1000–1015.

Chen Z, Font MP, Loiseau P, Bories JC, Duparc N, Degos L, Lefranc MP, Sigaux F (1988): The Vγ locus: Cloning of new segments and study of Vγ rearrangements in neoplastic B and T cells. *Blood* 72:776–783.

d'Auriol L, Macintyre E, Galibert F, Sigaux F (1989): In vitro amplification of T cell γ gene rearrangements: A new tool for the assessment of minimal residual disease in acute lymphoblastic leukemias. *Leukemia* 3:155–158.

Delfau M, Hance A, Leossier D, Vilmer E, Grand-champs B (1992): Restricted diversity of Vγ9-JP rearrangements in unstimulated human γ/δ T lymphocytes. *Eur J Immunol* 22:2437–2443.

Font MP, Chen Z, Bories JC, Duparc N, Loiseau P, Degos L, Cann H, Cohen D, Dausset J, Sigaux F (1988): The Vγ locus of the human T-cell receptor γ gene: Repertoire polymorphism of the first variable gene segment subgroup. *J Exp Med* 168:1383–1394.

Gu Y, Nakamura H, Alder R, Prasad R, Canaani O, Cimino G, Croce C, Canaani E (1992): The t(4;11) chromosome translocation of human acute leukemias fuse the ALL-1 gene, related to Drosophila trithorax, to the AF4 gene. *Cell* 71:701–708.

Hansen-Hagge TE, Yokota S, Bartram CR (1989): Detection of minimal residual disease in acute lymphoblastic leukemia by in-vitro amplification of rearranged T-cell receptor δ chain sequences. *Blood* 74:1762–1767.

Hansen-Hagge T, Yokota S, Reuter H, Schwarz K, Bartram C (1992): Human common acute lymphoblastic leukemia-derived cell lines are competent to recombine their T-cell receptor δ/α regions along a hierarchically ordered pathway. *Blood* 80:2353–2362.

Hata S, Clabby M, Devlin P, Spits H, de Vries J, Krangel M (1989): Diversity and organization of human T cell receptor delta variable gene segments. *J Exp Med* 169:41–57.

Huck S, Lefranc MP (1987): Rearrangements to the JP1, JP and JP2 segments in the human T-cell rearranging gamma gene (TRG) locus. *FEBS Lett* 224:291–295.

Huck S, Dariavach P, Lefranc MP (1988): Variable region genes in the human T-cell rearranging gamma (TRG) locus: V-J junction and homology with the mouse genes. *EMBO J* 7:719–726.

Kamps M, Murre C, Sun X, Baltimore D (1990): A new homeobox gene contributes the DNA binding domain of the t(1;19) translocation protein in pre-B ALL. *Cell* 60:547–555.

Lafaille J, DeCloux A, Bonneville M, Takagaki Y, Tonegawa S (1989): Junctional sequences of T cell receptor gd genes: Implications for γδ T cell lineages and for a novel intermediate of V(D)J joining. *Cell* 59:859–870.

Lefranc MP, Rabbits TH (1985): Two tandemly organized human genes encoding the T-cell constant region sequences show multiple rearrangement in different T-cell types. *Nature (London)* 316:464–466.

Lefranc MP, Forster A, Baer R, Stinson M, Rabbitts TH (1986a). Diversity and rearrangement of the human T cell rearranging gamma genes: Nine germ-line variable genes belonging to two subgroups. *Cell* 45:237–246.

Lefranc MP, Forster A, Rabbitts T (1986b): Rearrangement of two distinct T-cell gamma chain variable region genes in human DNA. *Nature (London)* 319:420–422.

Loh EY, Cwirla S, Serafini AT, Philips JH, Lanier LL (1988): Human T-cell receptor δ chain: Genomic organization, diversity and expression in populations of cells. *Proc Natl Acad Sci USA* 85:9714–9718.

Loiseau P, Guglielmi P, Le Paslier D, Macintyre E, Gessain A, Bories J, Flandrin G, Chen Z, Sigaux F (1989): Rearrangements of the T cell receptor δ gene in T acute lymphoblastic leukemia cells are distinct from those occurring in B lineage acute lymphoblastic leukemia and preferentially involve one Vδ gene segment. *J Immunol* 142:3305–3311.

Macintyre E, d'Auriol L, Amesland F, Loiseau P, Chen Z, Boumsell L, Galibert F, Sigaux F (1989): Analysis of junctional diversity in the preferential Vδ1-Jδ1 rearrangement of fresh T-acute lymphoblastic leukemia cells by in vitro gene amplification and direct sequencing. *Blood* 74:2053–2061.

Macintyre E, d'Auriol L, Duparc N, Leverger G, Galibert F, Sigaux F (1990): Use of oligonucleotide probes directed against T cell antigen receptor gamma delta variable-(diversity)-joining junctional sequences as a general method for detecting minimal residual disease in acute lymphoblastic leukemias. *J Clin Invest* 86:2125–2135.

McVay L, Carding S, Bottomly K, Hayday A (1991): Regulated expression and structure of T cell receptor γ/δ transcripts in human thymic ontogeny. *EMBO J* 10:83–91.

Neale G, Menarguez J, Kitchingman G, Fitzgerald T, Koehler M, Mirro J, Goorha R (1991): Detection of minimal residual disease in T-cell acute lymphoblastic leukemia using polymerase chain reaction predicts impending relapse. *Blood* 78:739–747.

Nizet Y, Martiat P, Vaerman J, Philippe M, Wildmann C, Staelens J, Cornu G (1991): Follow-up residual disease (MRD) in B lineage acute leukaemias using a simplified PCR strategy: Evolution of MRD rather than its detection is correlated with clinical outcome. *Br J Haematol* 79:205–210.

Nourse J, Mellentin J, Galili N, Wilkinson J, Stanbridge E, Smith S, Cleary M (1990): Chromosomal translocation t(1;19) results in synthesis of a homeobox fusion mRNA that codes for a potential chimeric transcription factor. *Cell* 60:161–171.

Potter M (1992): The detection of minimal residual disease in acute lymphoblastic leukaemia. *Blood Rev* 6:68–82.

Schatz D (1992): V(D)J recombination: Molecular biology and regulation. *Annu Rev Immunol* 10:359–383.

Takiyara Y, Tkachuk E, Michalopulos E, Champagne E, Reiman J, Minden M, Mak T (1988): Sequence and organization of the diversity, joining and constant region genes of the human T-cell δ chain locus. *Proc Natl Acad Sci USA* 85:6097–6101.

Takiyara Y, Reiman J, Michalopoulos E, Ciccone E, Moretta L, Mak T (1989): Diversity and structure of human T cell receptor δ chain genes in peripheral blood γδ bearing T lymphocytes. *J Exp Med* 169:393–406.

Tkachuk D, Kohler S, Cleary M (1992): Involvement of an homolog of Drosophila trithorax by 11q23 chromosomal translocations in acute leukemias. *Cell* 71:691–700.

Tycko B, Palmer JD, Link MP, Smith SD, Sklar J (1989): Polymerase chain reaction amplification of rearranged antigen receptor genes: Possible application for detection of minimal residual disease in acute lymphoblastic leukemia. In *Molecular Diagnosis of Human Cancer*. Cold Spring Harbor: Cold Spring Harbor Laboratory Press.

Van Dongen J, Breit T, Adriaansen H, Beishuizen A, Hooijkaas H (1992): Detection of minimal residual disease in acute leukemia by immunological marker analysis and polymerase chain reaction. *Leukemia* 6 (suppl 1):47–59.

Veelken H, Tycko B, Sklar J (1991): Sensitive detection of clonal receptor gene rearrangements for the diagnosis and monitoring of lymphoid neoplasms by a polymerase chain reaction-mediated ribonuclease protection assay. *Blood* 78:1318–1326.

Wasserman R, Galili N, Ito Y, Silber J, Reichard B, Shane S, Womer R, Lange B, Rovera G (1992a): Residual disease at the end of induction therapy as a predictor of relapse during therapy in childhood B-lineage acute lymphoblastic leukemia. *J Clin Oncol* 10:1879–1888.

Wasserman R, Yamada M, Ito Y, Finger L, Reichard B, Shane S, Lange B, Rovera G (1992b): V_H gene rearrangement events can modify the immunoglobulin heavy chain during progression of B-lineage acute lymphoblastic leukemia. *Blood* 79:223–228.

Yamada M, Hudson S, Tournay O, Bittenbender S, Shane S, Lange B, Tsujimoto Y, Caton A, Rovera G (1989): Detection of minimal disease in hematopoietic malignancies of the B-cell lineage by using third-complementarity-determining region (CDR-III)-specific probes. *Proc Natl Acad Sci USA* 86:5123–5127.

Yamada M, Wasserman R, Lange B, Reichard B, Womer R, Rovera G (1990): Minimal residual disease in childhood B-lineage lymphoblastic leukemia: Persistence of leukemic cells during the first 18 months of treatment. *N Engl J Med* 323:448–455.

Yokota S, Hansen-Hagge T, Ludwig W, Reiter A, Raghavachar A, Kleihauer E, Bartram C (1991): Use of polymerase chain reactions to monitor minimal residuals disease in acute lymphoblastic leukemia patients. *Blood* 77:331–339.

29

Assessment of Therapy Effectiveness: Infectious Disease

Salvatore J. Arrigo

Introduction

The ability of the polymerase chain reaction (PCR) to quantitatively detect both RNA and DNA at the single copy level has exponentially amplified our ability to examine low level molecular events using limited amounts of sample. Nucleic acids that were previously undetectable can now be examined using only minute amounts of material. One obvious utilization of this technique is the detection of RNA and DNA species that are specific to an infectious organism. In this way, diagnosis of the presence of a disease-causing organism can be rapidly and conclusively determined. Beyond determining the presence of an organism, the amount of nucleic acids specific for this infectious agent can be quantitated to assess the level of infection, replication, and expression by this organism. Thus, PCR allows the analysis, at the molecular level, of the progression of infectious diseases *in vivo*.

An example of an infectious disease that is readily detected by PCR is acquired immune deficiency syndrome (AIDS), for which the etiological agent is human immunodeficiency

virus type 1 (HIV-1) (Barre et al., 1983; Broder and Gallo, 1984; Gallo et al., 1984; Levy et al., 1984; Popovic et al., 1984). The replication of this virus within the immune system leads to a devastation of immune function by both direct and indirect mechanisms (for review see Levy, 1993). Therefore detection of the virus and assessment of its replication over time provide an excellent marker for disease progression. Since this virus employs both DNA and RNA as intermediates in its replication process, both of these nucleic acids are available as substrates for detection using PCR. Infection with HIV-1 will be discussed as a model system in this chapter to examine the use of PCR in the assessment of therapy effectiveness and disease progression.

Alternatives to PCR

To assess therapy effectiveness, an accurate calculation of the extent of viral infection and the level of viral replication must be made. Alternate methods to PCR for the detection of HIV-1 involve direct detection of viral proteins, screening for antibodies produced

The Polymerase Chain Reaction
K.B. Mullis, F. Ferré, R.A. Gibbs, editors
© 1994 Birkhauser Boston

against the virus by the infected individual, or coculture of infected patient serum with susceptible cells and subsequent amplification of the virus *in vitro* (Allain et al., 1986; Brun et al., 1984; Goudsmit et al., 1986; Ho et al., 1989; Kalyanaraman et al., 1984; Salahuddin et al., 1985; Sarngadharan et al., 1984). Direct detection of viral proteins is successful only in a small number of infected individuals and therefore would be of use only in those patients that exhibit high enough levels to allow for a measurable decrease in this level after commencement of therapy. Screening for antibody production in infected individuals is a reasonably accurate method for detection of the presence of virus, but due to the fact that it does not directly measure virus, does not allow for a quantitative analysis of viral load over time. Therefore, this technique of virus detection would be of only limited value in assessing a given therapy. Coculture is an extremely sensitive method of viral detection. This method is important in assessing the infectious nature of any virus in the serum, as well as within a particular cell type. However, due to stimulation of infected cells, even latent virus within cells may be induced to replicate in this assay system, giving an inaccurate assessment of viral replication within the patient. This method involves substantial expense and involves a considerable waiting period before results are obtained. Additionally, quantitation of virus by this method is difficult, of indeterminate accuracy, and costly. Since only the final product of successful viral replication is measured, no insight can be gained by this method into the specific stage at which replication might be blocked by a given therapy. None of the above methods is capable of determining the immediate effect of a given therapy on an HIV-1 gene expression. Therefore, although the above methods might be well suited for the diagnosis of most cases of HIV-1 infection, a more powerful approach is necessary to more accurately assess the effectiveness of disease therapy in an infected individual over an extended period of time.

PCR to Assess Therapy Effectiveness

PCR provides an excellent method with which to analyze the extent to which a certain therapy is effective, by allowing a direct analysis of HIV-1 RNA and DNA levels within a given individual. Using a variety of techniques to separate cell populations and serum, assessment of the extent of viral infection, type of cells infected, amount of extracellular virus, level of viral transcription, and extent of processing of the various viral RNAs are all possible using only a small sample of material from the infected individual. At present, a large number of drugs are being developed that interfere with various stages in the virus life cycle (Palca, 1991). The multiple steps involved in the HIV-1 life cycle offer a large spectrum of molecular events that might serve as targets for therapy. These include viral binding, entry, uncoating, reverse transcription, nuclear migration, integration, transcription, RNA processing, RNA transport, translation/protein processing, assembly, and budding. A schematic representation of these steps in the HIV-1 life cycle is shown in Figure 29.1. The drugs that might serve in potential therapies include reverse transcriptase inhibitors, protease inhibitors, myristolation inhibitors, and other inhibitors that block the replication of HIV-1. Presumably all effective therapies for AIDS will involve inhibition of HIV-1 viral replication, either through specific killing of infected cells or inhibition of a specific viral protein function. Therefore, potential therapies against HIV-1 infection might be directed against the Gag, Pol, Env, Tat, Rev, Vif, Vpr, Vpu, or Nef proteins of HIV-1. Additional therapies might also be directed against the viral RNA or DNA species in order to prevent the expression of various HIV-1 proteins. Each of the HIV-1 protein functions will be addressed separately, in terms of potential inhibitors of these functions and the analysis of the effects of these inhibitors *in vivo*. The extent to which a given therapy, directed against one or more viral functions, can potentially be assayed by PCR will be discussed.

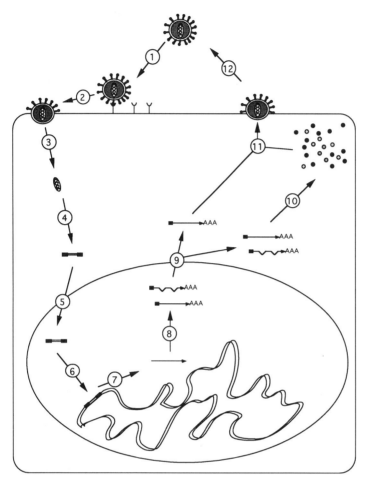

FIGURE 29.1. Schematic representation of HIV-1 life cycle. The nuclear and cytoplasmic subcellular compartments are shown. The following steps involved in the replication of HIV-1 are shown: (1) Binding of the virus to the cell; (2) entry of the virus into the cell; (3) uncoating of the virus; (4) reverse transcription of the viral RNA into a double-stranded DNA copy; (5) migration of the viral DNA to the nucleus; (6) integration of the viral DNA into the host chromosome to form the provirus; (7) transcription of a viral primary RNA transcript; (8) processing of this RNA; (9) transport of the RNA from the nucleus to the cytoplasm; (10) translation of mRNA into protein and processing of these proteins; (11) assembly of viral proteins with genomic viral RNA. Release of infectious virus. For simplicity, these steps are represented as independent functions, although coupling may exist between them.

Specific Cell Killing

Since cells infected by HIV-1 should express viral proteins on their surfaces and may also exhibit variations in normal responses to extracellular factors, specific targeting of infected cells may prove to be a reasonable therapy for HIV-1 infection at early stages in the infection. The targeting of infected cells by an interleukin-2 (IL-2) receptor-specific cytotoxin (Finberg et al., 1991) has recently been demonstrated to be effective at selective cell killing of infected cells *in vitro*. The use of such cytotoxin *in vivo*, by selectively killing infected cells, should theoretically reduce the total levels of both intracellular HIV-1 RNA and DNA in the infected individual. Analysis of these levels could be accomplished using whole blood or specific cell fractions (such as CD4-positive lymphocytes). PCR could be used on samples taken from a patient before and during treatment to determine whether a reduction in HIV-1 specific RNA or DNA is detectable. Concurrent cell counting of various lymphoid cell types would determine the extent of any cell death of specific and nonspecific cell types. Since RNA is present as the genetic material in free virions, these patients could be examined further for the amount of free virus in the serum by PCR for genomic HIV-1 RNA. Any substantial reduction in the viral DNA and RNA copy number within an individual in the absence of any extraneous cell death would be considered a promising aspect of that therapy. In the particular case mentioned above, since cells that express high affinity IL-2 receptors are killed, it may also be possible to use PCR to examine the level of IL-2 receptor RNA within a given cell population. After therapy has commenced, one would expect a reduction in the level of IL-2 receptor RNA being produced in T cells and monocytes. Any therapies directed against other cellular products that are elevated by HIV-1 infection could potentially be monitored in a similar fashion.

Gag

The Gag proteins of HIV-1 assemble to form the internal structural core of the virus. These proteins are produced at high levels during a viral infection and antibodies raised against them are common in the serum of infected individuals. These proteins are translated as a 55-kDa precursor molecule that is subsequently cleaved by a viral protease, encoded by the *pol* gene, into mature viral proteins (step 10 of Fig. 29.1). Multimers of these mature proteins are assembled into a virion core particle (step 11 of Fig. 29.1). One potential therapy involves the use of transdominant Gag mutants to block the infectious assembly of the virus. Several mutants of the Gag proteins have been demonstrated to be capable of interfering *in trans* with the production of infectious virus *in vitro* (Trono et al., 1989). Presumably these mutants interfere with the normal assembly of the viral core particle by creating mixed multimers of wild-type and mutant proteins (at step 11 in Fig. 29.1). These mutated Gag proteins would presumably be administered as synthetic peptides that would be incorporated into the assembly of the virus and block subsequent steps in the process. To assess the effectiveness of such inhibitors in an infected individual, PCR could be used to examine the level of HIV-1 infection by determining the number of permissive cells that are infected. Quantitative PCR specific for HIV-1 DNA, as well as a cellular DNA control, could be used to determine whether the percent of infected cells was increasing or decreasing over time. If viral assembly were blocked, no increase in the number of infected cells should occur. If cell death affects those cells that were previously infected, then a decrease in the number of infected cells should occur. Examination of the level of free virus in the serum by PCR of HIV-1 RNA might not give an accurate estimation of infectious virus production, since non-

infectious virus particles might still be shed from infected cells. These particles might contain viral RNA that could not be discriminated from the RNA of infectious virus. However, if a concomitant assay of the serum by coculture is performed, the infectivity of these particles could be ascertained by comparison of the number of infectious units to the amount of RNA. Any difference in the level of free infectious virus in the serum would be considered a promising aspect of this therapy. Utilizing a combination of PCR and other standard techniques, a reasonable idea of the promise of such a therapy would be forthcoming.

Pol

The *pol* gene of HIV-1 encodes reverse transcriptase, RNase H, integrase, and protease proteins. Each of these functions offers an attractive prospect for drug therapy (steps 4, 6, and 10 in Fig. 29.1). The *pol* gene is translated as a 160-kDa gag–pol fusion protein that is cleaved by the HIV-1-encoded protease. The reverse transcriptase function of the *pol* gene creates a cDNA copy from the RNA genome of the virus. Presently, various nucleoside analogs, such as azidodideoxythimidine (AZT), dideoxyinosine (ddI), and dideoxycytosine are being employed as substrates for the reverse transcriptase due to the high affinity of the enzyme for this substrate and the low affinity of host DNA polymerases. By interfering with the production of proviral DNA from genomic RNA, specific inhibition of all subsequent steps in viral replication is achieved. The proviral copy number in peripheral blood mononuclear cells of AIDS patients undergoing therapy with AZT or ddI has been examined using quantitative PCR (Aoki et al., 1990; Donovan et al., 1991). However, these studies came to different conclusions about the efficacy of nucleoside inhibitors in reducing proviral copy numbers in these cells. The use of chain terminating nucleoside analogs should result in the appearance of aborted reverse transcripts within newly infected cells. It may be possible to use PCR to detect these transcripts by determining the ratio of nascent short transcripts to full length transcripts, using PCR primers specific for various steps in the reverse transcription process. Primers have been successfully used *in vitro* to examine these steps and have demonstrated that AZT does not block the initiation of reverse transcription, but does block the extension of the DNA to a full-length copy of proviral DNA (Zack et al., 1990). Inhibition of the RNase H function would lead to aborted transcripts that might also be detected by this method. Inhibitors of the integrase function of pol would lead to an increase in the ratio of unintegrated to integrated viral DNA and it may be possible to use PCR to detect this difference by PCR analysis of high- and low-molecular-weight fractions. This approach has been previously used successfully with both brain and blood samples from AIDS patients (Bukrinsky et al., 1991; Pang et al., 1990).

Another potential way to interfere with viral replication is the use of specific inhibitors of the HIV-1 protease (for review see Huff, 1991). These inhibitors interact directly with the protease and inactivate cleavage of the Gag and Gag–Pol precursor molecules, interfering with production of infectious virus at a step near the end of the virus life cycle. Without cleavage of the precursor molecules, infectious viral particles would not be assembled. Blocking this function, or any of the other pol functions, should lead to a decrease in virus production. This decrease could most readily be detected by analysis of free virus by PCR for genomic viral RNA in the serum. With all types of pol inhibitors, PCR could be used to determine the percent of infected permissible cells by examining the level of HIV-1 DNA. One could also use PCR to detect changes in the ratio of HIV-1 DNA to RNA with the protease inhibitors. Since the reverse transcriptase function of the virus is affected by these inhibitors, as well as the production of functional gag proteins, one would expect that the level of HIV-1 DNA found in permissive cells should not increase; however, the level of total intracellular HIV-1 RNA might increase due to a reduction of packaging (and hence release) of the virus. This might result in a decrease in the HIV-1 DNA:RNA ratio in the treated individual. The effect of cell death should not affect this ratio, although any reduction in the stability of HIV-1 RNAs or production of noninfectious RNA-containing particles in the absence of functional Gag proteins might increase this ratio and interfere with interpretation. One might also expect a decrease in the ratio of extracellular to intracellular genomic RNA due to inefficiency of packaging of the virus, which could be assayed by PCR.

Env

The Env proteins of HIV-1 provide the outer envelope of the virus necessary for attachment and entry into the host cell (steps 1 and 2 in Fig. 29.1). Since the entry of the virus into a cell is mediated through the CD4 receptor, various compounds that interfere with the binding of the virus to this receptor might prove successful in decreasing the spread of the virus. Also, since CD4 does not seem to be sufficient for infection of all cell-types by all HIV-1 strains, it may be feasible to block viral entry at a level independent of CD4 binding (Liu et at., 1990; O'Brien et al., 1990). The binding of the virus to a target cell could be inhibited by a direct interaction with the virus, such as a neutralizing antibody, or by an indirect interaction with cellular receptors for the virus. Certainly, a direct interaction provides much more specificity than an indirect one and therefore a therapy directed against the virus itself is much more likely to be successful. Passive immunization of symptomatic patients with hyperimmune plasma from asymptomatic patients has been attempted as a therapy in order to provide neutralizing antibodies to the virus (Karpas et al., 1990). Since env is present on the outside of the virus, this therapy presumably acts by interactions with env. In this case PCR of HIV-1 DNA and RNA analysis has shown that the level of extracellular virus was reduced to an undetectable level. Other similar therapies could similarly be examined by PCR for the percent of infected cells and the level of extracellular virus to determine any change in the infected cell population and virus production. A compound that interferes with the binding of HIV-1 to a cell may actually ' increase the amount of extracellular virus in the serum.

Any compounds that interfere with internalization of virus that has bound to infectible cells might result in an increase in virus on the surface of cells. It might be possible to measure this level by proteolitically treating isolated cells and preparing RNA from the released and cell associated fractions. PCR analysis of these fractions might reveal an increase in the ratio of this externally bound to intracellular genomic RNA or an increase in the total level of externally bound RNA after commencement of therapy with this compound.

Tat

The Tat protein of HIV-1 is required for high levels of HIV-1 LTR-driven gene expression (Rosen et al., 1986a,b). Tat acts through binding to a stem–loop structure, TAR, located within the leader sequence of all HIV-1 RNAs to increase transcription and translation (steps 7 and 10 in Fig. 29.1) of these RNAs (Hauber and Cullen, 1988; Cullen, 1986). The effect of this protein on gene expression appears to be many orders of magnitude and consequently this protein is absolutely required for viral replication (Dayton et al., 1986). Compounds that interfere with the Tat protein could have very large effects on viral replication. One such compound is RO 24-7429, which apparently interferes with the ability of Tat to bind RNA (Palca, 1991). Since these effects would result in decreases in gene expression, PCR analysis of the ratio of intracellular RNA to DNA should indicate a decrease in this ratio in patients receiving these compounds. Analysis of the total level of HIV-1 RNA over the period of treatment with these compounds should also demonstrate a reduction in the level of this RNA. The level of extracellular virus should also be decreased with these compounds and could be detected by PCR for genomic viral RNA. Due to the large effects of this protein on RNA production, the success of a particular compound directed against the Tat protein should be apparent soon after it is administered.

Rev

The Rev protein of HIV-1 is another transactivator protein of HIV-1, absolutely required for HIV-1 replication (Feinberg et al., 1986; Sodroski et al., 1986). This protein is necessary for the expression of HIV-1 Gag, Pol, and Env proteins. It appears to act to regulate the ratio of unspliced to completely spliced RNA (Emerman et al., 1989; Hadzopoulou et al., 1989; Hammarskjold et al., 1989; Malim et al., 1988, 1989; Sadaie et al., 1988; Arrigo et al., 1989) and to be necessary for the translation of unspliced and partially spliced RNAs (Arrigo and Chen, 1991). Compounds targeted against this protein should demonstrate effects on the ratio of full-length *gag/pol* RNA to the completely spliced RNAs that code for Tat, Rev, and Nef. PCR analysis of the intracellular cellular RNA levels of specific RNAs should show a change in this ratio, demonstrating an increase in the completely spliced RNAs and a decrease in the accumulation of *gag/pol* RNA. Similarly, the amount of extracellular genomic viral RNA should be reduced. Due to the inherent liability of RNA, these effects should be observable soon after treatment has commenced.

Other Potential Therapies

Other therapies against Vif or Vpu proteins, both of which affect the production of infectious virus, could be assessed by previously described techniques. Therapies against nef or vpr proteins are difficult to discuss due to the uncertain nature of the function of these proteins. It is also feasible to design therapies against the DNA or RNA constituents of the virus. For example, antisense RNA or ribozymes could be used to interfere with protein expression from specific HIV-1 RNAs (Sarver et al., 1990; Vickers et al., 1991). In these cases, previously described techniques for the detection of viral replication would also be applicable, dependent on the gene function(s) affected by the therapy. The use of antisense RNA or ribozymes would further allow their detection by PCR. By analysis of the specific uptake of these therapeutic nucleic acids, the delivery of these agents to individual cell types can be directly assessed. The ability to trace the delivery of a compound at the level of a single molecule potentially might even be exploited to allow tagging of compounds with a stable nucleic acid moiety that could subsequently be followed by PCR.

Feasability of Detection by PCR

Detection of DNA

The feasibility of these applications of PCR to the detection of viral DNA depends on many criteria. The number of initially infected cells will affect the detection of nucleic acids at all subsequent times after commencement of disease therapy. The sample size must be large enough to allow for the detection of a reasonable number of copies of HIV-1 DNA both before and during therapy. The sensitivity of the specific PCR protocol will determine what constitutes a reasonable number of molecules of HIV-1 DNA. PCR has been used in the analysis of HIV-1 DNA in patient samples of peripheral blood, cerebrospinal fluid, brain tissue, saliva, skin, feces, and fetal tissue (Courgnaud et al., 1991; Goto et al., 1991; Kanitakis et al., 1991; Mano et al., 1991; Pang et al., 1990; Simmonds et al., 1990; Sonnerborg et al., 1991; Weintrub et al., 1991; Yolken et al., 1991; Young et al., 1990). Using PCR it has been demonstrated that detection of HIV-1 DNA in peripheral blood of seropositive individuals approaches 100%. Since the quantitative analysis of as few as 10 copies of HIV-1 DNA has previously been demonstrated (Ferre et al., 1992; Zack et al., 1990), detection of single copies of proviral DNA seems to be a realistic goal. Reproducible detection of single copies of proviral DNA by varying the number of cells that are harvested such that DNA from only a single infected cell is assayed has also been demonstrated (Bukrinsky et al., 1991). Although not strictly a quantitative PCR protocol, quantitative assessments of proviral copy number can be made using this type of approach. Since quantitative analysis of proviral DNA by PCR has been performed in the range

of single copies of DNA, it seems likely that if a large enough number of cells are examined, a precise measurement of the proviral copy number can be made. The collection of samples must be sufficient for examination, but not hazardous to the patient. Therefore, the easiest procedure would involve the collection of a small blood sample from the patient and separation of the sample into various cell fractions. Since lymphocytes seem to contain approximately one copy of HIV-1 DNA for each 1000 cells in infected individuals at late stages in the disease and these numbers agree well with the number of cells harboring infectious virus (Ho et al., 1989), quantitative analysis of HIV-1 DNA in lymphocytes should be potentially straightforward using a relatively small draw of blood. Up to two million cell equivalents of DNA have been used in a single PCR (Lee et al., 1991a). Purification of CD4 positive T-lymphocytes would increase the proviral copy number for a given number of cells (or amount of DNA) (Hsia et al., 1991). Since one would be initially examining hundreds or thousands of copies of HIV-1 DNA, any reduction in this number after commencement of drug therapy should be readily apparent.

Evaluation of the DNA copy number in asymptomatic infected individuals is more difficult since one is dealing with levels of viral DNA that are 10–100 times lower than in symptomatic patients. In these patients, the sensitivity of the PCR would need to be such that as little as one copy of HIV-1 DNA could be quantitatively detected. The quantitive aspects of PCR would need to be optimized so that as little as 2-fold difference in copy number could be detected in order to accurately judge reductions in proviral copy number. The inclusion of a control for a cellular gene would need to be included to provide an internal control for the amount of DNA in each sample (Lee et al., 1991b). Obviously, with individuals who only have low levels of proviral DNA this reduction may put the level of DNA below the detection limit. The easiest use of PCR would be to assess the ability of a given therapy to halt the progression of the disease at some point before the induction of high levels of proviral DNA and retain the lower levels found in the asymptomatic patient. Within these constraints, the analysis of HIV-1 copy number over time, in a given individual, should be achieved. This copy number could be expressed in terms of the number of CD4 positive or total lymphocytes. Many reports have attempted to express HIV-1 viral load in precisely these terms with numbers ranging from 1 in 10 to 1 in 26,000 (Brinchmann et al., 1991; Hsia and Spector, 1991; Jurriaans et al., 1992; Poznansky et al., 1991; Schnittman et al., 1989). Consequently, the effectiveness of disease therapy in decreasing the number of proviral genomes present in a patient might be assessed using PCR.

Detection of RNA

Over the last few years quantitative RNA PCR has been developed to detect low abundance RNAs in a variety of systems, although its use has not been as widespread as that of DNA PCR (Arrigo and Chen, 1991; Arrigo et al., 1989, 1990; Becker and Hahlbrock, 1989; Cann et al., 1990; Funk and FitzGerald, 1991; Gilliland et al., 1990; Henco and Heibey, 1990; Wang et al., 1989). The feasibility of employing PCR in the assessment of the effect of treatment on the level of viral RNA is more complex than the application of DNA PCR. Theoretically, each intact copy of HIV-1 DNA is capable of producing many copies of HIV-1 RNA. These RNA copies may be apparent as multiple spliced or unspliced species of RNA. Therefore, the choice of PCR primers affects the copy number and species of RNA that are detected. Additionally, a proviral DNA molecule may exist in a latent state in which no RNA or only a few species of RNA are produced. In these cells, proviral DNA may be found in the absence of detectable RNA.

The most difficult problem to overcome in the detection of viral RNA is the inherent instability of RNA and the additional step required to convert RNA into cDNA for PCR analysis. Any degradation of the RNA or an efficiency of less than 100% in the reverse transcription process will provide less substrate in the PCR analysis. Degradation of the RNA should be avoidable through the use of RNase-free reagents and strong denaturants during the preparation of RNA. The efficiency of the reverse transcription process can be optimized in many ways. The primers for PCR should be chosen so that the reverse transcriptase will have to traverse the shortest distance possible to generate a product that can be detected by PCR. This fragment of the RNA should not contain any complex secondary structure that might interfere with the procession of the reverse transcriptase. Different reverse transcriptase preparations and temperatures of extension should be attempted to optimize cDNA production. The extent of time of reverse transcription can also be altered. Various salt and pH conditions may also affect the amount of product. This maximization of PCR signal would be best accomplished with *in vitro* synthesized RNA that can be quantitated such that the lower limit of detection can be determined in terms of precise numbers of RNA molecules. This would necessitate cloning of cDNAs for each RNA that was to be examined, however, this could readily be accomplished by cloning of the PCR products specific for these RNAs. These RNA standards could then be used in the direct quantitation of that specific viral RNA from patient samples to provide an accurate estimation of the number of copies of that RNA before and during therapy.

The additional limitations imposed on PCR analysis of viral DNA from infected individuals, such as sample size and the number of infected cells, also apply to the detection of RNA from these individuals. Since the sample obtained from symptomatic patients should contain an average of 100–1000 infected cells, analysis of the production of RNA from these cells should potentially be feasible. Although the detection of HIV-1 RNA in patient samples has not yet been optimized to the extent that the detection of HIV-1 DNA has been, specific viral RNA has been detected in the majority of infected patients by PCR (Schnittman et al., 1991). Additionally, *in situ* hybridization experiments have shown that less than 1 in 10,000 cells from symptomatic patients are positive for HIV-1 RNA and that the RNA is expressed at 20–300 copies per cell (Harper et al., 1986). If 100,000 cell equivalents of RNA from these patients are assayed using PCR, 200–3000 copies of RNA should be available as substrate. This seems to be a reasonable number of copies for quantitative detection since less than 100 copies of specific RNA have been previously detected by quantitative RNA PCR (Becker and Hahlbrock, 1989; Cann et al., 1990). The analysis of RNA from asymptomatic patients will be more difficult since there may be 10–100 times less RNA as substrate. In certain asymptomatic patients, the analysis of RNA may be below the limits of detection. However the inability to detect RNA in an infected individual over time may prove to be an excellent indication of the success of a particular therapy. As can be done with PCR for HIV-1 DNA, standardization of results can be accomplished by the inclusion of an internal standard in the reaction (Becker and Hahlbrock, 1989; Funk and FitzGerald, 1991; Gilliland et al., 1990; Wang et al., 1989; Henco and Heibey, 1990). Recent quantitative PCR analysis of RNA from infected patients supports the utility of RNA PCR detection as a useful tool in the assessment of therapy effectiveness (Menzo et al., 1992).

The analysis of extracellular virus from infected individuals will be subject to many of the same problems as the detection of intracellular RNA. However, if these problems can be overcome, PCR analysis of genomic HIV-1 RNA should provide a relatively good guide as to the extent of virus replication in an individual. One potential problem with this type of analysis might be the extremely low levels of free virus at any given point in time. In infected individuals, the level of infectious virus has been shown to average 30 to greater than 3000 tissue culture infectious particle per millimeter of serum (Ho et al., 1989). If one includes the number of noninfectious particles containing viral RNA, a reasonable number of RNA molecules should be present in a relatively small sample of blood from most infected individuals to allow a quantitative assessment of RNA copy number before and during therapy. Recent accomplishments in the absolute quantitation of HIV-1 viral RNAs in infected patients has demonstrated the feasibility of this approach (Menzo et al., 1992) as well as demonstrating a significant decrease in the level of HIV-1 RNA in viral particles from patients undergoing ddI therapy (Aoki et al., 1992). Although the detection of viral RNA in the serum does not directly measure the level of infectious virus, this can be determined by alternate methods as mentioned previously.

Summary

PCR has opened up new realms of experimentation in the area of infectious disease. Not only has the detection of infectious organisms been improved, but the progression of disease caused by that organism can be followed and quantitated in precise terms of the level of replication of that organism. Organisms that have been historically difficult to detect can now be detected in a very short period of time with unrivaled sensitivity. This potentially allows for improvements in the way that therapies against these organisms are assessed. The immediate effect of a specific compound on specific functions of the virus can be detected and quantitated at the molecular level. If a compound is not providing the desired effect *in vivo*, a quick decision can be made to discontinue the therapy or to attempt an alternate one. The analysis of the levels RNA and DNA specific for that organism allows for direct examination of the molecular events responsible for its replication. In this way, a more complete understanding of the direct effects of a compound on the organism can be elucidated. The ability to perform this analysis with limited amounts of patient material permits the repeated examination of a patient's response to a given therapy over time.

Whether or not PCR becomes a standard method in the assessment of disease therapy depends on a large number of unknown parameters. Certain improvements in the present technology will certainly aid in this goal. Enhancement of the sensitivity as well as quantitative aspects of PCR will contribute to its widespread use. The use of nonisotopic detection methods, improved methods for sample preparation, and simplification of the number of manipulations involved in PCR, in particular RNA PCR, will allow for a more general use in a clinical setting. Certainly, PCR is already being successfully used to examine the presence of HIV-1 RNA and DNA in patients undergoing various anti-HIV-1 therapies (Aoki et al., 1990, 1992; Boucher et al., 1992; Donovan et al., 1991; Edlin et al., 1992; Karpas et al., 1990; Larder et al., 1991; Richman et al., 1991; Saag et al., 1991; Wahlberg et al., 1992). Judging from these results, and due to the lack of comparable alternatives, PCR will likely be used in the evaluation of many future therapies designed against infectious organisms. The precise limits to which PCR can be pushed will likely become clear within the next few years. If PCR can be performed easily and quantitatively at the level of single copies of RNA and DNA, it will undoubtably become the obvious choice for the testing of various therapies against infectious agents.

References

Allain JP, Laurian Y, Paul DA, Senn D (1986): Serological markers in early stages of human immunodeficiency virus infection in haemophiliacs. *Lancet* 2(8518):1233–1236.

Aoki S, Yarchoan R, Thomas RV, Pluda JM, Marczyk K, Broder S, Mitsuya H (1990): Quantitative analysis of HIV-1 proviral DNA in peripheral blood mononuclear cells from patients with AIDS or ARC: Decrease of proviral DNA content following treatment with 2′,3′-dideoxyinosine (ddI). *Aids Res Hum Retrovirus* 6(11):1331–1339.

Aoki SS, Yarchoan R, Kageyama S, Hoekzema DT, Pluda JM, Wyvill KM, Broder S, Mitsuya H (1992): Plasma HIV-1 viremia in HIV-1 infected individuals assessed by polymerase chain reaction. *Aids Res Hum Retrovirus* 8(7):1263–1270.

Arrigo SJ, Chen ISY (1991): Rev is necessary for translation but not cytoplasmic accumulation of HIV-1 vif, vpr, and env/vpu-2 RNAs. *Genes Dev* 5(5):808–819.

Arrigo SJ, Weitsman S, Rosenblatt JD, Chen IS (1989): Analysis of rev gene function on human immunodeficiency virus type 1 replication in lymphoid cells by using a quantitative polymerase chain reaction method. *J Virol* 63(11):4875–4881.

Arrigo SJ, Weitsman S, Zack JA, Chen IS (1990): Characterization and expression of novel singly spliced RNA species of human immunodeficiency virus type 1. *J Virol* 64(9):4585–4588.

Barre SF, Chermann JC, Rey F, Nugeyre MT, Chamaret S, Gruest J, Dauguet C, Axler BC, Vezinet BF, Rouzioux C, Rozenbaum W, Montagnier L (1983): Isolation of a T-lymphotropic retrovirus from a patient at risk for acquired immune deficiency syndrome (AIDS). *Science* 220(4599):868–871.

Becker AM, Hahlbrock K (1989): Absolute mRNA quantification using the polymerase chain reaction (PCR). A novel approach by a PCR aided transcript titration assay (PATTY). *Nucl Acids Res* 17(22):9436–9446.

Boucher CA, O'Sullivan E, Mulder JW, Ramautarsing C, Kellam P, Darby G, Lange JM, Goudsmit J, Larder BA (1992): Ordered appearance of zidovudine resistance mutations during treatment of 18 human immunodeficiency virus-positive subjects. *J Infect Dis* 165(1):105–110.

Brinchmann JE, Albert J, Vartdal F (1991): Few infected CD4 + T cells but a high proportion of replication-competent provirus copies in asymptomatic human immunodeficiency virus type 1 infection. *J Virol* 65(4):2019–2023.

Broder S, Gallo RC (1984): A pathogenic retrovirus (HTLV-III) linked to AIDS. *N Engl J Med* 311(20):1292–1297.

Brun VF, Rouzioux C, Montagnier L, Chamaret S, Gruest J, Barre SF, Geroldi D, Chermann JC, McCormick J, Mitchell S, et al. (1984): Prevalence of antibodies to lymphadenopathy-associated retrovirus in African patients with AIDS. *Science* 226(4673):453–456.

Bukrinsky MI, Stanwick TL, Dempsey MP, Stevenson M (1991): Quiescent T lymphocytes as an inducible virus reservoir in HIV-1 infection. *Science* 254(5030):423–427.

Cann AJ, Zack JA, Go AS, Arrigo SJ, Koyanagi Y, Green PL, Koyanagi Y, Pang S, Chen IS (1990): Human immunodeficiency virus type 1 T-cell tropism is determined by events prior to provirus formation. *J Virol* 64(10):4735–4742.

Courgnaud V, Laure F, Brossard A, Bignozzi C, Goudeau A, Barin F, Brechot C (1991): Frequent and early in utero HIV-1 infection. *Aids Res Hum Retrovirus* 7(3):337–341.

Cullen BR (1986): Trans-activation of human immunodeficiency virus occurs via a bimodal mechanism. *Cell* 46(7):973–982.

Dayton AI, Sodroski JG, Rosen CA, Goh WC, Haseltine WA (1986): The trans-activator gene of the human T cell lymphotropic virus type III is required for replication. *Cell* 44(6):941–947.

Donovan RM, Dickover RE, Goldstein E, Huth RG, Carlson JR (1991): HIV-1 proviral copy number in blood mononuclear cells from AIDS patients on zidovudine therapy. *J Acquir Immune Defic Syndr* 4(8):766–769.

Edlin BR, Weinstein RA, Whaling SM, Ou CY, Connolly PJ, Moore JL, Bitran JD (1992): Zidovudine-interferon-alpha combination therapy in patients with advanced human immunodeficiency virus type 1 infection: Biphasic response of p24 antigen and quantitative polymerase chain reaction. *J Infect Dis* 165(5):793–798.

Emerman M, Vazeux R, Peden K (1989): The rev gene product of the human immunodeficiency virus affects envelope-specific RNA localization. *Cell* 57(7):1155–1165.

Feinberg MB, Jarrett RF, Aldovini A, Gallo RC, Wong SF (1986): HTLV-III expression and production involve complex regulation at the levels of splicing and translation of viral RNA. *Cell* 46(6):807–817.

Ferre F, Marchese A, Duffy PC, Lewis DE, Wallace MR, Beecham HJ, Burnett KG, Jensen FC, Carlo DJ (1992): Quantitation of HIV viral burden by PCR in HIV seropositive Navy personnel representing Walter Reed stages 1 to 6. *Aids Res Hum Retrovirus* 8(2):269–275.

Finberg RW, Wahl SM, Allen JB, Soman G, Strom TB, Murphy JR, Nichols JC (1991): Selective elimination of HIV-1-infected cells with an interleukin-2 receptor specific cytotoxin. *Science* 252(5013):1703–1705.

Funk CD, FitzGerald GA (1991): Eicosanoid forming enzyme mRNA in human tissues. Analysis by quantitative polymerase chain reaction. *J Biol Chem* 266(19):12508–12513.

Gallo RC, Salahuddin SZ, Popovic M, Shearer GM, Kaplan M, Haynes BF, Palker TJ, Redfield R, Oleske J, Safai B, et al. (1984): Frequent detection and isolation of cytopathic retroviruses (HTLV-III) from patients with AIDS and at risk for AIDS. *Science* 224(4648):500–503.

Gilliland G, Perrin S, Blanchard K, Bunn HF (1990): Analysis of cytokine mRNA and DNA: Detection and quantitation by competitive polymerase chain reaction. *Proc Natl Acad Sci USA* 87(7):2725–2729.

Goto Y, Yeh CK, Notkins AL, Prabhakar BS (1991): Detection of proviral sequences in saliva of patients infected with human immunodeficiency virus type 1. *Aids Res Hum Retrovirus* 7(3):343–347.

Goudsmit J, de WF, Paul DA, Epstein LG, Lange JM, Krone WJ, Speelman H, Wolters EC, Van dNJ, Oleske JM, et al. (1986): Expression of human immunodeficiency virus antigen (HIV-Ag) in serum and cerebrospinal fluid during acute and chronic infection. *Lancet* 2(8500):177–180.

Hadzopoulou CM, Felber BK, Cladaras C, Athanassopoulos A, Tse A, Pavlakis GN (1989): The rev (trs/art) protein of human immunodeficiency virus type 1 affects viral mRNA and protein expression via a cis-acting sequence in the env region. *J Virol* 63(3):1265–1274.

Hammarskjold ML, Heimer J, Hammarskjold B, Sangwan I, Albert L, Rekosh D (1989): Regulation of human immunodeficiency virus env expression by the rev gene product. *J Virol* 63(5):1959–1966.

Harper ME, Marselle LM, Gallo RC, Wong SF (1986): Detection of lymphocytes expressing human T-lymphotropic virus type III in lymph nodes and peripheral blood from infected individuals by in situ hybridization. *Proc Natl Acad Sci USA* 83(3):772–776.

Hauber J, Cullen BR (1988): Mutational analysis of the trans-activation-responsive region of the human immunodeficiency virus type I long terminal repeat. *J Virol* 62(3):673–679.

Henco K, Heibey M (1990): Quantitative PCR: The determination of template copy numbers by temperature gradient gel electrophoresis (TGGE). *Nucl Acids Res* 18(22):6733–6734.

Ho DD, Moudgil T, Alam M (1989): Quantitation of human immunodeficiency virus type 1 in the blood of infected persons [see comments]. *N Engl J Med* 321(24):1621–1625.

Hsia K, Spector SA (1991): Human immunodeficiency virus DNA is present in a high percentage of CD4 + lymphocytes of seropositive individuals. *J Infect Dis* 164(3):470–475.

Huff JR (1991): HIV protease—A novel chemotherapeutic target for AIDS. *J Med Chem* 34(8):2305–2314.

Jurriaans S, Dekker JT, de Ronde A (1992): HIV-1 viral DNA load in peripheral blood mononuclear cells from seroconverters and long-term infected individuals. *Aids* 6(7):635–641.

Kalyanaraman VS, Cabradilla CD, Getchell JP, Narayanan R, Braff EH, Chermann JC, Barre SF, Montagnier L, Spira TJ, Kaplan J, et al. (1984): Antibodies to the core protein of lymphadenopathy-associated virus (LAV) in patients with AIDS. *Science* 225(4659):321–323.

Kanitakis J, Escaich S, Trepo C, Thivolet J (1991): Detection of human immunodeficiency virus-

DNA and RNA in the skin of HIV-infected patients using the polymerase chain reaction. *J Invest Dermatol* 97(1):91–96.

Karpas A, Hewlett IK, Hill F, Gray J, Byron N, Gilgen D, Bally V, Oates JK, Gazzard B, Epstein JE (1990): Polymerase chain reaction evidence for human immunodeficiency virus 1 neutralization by passive immunization in patients with AIDS and AIDS-related complex. *Proc Natl Acad Sci USA* 87(19):7613–7617.

Larder BA, Kellam P, Kemp SD (1991): Zidovudine resistance predicted by direct detection of mutations in DNA from HIV-infected lymphocytes. *Aids* 5(2):137–144.

Lee TH, el AZ, Reis M, Adams M, Donegan EA, O'Brien TR, Moss AR, Busch MP (1991a): Absence of HIV-1 DNA in high-risk seronegative individuals using high-input polymerase chain reaction. *Aids* 5(10):1201–1207.

Lee TH, Sunzeri FJ, Tobler LH, Williams BG, Busch MP (1991b): Quantitative assessment of HIV-1 DNA load by coamplification of HIV-1 gag and HLA-DQ-alpha genes. *Aids* 5(6):683–691.

Levy JA, Hoffman AD, Kramer SM, Landis JA, Shimabukuro JM, Oshiro LS (1984): Isolation of lymphocytopathic retroviruses from San Francisco patients with AIDS. *Science* 225(4664): 840–842.

Levy JA (1993): Pathogenesis of human immunodeficiency virus infection. *Microbiol Rev* 57(1): 183–289.

Liu ZQ, Wood C, Levy JA, Cheng MC (1990): The viral envelope gene is involved in macrophage tropism of a human immunodeficiency virus type 1 strain isolated from brain tissue. *J Virol* 64(12):6148–6153.

Malim MH, Hauber J, Fenrick R, Cullen BR (1988): Immunodeficiency virus rev trans-activator modulates the expression of the viral regulatory genes. *Nature (London)* 335(6186):181–183.

Malim MH, Hauber J, Le SY, Maizel JV, Cullen BR (1989): The HIV-1 rev trans-activator acts through a structured target sequence to activate nuclear export of unspliced viral mRNA. *Nature (London)* 338(6212):254–257.

Mano H, Chermann JC (1991): Fetal human immunodeficiency virus type 1 infection of different organs in the second trimester. *Aids Res Hum Retrovirus* 7(1):83–88.

Menzo S, Bagnarelli P, Giacca M, Manzin A, Varaldo PE, Clementi M (1992): Absolute quantitation of viremia in human immunodeficiency virus infection by competitive reverse transcription and polymerase chain reaction. *J Clin Microbiol* 30(7):1752–1757.

O'Brien WA, Koyanagi Y, Namazie A, Zhao JQ, Diagne A, Idler K, Zack JA, Chen IS (1990): HIV-1 tropism for mononuclear phagocytes can be determined by regions of gp120 outside the CD4-binding domain. *Nature (London)* 348(6296):69–73.

Palca J (1991): The growing anti-HIV armamentarium. *Science* 253(5017):263.

Pang S, Koyanagi Y, Miles S, Wiley C, Vinters HV, Chen IS (1990): High levels of unintegrated HIV-1 DNA in brain tissue of AIDS dementia patients. *Nature (London)* 343(6253):85–89.

Popovic M, Sarngadharan MG, Read E, Gallo RC (1984): Detection, isolation, and continuous production of cytopathic retroviruses (HTLV-III) from patients with AIDS and pre-AIDS. *Science* 224(4648):497–500.

Poznansky MC, Walker B, Haseltine WA, Sodroski J, Langhoff E (1991): A rapid method for quantitating the frequency of peripheral blood cells containing HIV-1 DNA. *J Acquir Immune Defic Syndr* 4(4):368–373.

Richman DD, Guatelli JC, Grimes J, Tsiatis A, Gingeras T (1991): Detection of mutations associated with zidovudine resistance in human immunodeficiency virus by use of the polymerase chain reaction. *J Infect Dis* 164(6):1075–1081.

Rosen CA, Sodroski JG, Campbell K, Haseltine WA (1986a): Construction of recombinant murine retroviruses that express the human T-cell leukemia virus type II and human T-cell lymphotropic virus type III trans activator genes. *J Virol* 57(1):379–384.

Rosen CA, Sodroski JG, Goh WC, Dayton AI, Lippke J, Haseltine WA (1986b): Post-transcriptional regulation accounts for the trans-activation of the human T-lymphotropic virus type III. *Nature (London)* 319(6054):555–559.

Saag MS, Crain MJ, Decker WD, Campbellhill S, Robinson S, Brown WE, Leuther M, Whitley RJ, Hahn BH, Shaw GM (1991): High-level viremia in adults and children infected with human immunodeficiency virus—Relation to disease stage and CD4+ lymphocyte levels. *J Infect Dis* 164(1):72–80.

Sadaie MR, Benter T, Wong SF (1988): Site-directed mutagenesis of two trans-regulatory genes (tat-III,trs) of HIV-1. *Science* 239(4842): 910–913.

Salahuddin SZ, Markham PD, Popovic M, Sarngadharan MG, Orndorff S, Fladagar A, Patel A, Gold J, Gallo RC (1985): Isolation of infectious human T-cell leukemia/lymphotropic virus type III (HTLV-III) from patients with acquired immunodeficiency syndrome (AIDS) or AIDS-related complex (ARC) and from healthy carriers: A study of risk groups and tissue sources. *Proc Natl Acad Sci USA* 82(16):5530–5534.

Sarngadharan MG, Popovic M, Bruch L, Schupbach J, Gallo RC (1984): Antibodies reactive with human T-lymphotropic retroviruses (HTLV-III) in the serum of patients with AIDS. *Science* 224(4648):506–508.

Sarver N, Cantin EM, Chang PS, Zaia JA, Ladne PA, Stephens DA, Rossi JJ (1990): Ribozymes as potential anti-HIV-1 therapeutic agents. *Science* 247(4947):1222–1225.

Schnittman SM, Psallidopoulos MC, Lane HC, Thompson L, Baseler M, Massari F, Fox CH, Salzman NP, Fauci AS (1989): The reservoir for HIV-1 in human peripheral blood is a T cell that maintains expression of CD4 [published erratum appears in *Science* 1989 Aug 18;245(4919):preceding 694]. *Science* 245(4915):305–308.

Schnittman SM, Greenhouse JJ, Lane HC, Pierce PF, Fauci AS (1991): Frequent detection of HIV-1-specific messenger RNAs in infected individuals suggests ongoing active viral expression in all stages of disease. *AIDS Res Human Retrovirus* 7(4):361–367.

Simmonds P, Balfe P, Peutherer JF, Ludlam CA, Bishop JO, Brown AJ (1990): Human immunodeficiency virus-infected individuals contain provirus in small numbers of peripheral mononuclear cells and at low copy numbers. *J Virol* 64(2):864–872.

Sodroski J, Goh WC, Rosen C, Dayton A, Terwilliger E, Haseltine W (1986): A second post-transcriptional trans-activator gene required for HTLV-III replication. *Nature* (*London*) 321(6068):412–417.

Sonnerborg A, Johansson B, Strannegard O (1991): Detection of HIV-1 DNA and infectious virus in cerebrospinal fluid. *Aids Res Hum Retrovirus* 7(4):369–373.

Trono D, Feinberg MB, Baltimore D (1989): HIV-1 Gag mutants can dominantly interfere with the replication of the wild-type virus. *Cell* 59(1):113–120.

Vickers T, Baker BF, Cook PD, Zounes M, Buckheit RW, Germany J, Ecker DJ (1991): Inhibition of HIV-LTR gene expression by oligonucleotides targeted to the TAR element. *Nucl Acids Research* 19(12):3359–3368.

Wahlberg J, Albert J, Lundeberg J, Cox S, Wahren B, Uhlen M (1992): Dynamic changes in HIV-1 quasispecies from azidothymidine (AZT)-treated patients. *Faseb J* 6(10):2843–2847.

Wang AM, Doyle MV, Mark DF (1989): Quantitation of mRNA by the polymerase chain reaction [published erratum appears in *Proc Natl Acad Sci USA* 1990 Apr;87(7):2865]. *Proc Natl Acad Sci USA* 86(24):9717–9721.

Weintrub PS, Ulrich PP, Edwards JR, Boucher F, Levy JA, Cowan MJ, Vyas GN (1991): Use of polymerase chain reaction for the early detection of HIV infection in the infants of HIV-seropositive women. *AIDS* 5(7):881–884.

Yolken RH, Li S, Perman J, Viscidi R (1991): Persistent diarrhea and fecal shedding of retroviral nucleic acids in children infected with human immunodeficiency virus. *J Infect Dis* 164(1):61–66.

Young KK, Peter JB, Winters RE (1990): Detection of HIV DNA in peripheral blood by the polymerase chain reaction: A study of clinical applicability and performance. *Aids* 4(5):389–391.

Zack JA, Arrigo SJ, Weitsman SR, Go AS, Haislip A, Chen IS (1990): HIV-1 entry into quiescent primary lymphocytes: Molecular analysis reveals a labile, latent viral structure. *Cell* 61(2):213–222.

30

Gene Therapy

Richard A. Morgan and W. French Anderson

Introduction to Human Gene Therapy

A reporter once asked, "isn't it true that human gene therapy would not have been possible without the development of polymerase chain reaction?" The investigator said no. Afterward, the investigator realized that the reporter was partially correct. The power of PCR technology (Mullis and Faloona, 1987; Saiki et al., 1988) has allowed some remarkable accomplishments, e.g., the detection of one marked cell in a million unmarked cells (Crescenzi et al., 1988), direct gene isolation and sequencing from bulk cellular DNA (Engelke et al., 1988), the analysis of DNA from a single human sperm (Hoghua et al., 1988), and, perhaps, aspects of the development of human gene therapy. We must acknowledge that PCR was essential to the first human gene therapy experiments, not conceptually, but because only PCR permitted the unambiguous detection of gene-engineered cells from biological specimens and this technical ability was key to approval of the first gene therapy protocol.

The majority of the currently approved human gene therapy protocols use, as a gene transfer technique, retroviral-mediated gene transfer (Morgan and Anderson, 1993). Retroviral-mediated gene transfer (RMGT) is a process in which a replication-defective retrovirus is used as a biological vector to transfer genetic material, *ex vivo*, into an appropriate host cell. Because it allows highly efficient, stably integrated gene transfer in a variety of cell types, (Anderson, 1992; Eglitis and Anderson, 1988) RMGT is finding increased application in experimental gene therapy protocols (the term transduction will be used to denote the procedure of gene transfer into target cells by infection with a retroviral vector).

The clinical application of RMGT generally consists of four phases: construction of the retroviral vector packaging cell lines, *ex vivo* transduction of target cells by the retroviral vector preparation, transfer of the engineered cells to the patient, and analysis of posttransfer specimens for the transduced target cells. Several of the current RMGT systems in human clinical protocols call for the *ex vivo* transduction of primary culture lymphocytes by exposure to culture medium from retroviral vector producer cell lines. These procedures have been used for the gene marking (Rosenberg et al., 1990) of human tumor infiltrating lympho-

The Polymerase Chain Reaction
K.B. Mullis, F. Ferré, R.A. Gibbs, editors
© 1994 Birkhäuser Boston

cytes (TIL), and are further being used as a gene therapy for the treatment of adenosine deaminase (ADA) deficiency (Blaese, 1990) and in a TIL-based strategy for treating malignant melanoma by delivery of tumor necrosis factor (TNF) engineered TIL (Rosenberg, 1990). The uniqueness of these protocols, which were the first approved experiments in which genetically engineered cells were administered to human beings, necessitated the development of novel biological and physical testing procedures.

We sought to develop procedures that apply the technology of polymerase chain reaction (PCR) to rapidly evaluate and identify cells transduced by retroviral vectors. The majority of the retroviral vectors in general use contain selectable marker genes that greatly aid in obtaining pure transduced cell populations. One of the most versatile and efficient vectors is termed N2 and contains, as a selectable marker, the bacterial neomycin phosphotransferase (Neo^R) gene (Armentano et al., 1987; Eglitis et al., 1985). In order to identify Neo^R-transduced cells by PCR, several primer pair combinations were evaluated in a standard PCR reaction using both cloned and purified genomic DNA. Amplification of the region containing the entire 790-bp Neo^R gene yielded a consistently intense signal following gel analysis and was chosen as a standard primer pair for the detection of Neo^R-transduced cells (Morgan et al., 1990).

Lesson from TIL Transductions

The first federally approved experiment designed to transfer gene-engineered cells into human beings were the TIL gene marking experiments (Rosenberg et al., 1990). In this experiment, TIL were genetically marked by transduction with a retroviral vector that carries a selectable marker gene from bacteria, the neomycin phosphotransferase gene (Neo^R). The protocol entailed the transduction of TIL with a retroviral vector (the vector LNL6, is similar to N2, but with several added safety features, Bender et al., 1987), and transfer of these gene-marked cells into pa-

tients undergoing TIL adoptive immunotherapy for the treatment of advanced malignant melanoma (Rosenberg et al., 1989, see Fig. 30.1). The retroviral vector/packaging cell line system (PA317/LNL6) in use in this protocol has the ability to generate high titer vector preparations and has a low potential for the production of replication-competent helper virus.

Using gene marking, questions concerning TIL distribution and survival in circulation, lymph nodes, or tumor deposits could possibly be addressed. This is important because in current TIL therapy only 40% of patients show a measurable response to the therapy and any correlations between TIL trafficking and clinical outcome could potentially be used to increase efficacy. Labeling cells with a retroviral vector results in stable integration of the marker gene into the host cell chromosome. Integration ensures the transfer of the marker to the cells' descendants permitting long-term follow-up of tagged cells if detection procedures are sensitive enough. It was the enhanced sensitivity of PCR that permitted these experiments to become reality.

An additional reason for gene marking the TIL cells with a Neo^R-containing vector was the possibility of selection (via G418 resistance) of these cells from patients at later times following administration of the cells. The ability to specifically select TIL that had migrated to tumor deposits afforded the possibility to enrich for cells that traffic to tumors. A second infusion of selected TIL could return to patients cells with a high potential for tumor trafficking. In one of the five original patients administered marked TIL, engineered cells could be obtained from clinical samples following selection for the Neo^R gene (Aebersold et al., 1990).

Figure 30.2 shows representative data obtained from one of the first five TIL gene marking patients. Circulating peripheral blood mononuclear cells (PBMC) were isolated from the patient at the times indicated and DNA was isolated and subjected to PCR analysis for the Neo^R gene. Gene marked cells were readily detected up to day 19 postinfusion and to a very limited extent at day 60 (Fig. 30.3). In

FIGURE 30.1. TIL marking. Shown is a diagram of a typical TIL gene marking protocol. A culture of exponentially growing TIL is exposed three times to a retroviral vector preparation (here indicated as N7 supernatant) in the presence of protamine to enhance cell/virus binding. The culture can then be selected for 1 week in the neomycin analog G418 to enrich for gene-marked cells. The culture is then expanded before infusion into the patient. On the left side of the figure is shown a graph of a typical growth curve for unmarked TIL (solid line) and gene-marked TIL (dashed line).

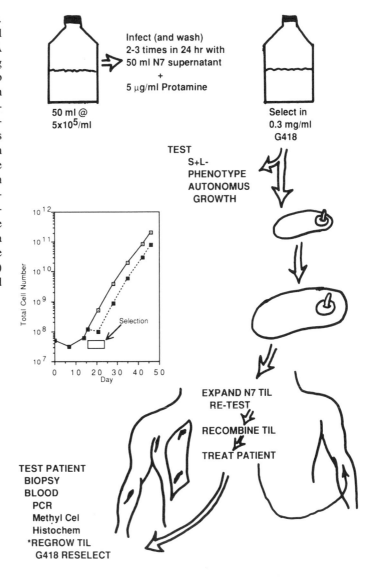

Figure 30.4, data are presented from a second TIL patient showing the distribution of TIL in peripheral blood as well as tumor biopsies. Again gene-marked TIL were easily detected in the blood for the first 3 weeks but then after, only rarely. The presence of marked TIL in tumor was unambiguously detected at day 2 after which time tumor regression occurred. Subsequent regrowth of tumor permitted a second resection of tumor at day 64. No gene-marked TIL were detected in the tumor biopsies but TIL regrown from that tumor were strongly PCR positive for the Neo[R] gene.

The major result from these studies was the consistent finding of gene-marked cells in the circulation during the first 21 days after cell infusion. Circulating gene-marked cells could occasionally be observed at later times (51 days in one patient and 60 days in a second). The 21 day cut-off for detection is associated with the ending of administration of interleukin-2 in some patients. As interleukin-2 (IL-2) is a necessary growth factor for TIL *in vitro*, these results suggest that IL-2 is also necessary for *in vivo* maintenance of TIL. The ability to regrow gene-marked TIL from the

DISTRIBUTION OF TIL IN PBL

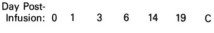

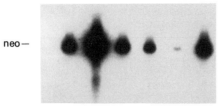

FIGURE 30.2. Detection of small numbers of gene-marked human TIL cells in patient PBL. LNL6 transduced and selected human TIL cells were mixed with untransduced TIL and infused into a patient on day 1. PBL were isolated at the indicated days and DNA extracted from each cell sample. DNA (2.0 μg) was subjected to PCR amplification for the Neo^R gene. The entire PCR reaction was analyzed by gel electrophoresis, followed by Southern blot transfer, and hybridization with a random prime NEO^R DNA probe. Shown is the resultant autoradiogram. The lane labeled C is a positive control representing approximately 1 gene marked cell per 1000 unmarked cells.

tumor biopsy from one patient at day 66 further suggests that TIL that are able to target to tumor sites may either directly possess or possibly be in an environment that permits long-term survival. These initial studies, although limited in scope and number of patients treated, were the first time in which genetically modified cells were introduced in human beings and they thus laid the ground work for all future gene therapy experiments.

Quantitation

An ability to quantitate the number of gene-engineered cells in patient samples can yield critical information about the biology of the transduced cell. In preliminary experiments, Neo^R PCR was observed to be roughly quantitative at levels of 5- to 10-fold differences (e.g., one can easily distinguish 10% transduction efficiency from 100% transduction by visualization of PCR reactions products on ethidium bromide-stained gels, data not

shown). To further examine the extent that PCR results are quantitative we set up a series of cell mixing experiments. This experiment was designed to duplicate the potential recovery of low numbers of gene-marked cells encountered in the analysis of clinical samples.

As a source of gene-marked cells, NIH/3T3 cells were transduced with the LASN vector, selected by growth in the presence of G418, then mixed with untransduced (PBMC). The LASN vector is a two-gene-containing vector in which the LTR promotes the expression of adenosine deaminase and the SV40 early region promoter is used to drive the expression of the Neo^R gene (Hock et al., 1989). LASN is the vector currently used to transduce lymphocytes from ADA-deficient SCID patients.

Cells were mixed in the ratio of transduced to untransduced ranging from 100,000 : 1 $\times$ 10^6 down to 10 : 1 $\times$ 10^6. The cell mixtures were collected, DNA was isolated, and 2 μg of DNA was mixed with 2 fg of plasmid pLASΔN and subjected to PCR amplification for the Neo^R gene. The pLASΔN plasmid contains a deletion in the NEO^R gene that generates a lower molecular weight band on agarose gel analysis following PCR amplification. The use of the pLASΔN plasmid (Palmer et al., 1991) introduces an internal control for experimental variation in amplification efficiency. Because the control plasmid is added as part of the master reaction mix, it should be amplified approximately equally in all reactions. The resultant cpm of the deleted NEO^R band can then be used to normalize the counts detected in the experimental band.

The level of radioactivity on the Southern blot filters from this experiment was directly measured using a betascope 603. This instrument is a gas proportional counter that directly measures beta particles. The results of this analysis are shown in Figures 30.5 and 30.6. Quantitation of gene copy number by PCR has been demonstrated in a number of systems (Bell and Ratner, 1989; Chelly et al., 1988; Guatelli et al., 1989). The ability to quantitate gene copy number is dependent on the amplification being in the exponential (linear) range. In practice, amplification is not 2^n (where n is the cycle number) but is $(1 + X)^n$, where X is

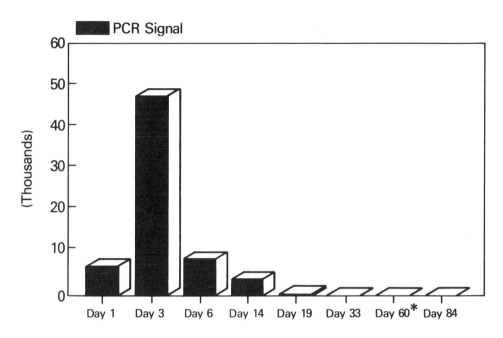

FIGURE 30.3. Distribution of TIL on PBL. The Southern blot filters (nylon membranes) from the experiments described in Figures 30.2 and subsequent gels were analyzed on a Betascope 603 instrument. The total number of counts (minus background) obtained in 30 min was plotted versus the days postinfusion. The sample at day 60 was visible on a 1 week autoradiogram but was not imaged on the 30 min scan on the betascope instrument.

the efficiency of amplification (Guatelli et al., 1989; Saiki et al., 1988). Our data indicate that Neo^R amplification was essentially linear from 10 to 10,000 marked cells per one million unmarked cells.

RNA PCR

Next to quantitation, the ability to detect the expression of gene engineered cells is an essential element in the analysis of the effectiveness of gene therapy. To measure expression by PCR, we must first isolate RNA from the relevant samples. As an example, PBMC were isolated from an ADA-deficient patient who had previously received lymphocytes engineered with the LASN retroviral vector. RNA isolation from PBMC is technically difficult to perform because the yield from 1×10^7 cells (a clinically relevant amount) is small (usually only a few micrograms). The meager amount of RNA obtained from PBMC also necessitates the use of PCR as a detection technique.

In the experiment presented in Figure 30.7, expression of the NEO^R gene was assayed by first subjecting RNA to reverse transcription followed by isolation of cDNA and then NEO^R PCR. We have found that cDNA synthesis using random hexamer primers results in greater end-point sensitivity for the detection of small numbers of gene-marked cells. An important option in this type of experiment is the choice of a control gene used to judge the quality and quantity of the starting RNA. The control gene should be present in a variety of lymphocytes

PCR DETECTION OF neo^R GENE IN BLOOD AND TUMOR

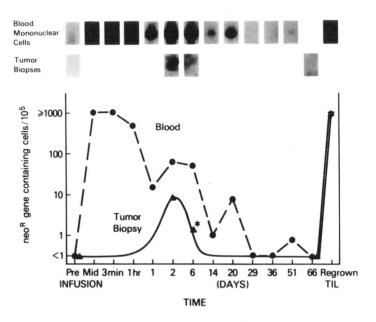

FIGURE 30.4. Detection of gene-marked TIL in blood and tumor. PCR was used to detect Neo^R gene-marked cells in PBMC and tumor biopsies at various times following infusion. DNA (2 μg) was extracted from each sample subjected to amplification, Southern blotting, autoradiography, and Betascope imaging. The areas of the autoradiograms corresponding to the indicated points are shown above a plot of the data obtained by analysis of the Southern blot filters on the Betascope instrument. Samples were obtained preinfusion, during infusion, 3 min, 1 hr postinfusion, and then on the indicated days postinfusion. The signal obtained from tumor biopsy on day 6 could not be unambiguously defined due to a hybridization artifact. TIL cultured from a tumor regrowth resected on day 66 were strongly positive while the signal from the original tumor was negative.

and be readily detectable. As the internal control for RNA PCR we have chosen to assay for the translation factor eIF-2β, which is a representative gene whose RNA is present even in quiescent lymphocytes. Results presented in Figure 30.7 indicate that in RNA isolated form PBMC of an ADA SCID patient, engineered cells were detected up to 6 weeks following infusion of transduced lymphocytes.

Safety Testing

The safety concerns in retroviral-mediated gene transfer can be divided into four categories: (1) general safety concerns relating to the production of a biological agent, (2) risks associated with the specific gene being transferred, (3) possible effects from the obligatory integration of the retroviral vector into the host cell genome, and (4) the potential contamination of the retroviral vector preparation with replication-competent retrovirus. PCR has been specifically applied to test concerns involving the fourth category, detection of replication-competent viral contaminations.

The major acute risk associated with RMGT is thought to be the possibility for the generation of replication-competent helper virus through recombination between the vector and the producer cell genome (Cornetta et al., 1991). Major advances in the design of packaging cell lines have led to systems that greatly

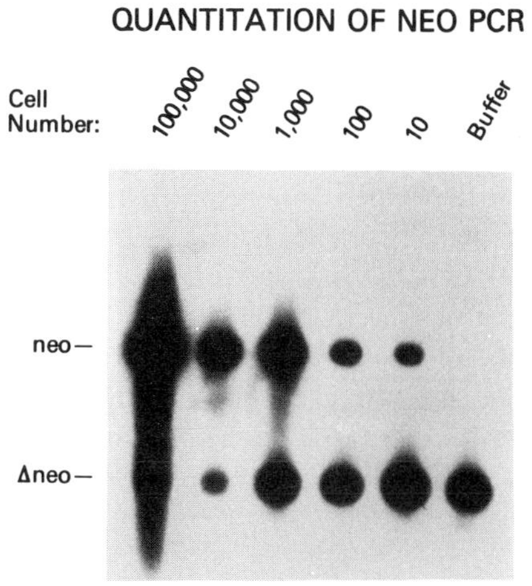

QUANTITATION OF NEO PCR

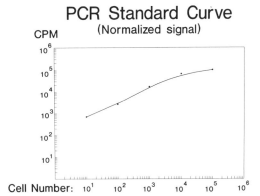

FIGURE 30.5. Quantitation of NEO[R] gene PCR analysis. In this experiment LASN-transduced 3T3 cells were mixed with normal human PBMC at the ratios of 10 to 100,000 Neo[R] containing cells per 10^6 total cells. DNA was extracted from each mixture and 2 µg subjected to PCR amplification for the Neo[R] gene. The master reaction mix contains 2 fg of the internal control plasmid pLASΔN that contains a 200-bp deletion in the Neo[R] gene. The entire reaction mix was analyzed by gel electrophoresis followed by Southern blotting and hybridization with a random prime NEO[R] DNA probe. Shown is the resultant autoradiogram. Cell number refers to the number of Neo[R]-containing cell equivalents per 10^6 total cell equivalents.

FIGURE 30.6. PCR standard curve. The southern blot filter from the experiment described in Figure 30.5 was analyzed on a Betascope 603 instrument to quantitate the radioactivity in each signal. The total counts obtained in a 30 min scan from the Δneo band in the negative control sample (buffer) was used to normalize sample values by the following formula: normalized sample counts = (neo sample counts) × (Δneo counts in buffer/Δneo counts in the sample). The data for the normalized counts were then plotted versus the number of marked cells per 10^6 total cells.

reduce the possibility of helper virus generation. Safety modifications in the current RMGT system include deletions in the 5′ LTR, and removal of 3′ LTR, in the molecular clone used to generate the PA317 packaging cell line (Miller and Buttimore, 1986). Further enhancements in safety come from the use of retroviral vectors that contain a mutated GAG gene start codon, substitution of MSV for Mo-MLV sequences, and the removal of noncritical 3′-end sequences (Bender et al., 1987). This and other similar systems require multiple recombinations (and possible correction of point mutations) in order to generate replication-competent helper virus.

Since the potential for the generation of recombinant helper virus in the currently used RMGT system is very small, extremely sensitive tests were required to screen vector prepa-

rations for what would be a very rare event. As part of the safety testing in the original TIL cell gene marking protocol, a PCR assay was developed for the analysis of transduced TIL cells for the presence of helper virus genomes (Morgan et al., 1990). As a target for PCR analysis, the ENV gene of the amphotropic packaging genome was chosen. The specific region of the ENV gene used determines the host range (and presumably receptor binding) of the virus and is thus less likely to mutate than other noncritical domains.

To test the sensitivity of this system, DNA from PA317 cells was mixed with untransduced TIL cell DNA in the ratio of 1 PA317 cell for 10^6 TIL cells to a ratio of 10,000 PA317 cell to 10^6 TIL cells. DNA from these mixtures is sufficient to permit detection of one cell in a million (the amount of DNA used, 8 µg, is equivalent to approximately 1,330,000 cells). The samples were subjected to PCR amplification (using both 25 and 30 cycles) for the ENV gene, followed by Southern blot analysis. Figure 30.8 shows the resulting autoradiogram

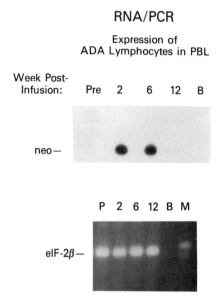

RNA/PCR

Expression of
ADA Lymphocytes in PBL

FIGURE 30.7. RNA PCR. RNA PCR was used to detect the expression of LASN engineered lymphocytes in the blood of an ADA SCID gene therapy patient. RNA was isolated from PBL at the indicated times post the first infusion of LASN engineered cells. One microgram of RNA was first reverse transcribed with Moloney murine leukemia virus reverse transcriptase using random hexamers as primers. The entire cDNA synthesis was then added to a PCR reaction mix containing primers to amplify either the Neo[R] gene or a control gene eIF-2β. The top panel is the resultant autoradiogram from Southern blot analysis of the Neo PCR reaction (Pre, preinfusion; B, buffer control). The bottom panel is a photograph of an ethidium bromide-stained gel used to analyze for the eIF-2β transcript (P, preinfusion; B, buffer; M, molecular weight marker).

from this Southern blot analysis. The data indicate that in the 30 cycle amplification, cells containing a helper virus can be detected at the level of 1 in 10^6 unmarked cells.

The polymerase chain reaction (PCR) protocols developed for the analysis of transduced TIL cells are essential components in gene transfer/therapy safety testing procedures. Standard PCR analysis for the helper virus genome can readily detect 1 cell containing a helper virus genome in 10^5 TIL cells (if the amount of DNA used is $> 10^6$ cell equivalents, 1 cell in 10^6 can be detected). Interest-

ingly, helper virus does not replicate well in human TIL cells. The lack of virus replication may account for the inability to detect helper virus genomes in all TIL cell populations exposed to helper virus-contaminated vector supernatant (Cornetta et al., 1993). This observation points out a clear example where physical testing methods such as PCR would detect a helper virus contamination in cell samples that would be negative by biological assays (i.e., because the helper virus was not replicating).

Summary

Retroviral vector-mediated gene transfer is now being used for the treatment of both rare genetic diseases and common place maladies such as cancer. At present, the ability to perform the gene transfer is not in itself a complex or technically elaborate procedure. Gene transfer has now been performed on several dozen patients with no detectable side effects. PCR analysis is an indispensable technique in human gene therapy protocols. It permits the rapid detection and quantitation of small numbers of gene-engineered cells in clinical specimens. It can also be used to assay for the expression of the transduced gene and is an important part of safety testing procedures. Without the advent of PCR it is possible that the initial gene therapy protocols would have been substantially delayed or not approved at all.

In the future, if gene therapy is to become a widely used medical therapy, three technical hurdles need to be overcome. First, gene transfer vectors are needed that can be directly injected into the patient. In addition, the injected vector would need to specifically target to and enter the particular tissue or organ. Second, once the gene vector has reached the cell of interest, it needs to safely integrate into a noncritical site on the chromosome, or homologously recombine with the defective gene it is trying to replace. This would decrease the potential for initiating events leading to malignancy. Third, the introduced gene needs to have the ability to respond to physiological

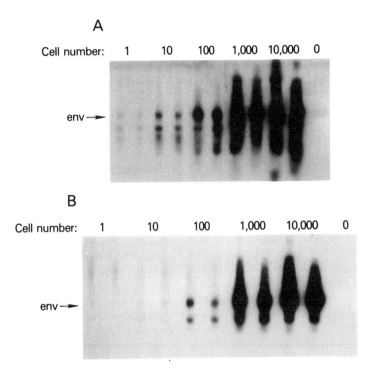

Figure 30.8. Sensitivity of helper virus envelope PCR assays. DNA from the PA317 packaging cell line was mixed with DNA from TIL cells at the equivalent of one PA317 cell per 10^6 total cells, to 10^4 PA317 cell per 10^6 total cells. Eight micrograms of each DNA mix was then subject to PCR amplification for the envelope gene of the amphotropic 4070A virus using 30 cycles (**A**) and 25 cycles (**B**). The entire reaction mix was loaded onto an agarose gel, and following electrophoresis, subjected to Southern blot analysis with a random primed env DNA probe. The resulting autoradiogram detects the amplified region of the helper virus envelope that is 375 bp (arrow). The lower molecular weight band is an artifact resulting from internal priming of one of the PCR primers used in this specific experiment.

changes in blood or cellular metabolites. For example, in gene therapy for diabetes, the rise and fall in glucose levels would be sensed and responded to by an appropriately engineered insulin gene. The future for gene therapy is promising and it is likely that PCR technology will continue to be an indispensable part of the analysis of this rapidly developing area of molecular medicine.

References

Aebersold P, Kasid A, Rosenberg SA (1990): Selection of gene-marked tumor infiltrating lymphocytes from post-treatment biopsies: A case study. *Human Gene Ther* 1:373–384.

Anderson WF (1992): Human gene therapy. *Science* 256:808–813.

Armentano D, Yu SF, Kantoff PW, von Ruden T, Anderson WF, Gilboa E (1987): Effects of internal viral sequences on the utility of retroviral vectors. *J Virol* 61:1647–1650.

Bell J, Ratner L (1989): Specificity of polymerase chain amplification reactions for human immunodeficiency virus type 1 DNA sequences. *AIDS Res Human Retrovirus* 5:87–95.

Bender MA, Palmer TD, Gelinas RE, Miller AD (1987): Evidence that the packaging signal of Moloney leukemia virus extends into the gag region. *J Virol* 61:1639–1646.

Blaese RM (1990): The ADA human gene therapy clinical protocol. *Human Gene Ther* 1:327–329.

Chelly JJ, Kaplan JC, Maire P, Gautron S, Kahn A (1988): Transcription of the dystrophin gene in human muscle and non-muscle tissues. *Nature (London)* 333:858–860.

Crescenzi M, Seto M, Herzig GP, Weiss PD, Griffith RC, Korsmeyer SJ (1988): Thermostable DNA polymerase chain amplification of t(14;18) chromosomal breakpoints and detection of minimal residual disease. *Proc Natl Acad Sci USA* 85: 4869–4873.

Cornetta K, Morgan RA, Anderson WF (1991): Safety issues related to retroviral-mediated gene transfer in humans. *Human Gene Ther* 2:5–14.

Cornetta K, Nguyen N, Morgan RA, Muenchau DD, Hartley JW, Blaesa RM, Anderson WF (1993): Infection of human cells with marine amphrotropic replication competent retrovirus. *Human Gene Ther* 4:579–588.

Eglitis MA, Anderson WF (1988): Retroviral vectors for introduction of genes into mammalian cells. *Biotechniques* 6:608–614.

Eglitis MA, Kantoff P, Gilboa E, Anderson WF (1985): Gene expression in mice after high efficiency retroviral-mediated gene transfer. *Science* 230:1395–1398.

Engelke DR, Hoener PA, Collins FS (1988): Direct sequencing of enzymatically amplified human genomic DNA. *Proc Natl Acad Sci USA* 85:544–548.

Guatelli JC, Gingeras TR, Richman DD (1989): Nucleic acid amplification in vitro: Detection of sequences with low copy numbers and applications to diagnosis of human immunodeficiency virus type 1 infection. *Clin Microbiol Rev* 2:217–226.

Hock RA, Miller AD, Osborne WRA (1989): Expression of human adenosine deaminase from various strong promoters after gene transfer into human hematopoietic cell lines. *Blood* 74:876–881.

Honghua L, Gyllensten UB, Cui X, Saiki RK, Erlich HA, Arnheim N (1988): Amplification and analysis of DNA sequences in single human sperm and diploid cells. *Nature (London)* 335: 414–417.

Miller AD, Buttimore C (1986): Redesign of retrovirus packaging cell lines to avoid recombination leading to helper virus production. *Mol Cel Biol* 6:2895–2902.

Morgan RA, Anderson WF (1993): Human gene therapy. *Ann Rev Biochem* 62:191–217.

Morgan RA, Cornetta K, Anderson WF (1990): Application of polymerase chain reaction in retroviral mediated gene transfer and the analysis of gene marked human TIL cells. *Human Gene Ther* 2:135–150.

Mullis KB, Faloona FA (1987): Specific synthesis of DNA in vitro via a polymerase-catalyzed chain reaction. *Methods Enzymol* 155:335–350.

Palmer TD, Rosman GJ, Osborne WR, Miller AD (1991): Genetically modified skin fibroblasts persist long after transplantations but gradually inactivate introduced genes. *Proc Natl Acad Sci USA* 88:1330–1334.

Rosenberg SA et al. (1989): Use of tumor-infiltrating lymphocytes and interleukin-2 in the immunotherapy of patients with metastatic melanoma. *New England J Med* 319:1676–1680.

Rosenberg SA (1990): TNF/TIL human gene therapy clinical protocol. *Human Gene Ther* 1:443–462.

Rosenberg SA, Aebersold P, Kasid A, Morgan RA, Cornetta K, Karson E, Lotze MT, Yang JC, Toplain S, Moen R, Culver K, Blaese M, Anderson WF (1990): Gene transfer in humans: Immunotherapy of patients with advanced melanoma using tumor infiltrating lymphocytes modified by retroviral gene transduction. *N Engl J Med* 323: 570–578.

Saiki RK, Gelfand DH, Stoffel S, Scharf SJ, Higuchi R, Horn GT, Mullis KB, Erlich HA (1988): Primer-directed enzymatic amplification of DNA with a thermostable DNA polymerase. *Science* 239:487–491.

PART TWO
Applications

SECTION IV
Diagnostics

31

PCR and Cancer Diagnostics: Detection and Characterization of Single Point Mutations in Oncogenes and Antioncogenes

Manuel Perucho

Introduction

The theory that the accumulation in a single cell of genetic alterations in some critical genes, the oncogenes and the tumor suppressor genes, is the underlying cause of neoplastic transformation is becoming generally accepted (Fearon and Vogelstein, 1990; Bishop, 1991). Cellular genes whose products are involved in any of the steps of signal transduction leading to cell replication are potential candidates for oncogenes and for tumor suppressor genes. For an extensive review on oncogenes, see Pimentel (1989). For recent reviews on tumor suppressor genes or antioncogenes, see Weinberg (1991) and Marshall (1991a). The balanced interplay between protooncogenes and tumor suppressor genes in cell growth and differentiation is disrupted by cumulative genetic damage and, despite the fail-safe mechanisms provided by natural selection, neoplastic transformation occurs.

The genetic alterations that are responsible for the activation and inactivation of the function of oncogenes and tumor suppressor genes are schematized in Figure 31.1. Although with differences in their relative proportions, the same alterations occur in both types of genes in tumorigenesis. Gene amplification (Collins and Groudine, 1982; Schwab et al., 1983; Alitalo et al., 1983; Kohl et al., 1983), chromosomal translocations (Taub et al., 1982; de Klein et al., 1982; Klein, 1983), and proviral insertion (Hayward et al., 1981; Payne et al., 1982; Nusse and Varmus, 1982; Peters et al., 1983) mediate oncogene activation. Intragenic deletions have been also described to activate protooncogenes in a few instances (Meijlink et al., 1985; Luscher et al., 1990). Finally, point mutations (Tabin et al., 1982; Reddy et al., 1982; Taparowski et al., 1982; Bargmann et al., 1986; Roussell et al., 1988; Landis et al., 1989) are responsible for the activation of the oncogenic potential of some protooncogenes (see Table 31.1).

Similarly, chromosomal translocations have been involved in the inactivation of tumor suppressor genes (Bodmer et al., 1987; Viskochil et al., 1990; Xu et al., 1990; Wallace et al., 1990) as well as intragenic insertions (Fearon et al., 1990; Wallace et al., 1990). Gene amplification also can lead to the inactivation of tumor suppressor genes, albeit in an indirect manner, by overexpressing a cellular protein that binds and inactivates the p53 gene product

The Polymerase Chain Reaction
K.B. Mullis, F. Ferré, R.A. Gibbs, editors
© 1994 Birkhauser Boston

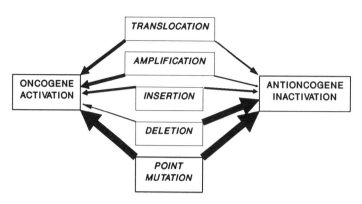

FIGURE 31.1. Genetic alterations in neoplastic transformation.

(Momand et al., 1992; Oliner et al., 1992). Deletions at the genic or chromosomal levels are very frequently responsible for the functional loss of tumor suppressor genes (reviewed in Marshall, 1991a; Weinberg, 1991). In addition, in many tumors where the normal allele of several tumor suppressor genes has been lost by deletion, point mutations are often present in the remaining allele (Dunn et al., 1988, 1989; Horowitz et al., 1989; Lee et al.,

1988b; Baker et al., 1989; Nigro et al., 1989; Takahashi et al., 1989).

The development of technologies for the detection and characterization of these genetic alterations is having a great impact in the genetic analysis of malignancy. The classification of neoplasias based on the presence and nature of these tumor-specific mutations is finding applications for cancer diagnosis at the molecular genetic level (Furth and Greaves, 1989) and

TABLE 31.1. Somatic point mutations[a] in oncogenes.

	Activity[b]	Other alterations[c]	Tumor[d]	Method[e]	References
Tyrosine kinases					
erbB/neu	+	Amplification	Breast, ovary	SEQ	Bargman et al., 1986
fms	+	?	Preleukemia	SEQ	Roussell et al. (1988), Ridge et al. (1990), reviewed in Carter et al. (1992)
GPTase proteins					
ras	+	Amplification	Carcinomas, sarcomas, leukemias	ASO, RNase RFLP, SSCP ASA, SEQ	Reviewed in van Mansfeld and Bos (1992)
gsp/gip	+	?	Pituitary, ovary, thyroid, adrenal	SEQ, ASO	Landis et al. (1989), Lyons et al. (1990)
Nuclear factors					
myc	−	Translocation/ amplification	Lymphomas, carcinomas	RNase SEQ	Cesarman et al. (1987)

[a]Single base substitutions leading to missense mutations in the gene product, unless otherwise specified.
[b]Functionality of these missense mutations demonstrated because they confer transforming activity in transfection assays (+). (−): Somatic mutations detected in the noncoding region are associated with altered transcription. However, the role of these mutations in myc transcription regulation has not been demonstrated (Richman and Hayday, 1989).
[c]Other genetic alterations involved in the activation of these oncogenes. In the erbB2/neu oncogene, these activating missense point mutations have not been found in spontaneous tumors, and the common mechanism of activation resides in low to moderate levels of gene amplification. Similarly, the most frequent alterations in the myc oncogene are chromosomal translocations and moderate to high levels of gene amplification.
[d]Tumors where mutations have been consistently detected.
[e]Diagnostic method used for the detection of these mutations (see text and Fig. 31.2). SEQ, sequencing.

also provides additional avenues for cancer prognosis (Little et al., 1983; Brodeur et al., 1984; Slamon et al., 1987; Slebos et al., 1990). The exponential *in vitro* amplification of genomic sequences by the polymerase chain reaction (PCR) (Saiki et al., 1985; Mullis and Faloona, 1987) has facilitated enormously the detection of oncogenic genetic alterations and the analysis of their role in tumorigenesis. The PCR has found applications in the detection of chromosomal translocations, gene amplifications, integration of viral sequences, and intragenic deletions and insertions (reviewed in McCormick, 1989a). Here we will focus in reviewing its applications for the diagnostic detection and characterization of single point mutations involved in cancer, of which the mutations activating the *ras* oncogenes and inactivating the p53 antioncogene can be taken as paradigmatic examples.

Oncogenic Point Mutations

The differences in the thickness of the arrows of Figure 31.1 are intended to illustrate the relative extent of involvement of the different alterations in neoplastic transformation. I propose that the types of mutation more often implicated in cancer are the point mutations. I make a few comments in support of this hypothesis. Tables 31.1 and 31.2 list the oncogenes and tumor suppressor genes where somatic point mutations have been characterized. Due to the intrinsic difficulty in detecting these subtle mutations, it is reasonable to assume that their involvement in tumorigenesis is even more widespread than currently known. While all other alterations (translocations, amplifications, insertion, and deletions) can be detected by cytogenetics and/or by Southern blot hybridization, the point mutations are undetectable by these methods, and the development of more sensitive and sophisticated techniques has been necessary for their systematic identification. The point mutations characterized to date in cancers are probably like the tip of the iceberg, and there are likely many more still unknown in the same or other genes.

To illustrate this point, I mention two examples. The first is the initial discovery of point mutations in the α chain of the Gs proteins in pituitary tumors (Landis et al., 1989). The presence of these mutations was predicted based on the homology of these proteins with the *ras* oncogenic proteins. The transforming activity of these mutant genes was demonstrated after the discovery of somatic point mutations in tumors (Pace et al., 1991; Gupta et al., 1992). Therefore, the involvement of these genes in tumorigenesis was identified before their possible oncogenic potential was recognized, and their classification as oncogenes was done precisely because of the presence in them of point mutations. The second example is the initial discovery of somatic point mutations in the p53 gene in two colorectal tumors (Baker et al., 1989). For 10 years, the p53 gene was thought to be an oncogene. However, the observation of allelic losses in the chromosome 17p region (where the p53 gene was known to be located) in a vast majority of colorectal tumors (Vogelstein et al., 1988) led to the insightful prediction that the remaining p53 allele would not be normal, but, on the contrary, would have undergone subtle mutations inactivating the gene product. In the few years that have lapsed since this seminal observation, it has become clear that somatic single point mutations in the p53 gene are the most common genetic alterations in human cancer. The fact that the oncogenes most frequently involved in human cancer, the *ras* oncogenes, are activated by single amino acid substitutions, underscore the relative importance of the point mutations in cancer development and progression.

ras Oncogenes

The *ras* genes pertain to a large and complex multigene family encoding small GTPase proteins (reviewed in Bourne et al., 1991; Cox and Der, 1992). The three members of the highly conserved *ras* gene family (c-K-*ras*, c-H-*ras*, and N-*ras*) encode membrane-bound proteins, which possess great affinity for GTP and GDP and are involved in signal transduc-

TABLE 31.2. Somatic point mutations[a] in tumor suppressor genes.

Gene	Functionality[b]	Tumor type[c]	Method[d]	References
p53	+	Carcinomas,	SEQ, RFLP	Baker et al. (1989), Nigro et al. (1989)
		sarcomas,	RNase	Takahashi et al. (1989)
		brain tumors,	MCC	Rodrigues et al. (1990)
		leukemias	SSCP	Mashiyama et al. (1991)
			DGGE, ASO	Shirasawa et al. (1991)
				Reviewed in Tominaga et al. (1992)
RB	+	Retinoblastoma,	RNase	Dunn et al. (1988, 1989)
		sarcomas,	SSCP	Murakami et al. (1991)
		carcinomas	SEQ	Reviewed in Bookstein and Lee (1990)
MCC	–	Colon carcinoma	RNase	Kinzler et al. (1991)
APC	–	Gastrointestinal	RNase	Nishisho et al. (1991)
		carcinomas	SSCP	Groden et al. (1991)
			SEQ	Powell et al. (1992)
NF1	+	Neurofibromatosis	SSCP	Cawthon et al. (1990)
			ASO	Li et al. (1992)
WT	–	Wilms' tumor	MCC	van Heyningen and Hastie (1992)
DCC	–	Colon carcinoma	SEQ	Fearon et al. (1990)

[a]In addition to single base deletions, insertions, and substitutions, insertions/deletions of a few nucleotides are included. Germ line single point mutations have been described already for the RB (Yandell et al., 1989), p53 (Malkin et al., 1990, 1992; Srivastava et al., 1990), APC (Groden et al., 1991; Nishisho et al., 1991; Miyoshi et al., 1992b), and NF1 (Cawthon et al., 1990) tumor suppressor genes.

[b]Functionality of many of these point mutations demonstrated because they are frameshift insertions or deletions of one or two nucleotides, and many of the single base substitutions destroy the correct splicing or introduce stopping codons. The functionality of missense mutations is demonstrated in some cases. Transfection assays have been used for p53, by cooperating with *ras* oncogenes for transformation of primary fibroblasts, (Eliyahu et al., 1994; Parada et al., 1994) or by failing to revert the transformed phenotype of tumor cells (reviewed in Vogelstein and Kinzler, 1992a). More indirect biochemical assays have been used for RB, by inhibiting phosphorylation of the gene product (Kaye et al., 1990; Templeton et al., 1991) and for NF1, by inhibiting the GTPase activity (Li et al., 1992). The functionality of missense mutations in the other tumor suppressor genes (MCC, APC, WT, DCC) can be inferred only indirectly in the absence of assays for protein function.

[c]Type of tumor where these mutations are consistently found.

[d]In all cases, sequencing was used to characterize the mutations.

tion across the cell membrane (reviewed in Barbacid, 1987; Santos and Nebreda, 1989). The active conformation of *ras* is that bound to GTP while the protein is inactive when bound to GDP (Trahey and McCormick, 1987; Field et al., 1987). The GTP-bound state is downregulated by another protein, termed GAP (Trahey and McCormick, 1987), which stimulates the intrinsic GTPase activity of *ras* proteins (Gibbs et al., 1984; McGrath et al., 1984; Sweet et al., 1984). Many mutant *ras* proteins are independent on GAP regulation and are therefore constitutively activated (reviewed in McCormick, 1989b). The *ras* gene products are also regulated *in vivo* by at least another GTPase activating protein, the product of the neurofibromatosis (NF1) gene (reviewed in Marshall, 1991b).

Activation of the oncogenic potential of *ras* proteins by single amino acid substitutions is sufficient to induce malignant transformation of some cultured established cells in a dominant but dose-dependent manner (reviewed in Spandidos and Lang, 1989). The dramatic changes in cell physiology observed immediately after introduction of mutant *ras* proteins, leading to the manifestation of the phenotypic alterations characteristic of malignancy, strongly suggest that *ras* play a pivotal role in the metabolic pathways controlling cell proliferation. Somatic mutational activation of *ras* oncogenes reproducibly occurs in many human malignancies (reviewed in Bos, 1989). The importance of the role of *ras* activation in oncogenesis is underscored by the continued presence and increased frequency of mutated genes along the entire tumorigenesis process (Perucho et al., 1989). Thus, *ras* genes are found mutated from the early and benign stages of tumor development, like colorectal adenomatous polyps (Bos et al., 1987; Forrester et al., 1987), to the most advanced stages of tumor progression, like metastases of pancreatic carcinomas (Almoguera et al., 1988).

The p53 Tumor Suppressor Gene

While *ras* activation has been until recently the most prevalent genetic alteration involved in human tumors, the inactivation of the p53 tumor suppressor gene has rapidly become the primary gene mutation associated with human cancer. Since the initial report describing the presence of somatic point mutations in the p53 gene accompanying the allelic loses of chromosome 17p sequences in two distinct colorectal carcinomas (Baker et al., 1989) and their extension to other tumors (Takahashi et al., 1989; Nigro et al., 1989), there has been an explosive growth of papers reporting the presence of p53 mutations in numerous types of tumors (reviewed in Hollstein et al., 1991; Tominaga et al., 1992).

The p53 gene product (Lane and Cradford, 1979; Linzer and Levine, 1979) is a nuclear phosphoprotein with specific DNA binding activity, constitutively expressed at low levels in most normal tissues and involved in cell proliferation (reviewed in Levine et al., 1991; Vogelstein and Kinzler, 1992a). Although mutant p53 can cooperate with activated *ras* to transform primary fibroblasts (Parada et al., 1984; Eliyahu et al., 1984), like the oncoproteins from DNA viruses and the nuclear *myc* oncogene family proteins (reviewed in Hunter, 1991), the wild-type protein suppresses the transformation of normal cells by *ras* and other oncogenes (Finlay et al., 1989; Eliyahu et al., 1989), and the growth of transformed cells *in vitro* (Baker et al., 1990; Michalowitz et al., 1990; Mercer et al., 1990) and *in vivo* (Chen et al., 1990).

In contrast with the point mutations that activate the *ras* genes, which are concentrated in a few positions (codons 12, 13, 61, 117, and 146), diverse types of structural alterations occur in the p53 gene, of which the most common, the missense mutations, are dispersed in a large portion of the gene coding region. This is probably a reflection of the different mechanisms of action of these mutations, in the first case activating a dominant oncogene, and in the second inactivating a recessive tumor suppressor gene. In support of this interpretation, while all oncogenic *ras* mutations are somatic, germ line mutations in the p53 gene have been described in some patients of the Li-Fraumeni familial cancer syndrome (Malkin et al., 1990, 1992; Srivastava et al., 1990). Moreover, while tumor cells can be heterozygous for the mutant *ras* allele (Winter et al., 1985; Perucho et al., 1989), mutations in the p53 gene are usually accompanied by deletion of the other allele (Baker et al., 1989, 1990; Takahashi et al., 1989; Nigro et al., 1989).

The high frequency and wide spectrum of mutations in *ras* and p53 genes make them very appropriate for a descriptive molecular analysis of mammalian mutagenesis and its relationship with carcinogenesis (Vogelstein and Kinzler, 1992b). These studies have already shown a clear association between the type of mutations and the tissue of origin of the tumors. For instance, in human tumors, G:C to A:T transitions at codons 12 and 13 of the c-K-*ras* gene are the most frequent mutations in colorectal adenomas and carcinomas (Bos et al., 1987; Vogelstein et al., 1988; Delattre et al., 1989; Miyaki et al., 1990; Capella et al., 1991), while G:C to T:A transversions predominate in lung carcinomas (Rodenhuis et al., 1988; Slebos et al., 1990; Mitsudomi et al., 1991; Capella et al., 1991). Similarly, p53 gene transitions at CpG sequences are the most frequent mutations in colorectal carcinomas while G to T transversions are more prevalent in lung carcinomas (reviewed in Hollstein et al., 1991). These are examples of how the molecular genetics of oncogenes and tumor suppressor genes offers direct applications for the molecular epidemiology of cancer (reviewed in Harris, 1991).

Methods of Detection of Single Point Mutations

Due to their subtle nature, the point mutations are the most difficult to detect of all the genetic alterations involved in cancer. Nevertheless, there are quite a few techniques capable of recognizing the presence of single base changes in mammalian genes. A diagram of the methods currently utilized for detection and characterization of single base substitutions, deletions, and insertions is shown in Figure 31.2. In the first row (A) are listed the methods for detection of the presence of the mutation. In (B) are the methods that permit characterization of the molecular nature of the mutation. While detection of the presence of a mutation might be sufficient for some diagnostic and prognostic purposes, characterization of the single base substitutions is also important for several reasons. In addition to be useful for understanding the etiology of mammalian mutations (see above), oncogene and tumor suppressor gene products may exhibit different biological properties depending on the amino acid substitutions (Seeburg et al., 1984; Der et al., 1986; Halevy et al., 1990). These differences may be associated with distinct clinical manifestations of potential prognostic value. For instance, we have found that c-K-*ras* gene products with aspartic acid substitutions at codon 13 are differentially associated with colorectal tumors of less aggressive neoplastic phenotype and of delayed cancer onset, relative to those with mutations at codon 12 (Capella et al., 1991; Malkhosyan et al., in preparation).

The RNase A mismatch cleavage method is based on the ability of pancreatic ribonuclease to recognize and cleave single base mismatches in RNA:RNA (Winter et al., 1985) and RNA:DNA heteroduplexes (Myers et al., 1985a). The method is performed by hybridization of the target sequence to a labeled complementary riboprobe, digestion with RNase A, and analysis of the resistant products by polyacrylamide electrophoresis in denaturing gels. Mutations are detected and localized by the presence and size of the RNA fragments generated by cleavage at the mismatches. Single nucleotide mismatches in DNA heteroduplexes are also recognized and cleaved by some chemicals, providing another strategy to detect single base substitutions, the mismatch chemical cleavage (MCC) generic denomination (Cotton et al., 1988; Montandon et al., 1989; Gogos et al., 1990).

The single strand conformation polymorphism (SSCP) is another method developed by Hayashi, Sekiya, and colleagues (Orita et al., 1989a,b; reviewed by Hayashi, 1991). It is based on the differences in the secondary structure of single-strand DNA molecules differing in a single nucleotide, which also is frequently reflected in an alteration of their electrophoretic mobility in nondenaturing gel electrophoresis. Mutations are detected by comparing side by side the electrophoretic patterns of tumor versus normal tissue DNAs after denaturation. The denaturing gradient gel electrophoresis (DGGE) method (Fischer and Lerman, 1983) uses electrophoresis in the presence of a gradient of a denaturing reagent like urea or formamide. Differences in melting properties of homoduplexes versus heteroduplexes differing in a single nucleotide can detect the presence of mutations in the target sequences because of the corresponding changes in their electrophoretic mobilities. The attachment of a GC "clamp" to the DNA fragments increases the fraction of mutations that can be recognized by DGGE (Myers et al., 1985b; Abrams et al., 1990). Modifications of the technique have been developed, using temperature gradients (Wartell et al., 1990), and the method can be also applied to RNA:RNA duplexes (Smith et al., 1988).

Hybridization with radioactively labeled allelic specific oligonucleotides (ASO) also has been applied to the detection of specific point mutations (Conner et al., 1983). The method is based on the differences in the melting temperature of short DNA fragments differing by a single nucleotide. Stringent hybridization and washing conditions can differentiate between mutant and wild-type alleles. Single point mutations have been also detected by the creation or destruction of restriction fragment length polymorphisms (RFLP).

FIGURE 31.2. Methods for the detection (**A**) and characterization (**B**) of point mutations.

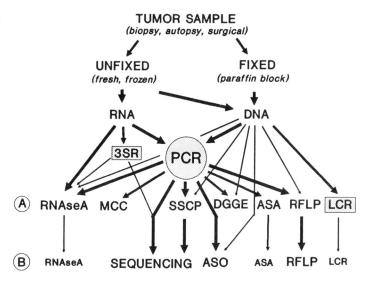

With the exception of the MCC, all these methods have been successfully utilized with total genomic DNA or total cellular RNA. The RNase A mismatch cleavage method has been used for detecting point mutations in oncogenes, in genes involved in hereditary diseases, and in RNA viruses (reviewed in Perucho, 1989; Lopez-Galindez et al., 1991) using total cellular RNA. This method was also successfully used for the detection of a few point mutations in total genomic DNA (Myers et al., 1985a). Similarly, single base substitutions can be detected using total genomic DNA by ASO hybridization (Conner et al., 1982; Bos et al., 1984, 1986; Guerrero et al., 1984; Zarbl et al., 1985; Valenzuela and Groffen, 1986). RFLP and Southern blot hybridization have also been applied to detect point mutations in *ras* genes using total genomic DNA (Feinberg et al., 1983; Santos et al., 1984; Kraus et al., 1984), and detection of point mutations by the DGGE and the SSCP methods was initially achieved with total genomic DNA (Myers et al., 1985c; Orita et al., 1990a, respectively). However, all these techniques have been greatly simplified by their application to genomic sequences previously amplified by *in vitro* enzymatic techniques, especially the PCR.

There are other techniques that can amplify genomic sequences *in vitro* besides the PCR.

The self-sustained sequence replication (3SR) (Guatelli et al., 1990) is a transcription-based *in vitro* amplification system (Kwoh et al., 1989) that can exponentially amplify RNA sequences at a uniform temperature. The amplified RNA can then be utilized for mutation detection (Fahy et al., 1991). Another technique that can achieve *in vitro* exponential amplification of cellular DNA sequences is the ligase amplification reaction (LAR) (Wu and Wallace, 1989) or ligase chain reaction (LCR) (Barany, 1991). This approach can amplify short DNA fragments by cycles of ligation/denaturation and can simultaneously identify the presence of single base mutations at the junction point of the oligonucleotides. The LAR, LCR, or oligonucleotide ligation assays (OLA) can be coupled to the PCR, and used for mutation detection (Landegren et al., 1988b; Wu and Wallace, 1989; Barany, 1991).

Besides the facilitation of the diagnostic techniques described before, the PCR has generated exclusive methods for single point mutation detection, based on the selective amplification of specific alleles. Again, the acronyms are numerous for a series of techniques based on the presence of mismatches at, or near, the 3'-end of the PCR primers. The mismatch between the primer and the wild-type sequence may impede the extension by *Taq* polymerase and little or no amplification occurs. On the other hand, the presence of a particular mutation, complementary to the primer, allows efficient amplification (Kwok et al., 1990). Variations of this approach are called allelic-specific amplification (ASA) (Wu et al., 1989; Okayama et al., 1989), allelic-specific enzymatic amplification (ASEA) (Nichols et al., 1989), amplification refractory mutation system (ARMS) (Newton et al., 1989), mismatched PCR (Stork et al., 1991), polymerase allelic-specific amplification (PASA) (Sommer et al., 1992), mutation-specific PCR assay (MSPA) (Nelson et al., 1992), and mismatch amplification mutation assay (MAMA) (Cha et al., 1992).

Some methods such as the MCC, the DGGE, or the SSCP are able to detect the mutations, but not their characterization (Fig. 31.2). Although the characterization of mutations can be achieved with the RNase A mismatch cleavage method, by using batteries of mutant riboprobes (Winter et al., 1985; Forrester et al., 1987b), this is complicated and cumbersome. Other methods are applicable only when the nature and/or the position of the mutation is known, like the ASA or the LCR.

Detection and Characterization of Oncogenic Single Point Mutations

The RNase A mismatch cleavage method has been used frequently for detection of point mutations in oncogenes (Forrester et al., 1987a,b; Perucho et al., 1989; Cesarman et al., 1987) and tumor suppressor genes (Dunn et al., 1988, 1989; Takahashi et al., 1989; Chiba et al., 1990) using total cellular RNA. Mutations have also been detected by this method using DNA amplified by the PCR in ras oncogenes (Almoguera et al., 1988, 1989; Shibata et al., 1990a) and in the MCC (Kinzler et al., 1991) and the APC (Nishisho et al., 1991; Miyoshi et al., 1992a,b) tumor suppressor gene (see Tables 31.1 and 31.2). The major drawback of this approach is the inability of RNase A to recognize some mismatches and the variable

extent of cleavage of another mismatches (reviewed in Perucho, 1989).

The ASO approach applied to PCR products also has been extensively utilized by Bos, Mc-Cormick, Rodenhuis, Marshall, and colleagues to detect and characterize point mutations in ras genes (Verlaan-de Vries et al., 1986; Bos et al., 1987; Rodenhuis et al., 1987; Vogelstein et al., 1988; Farr et al., 1988) and gsp/gip oncogenes (Lyons et al., 1990). Because of the presence of various nucleotide changes in multiple positions, the ASO method requires the use of many oligonucleotides to cover all possible oncogenic mutations. For instance, there are six different oncogenic nucleotide substitutions at codon 12 of each of the three ras oncogenes, and another six at codons 13 and 61. The analysis is even much more laborious in the tumor suppressor genes, where the missense and other point mutations are widely scattered. Therefore, the ASO method has been infrequently used for mutation detection in tumor suppressor genes (Shirasawa et al., 1991; Li et al., 1992).

In contrast, the SSCP method is more appropriate to detect the dispersed mutations in tumor suppressor genes. Since its inception, the SSCP has been utilized very extensively for detection of point mutations in ras oncogenes (Orita et al., 1990a,b; Suzuki et al., 1990) and in the p53 (reviewed in Hayashi, 1991; Tominaga et al., 1992), the RB (Murakami et al., 1991), the NF1 (Cawthon et al., 1991), and the APC (Groden et al., 1991) tumor suppressor genes. The sensitivity of the SSCP is superior to that of the RNase A mismatch cleavage, and the fraction of mutations that is not detectable is much smaller (Hayashi, 1991). Although detection of alterations in electrophoretic mobility is strongly dependent on the size of the fragments, this limitation can be circumvented by digesting with a restriction endonuclease the PCR products prior to SSCP analysis (Peinado et al., 1993).

Sequencing has been universally utilized to directly detect oncogenic point mutations or to characterize the mutations previously identified by other scanning methods, like the RNase A mismatch cleavage, the DGGE, or the SSCP. There are various methods for the sequencing of the PCR products, using both single- and double-strand DNA molecules (reviewed in Gyllensen, 1989; Bevan et al., 1992), and more recent protocols that use coupled amplification and sequencing, taking advantage of the amplification and sequencing capabilities of *Taq* DNA polymerase (Ruano and Kidd, 1991; Tracy and Mulcahy, 1991). *Ras* and p53 gene mutations have been characterized by direct sequencing protocols (McMahon et al., 1987; Collins et al., 1988) or after cloning the PCR products (Mariyama et al., 1989; Baker et al., 1989; Nigro et al., 1989). Cycle sequencing has also been utilized for the detection of p53 gene mutations, directly from total cellular RNA, using a reverse transcriptase-PCR approach (Peinado et al., 1993). The main limitation of the direct sequencing approach is its low sensitivity. Only when the mutant alleles are well represented in the tumor sample can they be readily identified. Because of the misincorporation rate of *Taq* polymerase, the mutations have to be confirmed by an independent amplification. In addition, the approach represents a formidable task when many mutations in many samples or large gene regions need to be analyzed (Powell et al., 1992).

Detection of Point Mutations by RFLP of PCR Amplified DNA Sequences

In contrast with the scanning detection methods (RNase A, MCC, DGGE, SSCP) that cannot characterize the mutations, the PCR/RFLP approach combines detection and characterization capabilities. The method has been used mainly for detection of *ras* mutations. The generation or destruction of restriction sites allows the rapid detection of point mutations after the genomic sequences are amplified by the PCR. In the former case, the mutation is cleaved by the specific restriction endonuclease, while the wild-type sequence is not. Gel electrophoresis easily identifies the mutations, since they generate smaller DNA fragments (Kumar and Barbacid, 1988). The situation is reversed when the mutation de-

stroys the restriction site previously present in the wild-type sequence. In this case the mutations are evidenced by the presence of undigested DNA fragments (Deng, 1988; Jiang et al., 1989).

Although many point mutations do not create or destroy a restriction site and therefore cannot be detected by this straightforward approach, the use of PCR primers containing mismatches relative to the target sequences can circumvent this limitation. The DNA fragments incorporate the sequence of the primers that can be designed to create a new RFLP (Kumar and Barbacid, 1988; Jiang et al., 1989; Haliassos et al., 1989). There are several compilations of mutant PCR primers designed to create new restriction sites in codons 12 and 61 of the *ras* oncogenes (Kumar and Dunn, 1989; Jacobson and Moskovits, 1991; Mitsudomi et al., 1991). The main advantage of this approach is that it does not require the use of radioactive isotopes and is more amenable therefore to analyses in clinical settings.

Figure 31.3 shows an example of the RFLP approach that we use for detection (top panel) and characterization (bottom panel) of *ras* mutations (Shibata et al., 1990b; Capella et al., 1991). Specifically, the aspartic acid substitution at codon 12 of the c-K-*ras* protooncogene (GGT→GAT, GLY→ASP). Replacement of the second G at codon 13 by an A generates an *Hph*I site (*GGT*GA) that is destroyed by any mutation at any of the two Gs of codon 12. Mutations of the T (third base of triplet 12) and G (first base of codon 13) are not considered, because after amplification they would be "erased" by the PCR primers. After a first round of PCR, using external primers, the amplified DNA fragments are reamplified with mutant primers that incorporate an *Hph*I site at codon 12. Mutations are detected by the presence of undigested DNA fragments with this enzyme. The other *Hph*I site introduced by the downstream primer is used as internal control to test for the completion of digestion (Fig. 31.3, top).

The sensitivity of this method is high initially, because the mutation is detected by the presence of nondigested DNA fragments, which includes not only the mutant sequences,

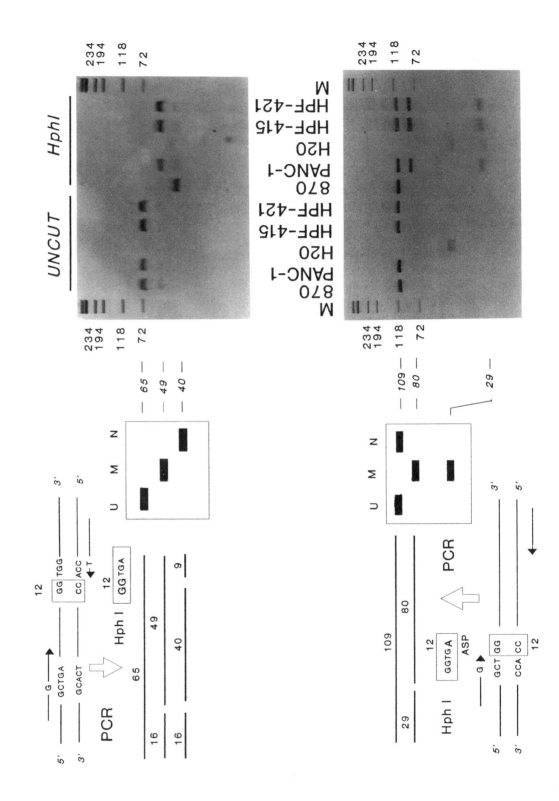

FIGURE 31.3. Detection and characterization of c-K-ras codon 12 point mutations by PCR/RFLP. Left panel: DNA sequences of the first coding exon of the c-K-ras gene were amplified by a first PCR as described in Capella et al. (1991). The amplified DNA was reamplified in a second, nested PCR, with primers designed to change the C to a T in the noncoding strand of codon 13 (top), or to change the G to a C at the coding strand of codon 11 (bottom). In the first case, an HphI site is present in wild-type sequences and in the second case only in mutant sequences containing the aspartic acid substitution at codon 12. The numbers indicate the sizes (in base pairs) of the restriction fragments.

Right panel: The PCR products were digested with HphI and analyzed in nondenaturing gel electrophoresis and stained with ethidium bromide. The numbers at the sides indicate the size in base pairs of HaeIII digested ΦX174 DNA fragments (M). 870, DNA from a normal tissue; Panc-1, a pancreatic carcinoma cell line. HPF-415 and 421 are cultures of human normal pancreatic cells at different passages after treatment with methyl nitroso urea, which turned out to be contaminated by cells of the Panc-1 tumor cell line (Perucho, unpublished observations). H2O is a blank lane with no DNA added to the PCR.

but also the hybrid DNA molecules between wild-type and mutant DNA strands (Fig. 31.4). This easily occurs, especially if the PCR is carried out for a high number of cycles, during the melting and annealing steps of the last cycles (Erlich and Arnheim, 1992). The reverse situation is also true: when a heterozygous mutant gene is detected by cleavage with a polymorphic enzyme, the mutant allele is underrepresented in the gel because the heteroduplexes between mutant and normal sequences are not cleaved (Figs. 31.4 and 31.3, bottom). This experiment illustrates the problem of the differential representation of mutant versus normal alleles depending on the cleavage or resistance to digestion: the apparent ratio of mutant/normal *ras* allele is higher in the top panel than in the lower panel, despite the fact that the analysis was carried out with DNA from the same cells. This problem can make difficult the estimation of the real ratio of mutant/normal alleles. The problem is exacerbated when the initial ratio of mutant/normal allele is less than 1:1. In contrast with hereditary diseases, this is a very frequent situation in the oncogenic somatic mutations occurring in tumors, due to the presence of contaminating normal tissue or to the absence of the mutation in some tumor cell subclones (Sidransky et al., 1992a; Shibata et al., 1993).

Detection of Point Mutations Present in Minor Proportions

Mutant alleles present between 3 and 10% of the molecules in the DNA preparation can be detected by the SSCP (Suzuki et al., 1991; Mitsudomi et al., 1991), RFLP (Jiang et al., 1989), RNase A (Almoguera et al., 1989), and ASO (Lyons, 1990) methods previously described, in decreasing order of sensitivity. This sensitivity is sometimes not sufficient when analyzing tumors where the neoplastic cells can be only a minor fraction of the tissue, for instance, in the initial stages of tumor development. In addition, in advanced tumors, the detection of cell subclones exhibiting higher malignant potential may be desirable (Sidransky

et al., 1992a). The detection of mutant *ras* genes in residual disease also has clear diagnostic and prognostic implications (reviewed in McCormick, 1989a).

The RFLP approach has been modified to increase the sensitivity of detection of *ras* point mutations in a minor fraction of cells in the tumor samples. This is achieved by digesting the amplified DNA with an enzyme (e.g., *Hph*I in Fig. 31.3, top panel) that cuts the wild-type but not the mutant allele, and reamplifying the digested products. In principle, only the mutant (noncleaved) DNA fragments would be amplified. This approach has been utilized for detecting mutant *ras* genes in human tumors (Kahn et al., 1991; Levi et al., 1991). However, the sensitivity can be increased only to about 1 mutant allele among 1000 wild-type alleles because of the fidelity of *Taq* polymerase (van Mansfeld and Bos, 1992) and because of the presence of DNA

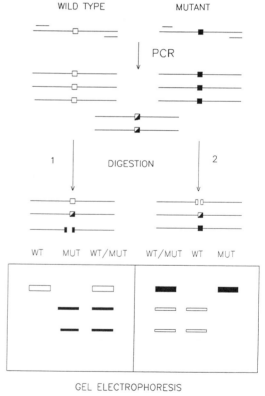

FIGURE 31.4. Mutant/wild-type allelic ratio bias in the PCR/RFLP mutation detection approach.

applications (Kirby, 1990). DNA fingerprinting using the highly polymorphic VNTRs (Jeffreys et al., 1985) has also been applied for the detection of polymorphisms during malignant transformation (Thein et al., 1987; de Jong et al., 1988). These polymorphisms have been useful for studies of clonality of tumors, both primary and metastatic (Smit et al., 1988; Fey et al., 1988; Wainscoat and Fey, 1988). DNA fingerprinting of minisatellite loci has also been applied to the analysis of somatic genetic alterations in transformation and both quantitative and qualitative genetic alterations have been detected in gastrointestinal tumors (Thein et al., 1987; Armour et al., 1989; Vogelstein et al., 1989). DNA fingerprinting has also benefited from the advent of the PCR (Jeffreys et al., 1990a,b).

A PCR-based DNA fingerprinting technique, the arbitrary primer PCR or AP-PCR (Welsh and McClelland, 1990) can also be applied for studying genetic alterations occurring in tumor cells (Peinado et al., 1992). This approach utilizes PCR amplification with a single arbitrary primer generating a large number of anonymous DNA bands that provide a fingerprint of the cell genome (see accompanying chapters). For a determined set of experimental conditions the pattern of DNA bands that is amplified is quite reproducible. This property of the method is fundamental in its demonstrated application for fingerprinting and mapping of DNA polymorphisms in various prokaryotic and eukaryotic systems (Welsh and McClelland, 1990, 1991; Welsh et al., 1991).

When applied to DNA from tumor and normal tissue of the same individual, changes in these genomes can be easily detected by comparison of their AP-PCR fingerprints (Fig. 31.6). Because the priming events during the initial low stringency cycles are random events, which depend on the nucleotide sequence of the PCR primer that is arbitrarily chosen, the amplified sequences are in principle a representative random small sample of the donor DNA cell genome. We have found that there is no apparent bias for the chromosomal origins of the amplified bands and that most bands represent single copy sequences (Peinado et al., 1992; Ionov et al., 1993).

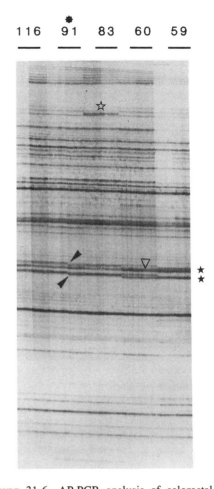

FIGURE 31.6. AP-PCR analysis of colorectal tumors. AP-PCR fingerprints of matched pairs of normal-tumor tissue DNA from colorectal carcinomas. Numbers on top indicate the case number. Normal and tumor tissue (left and right, respectively) were analyzed using 50 ng of genomic DNA with 125 μM each nucleotide, 2 μM arbitrary primer LH2: 5' GGATGGAAAAGTTGTATCAT 3', 5 μCi [α-^{32}S]dATP, and 2 units of *Taq* polymerase. The reaction consisted of 5 low-stringency cycles (1 min 95°C, 1 min 50°C, 1.5 min 72°C) and 30 high stringency cycles (30 sec 95°C, 30 sec 60°C, 1.5 min 72°C). The APPCR product was diluted with formamide-loading buffer, denatured at 90°C for 3 min, and analyzed in a sequencing gel for 6 hr at 50 W.

Therefore, it follows that a band pattern representing a near full complement of chromosomes can be obtained in a single amplification experiment. Also because the amplification levels of these bands are quantitative (Peinado et al., 1992), fluctuations in the intensities of the bands reflect changes in the relative amounts of these sequences. Thus, allelic losses and gains have been readily detected in colorectal tumors (Peinado et al., 1992). Therefore, the AP-PCR provides an alternative molecular approach for cancer cytogenetics.

In contrast with the VNTR DNA fingerprinting approach, the AP-PCR method permits the molecular cloning in a single step of altered DNA sequences, including those lost in tumor cells. Genomic sequences, initially identified by AP-PCR because they had undergone recurrent losses in colorectal tumors, were cloned and their localization at chromosome 17p was determined using amplification by PCR of somatic human/hamster cell hybrids (Peinado et al., 1992). These experiments showed that these sequences were linked to the p53 tumor suppressor gene, thus demonstrating the feasibility of the AP-PCR approach to detect, isolate, and characterize genomic sequences that by their linkage to tumor suppressor genes are useful markers for tumorigenesis. The chromosomal localization of many of the AP-PCR bands amplified with a specific arbitrary primer can be simultaneously determined by AP-PCR of the somatic cell hybrids (Peinado et al., 1992; Velazquez et al., in preparation). This is done by comparison of the AP-PCR pattern of cell hybrids containing only one human chromosome with those of human and hamster DNA. The presence in the cell hybrid DNA of extra bands with identical mobilities to human bands can assign the chromosomal origin for many bands specific for the arbitrary primer. This simplifies considerably the approach since allelic losses and gains of several known chromosomes simultaneously for many a single AP-PCR experiment a single step of sequences ymorphisms from characac l origins also has potential e mapping purposes.

The application of the AP-PCR approach to the analysis of colorectal tumorigenesis also has revealed the surprising existence of a subset of tumors (of which tumor 91 of Fig. 31.6 is a representative example) containing an enormous number of somatic mutations. These tumors, which show distinctive phenotypic, biological, and insertions, and clinical properties, contain deletions of one or a few nucleotides in simple repeated sequences that we calculate by extrapolation, can surpass the millions (Ionov et al., 1993). Although some of these somatic alterations are not strictly point mutations, they can be included in the category of cancer-specific mutations and due to the intrinsic difficulty in their detection, we postulated at the beginning that their frequency in tumors was underestimated. Therefore, the application of the AP-PCR approach to the analysis of genetic alterations in colorectal tumors has permitted the detection of these mutations that had passed inadverted by other methods, and has added further support to our hypothesis. These findings also strongly suggest that these tumors with ubiquitous somatic mutations represent a novel pathway for colorectal cancer, involving a profound subversion of the fidelity of the cell machinery for DNA replication or repair, possibly as a result of a somatic mutation in a gene controlling one of the steps in this process. Figure 31.6 shows a representative AP-PCR experiment where several of these somatic genetic alterations are exemplified. An interindividual polymorphic band is shown by an open star, and two bands representing length polymorphisms with solid stars. Allelic loss is shown by an empty triangle, and intragenic deletions by arrowheads.

Summary and Future Perspectives

The advent of the PCR has represented a revolution in many fields, including cancer research, because of the extraordinary facilitation achieved in the detection of somatic genetic alterations associated with tumorigenesis. The high analytical power of the PCR has had an important impact, especially in the analysis of point mutations activating onco-genes and inactivating tumor suppressor genes. Several techniques and combinations of techniques have been developed that allow the reliable and routine detection and characteriza-tion of these oncogenic mutations. The choice of these techniques depends on the specific type of mutations. For example, the localized and therefore predictable mutations in *ras* on-cogenes can be adequately detected and char-acterized by the ASO method, or by the RFLP approach, or by a combination of RFLP fol-lowed by ASO (Hruban et al., 1993). On the other hand, detection of the more scattered point mutations in tumor suppressor genes is more easily approached by scanning methods. To date, the most convenient and sensitive ap-proach probably is the SSCP method, followed by sequencing of the positive tumors. The coupling of amplification and sequencing also is attractive, although its sensitivity is not very high and mutations can be missed if the extent of contamination by normal tissue in tumor samples is considerable.

The ability of the PCR to amplify DNA seg-ments from tissues fixed in formalin and stored at room temperature for many years has also represented a great advance in the analysis of neoplastic diseases of rare incidence or poor prognosis. In addition, the power of PCR to amplify minute amounts of DNA offers a great opportunity as a molecular diagnostic tool for malignant disease (Shibata et al., 1990; Si-dransky et al., 1991, 1992b). These assays also have potential applications for risk assess-ment and for early cancer detection. Retro-spective studies can also readily be performed that facilitate the prognostic applications of mutations in oncogenes and tumor suppressor genes. The detection of oncogenic point muta-tions can be achieved without radioactivity (Fig. 31.3; van Mansfield and Bos, 1992), and by direct incorporation of fluorescent markers during the amplification reaction (Chebab and Kan, 1989; Makino et al., 1992) and some procedures are amenable to automation (Lan-degren et al., 1988a). These advances will un-doubtedly lead to the application of diagnostic tests in clinical environments.

The quantitative properties of PCR (Ferre, 1992), in concert with the ability of PCR for DNA fingerprinting with arbitrary primers (Welsh and McClelland, 1990), provides a complementary and alternative molecular ap-proach to the cytogenetics of solid tumors (Peinado et al., 1992). It also provides a pow-erful tool to estimate the spontaneous mutation rate of unstable sequences and to analyze so-matic genetic variation. The opportunity that AP-PCR offers to delve in the cancer cell genome from an unbiased perspective may also have applications for the understanding of the genomic instability of cancer cells (Ionov et al., 1993). Finally, the possibility of finger-printing RNA in a quantitative manner by AP-PCR (Liang and Pardee, 1992; Welsh et al., 1992) will undoubtedly open a new field of research to study differential gene expres-sion in many situations, of which malignant transformation is an obvious and important example.

References

Abrams ES, Murdaugh SE, Lerman LS (1990): Comprehensive detection of single base changes in human genomic DNA using denaturing gradi-ent gel electrophoresis and a GC-clamp. *Genom-ics* 7:463–475.

Alitalo K, Schwab M, Lin CC, Varmus HE, Bishop JM (1983): Homogeneously staining chromo-somal regions contain amplified copies of an abundantly expressed cellular oncogene (c-*myc*) in malignant neuroendocrine cells from a human colon carcinoma. *Proc Natl Acad Sci USA* 80:1707–1711.

Almoguera C, Shibata D, Forrester K, Martin J, Arnheim N, Perucho M (1988): Most human car-cinomas of the exocrine pancreas contain mutant c-K-*ras* genes. *Cell* 53:549–554.

Almoguera C, Forrester K, Perucho M (1989): Ap-plication of the polymerase chain reaction for the detection of single-base substitutions by the RNAse A mismatch cleavage method. In *Current Communications in Molecular Biology.* Erlich HA, Gibbs R, Kazazian HH, eds. Cold Spring Harbor, NY: Cold Spring Harbor Laboratory, pp. 37–45.

Armour JAL, Patel I, Thein SL, Fey MF, Jeffreys AJ (1989): Analysis of somatic mutations at human minisatellite loci in tumors and cell lines. *Genomics* 4:328–334.

Baker SJ, Fearon ER, Nigro JM, Hamilton SR, Preisinger AC, Jessup JM, van Tuinen P, Ledbetter DH, Barker DF, Nakamura Y, White R, Vogelstein B (1989): Chromosome 17 deletions and p53 gene mutations in colorectal carcinomas. *Science* 244:217–221.

Baker SJ, Markowitz S, Fearon ER, Wilson JKV, Vogelstein B (1990): Suppression of human colorectal carcinoma cell growth by wild-type p53. *Science* 249:912–915.

Barany F (1991): Genetic disease detection and DNA amplification using cloned thermostable ligase. *Proc Natl Acad Sci USA* 88:189–193.

Barbacid M (1987): *ras* genes. *Ann Rev Biochem* 56:779–827.

Bargmann CI, Hung M-C, Weinberg RA (1986): Multiple independent activations of the *neu* oncogene by a point mutation altering the transmembrane domain of p185. *Cell* 45:649–657.

Bennet WP, Hollstein MC, He A, Zhu SM, Reasau JH, Trump BF, Metcalf RA, Welsh JA, Midgley C, Lane DP, Harris CC (1991): Archival analysis of p53 genetic and protein alterations in Chinese esophageal cancer. *Oncogene* 6:1779–1784.

Bevan IS, Rapley R, Walker MR (1992): Sequencing of PCR-amplified DNA. *PCR Methods Applic* 1:222–228.

Bishop JM (1991): Molecular themes in oncogenesis. *Cell* 64:235–248.

Bodmer WF, Bailey CJ, Bodmer J, Bussey HJ, Ellis A, Gorman P, Lucibello FC, Murday VA, Rider SH, Scambler P, Sheer D, Solomon E, Spurr NK (1987): Localization of the gene for familial adenomatous polyposis on chromosome 5. *Nature (London)* 328:617–616.

Bookstein R, Lee W-H (1991): Molecular genetics of the retinoblastoma suppressor gene. *Crit Rev Oncogen* 2:211–228.

Bos JL (1989): *ras* Oncogenes in human cancer: A review. *Cancer Res* 49:4682–4689.

Bos JL, Verlaan-de Vries M, Jansen AM, Veeneman GH, van Boom JH, van der Eb AJ (1984): Three different mutations in codon 61 of the human N-*ras* gene detected by synthetic oligonucleotide hybridization. *Nucl Acids Res* 12:9155–9163.

Bos JL, Verlaan-de Vries M, Marshall CJ, Veeneman GH, van Boom JH, van der Eb AJ (1986): A human gastric carcinoma contains a single mutated and an amplified normal allele of the Ki-*ras* oncogene. *Nucl Acids Res* 14:1209–1217.

Bos JL, Fearon ER, Hamilton SR, Verlaan-de Vries M, van Boom J, van der Eb A, Vogelstein B (1987): Prevalence of *ras* gene mutations in human colorectal cancer. *Nature (London)* 327:293–297.

Bourne HR, Sanders D, McCormick F (1990): The GTPase superfamily: A conserved switch for diverse cell functions. *Nature (London)* 348:125–132.

Brodeur J, Seeger RC, Schwab M, Varmus HE, Bishop JM (1984): Amplification of N-*myc* in untreated human neuroblastoma correlates with advanced disease stage. *Science* 224:1121–1124.

Capella G, Cronauer-Mitra S, Peinado MA, Perucho M (1991): Frequency and spectrum of mutations at codons 12 and 13 of the c-K-*ras* gene in human tumors. *Environ Health Perspect* 93:125–131.

Carter G, Ridge S, Padula RA (1992): Genetic lesions in preleukemia. *Crit Rev Oncogen* 3:339–364.

Cawthon RM, Weiss R, Xu G, Viskochil D, Culver M, Stevens J, Robertson M, Dunn D, Gesteland R, O'Connell P, White R (1990): A major segment of the neurofibromatosis type 1 gene: cDNA sequence, genomic structure and point mutations. *Cell* 62:193–201.

Cesarman E, Dalla Favera R, Bentley D, Groudine M (1987): Mutations in the first exon are associated with altered transcription of c-*myc* in Burkitt lymphoma. *Science* 238:1272–1275.

Cha RS, Zarbl H, Keohavong P, Thilly WG (1992): Mismatch amplification mutation assay (MAMA): Application to the c-H-*ras* gene. *PCR Methods Applic* 2:14–20.

Chehab FF, Kan YW (1989): Detection of specific DNA sequences by fluorescence amplification: A color complementation assay. *Proc Natl Acad Sci USA* 86:9178–9182.

Chen P-L, Chen Y, Bookstein R, Lee W-H (1990): Genetic mechanisms of tumor suppression by the human p53 gene. *Science* 250:1576–1580.

Chiba I, Takahashi T, Nau MM, D'Amico DD, Curiel DT, Mitsudomi T, Bachhagen DL, Carbone D, Piantadosi S, Koga H, Reissman PT, Slamon DJ, Holmes EC, Minna JD (1990): Mutations in the p53 gene are frequent in primary, resected non-small cell lung cancer. *Oncogene* 5:1603–1610.

Collins S, Groudine M (1982): Amplification of endogenous *myc*-related DNA sequences in a human myeloid leukaemia cell line. *Nature (London)* 298:679–681.

Collins SJ (1988): Direct sequencing of amplified genomic fragments documents N-*ras* point mutations in myeloid leukemia. *Oncogene Res* 3:117–123.

Conner BJ, Reyes AA, Morin C, Itakura K, Teplitz RL, Wallace RB (1983): Detection of sickle cell β-S globin allele by hybridization with synthetic oligonucleotides. *Proc Natl Acad Sci USA* 80:278–282.

Cotton RG, Rodrigues NR, Campbell RD (1988): Reactivity of cytosine and thymine in single base pair mismatches with hydroxylamine as osmium tetroxide and its applications to study of mutations. *Proc Natl Acad Sci USA* 85:4397–4401.

Cox A, Der C (1992): The *ras*/cholesterol connection: Implications for *ras* oncogenicity. *Crit Rev Oncogen* 3:365–400.

Dal Cin P, Sandberg AA (1989): Chromosomal aspects of human oncogenesis. *Crit Rev Oncogen* 1:113–126.

de Jong D, Voetdijk BMH, Kluin-Nelemans JC, van Ommen GJB, Kluin PhM (1988): Somatic changes in B-lymphoproliferative disorders (B-LPD) detected by DNA-fingerprinting. *Br J Cancer* 58:773–775.

de Klein A, van Kessel AG, Grosveld G, Bartram CR, Hagemeijer A, Bootsma D, Spurr NK, Heisterkamp N, Groffen J, Stephenson JR (1982): A cellular oncogene is translocated to the Philadelphia chromosome in chronic myelocytic leukaemia. *Nature (London)* 300:765–767.

Delattre O, Law DJ, Remvikos Y, Sastre X, Feinberg AP, Olschwang S, Melot T, Salmon RJ, Validire P, Thomas G (1989): Multiple genetic alterations in distal and proximal colorectal cancer. *The Lancet* 11:353–355.

Deng G (1988): A sensitive non-radioactive PCR-RFLP analysis for detecting point mutations at 12th codon of oncogene c-Ha-*ras* in DNAs of gastric cancer. *Nucl Acids Res* 16:6231.

Der CJ, Finkel T, Cooper GM (1986): Biological and biochemical properties of human H-*ras* genes mutated at codon 61. *Cell* 44:167–176.

Dubeau K, Chandler LA, Gralow JR, Nichols PW, Jones PA (1986): Southern blot analysis of DNA extracted from formalin-fixed pathology specimens. *Cancer Res* 46:2964–2969.

Dunn JM, Phillips RA, Becker AJ, Gallie BL (1988): Identification of germline and somatic mutations affecting the retinoblastoma gene. *Science* 241:1797–1800.

Dunn JM, Phillips RA, Zhu X, Becker A, Gallie BL (1989): Mutations in the *RB1* gene and their effects on transcription. *Mol Cell Biol* 9:4596–4604.

Ehlen T, Dubeau L (1989): Detection of *ras* point mutations by polymerase chain reaction using mutation-specific, inosine-containing oligonucleotide primers. *Biochem Biophys Res Commun* 160:441–447.

Eliyahu D, Raz A, Gruss P, Givol D, Oren M (1984): Participation of p53 cellular tumor antigen in transformation of normal embryonic cells. *Nature (London)* 312:651–654.

Eliyahu D, Michalovitz D, Eliyahu S, Pinhasi-Kimi O, Oren M (1989): Wild-type p53 can inhibit oncogene-mediated focus formation. *Proc Natl Acad Sci USA* 86:8763–8767.

Erlich HA, Arnheim N (1992): Genetic analysis using the polymerase chain reaction. *Annu Rev Genet* 26:479–506.

Fahy E, Kwoh DY, Gingeras TR (1991): Self-sustained sequence replication (3SR): An isothermal transcription-based amplification system alternative to PCR. *PCR Methods Applic* 1:25–33.

Farr CJ, Saiki RK, Erlich HA, McCormick F, Marshall CJ (1988): Analysis of *RAS* gene mutations in acute myeloid leukemia by polymerase chain reaction and oligonucleotide probes. *Proc Natl Acad Sci USA* 85:1629–1633.

Fearon ER, Vogelstein B (1990): A genetic model for colorectal tumorigenesis. *Cell* 61:759–767.

Fearon ER, Cho KR, Nigro JM, Kern SE, Simons JW, Ruppert JM, Hamilton SR, Preisinger AC, Thomas G, Kinzler KW, Vogelstein B (1990): Identification of a chromosome 18q gene that is altered in colorectal cancers. *Science* 247:49–56.

Feinberg AP, Vogelstein B, Droller MJ, Baylin SB, Nelkin BD (1983): Mutation affecting the 12th amino acid of the c-H-*ras* oncogene product occurs infrequently in human cancer. *Science* 220:1175–1177.

Ferre F (1992): Quantitative or semi-quantitative PCR: Reality versus myth. *PCR Methods Applic* 2:1–9.

Fey MF, Wells RA, Wainscoat JS, Thein SL (1988): Assessment of clonality in gastrointestinal cancer by DNA fingerprinting. *J Clin Invest* 82:1532–1537.

Field J, Broek D, Kataoka T, Wigler M (1987): Guanine nucleotide activation of, and competition between, *RAS* proteins from *Saccharomyces cerevisiae*. *Mol Cell Biol* 7:2128–2133.

Finlay CA, Hinds PW, Levine AJ (1989): The p53 proto-oncogene can act as a suppressor of transformation. *Cell* 57:1083–1093.

Fischer SG, Lerman LS (1983): DNA fragments differing by single base pair substitutions separated in denaturing gradient gels: Correspondence with melting theory. *Proc Natl Acad Sci USA* 80:1579–1583.

Forrester K, Almoguera C, Han K, Grizzle WE, Perucho M (1987a): Detection of high incidence of K-*ras* oncogenes during human colon tumorigenesis. *Nature* (*London*) 327:298–303.

Forrester K, Almoguera C, Jordano J, Grizzle WE, Perucho M (1987b): High incidence of c-K-*ras* oncogenes in human colon cancer detected by the RNAse A mismatch cleavage method. *J Tumor Marker Oncol* 2:113–123.

Furth M, Greaves M (eds.) (1989): *Molecular Diagnostics of Human Cancer. Cancer Cells 7.* Cold Spring Harbor, NY: Cold Spring Harbor Laboratory.

Gibbs JB, Sigal IS, Poe M, Scolnick EM (1984): Intrinsic GTPase activity distinguishes normal and oncogenic *ras* p21 molecules. *Proc Natl Acad Sci USA* 81:5704–5708.

Goelz SE, Hamilton SR, Vogelstein B (1985): Purification of DNA from formaldehyde fixed and paraffin embedded human tissue. *Biochem Biophys Res Commun* 130:118–126.

Gogos JA, Karayiorgou M, Aburatani H, Kafatos FC (1990): Detection of single base mismatches of thymine and cytosine residues by potassium permanganate and hydroxylamine in the presence of tetrakylammonium salts. *Nucl Acids Res* 18:6807–6814.

Groden J, Thilveris A, Samowitz W, Carlson M, Gelbert L, Albertsen H, Joslyn G, Stevens J, Spirio L, Robertson M, Sargeant L, Krapcho K, Wolf E, Burt R, Hughes JP, Warrington J, McPherson J, Wasmuth J, Le Paslier D, Abderrahim H, Cohen D, Leppert M, White R (1991): Identification and characterization of the familial adenomatous polyposis coli gene. *Cell* 66:589–600.

Guatelli JC, Whitfield DY, Kwow KJ, Barringer DD, Richman DD, Gingeras TR (1990): Isothermal, in vitro amplification of nucleic acids by a multienzyme reaction modeled after retroviral replication. *Proc Natl Acad Sci USA* 87:1874–1878.

Guerrero I, Villasante A, Corces V, Pellicer A (1984): Activation of a c-K-*ras* oncogene by somatic mutation in mouse lymphomas induced by gamma radiation. *Science* 225:1159–1162.

Gupta S, Gallego C, Lowndes JM, Pleiman CM, Sable C, Eisfelder BJ, Johnson GL (1992): Analysis of the fibroblast transformation potential of GTPase-deficient gip2 oncogenes. *Mol Cell Biol* 12:190–197.

Gyllensen U (1989): Direct sequencing of in vitro amplified DNA. In *PCR Technology: Principles and Applications for DNA Amplification.* New York: Stockton Press, pp. 45–60.

Halevy O, Michalowitz D, Oren M (1990): Different tumor-derived p53 mutants exhibit distinct biological activities. *Science* 250:113–116.

Haliassos A, Chomel JC, Grandjouan S, Druh J, Kaplan JC, Kitzis A (1989): Detection of minority point mutations by modified PCR technique: A new approach for a sensitive diagnosis of tumor progression markers. *Nucl Acids Res* 17: 8093–8099.

Harris CC (1991): Chemical and physical carcinogenesis. Advances and perspectives for the 1990s. *Cancer Res* 51:5023–5044.

Harwood J, Tachibana A, Meuth M (1991): Multiple dispersed spontaneous mutations: A novel pathway of mutation in a malignant human cell line. *Mol Cell Biol* 11:3163–3170.

Hayashi K (1991): PCR-SSCP: A simple and sensitive method for detection of mutations in the genomic DNA. *PCR Methods Applic* 1:34–38.

Hayward WS, Neel BG, Astrin SM (1981): Activation of a cellular *onc* gene by promoter insertion in ALV-induced lymphoid leukosis. *Nature* (*London*) 290:475–480.

Heim S, Mitelman F (1987): *Cancer Cytogenetics.* New York: Alan Liss.

Hollstein M, Sidransky D, Vogelstein B, Harris CC (1991): p53 mutations in human cancers. *Science* 253:49–53.

Horowitz JM, Yandell DW, Park S, Canning S, Whyte P, Buchkovich K, Harlow E, Weinberg RA, Dryja TP (1989): Point mutational inactivation of the retinoblastoma antioncogene. *Science* 243:937–940.

Hruban RH, van Mansfeld AD, Offerhaus GJ, van Weering, Allison DC, Goodman SN, Kensler TW, Bose KK, Cameron JL, Bos JL (1993): K-ras oncogene activation in adenocarcinoma of the human pancreas: A study of 82 carcinomas using a combination of mutant-enriched polymerase chain reaction analysis and allele specific oligonucleotide hybridization. *Am J Pathol* 143: 545–554.

Hunter T (1991): Cooperation between oncogenes. *Cell* 64:249–270.

Impraim CC, Saiki RK, Erlich HA, Teplitz RL (1987): Analysis of DNA extracted from formalin-fixed, paraffin-embedded tissues by enzyme amplification and hybridization with sequence-specific oligonucleotides. *Biochem Biophys Res Commun* 142:710–716.

Ionov J, Peinado MA, Malkhosyan S, Shibata D, Perucho M (1993). Ubiquitous somatic mutations in simple repeated sequences reveal a new mechanism for colonic carcinogenesis. *Nature* 363:558–561.

Jacobson DR, Moskovits T (1991): Rapid, nonradioactive screening for activating *ras* mutations using PCR-primer introduced restriction analysis (PCR-PIRA). *PCR Methods Applic* 1:146–148.

Jeffreys AJ, Wilson V, Thein SL (1985): Hypervariable "minisatellite" regions in human DNA. *Nature (London)* 314:67–72.

Jeffreys AJ, Neumann R, Wilson V (1990a): Repeat unit sequence variation in minisatellites: A novel source of DNA polymorphism for studying variation and mutation by single molecule analysis. *Cell* 60:473–485.

Jeffreys AJ, Wilson V, Neumann R, Keyte J (1990b): Amplification of human minisatellites by the polymerase chain reaction; towards DNA fingerprinting of single cells. *Nucl Acids Res* 16:10953–10971.

Jiang W, Kahn SM, Guillem JG, Lu S-H, Weinstein IB (1989): Rapid detection of *ras* oncogenes in human tumors: Applications to colon, esophageal, and gastric cancer. *Oncogene* 4:923–928.

Kahn S, Jiang W, Culberston T, Weinstein IB, Williams GM, Tomita N, Ronai Z (1991): Rapid and sensitive nonradioactive detection of mutant K-*ras* genes via 'enriched' PCR amplification. *Oncogene* 6:1079–1083.

Kaye FJ, Kratzke RA, Gerster JL, Horowitz JM (1990): A single amino acid substitution results in a retinoblastoma protein defective in phosphorylation and oncoprotein binding. *Proc Natl Acad Sci USA* 87:6922–6926.

Kern SE, Fearon ER, Tersmette KWF, Enterline JP, Leppert M, Nakamura Y, White R, Vogelstein B, Hamilton SR (1989): Allelic loss in colorectal carcinoma. *J Am Med Assoc* 261:3099–3103.

Kinzler K, Nilbert M, Vogelstein B, Bryan T, Levy D, Smith K, Preisinger A, Hamilton S, Hedge P, Markham A, Carlson M, Joslyn G, Groden J, White R, Miki Y, Miyoshi Y, Nishisho I, Nakamura Y (1991): Identification of a gene located at chromosome 5q21 that is mutated in colorectal cancers. *Science* 251:1366–1370.

Kirby L (1990): *DNA Fingerprinting. An Introduction.* New York: Stockton Press.

Klein G (1983): Specific chromosomal translocations and the genesis of B-cell-derived tumors in mice and men. *Cell* 32:311–315.

Kohl NE, Kanda N, Schreck RR, Bruns G, Latt SA, Gilbert F, Alt FW (1983): Transposition and amplification of oncogene-related sequences in human neuroblastomas. *Cell* 35:359–367.

Kraus MH, Yuasa Y, Aaronson S (1984): A position 12-activated H-*ras* oncogene in all HS578T mammary carcinosarcoma cells but not normal mammary cells of the same patient. *Proc Natl Acad Sci USA* 81:5384–5388.

Kumar R, Barbacid M (1988): Oncogene detection at the single cell level. *Oncogene* 3:647–651.

Kumar R, Dunn L (1989): Designed diagnostic restriction fragment length polymorphisms for the detection of point mutations in *ras* oncogenes. *Oncogene Res* 1:235–241.

Kumar R, Sukumar S, Barbacid M (1990): Activation of *ras* oncogenes preceding the onset of neoplasia. *Science* 248:1101–1104.

Kwoh DY, Davis GR, Whitfield KM, Chappelle HL, DiMichele LJ, Gingeras TR (1989): Transcription-based amplification system and detection of amplified human immunodeficiency virus type 1 with a bead-based sandwich hybridization format. *Proc Natl Acad Sci USA* 86:1173–1177.

Kwok S, Kellogg DE, McKinney N, Spasic D, Goda L, Sninsky (1990): Effect of primer-template mismatches on the polymerase chain reaction: Human immunodefficiency virus type 1 model studies. *Nucl Acid Res* 18:999–1005.

Landegren U, Kaiser R, Caskey CT, Hood L (1988a): DNA diagnostics. Molecular techniques and automation. *Science* 242:229–237.

Landegren U, Kaiser R, Sanders J, Hood L (1988b): A ligase-mediated gene detection technique. *Science* 241:1077–1080.

Landis CA, Masters SB, Spada A, Pace AM, Bourne HR, Vallar L (1989): GTPase inhibiting mutations activate the a chain of Gs and stimulate adenylyl cyclase in human pituitary tumours. *Nature (London)* 340:692–696.

Lane DP, Crawford LV (1979): T antigen is bound to a host protein in SV40-transformed cells. *Nature (London)* 278:261–263.

Lee EY, Bookstein R, Young LJ, Lin CJ, Rosenfeld MG, Lee WH (1988b): Molecular mechanism of retinoblastoma gene inactivation in retinoblastoma cell line Y79. *Proc Natl Acad Sci USA* 85:6017–6021.

Levi S, Urbano-Ispizua A, Gill R, Thomas D, Gilberston J, Foster C, Marshall CJ (1991): Multiple K-*ras* codon 12 mutations in cholangiocarcinomas demonstrated with a sensitive polymerase chain reaction technique. *Cancer Res* 51:3497–3502.

Levine AJ, Momand J, Finlay CA (1991): The p53 tumour suppressor gene. *Nature* (*London*) 351:453–456.

Li Y, Bollag G, Clark R, Stevens J, Conroy L, Fults D, Ward K, Friedman E, Samowitz W, Robertson M, Bradley P, McCormick F, White R, Crawthon R (1992): Somatic mutations in the neurofibromatosis 1 gene in human tumors. *Cell* 69:275–281.

Liang P, Pardee AB (1992): Differential display of eukaryotic messenger RNA by means of the polymerase chain reaction. *Science* 257:967–970.

Linzer DP, Levine AJ (1979): Characterization of a 54k dalton cellular SV40 tumor antigen present in SV40 transformed cells and uninfected embryonal carcinoma cells. *Cell* 17:43–52.

Little CD, Nau MM, Carney DN, Gazdar AF, Minna JD (1983): Amplification and expression of the c-*myc* oncogene in human lung cancer cell lines. *Nature* (*London*) 306:194–196.

Loeb LA, Springgate CF, Battula N (1974). Errors in DNA replication as a basis of malignant changes. *Cancer Res* 34:2311–2321.

Lopez-Galindez C, Rojas JM, Najera R, Richman DD, Perucho M (1991): Characterization of genetic variation and AZT resistance mutations of HIV by the RNAse A mismatch cleavage method. *Proc Natl Acad Sci USA* 88:4280–4284.

Luscher B, Christenson E, Litchfield DW, Krebs EG, Eisenman RN (1990): Myb DNA binding inhibited by phosphorylation at a site deleted during oncogenic activation. *Nature* (*London*) 344:517–522.

Lyons J (1990): Analysis of *ras* gene point mutations by PCR and oligonucleotide hybridization. In *PCR Protocols. A Guide to Methods and Applications*. Innis MA, Gelfand DH, Sninsky JJ, White TJ, eds. San Diego: Academic Press, pp. 386–391.

Lyons J, Landis C, Harsh G, Vallar L, Grunewald K, Feichtinger H, Duh Q-Y, Clark OH, Kawasaki E, Bourne HR, McCormick (1990): Two G protein oncogenes in human endocrine tumors. *Science* 249:655–659.

Makino R, Yazyu H, Kishimoto Y, Sekiya T, Hayashi K (1992): F-SSCP: Fluorescence-bases polymerase chain reaction-single strand conformation polymorphism (PCR-SSCP) analysis. *PCR Methods Applic* 2:10–13.

Malkin D, Li, Strong LC, Fraumeni JF, Nelson CE, Kim DH, Kassel J, Gryka MA, Bischoff FZ, Tainsky MA, Friend SH (1990): Germ line p53 mutations in a familial syndrome of breast cancer, sarcomas and other neoplasias. *Science* 250:1233–1238.

Malkin D, Jolly KW, Barbier N, Look T, Friend SH, Gebhardt MC, Andersen TI, Borresen AL, Li FP, Garber J, Strong LC (1992): Germline mutations of the p53 tumor suppressor gene in children and young adults with second malignant neoplasm. *N Engl J Med* 326:1309–1315.

Mariyama M, Kishi K, Nakamura K, Obata H, Nishimura S (1989): Frequency and types of point mutation at the 12th codon of the c-Ki-ras gene found in pancreatic cancers from Japanese patients. *Japan J Cancer Res* 80:622–626.

Marshall C (1991a): Tumor suppressor genes. *Cell* 64:313–326.

Marshall C (1991b): How does p21 *ras* transform cells? *Trends Genet* 7:91–95.

Mashiyama S, Murakami Y, Yoshimoto T, Sekiya T, Hayashi K (1991): Detection of p53 gene mutations in human brain tumors by single-strand conformation polymorphism analysis of polymerase chain reaction products. *Oncogene* 6:1313–1318.

McCormick F (1989a): The polymerase chain reaction and cancer diagnosis. *Cancer Cells* (*a monthly review*) 1:56–61.

McCormick F (1989b): *ras* GTPase activating protein: Signal transmitter and signal terminator. *Cell* 56:5–8.

McGrath JP, Capon DJ, Goeddel DV, Levinson AD (1984): Comparative biochemical properties of normal and activated human *ras* p21 protein. *Nature* (*London*) 310:644–649.

McMahon G, Davis E, Wogan GN (1987): Characterization of c-Ki-*ras* oncogene alleles by direct sequencing of enzymatically amplified DNA from carcinogen-induced tumors. *Proc Natl Acad Sci USA* 84:4974–4978.

Meijlink F, Curran T, Miller AD, Verma IM (1985): Removal of a 67-base-pair sequence in the noncoding region of protooncogene *fos* converts it to a transforming gene. *Proc Natl Acad Sci USA* 82:4987–4991.

Mercer WE, Shields MT, Amin M, Sauve GJ, Appella E, Rommo J, Ullrich S (1990): Negative growth regulation in a glioblastoma tumor cell line that conditionally expresses human wild-type p53. *Proc Natl Acad Sci USA* 87:6166–6170.

Michalowitz D, Halevy O, Oren M (1990): Conditional inhibition of transformation and of cell proliferation by a temperature-sensitive mutant of p53. *Cell* 62:671–680.

Mitsudomi T, Viallet J, Mulshine JL, Linnoila RI, Minna JD, Gazdar AF (1991): Mutations of *ras* genes distinguish a subset of non-small cell lung cancer cell lines from small cell lung cancer cell lines. *Oncogene* 6:1353–1362.

Miyaki M, Seki M, Okamoto M, Yamanaka A, Maeda Y, Tanaka K, Kikuchi R, Iwama T, Ikeuchi T, Tonomura A, Nakamura Y, White R, Miki Y, Utsunomiya J, Koike M (1990): Genetic changes and histopathological types in colorectal tumors from patients with familial adenomatous polyposis. *Cancer Res* 50:7166–7173.

Miyoshi Y, Nagase H, Ando H, Horii A, Ichii S, Nakatsuru S, Aoki T, Miki Y, Mori T, Nakamura Y (1992a): Somatic mutations of the APC gene in colorectal tumors: Mutation cluster region in the APC gene. *Human Mol Genet* 1:229–234.

Miyoshi Y, Ando H, Nagase H, Nishisho I, Horii A, Miki Y, Mori T, Utsonomiya J, Baba S, Petersen G, Hamilton SR, Kinzler KW, Vogelstein B, Nakamura Y (1992b): Germ-line mutations of the APC gene in 53 familial adenomatous polyposis patients. *Proc Natl Acad Sci USA* 89:4452–4456.

Momand J, Zambetti GP, Olson DC, George D, Levine AJ (1992): The *mdm-2* oncogene product forms a complex with the p53 protein and inhibits p53-mediated transactivation. *Cell* 69:1237–1245.

Montandon AJ, Green PM, Giannelli F, Bentley DR (1989): Direct detection of point mutations by mismatch analysis: Application to hemophilia B. *Nucl Acids Res* 17:3347–3358.

Mullis KB, Faloona FA (1987): Specific synthesis of DNA *in vitro* via a polymerase catalyzed chain reaction. *Methods Enzymol* 155:335–350.

Murakami Y, Katahira M, Makino R, Hayashi K, Hirohashi S, Sekiya T (1991): Inactivation of the retinoblastoma gene in a human lung carcinoma cell line detected by single strand conformation polymorphism analysis of the polymerase chain reaction product of cDNA. *Oncogene* 6:37–42.

Myers RM, Larin Z, Maniatis T (1985a): Detection of single base substitutions by ribonuclease cleavage at mismatches in RNA:DNA duplexes. *Science* 230:1242–1246.

Myers RM, Fischer SG, Lerman LS, Maniatis T (1985b): Nearly all single base substitutions in DNA fragments joined to a GC-clamp can be detected by denaturing gradient gel electrophoresis. *Nucl Acids Res* 13:3131–3145.

Myers RM, Lumelsky N, Lerman L, Maniatis T (1985c): Detection of single base substitutions in total genomic DNA. *Nature (London)* 313:495–498.

Nelson MA, Futscher BW, Kinsella T, Wymer J, Bowden GT (1992): Detection of mutant Ha-*ras* genes in chemically initiated mouse skin epidermis before the development of benign tumors. *Proc Natl Acad Sci USA* 89:6398–6402.

Newton CR, Graham A, Heptinstall LE, Powell SJ, Summers C, Kalsheker N, Smith JC, Markham AF (1989): Analysis of any point mutation in DNA. The amplification refractory mutation system (ARMS). *Nucl Acids Res* 17:2503–2516.

Nichols WC, Liepnicks JJ, McKusick VA, Benson MD (1989): Direct sequencing of the gene for Maryland/German familial amyloidotic polyneuropathy type II and genotyping by allele-specific enzymatic amplification. *Genomics* 5:535–540.

Nigro JM, Baker SJ, Preisinger AC, Jessup JM, Hostetter R, Cleary K, Bigner SH, Davidson N, Baylin S, Devilee P, Glover T, Collins FS, Weston A, Modali R, Harris CC, Vogelstein B (1989): Mutations in the p53 gene occur in diverse human tumour types. *Nature (London)* 342:705–708.

Nishisho I, Nakamura Y, Miyoshi Y, Miki Y, Ando H, Horii A, Koyama K, Utsonomiya J, Baba S, Hedge P, Markham A, Krush AJ, Petersen G, Hamilton S, Nilbert MC, Levy DB, Bryan TM, Preisinger AC, Smith KJ, Su LK, Kinzler KW, Vogelstein B (1992): Mutations of chromosome 5q21 genes in FAP and colorectal cancer patients. *Science* 253:665–669.

Nusse RM, Varmus HE (1982): Many tumors induced by the mouse mammary tumor virus contain a provirus integrated in the same region of the host genome. *Cell* 31:99–109.

Okayama H, Curiel DT, Brantly ML, Holmes MD, Crystal RG (1989): Rapid, nonradioactive detection of mutations in the human genome by allele-specific amplification. *J Lab Clin Med* 114:105–113.

Oliner JD, Kinzler KW, Meltzer PS, George DL, Vogelstein B (1992): Amplification of a gene encoding a p53-associated protein in human sarcomas. *Nature (London)* 358:80–83.

Orita M, Iwahana H, Kanaqawa H, Hayashi K, Sekiya T (1989a): Detection of polymorphisms of human DNA by gel electrophoresis as single-strand conformation polymorphisms. *Proc Natl Acad Sci USA* 86:2766–2770.

Orita M, Suzuki Y, Sekiya T, Hayaski K (1989b): Rapid and sensitive detection of point mutations and DNA polymorphisms using the polymerase chain reaction. *Genomics* 5:874–879.

Pace AM, Wong YH, Bourne HR (1991): A mutant a subunit of G_{i2} induces neoplastic transformation of Rat-1 cells. *Proc Natl Acad Sci USA* 88:7031–7035.

Parada LF, Land H, Weinberg RA, Wolf D, Rotter V (1984): Cooperation between gene encoding p53 tumor antigen and *ras* in cellular transformation. *Nature (London)* 312:649–651.

Payne GS, Bishop JM, Varmus HE (1982): Multiple arrangements of viral DNA and an activated host oncogene in bursal lymphomas. *Nature (London)* 295:209–214.

Peinado MA, Malkhosyan S, Velazquez A, Perucho M (1992): Isolation and characterization of allelic losses and gains in colorectal tumors by arbitrarily primed polymerase chain reaction. *Proc Natl Acad Sci USA* 89:10065–10069.

Peinado MA, Fernandez-Renart, Capella G, Wilson L, Perucho M (1993): Mutations in the p53 suppressor gene do not correlate with c-K-*ras* oncogene mutations in colorectal cancer. *Int J Oncology* 2:123–134.

Perucho M (1989): Detection of single-base substitutions with the RNAse A mismatch cleavage method. *Strategies Mol Biol* 2:37–41.

Perucho M, Forrester K, Almoguera C, Kahn S, Lama C, Shibata D, Arnheim N, Grizzle WE (1989): Expression and mutational activation of the c-Ki-*ras* gene in human carcinomas. *Cancer Cells* 7:137–141.

Peters G, Brookes S, Smith R, Dickson C (1983): Tumorigenesis by mouse mammary tumor virus: Evidence for a common region for provirus integration in mammary tumors. *Cell* 33:369–377.

Pimentel E (1989): Oncogenes. Boca Raton, FL: CRC Press.

Powell SM, Zilz N, Beazer-Berclay Y, Bryan TM, Hamilton SR, Thibodeau SN, Vogelstein B, Kinzler KW (1992): APC mutations occur early during colorectal tumorigenesis. *Nature (London)* 359:235–237.

Reddy EP, Reynolds RK, Santos E, Barbacid M (1982): A point mutation is responsible for the acquisition of transforming properties by the T24 human bladder carcinoma oncogene. *Nature (London)* 300:149–152.

Richman A, Hayday A (1989): Normal expression of a rearranged and mutated c-myc oncogene after transfection into fibroblasts. *Science* 246:494–497.

Ridge SA, Worwood M, Oscier D, Jacobs A, Padua RA (1990): FMS mutations in myelodysplastic, leukemic and normal subjects. *Proc Natl Acad Sci USA* 87:1377–1381.

Rodenhuis S, Slebos RJC, Boot AJM, Evers SE, Mooi WJ, Wagenaar SSc, Van Bodegom PCh, Bos JL (1988): K-*ras* oncogene activation in adenocarcinoma of the lung: Incidence and possible clinical significance. *Cancer Res* 48:5737–5741.

Rodrigues NR, Rowna A, Smith ME, Kerr IB, Bodmer WF, Gannon JV, Lane DP (1990): p53 mutations in colorectal cancer. *Proc Natl Acad Sci USA* 87:7555–7559.

Roussel MF, Downing JR, Rettenmier CW, Sherr CJ (1988): A point mutation in the extracellular domain of the human CSF-1 receptor (c-fms) proto-oncogene product activates its transforming potential. *Cell* 55:979–988.

Ruano G, Kidd KK (1991): Coupled amplification and sequencing of genomic DNA. *Proc Natl Acad Sci USA* 88:2815–2819.

Saiki RK, Scharf S, Faloona F, Mullis GT, Erlich HA, Arnheim N (1985): Enzymatic amplification of β-globin genomic sequences and restriction site analysis for diagnosis of sickle cell anemia. *Science* 230:1350–1354.

Santos E, Nebreda A (1990): Structural and functional properties of *ras* proteins. *FASEB J* 3:2151–2163.

Santos E, Martin-Zanca D, Reddy E, Pierotti MA, Della Porta G, Barbacid M (1984): Malignant activation of a K-*ras* oncogene in lung carcinomas but not in normal tissue of the same patient. *Science* 223:661–664.

Schimke RT, Sherwood SW, Hill AB, Johnston RN (1986): Overreplication and recombination of DNA in higher eukaryotes: Potential consequences and biological implications. *Proc Natl Acad Sci USA* 83:2157–2161.

Schwab M, Alitalo K, Varmus HE, Bishop JM, George D (1983): A cellular oncogene (c-K-*ras*) is amplified, overexpressed and located within karyotypic abnormalities in mouse adrenocortical tumor cells. *Nature (London)* 303:497–501.

Seeburg P, Colby W, Capon DJ, Goeddel DV, Levinson A (1984): Biological properties of human c-H-*ras*1 genes mutated at codon 12. *Nature (London)* 312:71–75.

Shibata DK, Arnheim N, Martin WJ (1988): Detection of human polyoma virus in paraffin-embedded tissue using the polymerase chain reaction. *J Exp Med* 167:225–230.

Shibata D, Almoguera C, Forrester K, Dunitz J, Martin SE, Cosgrove M, Perucho M, Arnheim N (1990a): Detection of c-K-*ras* mutations in fine needle aspirates from human pancreatic adenocarcinomas. *Cancer Res* 50:1279–1283.

Shibata D, Capella G, Perucho M (1990b): Mutational activation of the c-K-*ras* gene in human pancreatic carcinoma. *Bailliere's Clin Gastroenterol* 4:151–169.

Shibata D, Hawes D, Li Z-H, Hernandez A, Spruck CHM, Nichols PW (1992): Specific genetic analysis of microscopic tissue after selective ultraviolet radiation fractionation and the polymerase chain reaction. *Am J Pathol* 141:1–5.

Shibata D, Schaeffer J, Li Z, Capella G, Perucho M (1993): Genetic heterogeneity of the c-K-ras locus in colorectal adenomas but not adenocarcinomas. *J Natl Cancer Inst* 85:1058–1063.

Shirasawa S, Urabe K, Yanagawa Y, Toshitani K, Iwama T, Sasazuki T (1991): p53 gene mutations in colorectal tumors from patients with familial polyposis coli. *Cancer Res* 51:2874–2878.

Sidransky D, Von Eschenbach A, Tsai YC, Jones P, Summerhayes I, Marshall F, Paul M, Green P, Hamilton SR, Frost P, Vogelstein B (1991): Identification of p53 gene mutations in bladder cancers and urine samples. *Science* 252:706–709.

Sidransky D, Mikkelsen T, Schwechheimer K, Rosenblum ML, Cavenee W, Vogelstein B (1992a): Clonal expansion of p53 mutant cells is associated with brain tumour progression. *Nature (London)* 355:258–260.

Sidransky D, Tokino T, Hamilton SR, Kinzler KW, Levin B, Frost P, Vogelstein B (1992b): Identification of ras oncogene mutations in the stool of patients with curable colorectal tumors. *Science* 256:102–105.

Slamon DJ, Clark GM, Wong SG, Levin WJ, Ullrich A, McGuire WL (1987): Human breast cancer: Correlation of relapse and survival with amplification of the HER-2/*neu* oncogene. *Science* 235:177–182.

Slebos RJ, Kibbelaar R, Dalesio O, Kooistra A, Stam J, Meijer C, Wagenaar S, Vanderschueren R, van Zandwijk N, Mooi W, Bos JL, Rodenhuis S (1990): K-*ras* oncogene activation as a prognostic marker in adenocarcinoma of the lung. *N Engl J Med* 323:561–565.

Smit V, Cornelisse CJ, de Jong D, Dijkshoorn NJ, Peters AAW, Fleuren GJ (1988): Analysis of tumor heterogeneity in a patient with synchronously occurring female genital tract malignancies by DNA flow cytometry, DNA fingerprinting, and immunohistochemistry. *Cancer* 62:1146–1152.

Smith FI, Latham TE, Ferrier JA, Palese P (1988): Novel method of detecting single base substitutions in RNA molecules by differential melting behavior in solution. *Genomics* 3:217–223.

Sommer SS, Goszbach AR, Bottema C (1992): PCR amplification of specific alleles (PASA) is a general method for rapidly detecting known single base changes. *Biotechniques* 12:82–87.

Spandidos DA, Lang JC (1989): *In vitro* transformation by ras oncogenes. *Crit Rev Oncogen* 1:195–209.

Srivastava S, Zou Z, Pirollo K, Blattner W, Chang EH (1990): Germ-line transmission of a mutated p53 gene in a cancer-prone family with Li-Fraumeni syndrome. *Nature (London)* 348:747–751.

Stork P, Loda M, Bosari S, Wiley B, Poppenhusen K, Wolfe H (1991): Detection of K-*ras* mutations in pancreatic and hepatic neoplasms by non isotopic mismatched polymerase chain reaction. *Oncogene* 6:857–862.

Suzuki Y, Orita M, Shiraishi M, Hayashi K, Sekiya T (1990): Detection of ras gene mutations in human lung cancers by single-strand conformation polymorphism analysis of polymerase chain reaction products. *Oncogene* 5:101–107.

Suzuki Y, Sekiya T, Hayashi K (1991): Allele-specific polymerase chain reaction: A method for amplification and sequence determination of a single component among a mixture of sequence variants. *Anal Biochem* 192:82–84.

Sweet RW, Yokoyama S, Kamata T, Feramisco JR, Rosenberg M, Gross M (1984): The product of ras is a GTPase and the T24 oncogenic mutant is deficient in this activity. *Nature (London)* 311:273–275.

Tabin CJ, Bradley SM, Bargmann CI, Weinberg RA, Papageorge AG, Scolnick EM, Dhar R, Lowy DR, Chang EH (1982): Mechanism of activation of a human oncogene. *Nature (London)* 300:143–149.

Takahashi T, Nau MM, Chiba I, Birrer MJ, Rosenberg RK, Vinocour M, Levitt M, Pass H, Gazdar AF, Minna JD (1989): p53: A frequent target for genetic abnormalities in lung cancer. *Science* 246:491–494.

Taparowsky E, Suard Y, Fasano O, Shimizu K, Goldfarb M, Wigler M (1982): Activation of the T-24 bladder carcinoma transforming gene is linked to a single amino acid change. *Nature (London)* 300:762–765.

Taub R, Kirsch I, Morton C, Lenoir G, Swan D, Tronick S, Aaronson SA, Leder P (1982): Translocation of the c-*myc* gene into the immunoglobulin heavy chain locus in human Burkitt lymphoma and murine plasmacytoma cells. *Proc Natl Acad Sci USA* 79:7837–7841.

Templeton DJ, Park SO, Lanier L, Weinberg RA (1991): Nonfunctional mutants of the retinoblastoma protein are characterized by defects in phosphorylation, viral oncogene association and nuclear tethering. *Proc Natl Acad Sci USA* 88:3033–3037.

Thein SL, Jeffreys AJ, Gooi HC, Cotter F, Flint J, O'Connor NTJ, Weatherall DJ, Wainscoat JS (1987): Detection of somatic changes in human cancer DNA by DNA fingerprint analysis. *Br J Cancer* 55:353–356.

Tominaga O, Hamelin R, Remvikos Y, Salmon RJ, Thomas G (1992): p53 from basic research to clinical applications. *Crit Rev Oncogen* 3:257–282.

Tracy TE, Mulcahy LS (1991): A simple method for direct automated sequencing of PCR fragments. *Biotechniques* 11:68–76.

Trahey M, McCormick F (1987): A cytoplasmic protein stimulates normal N-*ras* p21 GTPase, but does not affect oncogenic mutants. *Science* 238:542–545.

Valenzuela DM, Groffen J (1986): Four human carcinoma cell lines with novel mutations in position 12 of c-K-*ras* oncogene. *Nucl Acids Res* 14:843–852.

van Heyningen V, Hastie ND (1992): Wilms' tumor: Reconciling genetics and biology. *Trends Genet* 8:16–21.

van Mansfeld A, Bos JH (1992): PCR-based approaches for detection of mutated *ras* genes. *PCR Methods Applic* 1:211–216.

Verlaan-de Vries M, Boggard ME, Van den Elst H, van Boom JH, van der Eb AJ, Bos JL (1986): A dot-blot screening procedure for mutated *ras* oncogenes using synthetic oligodeoxynucleotides. *Gene* 50:313–320.

Viskochil D, Buchberg AM, Xu G, Cawthon RM, Stevens J, Woll RK, Culver M, Carey JC, Copeland NG, Jenkins NA, White R, O'Connell P (1990): Deletions and a translocation interrupt a cloned gene at the neurofibromatosis type 1 locus. *Cell* 62:187–192.

Vogelstein B, Kinzler KW (1992a): p53 function and dysfunction. *Cell* 70:523–526.

Vogelstein B, Kinzler KW (1992b): Carcinogens leave fingerprints. *Nature* (*London*) 355:209–210.

Vogelstein B, Fearon ER, Hamilton SR, Kern SE, Preisinger AC, Leppert M, Nakamura Y, White R, Smits AM, Bos JL (1988): Genetic alterations during colo-rectal tumor development. *N Engl J Med* 319:525–532.

Vogelstein B, Fearon ER, Kern SE, Hamilton SR, Preisinger AC, Nakamura Y, White R (1989): Allelotype of colorectal carcinomas. *Science* 244:207–211.

Wainscoat JS, Fey MF (1990): Assessment of clonality in human tumors: A review. *Cancer Res* 50:1355–1360.

Wallace MR, Marchuk DA, Andersen LB, Letcher R, Odeh HM, Saulino AM, Fountain JW, Brereton A, Nicholson J, Mitchell AL, Brownstein BH, Collins FS (1990): Type 1 neurofibromatosis gene: Identification of a large transcript disrupted in three NF1 patients. *Science* 249:181–186.

Wartell RM, Hosseini SH, Moran CJ (1990): Detecting base pair substitutions in DNA fragments by temperature gradient electrophoresis. *Nucl Acids Res* 18:2699–2701.

Weinberg RA (1991): Tumor suppressor genes. *Science* 254:1138–1146.

Welsh J, McClelland M (1990): Fingerprinting genomes using PCR with arbitrary primers. *Nucl Acis Res* 18:7213–7218.

Welsh J, McClelland M (1991): Genomic fingerprinting with AP-PCR using pairwise combinations of primers: Application to genetic mapping of the mouse. *Nucl Acids Res* 19:5275–5279.

Welsh J, Petersen C, McClelland M (1991): Polymorphisms generated by arbitrarily primed PCR in the mouse: Application to strain identification and genetic mapping. *Nucl Acids Res* 19:303–306.

Welsh J, Chada K, Dalal SS, Cheng R, Ralph D, McClelland M (1992): Arbitrarily primed PCR fingerprinting of RNA. *Nucl Acids Res* 20:4965–4970.

Williams JGK, Kubelik AR, Livak KJ, Rafalski JA, Tingey SV (1990): DNA polymorphisms amplified by arbitrary primers are useful as genetic markers. *Nucl Acids Res* 18:6531–6535.

Winter E, Yamamoto F, Almoguera C, Perucho M (1985): A method to detect and characterize point mutations in transcribed genes: Amplification and overexpression of the mutant c-Ki-*ras* allele in human tumor cells. *Proc Natl Acad Sci USA* 82:7575–7579.

Wu DY, Wallace RB (1989): The ligation amplification reaction (LAR): Amplification of specific DNA sequences using sequential rounds of template-dependent ligation. *Genomics* 4:560–569.

Wu DY, Ugozzoli L, Pal BK, Wallace RB (1989): Allele-specific enzymatic amplification of b-globin genomic DNA for diagnosis of sickle cell anemia. *Proc Natl Acad Sci USA* 86:2757–2760.

Xu G, O'Connell P, Viskovhil D, Cawthon R, Robertson M, Culver M, Dunn D, Stevens J, Gesteland R, White R, Weiss R (1990): The neurofibromatosis type 1 gene encodes a protein related to GAP. *Cell* 62:599–608.

Yandell DW, Campbell TA, Dayton SH, Petersen R, Walton D, Little JB, McConkie-Rosell A, Buckley EG, Dryja TP (1989): Oncogenic point mutations in the human retinoblastoma gene: Their application to genetic counseling. *N Engl J Med* 321:1689–1695.

Zarbl H, Sukumar S, Arthur AV, Martin-Zanca D, Barbacid M (1985): Direct mutagenesis of Ha-*ras*-1 oncogenes by N-nitroso-N-methylurea during initiation of mammary carcinogenesis in rats. *Nature* (*London*) 315:382–385.

32

Clinical Applications of the Polymerase Chain Reaction

Belinda J.F. Rossiter and C. Thomas Caskey

Introduction

The polymerase chain reaction (PCR), invented by Kary Mullis (Mullis and Faloona, 1987; Mullis, 1990), in only a few years has become a fundamental tool for the molecular biologist, wide-ranging in its application. The idea is simple and yet the PCR has revolutionized techniques available for the isolation and analysis of nucleic acids. Two major areas where the PCR is used for clinical applications are in the detection of disease gene mutations and in linkage analysis. Such analysis can be used to diagnose genetic diseases *after* occurrence of symptoms, *before* occurrence of symptoms, prenatally, or even before implantation during *in vitro* fertilization. The technique can also be used for detecting asymptomatic carriers of genetic diseases.

Use of the PCR for mutation detection in medical applications rapidly progressed from research settings to routine use in clinical laboratories, particularly after the innovation of using a thermostable DNA polymerase that need not be replenished after every cycle of the reaction (Saiki et al., 1988). The first uses of the PCR were in detecting sickle cell and β-thalas-

semia mutations in the β-globin gene (Saiki et al., 1985, 1986; Wong et al., 1987) but in less than 10 years there has been a considerable explosion in the clinical application of this technique. Not only is this method useful for any disease-causing gene for which sequence information is available, but various technical advances have broadened its applicability. For instance, it is even possible to amplify specific DNA sequences from single cells such as sperm (Li et al., 1988) or biopsied preimplantation embryos (Handyside et al., 1990).

Detection of Disease Gene Mutations

Old Methods of Mutation Detection

Traditionally, gene mutations have been detected by means of Southern analysis (restriction fragment length polymorphisms, large insertions, deletions, rearrangements), northern analysis (mRNA levels, splice mutations, insertions, deletions), or sequencing of cloned cDNA (point mutations and small rearrangements). Each of these methods takes several days to perform (particularly the synthesis and

The Polymerase Chain Reaction
K.B. Mullis, F. Ferré, R.A. Gibbs, editors
© 1994 Birkhauser Boston

sequencing of cDNA) and requires several micrograms of high-quality starting material (DNA or RNA). None of these methods is obsolete, but the PCR has frequently replaced older methods of DNA analysis in clinical laboratories because of greater specificity, increased speed, and reduced cost. Some of these new applications are described below.

Deletion Screening

The PCR was first reported as a method for deletion screening by Chamberlain et al. in 1988 for use with the dystrophin gene (Chamberlain et al., 1988). Several PCRs are performed simultaneously (a "multiplex" reaction) and the absence of one or more products within a multiplex PCR is taken to indicate a deletion in that portion of the gene (Fig. 32.1). In the dystrophin gene, the multiplex PCR is able to detect deletions that can also be visualized (more slowly) by Southern analysis (Multicenter Study Group, 1992), but there are also occasions where PCR can be used to detect deletions that are not detectable by Southern analysis. Such an example is that of

the most common cystic fibrosis gene mutation, a 3-bp deletion within the coding region resulting in the deletion of one amino acid from the protein (Kerem et al., 1989). The appropriate region of the gene may be amplified using the PCR and the size of the product directly determined by polyacrylamide gel electrophoresis without requiring hybridization (Rommens et al., 1990; Balnaves et al., 1991).

Point Mutation Detection

The amplification refractory mutation system (ARMS) (Newton et al., 1989a), or allele-specific amplification (Okayama et al., 1989; Ruano and Kidd, 1989; Wu et al., 1989), uses the PCR for detection of known point mutations without requiring endonuclease digestion or Southern hybridization (Fig. 32.2). A "constant" oligonucleotide primer is synthesized to correspond with one end of the portion of DNA to be amplified. At the other end, two or more oligonucleotide primers are synthesized with identical sequences except for their 3'-ends, which match the different alleles to be tested. For instance, primer "a" might match the normal sequence at that location and

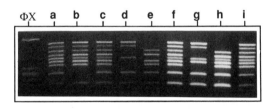

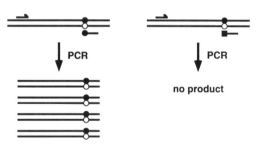

FIGURE 32.1. Multiplex PCR for the detection of Duchenne muscular dystrophy gene deletions. Nine regions of the Duchenne muscular dystrophy gene are amplified simultaneously using 18 oligonucleotide primers in a multiplex PCR, and then visualized after separation by gel electrophoresis. Samples in lanes a, c, f, and i show the normal pattern of nine bands; the other samples lack one or more bands according to the extent of the deletion. The lane marked ΦX contains size standards. Reproduced from Multicenter Study Group (1992) with permission. Copyright 1992, American Medical Association.

FIGURE 32.2. The amplification refractory mutation system (ARMS). A pair of PCRs is performed with a common primer at one end of the region to be amplified and different primers at the other end. The different primers are synthesized so that their 3'-ends match either the wild-type or mutant alleles at the point where the sequences differ (indicated by circles and squares). An allele will amplify only if both primers match the template, so whichever reaction generates a product indicates which allele was present in the original DNA.

primer "b" might match a particular point mutation. PCR amplification using the constant primer and primer "a" will generate a product only if there is a normal allele present and amplification using the constant primer and primer "b" will generate a product only if the mutant allele is present. DNA from heterozygote individuals would yield a product in both reactions. One use of this technique has been in prenatal diagnosis and carrier testing for cystic fibrosis (Newton et al., 1989b).

Competitive oligonucleotide priming PCR (COP PCR) (Gibbs et al., 1989) relies on the fact that when a mixture of priming oligonucleotides is present, the one matching the binding site exactly will be used in preference over others with mismatches. Thus, if two competing oligonucleotide primers are labeled differently and correspond to normal and mutant sequences at a particular location, it is possible to distinguish which sequence was present in the template by noting which primer is incorporated into the final product. Such reactions can be performed in pairs, with one or the other of the competing primers radiolabeled. However, a more elegant approach is to use different fluorescent tags so that the reaction can be performed in one tube. After unincorporated primers have been removed, the color of the final product indicates which primers were incorporated, without the need for electrophoresis (Chehab and Kan, 1989).

Detection of Expanded Unstable Repeats

In 1991 it was discovered that the mutation responsible for the fragile X syndrome is the expansion of an unstable triplet repeat (Kremer et al., 1991; Verkerk et al., 1991). It soon transpired that myotonic dystrophy, spinal and bulbar muscular atrophy, spinocerebellar ataxia type 1, and Huntington disease were also caused by similar repeat expansions, and it is probable that other diseases result from the same mechanism of mutation. These repeat regions are polymorphic in unaffected individuals, that is, the number of repeated triplets varies within a certain range. If the number of repeats exceeds the normal range, the phenom-

enon is called a "premutation" because there is a strong possibility of further expansion to a "full mutation" during inheritance from parent to child. Individuals with a full mutation have symptoms of the disorder with a rough correlation between the degree of expansion and the severity of the disease (Fu et al., 1991; Harley et al., 1992; la Spada et al., 1992; Yu et al., 1992; The Huntington's Disease Collaborative Research Group, 1993). Those with a premutation are usually mildly affected or have no symptoms, but have a high risk of bearing affected children.

Both the PCR and Southern analysis are currently used for detection of expanded unstable repeats. The PCR has the advantage of speed, convenience, and accurate measurement of normal and premutation alleles, but cannot reliably amplify full mutations. Failure to amplify a repeat region suggests that the number of repeats exceeds the limit of the PCR; this can be confirmed by Southern analysis (Fu et al., 1991, 1992).

Detection of Cancer Translocations

Several neoplasias are associated with chromosomal translocations that fuse two unrelated genes. One example of this is the chromosomal translocation in chronic myelogenous leukemia patients that fuses the c-*abl* gene on chromosome 9 to the breakpoint cluster region (BCR) gene on chromosome 22. The derivative chromosome 22 is called the "Philadelphia chromosome" and the hybrid bcr-abl protein is assumed to be responsible for the malignancy (Rowley, 1990). The PCR can detect mRNA generated from the *bcr-abl* fusion gene. With one primer in the BCR gene and the other in the c-*abl* gene, a product is generated only if a chromosomal translocation fusing the two genes has occurred (Dobrovic et al., 1988; Kawasaki et al., 1988). This method is useful for diagnosis of chronic myelogenous leukemia and for monitoring the effectiveness of treatment. It is rapid and more sensitive than other protocols, and can also be used for the detection of other chromosomal translocations when sequence information is available from the affected genes.

Material for Further Analysis

Many methods are available for the detection of mutations in DNA and RNA, and several have been used routinely in a clinical setting. The PCR has frequently been incorporated into these mutation detection assays as a way of providing ample amounts of material for analysis (often from minute amounts of starting material) and making the methods easier, quicker, and more accurate. Some of the more commonly used procedures are described here.

Restriction Endonuclease Digestion

The S allele of β-globin lacks a *Dde*I restriction site that is present in the wild-type and this property has been used in the detection of the mutant allele by Southern analysis (Geever et al., 1981). Presence or absence of a restriction endonuclease recognition sequence within a PCR product can be easily determined without the need for transfer and hybridization, simply by digestion, gel electrophoresis, and observation of an intact or cleaved product (Mullis and Faloona, 1987). An alternative method is to predigest the template DNA before the PCR and thus eliminate amplification from the allele retaining the restriction site. In this case a product is present or absent depending, respectively, on the absence or presence of a *Dde*I site (Mullis and Faloona, 1987).

Allele-Specific Oligonucleotide (ASO) Screening

Allele-specific oligonucleotide (ASO) screening was first used to detect the β-globin S allele responsible for sickle cell disease (Conner et al., 1983), and this was also one of the first clinical applications of the PCR (Saiki et al., 1986). Different short oligonucleotides (usually around 19 nucleotides), each complementary to a particular allele, are used as probes against sample DNA. The individual residues differing between the different alleles generally lie in the center of the oligonucleotides and hybridization conditions are chosen such that only those probes with a perfect match will hybridize to the sample. Thus, it is possible to distinguish by hybridization between alleles differing by only one nucleotide in sequence. The concentration of target sequence for hybridization with oligonucleotide probes is much higher with PCR-amplified material than with genomic DNA and therefore the result can be obtained by means of a dot-blot procedure instead of requiring digestion and electrophoresis of genomic DNA. Allele-specific oligonucleotides for this procedure have also been termed sequence-specific oligonucleotides (Scharf et al., 1988).

A technique termed "reverse ASO screening" has been developed to enable the detection of multiple alleles associated with a single locus, as is seen with the β-globin and HLA loci (Saiki et al., 1989). Oligonucleotides corresponding to the different alleles are immobilized on a nylon membrane and the appropriate region is amplified from genomic DNA using the PCR. The product is then given a radioactive or nonradioactive tag and used as a probe against the oligonucleotides on the nylon membrane. This method avoids multiple hybridizations for the detection of several alleles at one locus, is readily transferable between laboratories because the membranes can be prepared in large quantities and stored easily, and has the potential to be used for more than one locus if a multiplex PCR is performed initially.

Mismatch Cleavage

Several mutation detection methods have been described that are based on the hybridization of wild-type and mutant molecules, and then cleavage at the points of mismatch between the two. This cleavage may be achieved by enzymes or with chemical reagents. Since the enzymes used for cleavage generally act on RNA rather than DNA, the PCR has proved more useful in the generation of material for chemical cleavage mismatch detection (Fig. 32.3). In any event, chemical cleavage methods of mutation detection have the potential to detect all point mutations, which is not the case with the enzymatic methods (Myers et al., 1985c).

The hydroxylamine and osmium tetroxide cleavage method initially described by Richard Cotton (and therefore sometimes called the

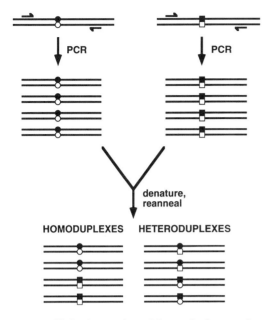

FIGURE 32.3. Generation of heteroduplexes using the PCR. Two PCRs are performed on different alleles of the same region of DNA; circles and squares represent sequence differences between the alleles. The products of these reactions, when mixed, denatured, and annealed (by heating and cooling), form heteroduplexes with sequence mismatches in addition to the original homoduplexes.

"HOT Cotton" method) (Cotton et al., 1988) modifies unpaired cytosine (with hydroxylamine) or thymidine (with osmium tetroxide) residues at points of mismatch between the two strands of DNA in a heteroduplex. Treatment with piperidine then results in cleavage at the modified bases and the reaction products are separated by gel electrophoresis. The PCR provides a convenient method for the generation of the DNA strands to be hybridized together. End-labeling of one of the PCR primers before the amplification yields a fragment labeled at one end, and the size of the cleaved product therefore indicates the approximate distance of the point mutation from the end of the molecule. Either the wild-type or the mutant strand can be labeled, and the heteroduplexes subjected to hydroxylamine or osmium tetroxide treatment, thus providing the potential for the detection of all possible point mutations. One example of this method

being used in a clinical setting is the detection of ornithine transcarbamylase mutations (Grompe et al., 1989).

Denaturing Gradient Gel Electrophoresis (DGGE)

A duplex of complementary DNA strands normally exists as a tightly associated double helix. In increasing concentrations of denaturant, for example, urea, the two strands begin to dissociate ("melt") starting with the region(s) most loosely held together. Since the bond between an AT nucleotide pair is weaker than that between a GC pair, AT-rich regions tend to separate first under such denaturing conditions. If a DNA duplex is being subjected to electrophoresis in a gradient of denaturant, at the point where the strands begin to separate the rate of migration is abruptly reduced because of the looser configuration of the duplex. If the fragment of DNA contains a mismatch in a region of the molecule that denatures early, the electrophoresis profile will be altered compared to a homoduplex of perfectly complementary strands. These properties form the basis of the denaturing gradient gel electrophoresis mutation detection assay (Myers et al., 1985d).

An initial drawback of the DGGE technique was its insensitivity to mutations in regions of the DNA that melt last in the gradient of denaturant, since at this point the strands separate and the resolution is lost. To overcome this limitation, a modification was designed that involved the addition of a GC-rich fragment at the end of the DNA to be analyzed, a so-called GC-clamp (Myers et al., 1985a,b). The clamp region then becomes the most stable part of the duplex, allowing variations in the melting profile of the remainder of the fragment to be detected. Such a GC-clamp is easily added to the DNA region to be studied by PCR amplification using two primers, one of which carries a GC-rich sequence at its 5'-end (Sheffield et al., 1989). This technique has been used in the detection of a number of mutations, including some in the β-globin gene (Abrams et al., 1990).

Single-Strand Conformational Polymorphism (SSCP)

The electrophoretic mobility of single-stranded nucleic acid depends not only on its size but also on its sequence. This property has been used in the analysis of DNA mutations and has been called single-strand conformational polymorphism (SSCP) (Orita et al., 1989). A PCR is performed with one or both primers radiolabeled, and the DNA product denatured and run out on an acrylamide gel, then viewed by autoradiography. DNA strands differing by only one nucleotide have different mobilities and can therefore be distinguished with this method. An example of the clinical use of this method is identification of a factor IX point mutation causing hemophilia B (Demers et al., 1990).

Direct Sequencing of PCR Products

The direct sequencing of PCR products without the need for subcloning is one of the most outstanding recent advantages in genetic technology, and several methods for this have been proposed. Previously, sequence analysis was something of a major undertaking, but with the improved methods now available it has become the method of choice for mutation detection in many cases. Further details of techniques for sequencing PCR products can be found in Chapters 17 and 18.

Linkage Analysis

The ability to distinguish between human beings has long had importance in forensic and medical applications. Before DNA analysis was possible, biochemical typing of blood group antigens offered a statistical probability that two samples could or could not have come from the same person. Analysis of the minisatellite repeat regions of DNA discovered by Jeffreys et al. (1985) opened the door for "DNA fingerprinting" methods of personal identification with much greater accuracy than the biochemical methods. Smaller tandem repeats in the genome, called microsatellites,

short tandem repeats, or simple sequence repeats, are very amenable to PCR amplification (Weber and May, 1989). Length variation (polymorphism) due to differences in the number of repeats at a particular locus is therefore easily and rapidly determined. Further details of the use of the PCR in genetic mapping and forensic analysis can be found in Chapters 21 and 25.

PCR amplification of polymorphic microsatellite repeats is useful for linkage analysis in families affected by a genetic disorder, especially when the gene responsible for that particular disorder has not yet been cloned. If a microsatellite repeat is sufficiently polymorphic to distinguish between the individual chromosomes within an affected family, inheritance of a closely associated disease gene can be tracked through that family (Fig. 32.4). For instance, if it is observed that one particular allele of a polymorphic microsatellite repeat is always present in family members affected with an inherited disease, inheritance of that microsatellite allele predicts the presence of the disease gene. It should be emphasized that linkage is a *family* study, and that the same disease gene may be associated with different microsatellite alleles in different families. It is also necessary to have sufficient genetic information from family members for the analysis to be successful.

Clinical Applications and Ethical Considerations

Mutation detection and linkage analysis not only provide or confirm a diagnosis of genetic disease in an affected individual, but can also be used in other clinical situations. The use of genetic analysis in these other circumstances may be accompanied by difficult social issues.

The genetic identity of an individual is determined at the time of conception, and it is therefore possible to provide a diagnosis of a genetic disease (caused by a known gene) before the appearance of symptoms. Such "presymptomatic diagnosis" can be performed before implantation of the embryo during *in vitro*

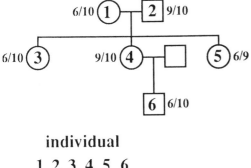

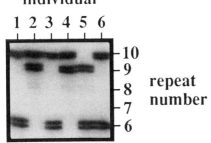

FIGURE 32.4. Linkage analysis using PCR amplification of polymorphic microsatellite repeats. In the pedigree shown above, circles indicate females and squares indicate males; the numbers within the symbols relate to the individuals shown in the panel below. The analysis shown here is PCR amplification of an autosomal $(AATG)_{6-10}$ repeat. The length of the radiolabeled amplification product varies according to the number of repeated units within it; the numbers shown alongside the pedigree symbols indicate the alleles detected in that individual. Reproduced from Rossiter and Caskey (1991) with permission.

fertilization, prenatally, or after birth. Examples of these would be the analysis of embryos for cystic fibrosis mutations before implantation (Handyside et al., 1992), prenatal diagnosis of β-thalassemia (Cai et al., 1989), and prediction of Huntington disease before the onset of symptoms (Fox et al., 1989). Despite the ability to predict a genetic disease before it occurs, this may not always be appropriate. In particular, there has been controversy in instances of incurable diseases with late onset, such as Huntington disease. A person at risk for Huntington disease, that is, with a family history, may not want to know whether the disorder will strike in later years and should not be forced to undergo testing. It has been generally accepted that children should not be tested

for the Huntington disease mutation, so that they can make their own decisions as adults (Bloch and Hayden, 1990). If such genetic testing is performed, it is not always clear who should have access to the results. Family members, potential employers, and insurance agencies may wish to know if someone will become sick in later years or pass on a genetic defect to his/her children. However, the widespread dissemination of such information may not be in the best interest of the individual. There are considerable concerns that the results of genetic testing may be used for the purposes of discrimination (Billings and Beckwith, 1992; Billings et al., 1992).

Where early intervention can be beneficial, presymptomatic diagnosis can provide an indication for treatment or lifestyle changes that can improve the outcome of a genetic disorder. One example of this is the detection of defects in the low-density-lipoprotein receptor gene that lead to familial hypercholesterolemia and a high likelihood of premature coronary artery disease (Humphries et al., 1988). This risk can be decreased with medication and lifestyle changes such as diet and exercise. Another example of the potential benefits of presymptomatic diagnosis is in familial breast cancer. Women who inherit the mutant *BRCA1* gene have an 85% lifetime risk of developing breast cancer but their prognosis can be greatly improved with aggressive monitoring for tumors. Some of these women also elect to undergo prophylactic bilateral mastectomy (King et al., 1993).

Not only are DNA-based tests able to diagnose a disorder before symptoms are apparent, but they can also identify unaffected individuals who are carrying a disease gene mutation, and who may therefore pass it on to a child. The diseases in question usually have a recessive inheritance, so that an affected individual inherits one copy of a disease gene mutation from each parent. There are two ways in which testing for carriers can be used. One situation is in a family where there is already at least one affected individual, and other family members wish to know whether they are carrying the gene for the same disorder. The other situation is where screening is offered to larger groups or the whole population, where people do not have a family history of the disorder.

There are a number of ways in which carrier screening can be offered to a community, and each has its advantages and disadvantages (Williamson, 1993). Testing could be done at birth, in school, before marriage, during pregnancy, or through primary healthcare services. Carrier screening has been very successful in reducing the incidence of β-thalassemia in Sardinia (Cao et al., 1991) and of Tay-Sachs disease in the Ashkenazi Jewish population (Blitzer and McDowell, 1992). Those who are identified as carriers have several options such as choosing a noncarrier mate, not having children, adopting children, sperm or egg donation, *in vitro* fertilization with selection of unaffected embryos, termination of affected pregnancies, or preparing to bear an affected child. Disadvantages of carrier screening include the potential problem of stigmatization and lack of education regarding the significance of the tests. A classic example of the misuse of carrier screening was compulsory testing of the black population for carriers of sickle cell anemia in the 1970s. This testing was accompanied by widespread misunderstanding and discrimination (Reilly, 1977).

The above examples show that DNA-based testing can be useful in a number of situations. It is also apparent that there is potential for inappropriate use of such tests or their results. It is not necessarily true that if a test *can* be done then it *should* be done. Conversely, it would be a tragedy if genetic tests were banned because of the potential for abuse. For these reasons, the Human Genome Project Working Group on Ethical, Legal and Social Implications (ELSI) has been charged with dealing with the ethical consequences of the acquisition and use of personal genetic information (Collins, 1991).

Conclusions

The PCR has found a multitude of clinical applications, particularly in the detection of disease gene mutations and in linkage analysis. The PCR can be used as a mutation detection assay in itself, or for the generation of DNA for further analysis. This procedure has proved superior to many older methods of genetic analysis because of its speed, specificity, low cost, and ease of use. It is now feasible on a routine basis to perform procedures, such as sequencing portions of disease genes, that were previously possible only in specialized research laboratories. One procedure that is now possible, but not yet routine, is the PCR amplification of DNA from single cells. The preimplantation diagnosis of *in vitro* embryos has been achieved (Handyside et al., 1992), and it should eventually be feasible to analyze fetal cells isolated from the maternal circulation without requiring amniocentesis or chorionic villus sampling (Holzgreve et al., 1992). The PCR has truly revolutionized the field of medical genetics and will probably continue to do so.

Acknowledgment. C.T.C. is a Howard Hughes Medical Institute Investigator.

References

Abrams ES, Murdaugh SE, Lerman LS (1990): Comprehensive detection of single base changes in human genomic DNA using denaturing gradient gel electrophoresis and a GC clamp. *Genomics* 7:463–475.

Balnaves ME, Nasioulas S, Dahl HHM, Forrest S (1991): Direct PCR from CVS and blood lysates for detection of cystic fibrosis and Duchenne muscular dystrophy deletions. *Nucl Acids Res* 19:1155.

Billings P, Beckwith J (1992): Genetic testing in the workplace: A view from the USA. *Trends Genet* 8:198–202.

Billings PR, Kohn MA, de Cuevas M, Beckwith J, Alper JS, Natowicz MR (1992): Discrimination as a consequence of genetic testing. *Am J Hum Genet* 50:476–482.

Blitzer MG, McDowell GA (1992): Tay-Sachs disease as a model for screening inborn errors. *Clin Lab Med* 12:463–480.

Bloch M, Hayden MR (1990): Opinion: Predictive testing for Huntington disease in childhood: Challenges and implications. *Am J Hum Genet* 46:1–4.

Cai SP, Chang CA, Zhang JZ, Saiki RK, Erlich HA, Kan YW (1989): Rapid prenatal diagnosis of β thalassemia using DNA amplification and non-radioactive probes. *Blood* 73:372–374.

Cao A, Rosatelli MC, Galanello R (1991): Population-based genetic screening. *Curr Opin Genet Dev* 1:48–53.

Chamberlain JS, Gibbs RA, Ranier JE, Nguyen PN, Caskey CT (1988): Deletion screening of the Duchenne muscular dystrophy locus via multiplex DNA amplification. *Nucl Acids Res* 16: 11141–11156.

Chehab FF, Kan YW (1989): Detection of specific DNA sequences by fluorescence amplification: a color complementation assay. *Proc Natl Acad Sci USA* 86:9178–9182.

Collins FS (1991): Medical and ethical consequences of the Human Genome Project. *J Clin Ethics* 2:260–267.

Conner BJ, Reyes AA, Morin C, Itakura K, Teplitz RL, Wallace RB (1983): Detection of sickle cell β^S-globin allele by hybridization with synthetic oligonucleotides. *Proc Natl Acad Sci USA* 80:278–282.

Cotton RGH, Rodrigues NR, Campbell RD (1988): Reactivity of cytosine and thymine in single-base-pair mismatches with hydroxylamine and osmium tetroxide and its application to the study of mutations. *Proc Natl Acad Sci USA* 85:4397–4401.

Demers DB, Odelberg SJ, Fisher LM (1990): Identification of a factor IX point mutation using SSCP analysis and direct sequencing. *Nucl Acids Res* 18:5575.

Dobrovic A, Trainor KJ, Morley AA (1988): Detection of the molecular abnormality in chronic myeloid leukemia by use of the polymerase chain reaction. *Blood* 72:2063–2065.

Fox S, Bloch M, Fahy M, Hayden MR (1989): Predictive testing for Huntington disease: I. Description of a pilot project in British Columbia. *Am J Med Genet* 32:211–216.

Fu YH, Kuhl DPA, Pizzuti A, Pieretti M, Sutcliffe JS, Richards S, Verkerk AJMH, Holden JJA, Fenwick RG Jr, Warren ST, Oostra BA, Nelson DL, Caskey CT (1991): Variation of the CGG repeat at the fragile X site results in genetic instability: Resolution of the Sherman paradox. *Cell* 67:1047–1058.

Fu YH, Pizzuti A, Fenwick RG Jr, King J, Rajnarayan S, Dunne PW, Dubel J, Nasser GA, Ashizawa T, de Jong P, Wieringa B, Korneluk P, Perryman MB, Epstein HF, Caskey CT (1992): An unstable triplet repeat in a gene related to myotonic muscular dystrophy. *Science* 255: 1256–1258.

Geever RF, Wilson LB, Nallaseth FS, Milner PF, Bittner M, Wilson JT (1981): Direct identification of sickle cell anemia by blot hybridization. *Proc Natl Acad Sci USA* 78:5081–5085.

Gibbs RA, Nguyen PN, Caskey CT (1989): Detection of single DNA base differences by competitive oligonucleotide priming. *Nucl Acids Res* 17: 2437–2448.

Grompe M, Muzny DM, Caskey CT (1989): Scanning detection of mutations in human ornithine transcarbamoylase by chemical mismatch cleavage. *Proc Natl Acad Sci USA* 86:5888–5892.

Handyside AH, Kontogianni EH, Hardy K, Winston RML (1990): Pregnancies from biopsied human preimplantation embryos sexed by Y-specific DNA amplification. *Nature (London)* 344:768–770.

Handyside AH, Lesko JG, Tarín JJ, Winston RML, Hughes MR (1992): Birth of a normal girl after in vitro fertilization and preimplantation diagnostic testing for cystic fibrosis. *N Engl J Med* 327:905–909.

Harley HG, Rundle SA, Reardon W, Myring J, Crow S, Brook JD, Harper PS, Shaw DJ (1992): Unstable DNA sequence in myotonic dystrophy. *Lancet* 339:1125–1128.

Holzgreve W, Garritsen HSP, Ganshirt-Ahlert D (1992): Fetal cells in the maternal circulation. *J Reprod Med* 37:410–418.

Humphries S, Taylor R, Jeenah M, Seed M (1988): The use of recombinant DNA techniques for the diagnosis of familial hypercholesterolaemia. *J Inherit Metab Dis 11 Suppl* 1:33–44.

Jeffreys AJ, Wilson V, Thein SL (1985): Hypervariable 'minisatellite' regions in human DNA. *Nature (London)* 314:67–73.

Kawasaki ES, Clark SS, Coyne MY, Smith SD, Champlin R, Witte ON, McCormick FP (1988): Diagnosis of chronic myeloid and acute lymphocytic leukemias by detection of leukemia-specific mRNA sequences amplified in vitro. *Proc Natl Acad Sci USA* 85:5698–5702.

Kerem BS, Rommens JM, Buchanan JA, Markiewicz D, Cox TK, Chakravarti A, Buchwald M, Tsui LC (1989): Identification of the cystic fibrosis gene: Genetic analysis. *Science* 245:1073–1080.

King MC, Rowell S, Love SM (1993): Inherited breast and ovarian cancer. What are the risks? What are the choices? *JAMA* 269:1975–1980.

Kremer EJ, Pritchard M, Lynch M, Yu S, Holman K, Baker E, Warren ST, Schlessinger D, Sutherland GR, Richards RI (1991): Mapping of DNA instability at the fragile X to a trinucleotide repeat sequence p(CCG)*n*. *Science* 252:1711–1714.

la Spada AR, Roling DB, Harding AE, Warner CL, Spiegel R, Hausmanowa-Petrusewicz I, Yee WC, Fischbeck KH (1992): Meiotic stability and genotype-phenotype correlation of the trinucleotide repeat in X-linked spinal and bulbar muscular atrophy. *Nature Genet* 2:301–304.

Li H, Gyllensten UB, Cui X, Saiki RK, Erlich HA, Arnheim N (1988): Amplification and analysis of DNA sequences in single human sperm and diploid cells. *Nature (London)* 335:414–417.

Mullis KB (1990): The unusual origin of the polymerase chain reaction. *Sci Am* 262(4):56–65.

Mullis KB, Faloona FA (1987): Specific synthesis of DNA in vitro via a polymerase-catalyzed chain reaction. *Methods Enzymol* 155:335–350.

Multicenter Study Group (1992): Diagnosis of Duchenne and Becker muscular dystrophies by polymerase chain reaction. A multicenter study. *JAMA* 267:2609–2615.

Myers RM, Fischer SG, Lerman LS, Maniatis T (1985a): Nearly all single base substitutions in DNA fragments joined to a GC-clamp can be detected by denaturing gradient gel electrophoresis. *Nucl Acids Res* 13:3131–3145.

Myers RM, Fischer SG, Maniatis T, Lerman LS (1985b): Modification of the melting properties of duplex DNA by attachment of a GC-rich DNA sequence as determined by denaturing gradient gel electrophoresis. *Nucl Acids Res* 13:3111–3129.

Myers RM, Larin Z, Maniatis T (1985c): Detection of single base substitutions by ribonuclease cleavage at mismatches in RNA:DNA duplexes. *Science* 230:1242–1246.

Myers RM, Lumelsky N, Lerman LS, Maniatis T (1985d): Detection of single base substitutions in total genomic DNA. *Nature (London)* 313:495–498.

Newton CR, Graham A, Heptinstall LE, Powell SJ, Summers C, Kalsheker N, Smith JC, Markham AF (1989a): Analysis of any point mutation in DNA. The amplification refractory mutation system (ARMS). *Nucl Acids Res* 17:2503–2516.

Newton CR, Heptinstall LE, Summers C, Super M, Schwarz M, Anwar R, Graham A, Smith JC, Markham AF (1989b): Amplification refractory mutation system for prenatal diagnosis and carrier assessment in cystic fibrosis. *Lancet* 2 (8678–8679):1481–1483.

Okayama H, Curiel DT, Brantly ML, Holmes MD, Crystal RG (1989): Rapid, nonradioactive detection of mutations in the human genome by allele-specific amplification. *J Lab Clin Med* 114:105–113.

Orita M, Suzuki Y, Sekiya T, Hayashi K (1989): Rapid and sensitive detection of point mutations and DNA polymorphisms using the polymerase chain reaction. *Genomics* 5:874–879.

Reilly P (1977): In *Genetics, Law, and Social Policy*. Cambridge, MA: Harvard University Press, pp. 65–86.

Rommens J, Kerem BS, Greer W, Chang P, Tsui LC, Ray P (1990): Rapid nonradioactive detection of the major cystic fibrosis mutation [letter]. *Am J Hum Genet* 46:395–396.

Rossiter BJF, Caskey CT (1991): Molecular studies of human genetic disease. *FASEB J* 5:21–27.

Rowley JD (1990): The Philadelphia chromosome translocation. A paradigm for understanding leukemia. *Cancer* 65:2178–2184.

Ruano G, Kidd KK (1989): Direct haplotyping of chromosomal segments from multiple heterozygotes via allele-specific PCR amplification. *Nucl Acids Res* 17:8392.

Saiki RK, Scharf S, Faloona F, Mullis KB, Horn GT, Erlich HA, Arnheim N (1985): Enzymatic amplification of β-globin genomic sequences and restriction site analysis for diagnosis of sickle cell anemia. *Science* 230:1350–1354.

Saiki RK, Bugawan TL, Horn GT, Mullis KB, Erlich HA (1986): Analysis of enzymatically amplified β-globin and HLA-DQα DNA with allele-specific oligonucleotide probes. *Nature (London)* 324:163–166.

Saiki RK, Gelfand DH, Stoffel S, Scharf SJ, Higuchi R, Horn GT, Mullis KB, Erlich HA (1988): Primer-directed enzymatic amplification of DNA with a thermostable DNA polymerase. *Science* 239:487–491.

Saiki RK, Walsh PS, Levenson CH, Erlich HA (1989): Genetic analysis of amplified DNA with immobilized sequence-specific oligonucleotide probes. *Proc Natl Acad Sci USA* 86:6230–6234.

Scharf SJ, Friedmann A, Brautbar C, Szafer F, Steinman L, Horn G, Gyllensten U, Erlich HA (1988): HLA class II allelic variation and susceptability to pemphigus vulgaris. *Proc Natl Acad Sci USA* 85:3504–3508.

Sheffield VC, Cox DR, Lerman LS, Myers RM (1989): Attachment of a 40-base-pair G+C-rich sequence (GC-clamp) to genomic DNA fragments by the polymerase chain reaction results in improved detection of single-base changes. *Proc Natl Acad Sci USA* 86:232–236.

The Huntington's Disease Collaborative Research Group (1993): A novel gene containing a trinucleotide repeat that is expanded and unstable on Huntington's disease chromosomes. *Cell* 72:971–983.

Verkerk AJMH, Pieretti M, Sutcliffe JS, Fu YH, Kuhl DPA, Pizutti A, Reiner O, Richards S, Victoria MF, Zhang F, Eussen BE, van Ommen GJB, Blonden LAJ, Riggins GJ, Chastain JL, Kunst CB, Galjaard H, Caskey CT, Nelson DL, Oostra BA, Warren ST (1991): Identification of a gene (*FMR-1*) containing a CGG repeat coincident with a breakpoint cluster region exhibiting length variation in fragile X syndrome. *Cell* 65:905–914.

Weber JL, May PE (1989): Abundant class of human DNA polymorphisms which can be typed using the polymerase chain reaction. *Am J Hum Genet* 44:388–396.

Williamson R (1993): Universal community carrier screening for cystic fibrosis? *Nature Genet* 3:195–201.

Wong C, Dowling CE, Saiki RK, Higuchi RG, Erlich HA, Kazazian HH Jr (1987): Characterization of β-thalassemia mutations using direct genomic sequencing of amplified single copy DNA. *Nature (London)* 330:384–386.

Wu DY, Ugozzoli L, Pal BK, Wallace RB (1989): Allele-specific amplification of β-globin genomic DNA for diagnosis of sickle cell anemia. *Proc Natl Acad Sci USA* 86:2757–2760.

Yu S, Mulley J, Loesch D, Turner G, Donnelly A, Gedeon A, Hillen D, Kremer E, Lynch M, Pritchard M, Sutherland GR, Richards RI (1992): Fragile-X syndrome: unique genetics of the heritable unstable element. *Am J Hum Genet* 50:968–980.

33

Infectious Diseases

W. John Martin

Introduction

PCR technology has helped catalyze the emergence of clinical molecular microbiology as one of the most promising recent advances in laboratory medicine. This technology can be applied to the detection of virtually any pathogen for which even limited DNA (or RNA) sequence information is known and in which a specimen of infected tissue or body fluid can be obtained. Beyond simple detection of a pathogen, PCR technology can potentially provide genetic information relating to the virulence, chemosensitivity, and epidemiological spread of a pathogen. The goal of this chapter is to provide an overview of the presently described diagnostic applications of PCR to infectious agents and to highlight anticipated new developments. These developments will likely establish PCR as an indispensable adjunct to more routine diagnostic methods and will likely facilitate the widespread introduction of molecular biology into the clinical microbiology laboratory.

Detection and Characterization of Specific Pathogens

PCR for infectious disease diagnosis has been primarily directed toward the detection of those pathogens for which conventional diagnostic techniques are either too insensitive, too slow, or cannot discriminate prognostic or therapeutically important subgroups. As with any new assay procedure, issues of sensitivity and specificity need to be carefully addressed. It is also important to define the type of clinical problems for which this type of assay offers unique advantages. Specific examples where PCR has shown promise in addressing a critical clinical need are as follows.

Viral Infections

Human Immunodeficiency Virus (HIV)

Early Detection of Infection

The vast majority of individuals infected with the human immunodeficiency virus (HIV) develop anti-HIV antibodies within 2–3 months of infection. A small percentage of individuals, however, may not seroconvert within this

The Polymerase Chain Reaction
K.B. Mullis, F. Ferré, R.A. Gibbs, editors
© 1994 Birkhauser Boston

time period. Because of the potential for false negative serology, PCR testing for HIV is frequently requested following occupational exposure to potentially contaminated blood, for example, after a needle stick injury. A negative PCR assay for HIV provides added reassurance that the source of the potentially contaminated blood is truly uninfected. PCR is also used to evaluate individuals suspected of being infected but in whom the HIV serology is negative or indeterminate (Coutlee et al., 1991; Yagi et al., 1991). A positive PCR assay, in the absence of serological confirmation, can, however, present a difficult diagnostic problem and caution is needed in advising PCR positive, seronegative patients. The most commonly used HIV primer set is reactive with a conserved sequence within the *gag* gene of HIV-1 (Jackson et al., 1990). The use of this primer set may occasionally yield a false positive response. For this reason, some authorities require a confirmatory positive PCR using an additional primer set reactive with either the *env* or the *pol* gene (Wages et al., 1991). Increasing the length and using inosine in positions of potential sequence ambiguity have reportedly improved the sensitivity of the commonly used *env* gene primer set (Cassol et al., 1991).

Detection of Neonatal Infection

PCR assays performed on blood of infants born to an infected mother can be used as a positive indicator of congenital infection (Laure et al., 1988). Unfortunately, a negative assay does not exclude infection and repeated testing is indicated during the first 6 months of life.

Quantitation of HIV Infection

Determinations of the amount of HIV proviral DNA (Gibson et al., 1991), unintegrated HIV DNA (Dickover et al., 1991), and viral RNA in cells (Bagnarel li et al., 1991a) or sera (Bagnarelli et al., 1991b; Holodniy et al., 1991; Ottmann et al., 1991) have been proposed for assessing disease progression and response to anti-HIV therapy (Oka et al., 1991). For meaningful quantitation, strict adherence

to standardized sample preparation and assay conditions must be followed. Preferably, direct comparisons within a single assay should be made between samples obtained at different time points from the same patient. A series of quantitative standards need also to be run in the same assay. A single time point study on an individual patient has yet to be shown to be clinically prognostic (Lee et al., 1991).

Detection of AZT Resistance

PCR can be used to screen for sequence changes within the polymerase gene of HIV (Fitzgibbon et al., 1991). It has been suggested that mutations within this gene may predict the emergence of AZT resistance (Richman et al., 1991). If this proves to be the case and as alternative therapies become available, PCR genotyping of the HIV polymerase gene will likely become a standard test in the management of AIDS patients.

Human T-Lymphocytotropic Viruses (HTLV)

Distinction between HTLV-1 and HTLV-II

HTLV-I infection is associated with the development of certain T cell neoplasms (Chadburn et al., 1991) and with the occurrence of tropical spastic paresis (Daenke et al., 1990). On the other hand, HTLV-II infection has yet to be associated with any well-defined disease process. There are only minor serological differences between HTLV-I and HTLV-II viruses and conventional serology does not discriminate between the two viruses. PCR provides a convenient method to distinguish the cause of infection in a seropositive individual (Ehrlich et al., 1989).

Detection of Latent Infection and Defective Viruses

The full range of diseases associated with HTLV viruses has yet to be determined. Of interest are the reported PCR findings of HTLV related sequences in various disease states (Greenberg et al., 1989; Reddy et al., 1989; DeFreitas et al., 1991). In several circumstances, only portions of the putative viral genomes appear to be present (Hall et al.,

1991; Korber et al., 1991). Because of DNA sequence homologies within certain regions of different classes of viruses, one cannot readily extrapolate a positive PCR using HTLV-reactive primers to the presence of this class of virus. Especially at low annealing temperatures in the presence of high concentrations of template DNA, cross-priming can be observed resulting in the production of spurious PCR products. The fidelity of the PCR can be assessed by the banding pattern of electrophoresed PCR products and by the results of high stringency secondary hybridization reactions.

Human Papillomaviruses (HPV)

Diagnosis

The sensitivity of PCR makes it an ideal approach to diagnose HPV infection in both female (Shibata et al., 1988a,b; Bauer et al., 1991) and male patients (Kataoka et al., 1991). PCR is readily applicable to cells scraped off a Papanicolaou-stained slide or to a thin section from a paraffin-embedded tissue block. Distinction between the various types of HPV can be readily made using generic primers (Snijders et al., 1990; Evander and Wadell, 1991; Williamson and Rybick, 1991) and type specific probes. PCR has been used to demonstrate HPV infection in nongenital lesions including conjunctival dysplasias (McDonnell et al., 1989) as well as squamous carcinomas of the head and neck region (Watts et al., 1991). It can also be used to study the epidemiology of virus spread (Ho et al., 1991). Of interest is the reported association between a failure to detect HPV infection in cervical cancer and poor prognosis. Some of these cases may reflect partial loss of the HPV genome, since positive PCR can be achieved using alternative primers sets (Stoler et al., 1991).

Human Herpesviruses

Cytomegalovirus (CMV)

PCR provides a rapid alternative to culture methods for the diagnosis of CMV infection (Shibata et al., 1988c; Gerna et al., 1991). It can be applied to blood, urine, and cerebro-spinal fluid (CSF) (Olive et al., 1989; Buffone et al., 1991; Brytting et al., 1991; Einsele et al., 1991). The assay can be made semiquantitative and used to assess disease progression and response to therapy. Because of the large size of the viral genome (225,000 nucleotide base pairs) there is an understandable reluctance to rely on a single primer set to exclude infection. It is incumbent on the investigators to establish the reliability of a single primer set to amplify all clinical isolates. One approach to avoid false negative PCR results has been to use at least two primer sets against conserved sequences. While genetic heterogeneity can lead to false negative PCR, it also holds promise for identifying the genetic basis for virulence and for potential drug resistance. It is important that clinical variants of CMV be saved and provided for detailed sequence analysis to help establish the next generation of PCR assays for this important infection.

Herpes Simplex Infection

PCR has been applied to detection and the typing of HSV-1 and HSV-2 infections (Cone et al., 1991; Piiparinen and Vaheri, 1991). Of considerable clinical value is the early and rapid detection of herpes simplex encephalitis (Rowley et al., 1990; Dennett et al., 1991).

Other Herpesviruses

PCR has been useful to distinguish between strains of Epstein–Barr virus (Sixbey et al., 1989) and to demonstrate this virus in some cases of Hodgkin's disease (Knecht et al., 1991) and in certain gastric cancers (Shibata et al., 1991). The definition of the role of human herpesvirus-6 in various lymphoproliferative lesions has been greatly aided by the use of PCR (Bushbinder et al., 1988; Collandre et al., 1991). PCR has also been used to assist in the diagnosis of varicella-zoster infection (Dlugosch et al., 1991; Kido et al., 1991) and central nervous system complications of varicella zoster infection (Puchhammer-Stockl et al., 1991). It is possible to identify several sequences more or less shared among the different types of human herpesviruses (Martin, 1991). By reducing the stringency of the PCR, such primers can serve as a useful screening method to rule out known herpesviral infection and to potentially identify new types of human pathogenic herpesviruses.

Hepatitis Viruses

PCR provides a sensitive method to detect the five hepatotropic viruses associated with hepatitis: HAV (Jansen et al., 1990), HBV (Kaneko et al., 1989; Sumazaki et al., 1989; Manzin et al., 1991), HCV (Brillanti et al., 1991; Widell et al., 1991), HDV (Luo et al., 1990), and HEV (McCaustland et al., 1991). Of particular interest has been the apparent association of genetic variants of HBV with more aggressive disease (Carman et al., 1989a). As with HIV, some infections with HBV and early infection with HCV may be present in the absence of seroconversion (Thiers et al., 1988; Widell et al., 1991). If this phenomenon is widespread, PCR will likely emerge as a critical diagnostic test for evaluating blood products to exclude unapparent HBV and HCV infections.

Polyomaviruses

Both BK and JC viruses can be readily detected using PCR methodology. These tests have proven useful in evaluating BK viruses in postrenal transplant patients (Marshall et al., 1990) and JC virus in cases of progressive multifocal encephalopathy (Arthur et al., 1989).

Parvovirus

A role has been established for B16 parvovirus infection in bone marrow aplasia and in unexpected abortions. PCR can provide solid evidence for the presence of this virus in the tissues and blood of infected individuals (Salimans et al., 1989; Kock and Adler, 1990).

RNA Viruses

Although an initial reverse transcription step is necessary, PCR has proven itself useful in identifying the presence of enteroviruses (Gow et al., 1991; Zoll et al., 1992), flaviviruses (Eldadah et al., 1991), rotavirus (Eiden et al., 1991; Gouvea et al., 1991), rubella virus (Car-

man et al., 1989b; Eggerding et al., 1991), influenza viruses (Yamada et al., 1991), dengue virus (Morita et al., 1991), and rabies viruses (Sacramento et al., 1991). PCR should prove especially useful in examination of CSF in cases of aseptic meningitis. Broadly reactive primers capable of recognizing a wide range of viral types will be needed to exclude viral involvement as a cause of CSF inflammation. Such broadly reactive primers should also prove useful in exploring the potential role of persistent viral infections in various chronic neurological and nonneurological illnesses.

Bacterial Infections

Mycobacteria

The increasing prevalence of mycobacterial infections has highlighted the need for a rapid sensitive direct assay on sputum and blood samples. *Mycobacteria tuberculosis* can be detected in sputum using PCR and distinguished from other mycobacterial species (Hance et al., 1989; Cousins et al., 1992; Srithanan and Barker, 1991). PCR has also been used to detect *Mycobacteria lepre* in skin lesions (de Wit et al., 1991).

Treponema pallidum

With the advent of AIDS, the previously accepted criteria required to establish syphilis infection of the CNS are not always met. Using PCR it is possible to detect *Treponema pallidum* organisms directly within CSF (Noordhoek et al., 1991). The PCR assay has also been applied to prenatal and neonatal infection (Grimprel et al., 1991).

Borrelia burgdorferi

Serology is not always positive in cases of Lyme disease. Conversely, the presence of antibodies does not distinguish a continuing infection from a previous infection that is no longer active. PCR assays have been established for this infection (Lebech et al., 1991; Rosa and Schwan, 1991; Wise and Weaver, 1991). Bacterial DNA has been detected in blood, cerebrospinal fluid (Krueger and Pulz,

1991), and urine (Goodman et al., 1991) of persistently infected individuals. As with any suggested new clinical application, the issue of genetic diversity between isolates as a possible cause of a false negative PCR must be considered and the diagnostic sensitivity and specificity parameters must be experimentally established.

Chlamydia

Although there are sensitive antibody based assays for the direct detection of *Chlamydia trachomatis,* molecular-based assays including PCR can offer major advantages (Claas et al., 1991). In particular, there is strong interest in the utility of PCR assays for the detection of infection in males partners of infected females. PCR assays for *Chlamydia pneumonis* and *Chlamydia psittacosis* (Kaltenboeck et al., 1991) have also been described.

Mycoplasma pneumonis

Relatively mild, persistent, respiratory infection in young adults is often attributed to mycoplasmal infection based solely on a therapeutic response to the appropriate antibiotics. Confirmation of infection by PCR would be diagnostically useful especially if the testing were to be coupled with testing for alternative pathogens capable of inducing a similar disease, e.g., *Chlamydia pneumonis* (Bernet et al., 1989; Kunita et al., 1990).

Toxigenic Bacteria

Staphylococcus

A major advance has been identification of the gene responsible for the production of the toxic shock syndrome. The presence of this gene can now be detected using PCR (Jaulhac et al., 1991; Johnson et al., 1991).

Escherichia coli

A limitation in the conventional bacteriological analysis of stool samples is the inability to readily distinguish normal *E. coli* flora from enteropathic and enterotoxic strains. The toxins responsible for these pathogenic effects

have recently been identified and specific PCR assays to detect these genes have been designed (Tyler et al., 1991; Victor et al., 1991).

Clostridium difficile

Infection with these bacteria can lead to severe diarrhea and a syndrome termed pseudomembranous colitis, which is caused by a bacterial toxin. The gene coding the *C. difficile* toxin has been sequenced and a PCR assay for its presence has been established (Kato et al., 1991).

Antibiotic Resistance

The major advantage of bacterial cultures is that it provides organisms for direct testing of antibiotic resistance. Given the potential of multiple pathways of antibiotic resistance, it was considered unlikely that simplified predictive molecular-based assay could be devised to define this function. This situation appears to be changing. An assay has been described for the detection of methicillin-resistant *Staphylococcus* (Murakami et al., 1991). The genetic basis for resistance to other antibiotics is becoming clearer as is the potential for PCR assays to replace routine bacterial cultures. In fact, the sensitivity of PCR in detecting DNA coding an antibiotic resistance gene in either an unexpressed form, or within a minor subpopulation of organisms, may better predict the emergence of drug sensitivity than does the current culture-based methods.

Parasitic and Fungal Infections

Malaria

Because of delay in technology transfer, PCR assays for the routine diagnosis of malaria in developing regions of the world is not currently feasible. PCR assays can be quite useful, however, for epidemiological purposes, especially since it can be readily applied to individual mosquitos. PCR has been used to define species variations in *Plasmodium vivax* (Rosenberg et al., 1989) and *P. falciparum* (Kain and Lanar, 1991). It has also proven useful in the detection of mutations within the gene coding the dihydrofolate reductase gene responsible for pyrimethamine resistance of *P. falciparum* (Peterson et al., 1988; Tanaka et al., 1990). The homolog of the mammalian multidrug resistance gene (mdr) has been implicated in chloroquine resistance in *P. falciparum*. This gene is amenable to quantitative and qualitative analysis using PCR (Foote et al., 1989; Wilson et al., 1989).

Pneumocystis carinii

Immunofluorescence and silver staining methods are generally more practical than PCR for the diagnosis of *P. carinii* infection in immunosuppressed patients. On the other hand, PCR-based assays have the potential of providing useful information concerning possible antibiotic resistance markers, etc. PCR is likely to be much more sensitive than current methods (Wakefield et al., 1991) and may help in deciding on the use of prophylactic therapy.

Toxoplasmosis gondii

PCR assays for *Toxoplasmosis* infection have been described (Burg et al., 1989; Savva et al., 1990). These assays offer particular promise in diagnosing central nervous system infection in immunosuppressed HIV-infected patients (Holliman et al., 1990). As with other types of opportunistic infections in patients with AIDS, there can be an absence of conventional serological and cellular inflammatory markers. PCR based toxoplasma assay is also useful in the detection of prenatal infections (Grover et al., 1990).

Entamoeba histolytica

While an experienced technologist can readily distinguish pathogenic *E. histolytica* from non-pathogenic *E. coli,* PCR-based assays can provide an alternative and much more sensitive approach (Tachibana et al., 1991; Tannich and Burchard, 1991; Zar and Fernandez, 1991). Furthermore, testing for amplification of the mdr-related gene may provide information concerning resistance to emetine therapy (Samuelson et al., 1990).

Trypanosoma cruzi

Chagas' disease, caused by *T. cruzi* infection, can present diagnostic difficulties when not clinically suspected. Serological assays are neither sensitive nor specific for diagnosing active infection. There is also a continuing concern for the possible spread of this disease by blood transfusion. For these reasons, there has been a recent surge in interest in applying PCR to the detection of *T. cruzi*. This effort appears to have been successful (Moser et al., 1989).

Fungi

Although not in widespread use, PCR assays have been designed to detect various fungal species including *Candida albicans* (Buchman et al., 1990), *Cryptococcus neoformans* (Vilgalys and Hester, 1990), etc.

Anticipated New Developments

In spite of its enormous potential in the clinical laboratory, PCR technology is still not widely utilized. Issues relating to the licensing of the technology and limitations in billing for investigational test procedures have discouraged many from exploring the use of PCR assays. There is a shortage of technologists trained in molecular procedures as well as a reluctance to work with radioisotopes. There is also the perception that contamination is so frequent that PCR assays are unreliable in a clinical setting. While all of these issues have a degree of validity, the rapid pace of progress currently being made should ensure a routine role for PCR-based assays in the near future.

Progress can be expected in improved and simplified methods for sample preparation. Although amplification can be achieved on crude lysates, such specimens show varying degrees of *Taq* enzyme inhibitory activity. On the other hand, more extensive purification adds time to the assay and increases the risk of sample contamination. Recombinant DNA synthesized polymerase enzymes that will be less susceptible to the common inhibitors in crude tissue and blood extracts offer a straightforward solution to this problem. Newer methods of DNA enrichment, e.g., the use of NaI (Loparev et al., 1991; Ishizawa et al., 1991), provide alternatives to organic extraction methods. Automated methods for dispensing reactants and microtiter plate format should allow for rapid assay set-up and amplification. Using recently introduced thermal cycling machines, 20 cycles of amplification can be achieved in less than an hour. With increasing knowledge of the kinetics of primer annealing and the use of optimal concentrations of reactants, the PCR assay conditions can be established such that a positive assay will result in the synthesis of essentially a single product. This improvement will greatly facilitate the development of automated methods of product analysis. Nonradioisotopic methods of detection, including the use of PCR-generated biotin labeled probes, are available for use in laboratories not experienced in the use of radioisotopes. Semiautomated methods for silver straining of polyacrylamide gel-separated PCR products can yield rapid results. Moreover, prior denaturation of the PCR products allows this nonisotopic technique to be used for single-strand conformation polymorphism (SSCP) analysis. SSCP is a very convenient method for qualitative analysis of PCR products, including the screening for minor differences in sequences (Moohabeer et al., 1991). Direct cloning and sequencing of PCR products can also be achieved within the space of several days and can help resolve difficult problems.

Even more optimism can be expressed concerning the rapid pace with which PCR technology is providing a new understanding into the molecular pathogenesis of infectious diseases. Sequencing of PCR products can help define the structural basis for variations in virulence and in chemosensitivity. As specific viral and bacterial genes become identified, new insights will be provided into the complexity of the host pathogen interactions and fresh areas for therapeutic intervention will become apparent. PCR-based assays can be particularly useful to test for persistent viral infections in the pathogenesis of many chronic illnesses. Detection of novel viruses that fail to evoke typical inflammatory reactions, or that may

have lost certain genes required for successful *in vitro* cultivation, is well within the current realm of PCR-based research. Finally, as sequence data are amassed, it will be easier to construct primer sets that will serve as screening reagents to detect broad categories of pathogens to assist in disease surveillance and prevention.

Acknowledgments. The author is especially grateful to the efforts of Anton Mayr, M.T., Peyman Javaherbin, M.T., and Li Cheng Zeng, M.D., for their tireless efforts to establish clinically informative PCR assays.

References

Arthur RR, Dogostin S, Shah KV (1989): Detection of BK virus and JC virus in urine and brain tissue by the polymerase chain reaction. *J Clin Microbiol* 27:1174–1179.

Bagnarelli P, Menzo S, Manzin A, et al. (1991a): Detection of human immunodeficiency virus type 1 transcripts in peripheral blood lymphocytes by the polymerase chain reaction. *J Virol Methods* 32:31–39.

Bagnarelli P, Menzo S, Manzin A, et al. (1991b): Detection of human immunodeficiency virus type 1 genomic RNA in plasma samples by reverse-transcription polymerase chain reaction. *J Med Virol* 34:89–95.

Bauer M, Yi T, Greer C, et al. (1991): Genital human papillomavirus infection in female university students as determined by a PCR-based method. *JAMA* 265:472–477.

Bernet C, Garret M, de Barbeyrac B, et al. (1989): Detection of mycoplasma pneumoniae by using the polymerase chain reaction. *J Clin Microbiol* 27:2492–2496.

Brillanti S, Garson JA, Tuke PW, et al. (1991): Effect of alpha interferon therapy on hepatitis C viremia in community-acquired chronic non-A, non-B hepatitis: a quantitative polymerase chain reaction study. *J Med Virol* 34:136–141.

Brytting M, Sundgvist VA, Stalhhandske P, et al. (1991): Cytomegaloviral DNA detection of an intermediate early protein gene with nested primer oligonucleotides. *J Virol Method* 32:127–138.

Buchman G, Timothy G, Rossier W, et al. (1990): Detection of surgical pathogens by in vitro DNA amplification. Part I. Rapid identification of Candida albicans by in vitro amplification of a fungus-specific gene. *Surgery* 108:338–346.

Buffone GJ, Demmler GJ, Schimbor CM, et al. (1991): Improved amplification of cytomegalovirus DNA from urine after purification of DNA with glass beads. *Clin Chem* 37:1945–1949.

Burg JL, Grover CM, Pouletty P, et al. (1989): Direct and sensitive detection of a pathogenic protozoan, Toxoplasma gondii, by polymerase chain reaction. *J Clin Microbiol* 27:1787–1792.

Bushbinder A, Josephs SF, Ablashi D, et al. (1988): Polymerase chain reaction amplification and in situ hybridization for the detection of human B-lymphotropic virus. *J Virol Methods* 21:191–197.

Carman WF, Jacyna MR, Hadziyannis S, et al. (1989a): Mutation preventing formation of hepatitis B antigen in patients with chronic hepatitis B infection. *Lancet* ii:588–590.

Carman WF, Williamson C, Cunliffe BA, et al. (1989b): Reverse transcription and subsequent DNA amplification of rubella virus RNA. *J Virol Methods* 25:21–29.

Cassol S, Salas T, Lapointe N, et al. (1991): Improved detection of HIV-1 envelope sequences using optimized PCR and inosine-substituted primers. *Mol Cell Probes* 5:157–160.

Chadburn A, Athan E, Wieczorek R, et al. (1991): Detection and characterization of human T-cell lymphotropic virus type I (HTLV-I) associated T-cell neoplasms in an HTLV-I nonendemic region by PCR. *Blood* 7:2419–2430.

Claas HC, Wagenvoort JH, Niesters HG, et al. (1991): Diagnostic value of the polymerase chain reaction for chlamydia detection as determined in a follow-up study. *J Clin Microbiol* 29:42.

Collandre H, Aubin JT, Agut H, et al. (1991): Detection of HHV-6 by the PCR. *J Virol Methods* 31:171–180.

Cone RW, Hobson AC, Palmer J, et al. (1991): Extended duration of herpes simplex virus DNA in genital lesions detected by the polymerase chain reaction. *J Infect Dis* 164:757–760.

Cousins DV, Wilton SD, Francis BR, et al. (1992): Use of polymerase chain reaction for rapid diagnosis of tuberculosis. *J Clin Microbiol* 30:255–258.

Coutlee F, Viscidi RP, Saint-Antoine P, et al (1991): The polymerase chain reaction: A new tool for the understanding and diagnosis of HIV-1 infection at the cellular level. *Mol Cell Probes* 5:241–259.

Daenke S, Nightingale S, Cruickshank JK, et al. (1990): Sequence variants from human t lymphotropic virus type I from patients with tropical paraparesis and adult T-cell leukemia do not distinguish neurological from leukemic isolates. *J Virol* 64:1278–1282.

DeFreitas E, Hilliard B, Cheney PR, et al. (1991): Retroviral sequences related to human T-lymphotropic virus type II in patients with chronic fatigue immune dysfunction syndrome. *Proc Natl Acad Sci USA* 88:2922–2926.

Dennett C, Klapper PE, Cleator GM, et al. (1991): CSF pretreatment and the diagnosis of herpes encephalitis using the polymerase chain reaction. *J Virol Methods* 34:101–104.

de Wit MY, Faber WR, Krieg SR, et al. (1991): Application of a polymerase chain reaction for the detection of Mycobacterium leprae in skin tissues. *J Clin Microbiol* 29:906–910.

Dickover RE, Donovan RM, Goldstein E, et al. (1991): Decreases in unintegrated HIV DNA are associated with antiretroviral therapy in AIDS patients. *J Aquir Imm Def Syn* 5:31–36.

Dlugosch D, Eis-Hubinger AM, Kleim J-P, et al. (1991): Diagnosis of acute and latent varicella-zoster virus infections using polymerase chain reaction. *J Med Virol* 35:136–141.

Eggerding FA, Peters J, Lee RK, et al. (1991): Detection of rubella virus gene sequences by enzymatic amplification and direct sequencing of amplified DNA. *J Clin Microbiol* 29:945–952.

Ehrlich GD, Glaser JB, LaVigne K, et al. (1989): Prevalence of human T-cell leukemia/lymphoma virus (HTLV) Type II infection among high-risk individuals: Type-specific identification of HTLVs by polymerase chain reaction. *Blood* 74:1658–1664.

Eiden JJ, Wilde J, Firoozmand F, et al. (1991): Detection of animal and human group B rotaviruses in fecal specimens by polymerase chain reaction. *J Clin Microbiol* 29:539–543.

Einsele H, Steindle M, Vallbracht A, et al. (1991): Early occurrence of human cytomegalovirus infection after bone marrow transplantation as demonstrated by PCR. *Blood* 77:1104–1110.

Eldadah ZA, Asher DM, Godec MS, et al. (1991): Detection of flaviviruses by reverse-transcriptase polymerase chain reaction. *J Med Virol* 33:260–267.

Evander M, Wadell G (1991): A general primer pair for amplification and detection of genital human papillomavirus types. *J Virol Methods* 31:239–250.

Fitzgibbon JE, Howell RM, Schwartzer TA, et al. (1991): In vivo prevalence of azidothymidine (AZT) resistance mutations in an AIDS patient before and after AZT therapy. *AIDS Res Hum Retrovirus* 7:265–269.

Foote SJ, Thompson JK, Cowman AF, et al. (1989): Amplification of the multidrug resistance gene in some chloroquine-resistant isolates of P. falciparum. *Cell* 57:921–930.

Gerna G, Zipeto D, Parea M, et al. (1991): Early viral isolation, early structural antigen detection and DNA amplification by the polymerase chain reaction in polymorphonuclear leukocytes from AIDS patients with human cytomegalovirus. *Mol Cell Probes* 5:365–374.

Gibson KM, McLean KA, Clewley JP (1991): A simple and rapid method for detecting human immunodeficiency virus by PCR. *J Virol Methods* 32:277–286.

Goodman JL, Jurkovich P, Kramber JM, et al. (1991): Molecular detection of persistent Borellia burgdorferi in the urine of patients with active Lyme disease. *Infect Immun* 59:269–278.

Gouvea V, Allen JR, Glass RI, et al. (1991): Detection of group B rotaviruses by polymerase chain reaction. *J Clin Microbiol* 29:519–523.

Gow JW, Behan WM, Clemments GB, et al. (1991): Enteroviral RNA sequences detected by polymerase chain reaction in muscle of patients with postviral fatigue syndrome. *Br J Med* 302: 692–696.

Greenberg SJ, Ehrlich GD, Abbott MA, et al. (1989): Detection of sequences homologous to human retroviral DNA in multiple sclerosis by gene amplification. *Proc Natl Acad Sci USA* 86: 2878–2882.

Grimprel E, Sanchez JP, Stortz J, et al. (1991): Use of polymerase chain reaction and rabbit infectivity testing to detect Treponema pallidum in amniotic fluid, fetal and neonatal sera and cerebrospinal fluid. *J Clin Microbiol* 29:1711–1718.

Grover CM, Thulliez P, Remington JS, et al. (1990): Rapid prenatal diagnosis of congenital Toxoplasma infection by using polymerase chain reaction and amniotic fluid. *J Clin Microbiol* 28:2297–2303.

Hance AJ, Grandchamp B, Levy-Frebault V, et al. (1989): Detection and identification of mycobacteria by amplification of mycobacterial DNA. *Mol Microbiol* 3:843–849.

Hall WW, Liu CR, Schneewind O, et al. (1991): Deleted HTLV-I provirus in blood and cutaneous lesions of patients with mycosis fungoides. *Science* 253:317–320.

Ho L, Chen S-Y, Chow V, et al. (1991): Sequence variants of human papillomavirus type 16 in clinical samples permit verification and extension of epidemiological studies and construction of a phylogenetic tree. *J Clin Microbiol* 29:1765–1772.

Holliman R, Johnson JD, Savva D (1990): Diagnosis of cerebral toxoplasmosis in association with AIDS using the polymerase chain reaction. *Scand J Infect Dis* 22:243–244.

Holodniy M, Katzenstein DA, Sengupta S, et al. (1991): Detection and quantitation of human immunodeficiency virus RNA in patient serum by use of the polymerase chain reaction. *J Infect Dis* 163:862–866.

Ishizawa M, Kobayashi Y, Miyamura T, et al. (1991): Simple procedure of DNA isolation from human serum. *Nucl Acids Res* 19:5792.

Jackson JB, Kwok SY, Sninsky JJ, et al. (1990): Human immunodeficiency virus type 1 detected in all seropositive symptomatic and asymptomatic individuals. *J Clin Microbiol* 28:16–19.

Jansen RW, Siegl G, Lemon SM (1990): Molecular epidemiology of human hepatitis A virus defined by an antigen-capture polymerase chain reaction method. *Proc Natl Acad Sci USA* 87:2867–2871.

Jaulhac B, Prevost G, Piemont Y (1991): Specific detection of the toxic shock syndrome Toxin-1 gene using PCR. *Mol Cell Probes* 5:281–284.

Johnson WM, Tyler SD, Ewan P, et al. (1991): Detection of genes for enterotoxins, exfoliative toxins and toxic shock syndrome Toxin 1 in Staph. aureus by PCR. *J Clin Microbiol* 29:426–430.

Kain KC, Lanar DE (1991): Determination of genetic variation within *Plasmodium falciparum* by using enzymatically amplified DNA from filter paper disks impregnated with whole blood. *J Clin Microbiol* 29:1171–1174.

Kaltenboeck B, Kousoulas KG, Stortz J (1991): Detection and strain differences of *Chlamydia psittaci* mediated by a two step polymerase chain reaction. *J Clin Microbiol* 29:1969–1975.

Kaneko S, Feinstone SM, Miller RH (1989): Rapid and sensitive method for the detection of serum hepatitis B virus DNA using the polymerase chain technique. *J Clin Microbiol* 27:1930–1933.

Kataoka A, Claesson U, Hansson BG, et al. (1991): Human papillomavirus infection of the male diagnosed by Southern-blot hybridization and PCR: Comparison between urethra samples and penile biopsy samples. *J Med Virol* 33:159–164.

Kato N, Ou CY, Kato H, et al. (1991): Identification of toxigenic *Clostridium difficile* by the polymerase chain reaction. *J Clin Microbiol* 29:33–37.

Kido S, Ozaka T, Asada H, et al. (1991): Detection of varicellazoster (VZV) DNA in clinical samples from patients with VZV by PCR. *J Clin Microbiol* 29:76–79.

Knecht H, Odermott BF, Bechmann E, et al. (1991): Frequent detection of Epstein-Barr virus DNA by the PCR in lymph node biopsies from patients with Hodgkin's disease without genomic evidence of B- or T-cell clonality. *Blood* 78:760–767.

Kock WC, Adler SP (1990): Detection of human parvovirus B19 by using the polymerase chain reaction. *J Clin Microbiol* 28:65–69.

Korber B, Okayama A, Donnelly R, et al. (1991): Polymerase chain reaction analysis of defective human T-cell leukemia virus type I proviral genomes in leukemia cells of patients with adult T-cell leukemia. *J Virol* 65:5471–5476.

Krueger WH, Pulz M (1991): Detection of Borrelia burgdorefi in cerebrospinal fluid by the polymerase chain reaction. *J Med Microbiol* 35:98–102.

Kunita S, Terada E, Goto K, et al. (1990): Sensitive detection of Mycoplasma pnumonis by using the polymerase chain reaction. *Jikken Dobutsu* 39:103–107.

Laure F, Courgnaud V, Rouzioux C, et al. (1988): Detection of HIV1 DNA in infants and children by means of the polymerase chain reaction. *Lancet* ii:538–541.

Lebech AM, Hindersson P, Vuust J, et al. (1991): Comparison of in vitro culture and PCR for detection of *Borrelia burgdorferi* in tissue from experimentally infected animals. *J Clin Microbiol* 29:731–737.

Lee TH, Sunzeri FJ, Tobler LH, et al. (1991): Quantitative assessment of HIV-1 DNA load by coamplification of HIV-1 gag and HLA-DQ-alpha genes. *AIDS* 5:683–691.

Loparev VN, Cartas MA, Monken CE, et al. (1991): An efficient and simple method of DNA extraction from whole blood and cell lines to identify infectious agents. *J Virol Methods* 34:105–112.

Luo GX, Chao M, Hsieh SY, et al. (1990): A specific base transition occurs on replicating hepatitis delta virus RNA. *J Virol* 64:1021–1027.

Manzin A, Salvoni G, Bagnarelli P, et al. (1991): A single-step DNA extraction procedure for the detection of serum hepatitis B virus sequences by the polymerase chain reaction. *J Virol Methods* 32:245–253.

Marshall WF, Telenti A, Proper J, et al. (1990): Survey of urine from transplant recipients for polyomaviruses JC and BK using the polymerase chain reaction. *Mol Cell Probes* 5:125–128.

Martin WJ (1991): Polymerase chain reaction: A tool for the modern pathologist. In *Modern Diagnostics in Pathology*. Fenogli-Preiser CM, Willman C, eds. Baltimore: Williams & Wilkins.

McCaustland KA, Bi S, Purdy MA, et al. (1991): Application of two RNA extraction methods prior to amplification of hepatitis E virus nucleic acid by the polymerase chain reaction. *J Virol Methods* 35:331–334.

McDonnell JM, Mayr AJ, Martin WJ (1989): DNA of human papillomavirus type 16 in dysplastic and malignant lesions of the conjunctiva and cornea. *N Engl J Med* 320:1442–1446.

Mohabeer AJ, Hiti AL, Martin WJ (1991): Non-radioactive single strand conformation polymorphism (SSCP) using the Pharmacia "Phast System." *Nucl Acids Res* 19:3154.

Morita K, Mariko T, Igarashi A (1991): Rapid identification of dengue virus serotypes by using the PCR. *J Clin Microbiol* 29:2107–2110.

Moser DR, Kirchhoff LV, Donelson JE (1989): Detection of Trypanosoma Cruzi by DNA amplification using the polymerase reaction. *J Clin Microbiol* 27:1477–1482.

Murakami K, Minamide K, Waden K, et al. (1991): Identification of methacillin-resistant strains of Staphylococci by PCR. *J Clin Microbiol* 29:2240–2244.

Noordhoek GT, Wolters EC, Marjolijn ES (1991): Detection by PCR of *Treponema pallidum* DNA in the cerebrospinal fluid from neurosyphilis patients before and after antibiotic treatment. *J Clin Microbiol* 29:1976–1984.

Oka S, Urayama K, Hirabayashi Y, et al. (1991): Quantitative estimation of human immunodeficiency virus type-1 provirus in CD4 + T lymphocytes using the polymerase chain reaction. *Mol Cell Probes* 5:137–142.

Olive DM, Simsek M, Al-Mufti S (1989): Polymerase chain reaction assay for detection of human cytomegalovirus. *J Clin Microbiol* 27:1238–1242.

Ottmann M, Innocenti P, Thenadey M, et al. (1991): The polymerase chain reaction for the detection of HIV-1 genomic RNA in plasma from infected individuals. *J Virol Methods* 31:273–284.

Peterson DS, Walker D, Wellens TE (1988): Evidence that a point mutation in dihydrofolate reductase-thymidylate synthase confers resistance to pyrimethamine in falciparum malaria. *Proc Natl Acad Sci USA* 85:9144–9188.

Piiparinen H, Vaheri V (1991): Genotyping of herpes simplex virus by polymerase chain reaction. *Arch Virol* 119:275–283.

Puchhammer-Stockl E, Popow-Kraupp T, Heinz FX, et al. (1991): Detection of varicella zoster virus DNA by polymerase chain reaction in the cerebrospinal fluid of patients suffering from neurological complications associated with chicken pox or herpes zoster. *J Clin Microbiol* 29:1513–1516.

Reddy EP, Sandberg-Wollheim M, Mettus RV, et al. (1989): Amplification and molecular cloning of HTLV-I sequences from DNA of multiple sclerosis patients. *Science* 243:529–533.

Richman DD, Guatelli JC, Grimes J, et al. (1991): Detection of mutation associated with Zidovudine resistance in human immunodeficiency virus by use of polymerase chain reaction. *J Infect Dis* 164:1075–1081.

Rosa PA, Schwan TG (1991): A specific and sensitive assay for the Lyme disease spirochete Borellia burgdorferi using the polymerase chain reaction. *J Infect Dis* 160:1018–1020.

Rosenberg R, Wirtz RA, Lanar DE, et al. (1989): Circumsporozoite protein heterogeneity in the human malaria parasite *Plasmodium vivax*. *Science* 245:973–976.

Rowley AH, Whitley RJ, Lakeman FD, et al. (1990): Rapid detection of herpes simplex-virus DNA in cerebrospinal fluid of patients with herpes simplex encephalitis. *Lancet* 335:440–441.

Sacramento D, Bourhy H, Tordo N (1991): PCR technique as an alternative method for diagnosis and molecular epidemiology of rabies virus. *Mol Cell Probes* 5:229–240.

Salimans MM, van de Ryke FM, Raap AK, et al. (1989): Detection of parvovirus B19 DNA in fetal tissue by in situ hybridization and polymerase chain reaction. *J Clin Pathol* 42:525–529.

Samuelson J, Ayala P, Orozco E, et al. (1990): Emetine-resistant mutants of Entamoeba histolytica overexpresses mRNAs for multidrug resistance. *Mol Biochem Parasitol* 38:281–290.

Savva D, Morris JC, Johnson JD, et al. (1990): Polymerase chain reaction for detection of Toxoplasma gondii. *J Med Microbiol* 32:25–31.

Shibata D, Arnheim N, Martin WJ (1988a): Detection of human papillomavirus in paraffin embedded tissue using the polymerase chain reaction. *J Exp Med* 158:225–230.

Shibata D, Fu YS, Gupta JW, et al. (1988b): Detection of human papillomavirus in normal and dysplastic tissue by the polymerase chain reaction. *Lab Invest* 59:555–559.

Shibata D, Martin WJ, Appleman M, et al. (1988c): Detection of cytomegaloviral DNA in peripheral blood of patients infected with human immunodeficiency virus. *J Infect Dis* 158:1185–1192.

Shibata D, Tokunaga M, Uemura Y, et al. (1991): Association of Epstein-Barr virus with undifferentiated gastric carcinomas with intense lymphoid infiltration. *Am J Surg Pathol* 139:469–474.

Sixbey JW, Shirley P, Chesney PJ, et al. (1989): Detection of a second widespread strain of Epstein-Barr virus. *Lancet* ii:761–765.

Snijders PJF, van den Brule AJC, Schrijnemakers HFJ, et al. (1990): The use of general primers in the polymerase chain reaction permits the detection of a broad spectrum of human papillomavirus genotypes. *J Gen Virol* 71:173–181.

Sritharan V, Barker RH (1991): A simple method for diagnosing M. Tuberculosis infection in clinical samples using PCR. *Mol Cell Probes* 5:385–395.

Stoler M, Stoerker J, Betsill WL (1991): A caveat for molecular biology diagnosis of papillomavirus. *Clin Chem* 37:2016–2017.

Sumazaki R, Motz M, Wolf H, et al. (1989): Detection of hepatitis B virus in serum using amplification of viral DNA by means of the polymerase chain reaction. *J Med Virol* 27:304–308.

Tachibana H, Ihara S, Kobayashi S, et al. (1991): Differences in genomic DNA sequences between pathogenic and non-pathogenic isolates of *Entamoeba histolytica* identified by PCR. *J Clin Microbiol* 29:2234–2239.

Tanaka M, Gu HM, Bzik DJ, et al. (1990): Dihydrofolate reductase mutations and chromosomal changes associated with pyrimethamine resistance in *Plasmodium falciparum*. *Mol Biochem Parasitol* 39:127–133.

Tannich E, Burchard GD (1991): Differentiation of pathogenic from nonpathogenic Entamoeba histolytica by restriction fragment analysis of a single gene amplified in vitro. *J Clin Microbiol* 29:250–255.

Thiers V, Nakajima E, Kremsdorf D, et al. (1988): Transmission of hepatitis B from hepatitis-B-seronegative subjects. *Lancet* ii:1273–1276.

Tyler SD, Johnson WM, Loir H, et al. (1991): Identification of verotoxic type 2 variant B subunit genes in *Escherichia coli* by the PCR and RFLP analysis. *J Clin Microbiol* 29:1339–1343.

Victor T, du Toit R, van Zyl J, et al. (1991): Improved method for the routine identification of toxigenic E. coli by DNA amplification of a conserved region of the heat-labile Toxin A subunit. *J Clin Microbiol* 29:158.

Vilgalys R, Hester M (1990): Rapid genetic identification and mapping of enzymatically amplified ribosomal DNA from several Cryptococcal species. *J Bacteriol* 172:4238–4246.

Wages JM Jr, Hamdallah M, Calabro MA, et al. (1991): Clinical performance of a polymerase chain reaction testing algorithm for diagnosis of HIV-1 infection in peripheral blood mononuclear cells. *J Med Virol* 33:58–63.

Wakefield AE, Guiver L, Miller RF, et al. (1991): DNA amplification on induced sputum samples for diagnosis of Pneumocystis carinii pneumonia. *Lancet* 337:1378–1379.

Watts SL, Brewer EE, Fry TL (1991): Human papillomavirus DNA types in squamous cell carcinomas of the head and neck. *Oral Surg Oral Med Oral Pathol* 71:701–707.

Widell A, Mansson A-S, Sundstrom G, et al. (1991): Hepatitis C virus RNA in blood donor sera detected by the polymerase chain reaction: Comparison with supplementary hepatitis C antibody assays. *J Med Virol* 35:253–258.

Williamson AL, Rybick EP (1991): Detection of genital HPV by PCR amplification with degenerate nested primers. *J Med Virol* 33:165–171.

Wilson CM, Serrano AE, Wasley A, et al. (1989): Amplification of a gene related to mammalian mdr genes in drug-resistant *Plasmodium falciparum. Science* 244:1184–1186.

Wise DJ, Weaver RE (1991): Detection of the Lyme disease bacterium Borellia burgdorferi by using PCR and a nonisotopic gene probe. *J Clin Microbiol* 29:1523–1526.

Yagi MJ, Joesten ME, Wallace J, et al. (1991): Human immunodeficiency virus type 1 (HIV-1) genomic sequences and distinct changes in CD8$^+$ lymphocytes precede detectable levels of HIV-1 antibodies in high-risk homosexuals. *J Infect Dis* 164:183–187.

Yamada A, Imanishi J, Nakajima E, et al. (1991): Detection of influenza viruses in throat swab by using polymerase chain reaction. *Microbiol Immunol* 35:259–265.

Zar FA, Fernandez M (1991): Distinguishing pathogenic isolates by *Entamoeba histolytica* by PCR. *J Infect Dis* 164:825.

Zoll GJ, Melchers WJG, Kopecke H, et al. (1992): General primer mediated polymerase chain reaction for detection of enteroviruses. Application for diagnostic routine and persistent infections. *J Clin Microbiol* 30:160–165.

PART THREE
PCR and the World of Business

34

PCR in the Marketplace

Ellen Daniell

Introduction

PCR is "a revolutionary new technology." PCR has "transformed molecular biological research." PCR "may soon replace gene cloning as the amplification method of choice for gene sequencing." PCR is "providing new options in molecular genetics." PCR has "allowed evolutionary biologists to study fragments of DNA from ancient specimens, and forensic scientists to analyze DNA in traces of biological fluids recovered from crime scenes."

These are just a few of the ways in which the power of the polymerase chain reaction is described in scientific and popular publications. Much of this volume is dedicated to describing applications and extensions of the basic PCR process and detailing aspects of these technical advances. This chapter looks at how the technical advances arising from PCR represent a business opportunity. By what means did those who owned the invention, supported development of the process, and pursued, obtained,

The views expressed in this article are those of the author and do not necessarily reflect those of Hoffmann-La Roche or any other party.

and defended the patent rights hope to recover their costs and reap financial benefit from the process? To answer this question, this chapter describes the businesses built around PCR and provides an historical account of how these businesses have developed.

The institution at the center of the story of establishing a PCR business was Cetus Corporation of Emeryville, California. Kary Mullis was employed by Cetus when he invented PCR. Mullis and other Cetus scientists developed the process and found numerous applications of it. Cetus filed patents on the basic process and on many applications, uses, improvements, and components used in the process. The first two of these patents were issued to Cetus in the United States in July 1987. Four additional patents on basic PCR methods, three patents on *Taq* DNA polymerase, patents on certain reagent kits and detection of specific genetic loci, and a thermal cycling instrument patent have issued as of March 1992.

The first, and critical, PCR business decisions Cetus made in 1985 were to publish the PCR method in the scientific literature and to permit scientists in academia, government, and industry to use it freely for noncommercial research purposes. Cetus could have kept the

The Polymerase Chain Reaction
K.B. Mullis, F. Ferré, R.A. Gibbs, editors
© 1994 Birkhäuser Boston

process a secret until patents and patent applications were made public, or asked for a royalty on revenues resulting from any discovery made using the process, as Stanford University did with the Cohen–Boyer recombinant DNA patent. These alternatives were debated internally, as the power of the PCR became apparent. In the autumn of 1985 and early in 1986, the PCR process and its application to the diagnosis of sickle cell anemia were presented in public talks by Randy Saiki and by Kary Mullis. Additional talks and publications (referenced throughout this volume) followed.

Cetus pursued PCR as a business in three major fields: human *in vitro* diagnostics, research and industrial quality assurance, and human identification. A different business strategy was selected for each of these fields. Rights to human diagnostics were licensed in conjunction with external support of Cetus research in that field; the research product market was developed in a joint venture with an instrument systems manufacturer; and human identity was approached as a fully integrated internal business. Other areas, such as veterinary diagnostics, were pursued as licensing opportunities.

In deciding how to commercialize PCR, Cetus management faced substantial resource allocation issues. Founded in 1971, Cetus was, at the time of the invention of PCR, a biotechnology company focused on building a pharmaceutical business. Efforts in diagnostics and instrumentation were looked on by top management as requiring resources that might detract from the main goal, so partial funding for those was sought from external sources. While basic PCR technology development was performed at Cetus, corporate strategy dictated that commercialization of the products utilizing the process would be done principally through other companies.

Human Diagnostics

When Kary Mullis conceived of PCR, on the fateful drive to Mendocino that he has described in lectures, in print, and in U.S. Federal Court proceedings (see Chapter 1), he was considering how to detect single base-pair changes in DNA. Interest in this problem was primarily related to potential diagnostic uses— a mutation may indicate that an individual has a genetic disease, or greater than average susceptibility to a disease. In the first publication demonstrating the utility of PCR, scientists in the Human Genetics Department at Cetus described the application of PCR to an ongoing project to develop an assay for the detection of the single base-pair change that causes sickle-cell anemia (Saiki et al., 1985). Half of the 20 papers on PCR published in the year following the Saiki et al. paper dealt specifically with human diagnostic applications.

PCR was immediately recognized as a powerful tool in the detection of genetic alterations because amplification of a specific segment of genetic material allowed direct analysis of the relevant region of DNA without the background of the entire complex genome. In addition, the potential of PCR in detecting one critical infectious disease target, human immunodeficiency virus (HIV), was quickly recognized. In 1984, HIV had been implicated as the causative agent of AIDS, and it was known that the viral DNA copies could be harbored in the genome of an infected individual in the absence of expression of viral proteins or clinical symptoms. A Cetus team, as well as other researchers in human molecular genetics, began to work on the use of PCR to detect the presence of HIV DNA in human blood. In June 1988 Cetus granted a license to Specialty Laboratories and to Pathology Institute, two clinical reference laboratories in California, to perform a PCR-based diagnostic assay for HIV. This assay, which had been developed at Cetus with extensive testing on clinical samples performed by Specialty Labs and Pathology Institute, was the first PCR-based service offered commercially. Cetus was cautious about more broadly licensing the technology in this area early on because reliable testing would require extensive optimization, controls to guard against false positives, and demonstration of clinical utility.

Other clinical research laboratories, based in universities, hospitals, and commercial reference laboratories, were applying the PCR process to a variety of infectious and genetic disease targets. By the middle of 1988, over 50 groups had inquired about the possibility of licensing the PCR process to perform diagnostic testing.

Selecting among a number of options for commercializing PCR in the diagnostic field, Cetus chose a close collaboration and licensing arrangement with Hoffmann-La Roche Inc. of Nutley, New Jersey and F. Hoffmann-La Roche Ltd. of Basel, Switzerland. The Cetus/Roche collaboration began in early 1989. Under the agreement, Roche agreed to fund research and development efforts by Cetus in PCR-based human *in vitro* diagnostics over a 5-year period and to engage in development of diagnostic products and services. Roche and its affiliated companies received exclusive worldwide rights to market the resulting products and services, and owed royalties to Cetus on net sales. Cetus would supply certain reagents for use in the clinical assays and diagnostic tests, an arrangement that complemented their manufacture and supply of similar reagents to the research market through a joint venture with Perkin-Elmer (see below). Roche provides diagnostic services through its reference lab network, Roche Biomedical Laboratories (RBL), and develops and sells diagnostic kits at Roche Diagnostic Systems (RDS). The reference lab capability makes it possible to commercialize complex PCR tests and make them available as a service to the medical community several years ahead of the FDA-licensed kits, which require greatly simplified formats.

At the time that the agreement with Roche went into effect, Cetus had licensed only Specialty Labs and Pathology Institute to provide PCR-based services for HIV-1 detection. Roche and Cetus together decided to expand this licensing to further encourage the development of PCR diagnostic testing. In the early months of the Roche arrangement, Cetus completed some 25 service licenses with certain of the academic institutions and companies who had been requesting PCR licenses for some time.

Early in 1991, Roche made a significant move to extend still further the availability of PCR technology to the medical field by entering into an agreement with SmithKline Beecham Clinical Laboratories, the largest clinical laboratory in North America. Under the agreement, SmithKline Beecham received broad rights to perform *in vitro* clinical laboratory testing services for PCR. The aim of this agreement was not only to provide a license, but to use the resources of the two companies to develop clinical PCR applications at a more rapid rate than would have been possible otherwise. Subsequent agreements with Metpath and Medigene were structured similarly.

Immediately after the establishment of the Cetus-Roche program in 1989, Roche established a group dedicated to PCR in Alameda, California, close to the research group at Cetus. The Alameda facility included a research effort as well as a group that was responsible for validating assays and procedures from research and transferring them to RBL and to the diagnostic kit development group in New Jersey.

The fruitful collaboration between Cetus and Roche culminated in the acquisition of the rights to PCR by Roche, described at the end of this chapter.

Research and Industrial QA/QC

While the potential of PCR for disease diagnosis was evident from its earliest stages, and human diagnostics was recognized as the largest single commercial opportunity, the process received even more immediate attention from the molecular biology research community. Scientists quickly recognized that a host of questions that were otherwise intractable because of lack of material or time constraints could be addressed in conjunction with precise, specific nucleic acid amplification. After Cetus scientists purified a heat-stable DNA polymerase from *Thermus aquaticus*, thereby simplifying the automation of PCR, demand for both the enzyme and thermal cycling instrumentation grew rapidly.

The vehicle for developing the PCR research products business was Perkin-Elmer Cetus Instruments (PECI), a joint venture between Cetus and The Perkin-Elmer Corporation that had been established in December 1985 to develop instrument systems and reagents for the biomedical research market. Although the joint venture was not established with PCR products as a principal objective, by November 1987 when the first PCR reagent products and the first DNA thermal cycler were introduced, interest in the technology and products was so great that managements of both parent companies viewed PECI as essentially PCR focused.

The joint venture first commercialized a system of PCR core reagents and the DNA thermal cycler that had been developed as a prototype by Cetus engineers in response to the in-house need for automation of PCR. As the PECI venture developed, the two partners each took responsibility for their own areas of greatest expertise, with instrument R&D and manufacturing being handled by Perkin-Elmer, and reagent R&D and manufacturing by Cetus. The venture, owned 49% by Cetus and 51% by Perkin-Elmer, benefitted from Perkin-Elmer's extensive worldwide sales, marketing, and customer service organization, with Perkin-Elmer being the exclusive distributor of venture products.

The objectives of the PECI business were to develop, manufacture, and supply instruments and reagents for use in bioanalytical research fields, focusing primarily on nucleic acid amplification and related procedures. Perkin-Elmer products for research laboratories had traditionally consisted of high-quality instrumentation; to address the needs of a different kind of market, the company added new sales people trained in molecular biology, and established new customer support teams to work with the scientific community to advance the development of PCR applications.

The first PECI reagents for PCR were native *Taq* DNA polymerase and a GeneAmp® PCR reagent kit containing that polymerase as well as buffers, deoxynucleoside triphosphates, target DNA, and primers to perform a "control" amplification. The following year, AmpliTaq® DNA polymerase, a recombinant polymerase produced in *E. coli*, and a GeneAmp® kit containing that enzyme were added. In the next year, more than 20 new products including an RNA PCR kit, a *Taq* polymerase-based sequencing kit, and numerous primer and probe products were introduced. Two new instrument systems along with specially designed consumables followed the first DNA thermal cycler, offering improved performance, ease of use, and an increased number of wells. PECI also developed products targeted for environmental testing, with the first kits in that field coming to market in early 1992.

PECI licensed a few companies to produce specific PCR products that had other proprietary components complementary to PCR. The first PECI licensee was Clontech, Inc., which sold a series of kits for the detection and analysis of oncogenes. Licenses were also granted to Applied Biosystems, Inc. for certain PCR-based DNA sequencing applications that incorporate ABI's own proprietary dye label technology.

Because PCR is such a basic technology, broadly used in research that might lead to commercially valuable products, there was some concern in the scientific community about what rights the patent holders might have to discoveries made through the use of PCR. To address this issue, Perkin-Elmer Cetus designed a licensing policy through which a license to use the PCR process for research and commercial development activities is passed on to customers through purchase and use of PECI PCR-related reagent and instrument products.

PECI's business strategy has been to build an organization that would provide a support network for users. The venture worked hard to establish a close relationship with the research community through development of applications, technical literature, seminars, and technical service information telephone lines. The wide variety of applications in which PCR is used demands that an organization providing products for those applications keep open communication with customers in order to fulfill new product needs as they develop. The very fact that PCR allows many types of experiments to be completed more quickly leads to a sense of urgency among users who want immediate answers to questions, immediate delivery of products, and rapid development of new products. Users have also enthusiastically shared ideas and suggested new applications based on their discoveries.

Human Identification Including Forensic Science

The use of PCR to analyze genetic differences between individuals is a basic demonstration of the power of this technology. A number of variable human genetic loci were known, which could be applied to human identification. These loci included the complex histocompatibility (HLA) region of the genome, which was already being studied at Cetus in the context of tissue typing and disease susceptibility. Biological materials such as blood, hair, semen, saliva, and skin all yield DNA for analysis. PCR is particularly appropriate to the requirements of forensic investigation, where samples are frequently size limited and/or damaged so that the DNA is degraded. The forensic and paternity testing markets had already been introduced to DNA analysis by the technique of restriction fragment length polymorphism (RFLP). A few laboratories had begun to adopt RFLP. The FBI, which led the evaluation of DNA technologies for crime laboratory use, was prepared to add DNA analysis methods to their existing programs. Since the process of getting RFLP methodologies adopted by the judicial system was under way, there was some reluctance to introduce the PCR process as a new technology. Cetus scientists worked closely with the FBI and other crime laboratories to develop PCR-based tests, to satisfy legal criteria, and ensure that the products were validated for use in casework.

Cetus chose to develop and market their PCR-based forensic products as a distinct business. A product manager was hired in 1989, and a marketing communication program established to address the specific needs of the forensic community. Cetus recognized the importance of providing legal as well as technical support to customers, assisting crime labs in assembling the information required for the admission of test results as evidence in court proceedings.

The first forensic kit was introduced by Cetus in February 1990, and distributed by Perkin-Elmer. The kit tests genetic variation at the HLA-DQα locus, and was the first commercial application of the "reverse dot-blot" PCR product detection format. Six different HLA-DQα alleles that determine 21 possible genotypes can be distinguished with this kit. In 1991, the FBI transferred the AmpliType® HLA-DQα assay from their research laboratory to their headquarters laboratory for implementation on casework.

Other types of identity products use amplified fragment length polymorphism or "AMP-FLP" technology, involving amplification of alleles that have variable numbers of tandem repeats (VNTR). Detection and sizing of alleles are accomplished by gel electrophoresis. A kit based on the human D1S80 locus, the first in a series of AMP-FLP products, was introduced in 1991.

Other applications for AmpliType and AMP-FLP products that greatly extend the value of the human identity business include parentage determination and large-scale personnel databanking for military identification.

Veterinary Diagnostics and Other Fields

In agricultural and veterinary fields, Cetus adopted a strategy of licensing services and products. Among the licenses for the provision of services in vet diagnostics are several for determining the sex of embryos in artificial breeding programs, and a broad license to Genmark Corporation of Salt Lake City, for diagnosis of disease in farm and companion animals. IDEXX Corporation of Portland, Maine, the market leader in veterinary diagnostics, obtained a license for the sale of PCR-based diagnostic products. IDEXX's kit for testing of Johne's disease, a devastating tuberculosis that affects dairy cattle, is the first PCR-based kit to be sold for an application outside of research.

In agriculture, PCR is being applied to detection of pets and to trace desirable genetic traits in plants through breeding programs. Ecologists and wildlife management experts have become interested in using PCR for identification and tracking of animal and plant populations.

PCR Is Purchased by Hoffmann-La Roche

Despite the dedication in November 1988 of a division to the PCR technology, Cetus continued to have difficulty devoting enough resources to fully expand the technology. A delayed FDA approval for its premier proprietary anticancer drug put Cetus in a precarious financial position, and the company reviewed a variety of options. On July 22, 1991, Cetus announced that it had agreed to sell the PCR technology to Hoffmann-La Roche for an aggregate cash price of $300 million, plus some additional royalties on future sales. (At the same time, Cetus and Chiron Corporation announced their agreement to merge, conditional on the completion of the sale of the PCR rights.)

The transaction closed on December 11, 1991, when regulatory and shareholder approvals were complete. Roche established a new company, Roche Molecular Systems, Inc., dedicated to the development and commercialization of PCR. Most of the employees of the Cetus PCR division were offered, and accepted, employment with the new company. The PECI joint venture was dissolved, and Perkin-Elmer and Roche entered into a strategic alliance under which Perkin-Elmer has the rights to the PCR process in research, environmental applications, forensic science, and certain other nondiagnostic fields and is the exclusive distributor of PCR reagent products developed and manufactured by Roche Molecular Systems for those fields. Perkin-Elmer also develops, manufactures, and sells instrument systems for the PCR process, and now solely owns the instrument business that was previously part of PECI.

At the time of this writing, early in 1992, PCR's place in the marketplace has begun a new chapter. Roche's diagnostic development efforts will soon be evaluated by the FDA for approval of the first PCR-based human diagnostic kit. Roche and Perkin-Elmer are establishing the new business relationship. Kits for specific applications in the environmental monitoring, human identity, and other markets will become a larger fraction of the nondiagnostic business.

PCR started as a complex generic procedure applied to basic research problems in molecular biology. It has developed into a simple, multipurpose procedure optimized for diverse applications in nearly every biological scientific discipline and commercial arena. It is certain that many uses of the PCR process have yet to be explored and, as they are developed, new business opportunities will follow.

35

PCR and Scientific Invention: The Trial of DuPont vs. Cetus

Kary B. Mullis

Part I

Had I known my way around in what they call the real world, I could have easily been bringing home a million dollars. I had no idea that my market value had soared temporarily to the level of a fairly good pitcher until the trial was over, and then it was too late.

Driving back from the courthouse to the offices of McCutchen, Doyle, Brown and Enersen in the Embarcadero Center downtown San Francisco with Lynn Pasahow, who led the defense against DuPont for Cetus and who had become over the last 2 years my friend, I learned how I had missed my chance for a cool million.

We were both elated by the clean victory, Cetus: 58, DuPont: 0. My patent had been upheld, Lynn's professional stature had been enhanced, and Cetus walked away with a fancy piece of parchment they would sell to Hofmann-La Roche for $300 million. We were feeling camaraderie at its most fun—when you have won big together. We had developed respect for each other over the past months. He had told me several days before that I had won his case for him with my testimony. I had assured him on multiple occasions that I was very impressed by his abilities. Lynn powered up one of San Francisco's famous hills. I lay back in the Toyota and suggested that it would have been a more interesting trial if he and I had been on opposite sides.

"I couldn't tell you this before, of course . . ." (and by now I was used to the "I couldn't of course tell you" kind of thing that keeps litigation from being too dull, like being in a long double-blind experiment), "but if you had gone in on DuPont's side, Cetus would have settled out of court. You could have negotiated for a lot more money."

"Oh yeah?"

"They needed you."

"Oh well."

It didn't dampen my enthusiasm. I figured someday my financial wagon would roll into the backyard regardless of how hard the idealistic scientist within me resisted it. And it did keep me from feeling any eruption of conscience when I sent in my bill for $74,000 for the last month or so of the trial. Most of that

The opinions expressed herein reflect those of the author only, not the publisher, or of the other contributors or editors to this volume.

last month I had just sat there and watched a show that has to rank with some of the best surfing movies I've ever seen.

It had all the ridiculous moments, the kind that make you look around to see if anybody's watching you see this. There were jurors, and the ones that were always awake seemed dead serious. There was one that slept shamelessly through the whole thing, but voted right in the end. He was the kind of a juror you might want to have if you were up for murder. There was the Very Honorable Marilyn Patel, who lived up to her somewhat medieval sounding appelation, by being just and fair and really, although she was never really tested in a serious crucible, very honorable. By the absent crucible I refer to the fact that nobody was in danger of being hung. I mean, as George Frank's smile had seemed to express when I first encountered him at the deposition of Ian Molineux in Austin early in the trial, "There should be no hard feelings here, son, don't take it personally, we're only in it for the money." George Frank was a general counsel for DuPont, who had taken a particular interest in the invalidation of my patent, Cetus' patent, that is, my name was on the wrong side of the "assigned to" phrase, and George's smile was right. We were all being paid by corporations, the fate of which no one should lament. After all, their founders have already sworn off any personal responsibility at the moment of incorporation. The corporate approach keeps business from being too scarey.

DuPont and Cetus were expected to put up a few million dollars each and we were expected to work long hours sometimes, but to eat well, live high off the hog, which in San Francisco is easy to do, and take it all with a grain of salt. Some heads might roll due to the outcome, but nobody was going to do time and probably any rolling heads would roll right into a new job with no less compensation. And being involved in something newsworthy, even if you do not do anything special, as long as you do not disgrace yourself, has its own reward. You have something to talk about at social gatherings.

The trial got off to an uncertain start. Within the week the curtain would come up on the war in Iraq. The tanks were lined up in the desert and last minute preparations and protests were being made on both sides; the Dow had fallen off since the first of the year, banks were collapsing in New England, and the airlines were once again in dire straits. The courthouse was shut for two or three days by antiwar demonstrations.

Arthur Kornberg from Stanford was called as a key witness for DuPont on account of his association with DNA polymerase. He was going to mystify a number of us in the next few days when he would testify for the plaintiff that, contrary to popular belief on several continents, the nearly grown-up former graduate student from Berkeley across the Bay presently sitting at the defense table in a blue suit and tie, did not really invent what was now called the polymerase chain reaction (PCR). It had not needed to be invented.

PCR, which Arthur Kornberg agreed to call it although he felt that the name was inappropriate, had been apparent since the late 1950s to him and anyone in the field who was blessed with an average wit. It was a simple logical extension, albeit an interesting one to some people, not necessarily to Arthur Kornberg, mind you, of the properties of DNA polymerase, which he had discovered.

In his declaration to the Patent Office during the reexamination proceedings of the previous year, Dr. Kornberg had stated that

In my opinion, either of the Kleppe et al. (1) or Panet et al. (2) references would have enabled a person of ordinary skill in March, 1984 to practice the process encompassed by the claims of the '202 patent (3). Indeed, as discussed in more detail below, the references were enabling at the time of their publication, but were not of practical utility, because ancillary technologies, such as nucleic acid synthesis methods and rapid DNA sequencing had not yet been discovered.

I thought this argument was weak enough to qualify as rather transparently motivated. It failed to account for the period of time, namely the late 1970s and the early 1980s, after which these ancillary technologies were developed and when PCR was introduced amid a great deal of excitement in 1985. I for one do not recall at the time of the first automated DNA synthesizers coming on line anybody sighing, "Good, now we'll be able to amplify DNA."

But when it came to the bright lights and sworn testimony of the trial itself, here was Arthur Kornberg going one further and claiming that even before Kleppe or Panet had supposedly shown the way to PCR, it was evident from the properties of polymerase, which he had described in the late 1950s.

What was it that drove him into this ridiculous position, I wondered?

He went on to say that post-docs in his lab or in similar labs anywhere could have done PCR anytime they wanted to once oligonucleotides were available. The need just never arose. Mullis was just the first person to need it. In Kornberg's deposition he had said in answer to, "I take it from that (referring to his written declaration) you believe that an ordinarily skilled nucleic acid enzymologist would have known it would be possible (prior to March 1984, when the patent was filed) to use the PCR reaction in human genomic DNA to pick out a rare sequence?"

Kornberg: "Yes. In fact it was done. The best illustration is Kary Mullis. He wasn't even a nucleic acid enzymologist, and he did it in a short time."
Pasahow: "And so you consider him as your ordinarily skilled person for that conclusion?"
Kornberg: "I would be generous in saying so."
Pasahow: "How would you describe his skills?"
Kornberg: "Well, as far as I know he never published a paper on nucleic acid enzymology. I didn't know his name. It doesn't make him persona non grata, but he had never trained in a laboratory that did nucleic acid enzymology, never published original work on the subject. So I would be hard put to call him a nucleic acid enzymologist. And I didn't notice until I read the description of his work in a deposition—and he certainly fooled around doing things that initially I never would have done, nor would any of my

students have done. And yet he, within a reasonable length of time, reasonably short length of time, was able to get amplification of a template."

Pasahow seemed to let him off easy, maybe in deference to his seemingly being from a distant planet. Lynn would take care of these issues later with another witness that DuPont was to call, Bruce Wallace. But just in case Arthur Kornberg wanted to go home thinking he had got away with it, Lynn let him tell the court about his textbook *DNA Replication*. Dr. Kornberg agreed that it was a standard textbook, probably *the* standard in the field, and that probably everything relevant to DNA replication was definitely in there. He kept up with the literature he assured us by reading about 10,000 papers a year. So then Lynn handed him a copy of *DNA Replication*, published conveniently in 1983, and asked if he could show us where it talks about amplifying DNA. His smile exuded condescension, robustly as from long years of practice and Dr. Kornberg informed us that there was nothing about amplifying DNA in there.

Then Lynn brought out Kornberg's manuscript for the new edition of *DNA Replication*. Tony Figg and company must surely have prepared him to testify about this; they had been obliged to turn it over during discovery, but he must not have been listening during their tutorial for he was in a terrible jam now. He could not have escaped it completely, but he at least could have lessened the impact a little. It looked as though he was secretly conspiring against DuPont. Well Doctor, do you recognize this document? and so on. Yes, the new edition did just happen to talk about DNA amplification; in fact there were a couple of pages describing this "astonishing and highly useful technique." And Arthur Kornberg had been in his right mind when he wrote that. It did not look too good for the doctor's testimony as he read to us from his manuscript. Lynn, in one of his better moves, left it quickly and let the jury form their own opinion.

Part II

In December 1983, when I first got PCR to work, I was pretty sure that I was the first person in recorded history to do so. By then for over six months I had been talking about it to anyone who would listen. I first had the idea in the spring when I was driving late at night in Mendocino County. It had been an exhilarating California buckeye-scented Eureka! moment, followed by a frantic episode of pacing around my cabin scribbling on every piece of paper and then every clean horizontal surface that would accept pencil, ink, or crayon until dawn when, with the aid of a last bottle of cabernet, I settled into a perplexed semiconsciousness.

Afternoon came, including new bottles of celebratory red fluids from Jack's Valley Store, but I was still puzzled, alternating between being absolutely pleased with my good luck and clever brain, and being mildly annoyed at myself and Jennifer Barnett for not seeing the flaw that must have been there. I had no phone at the cabin and there were no other biochemists besides Jennifer and me in Anderson Valley. The conundrum that lingered throughout the weekend and created an unprecedented desire in me to return to work early was compelling. If the cyclic reactions that by now were symbolized in various ways all over the cabin really worked, why had I never heard of them being used? If they had been used, I surely would have heard about it and so would everybody else including Jennifer, who was presently sunning herself by the pond taking no interest in the explosions that were rocking my brain. These simple reactions could solve the two most pressing problems in nucleic acid chemistry: abundance, because of the exponential growth of the chain reaction product, and distinction, because the products after the third cycle would have a distinct molecular size that could be arbitrarily set by the choice of primers.

Why wouldn't these reactions work? I could not rid myself of the suspicion that I was neglecting to account for some very simple and obvious property of nucleic acids. It was irritating, like a tick drilling into my dienceph-

alon, threatening to break my bubble, this glorious bubble, with its well-defined DNA molecules being called into existence by the logic of two primers out of the disgusting, viscous, hard-to-pipette solution of human DNA in the refrigerator. And I would be famous, the clever inventor of a method that would change DNA chemistry around the world. Amazing! I wanted to believe. But there was this creeping suspicion.

Monday morning I was in the library. The moment of truth. By afternoon it was clear. For whatever reasons, there was nothing in the abstracted literature about succeeding or failing to amplify DNA by the repeated reciprocal extension of two primers hybridized to the separate strands of a particular DNA sequence. By the end of the week I had talked to enough molecular biologists to know that I was not missing anything really obvious. No one could recall such a process ever being tried. My bubble was safe and still shimmering.

However, shocking to me, not one of my friends or colleagues would get excited over the potential for such a process. True, I was always having wild ideas, and this one maybe looked no different than last week's. But it *was* different. There was not a single unknown in the scheme. Every step involved had been done already. Everyone agreed that you could extend a primer on a DNA template, everyone knew you could melt double-stranded DNA. Everyone agreed that what you could do once, you could do again. Most people did not like to do things over and over, me in particular. If I had to do a calculation twice, I preferred to write a program instead. But no one thought it was impossible. It could be done, and there was always automation. The result on paper was so obviously fantastic, two to the tenth is a thousand, two to the twentieth is a million, that even I had little irrational lapses of faith that it would really work in a tube, and most everyone who would take a moment to talk about it with me felt compelled to come up with some reason why it would not work. It was not easy in that postcloning, pre-PCR year to accept the fact that you could have all the DNA you wanted. And that it would be easy.

I had a directory full of untested ideas in the computer. I opened a new file and named this one polymerase chain reaction. I didn't immediately try an experiment, but all summer I kept talking to people in and out of the company. I described the concept around August at an in-house seminar. Every Cetus scientist had to give a talk twice a year. But no one had to listen. Most of the talks were dry descriptions of labor performed and most of the scientists left early without comment. Michael Innis, who would later edit a book on PCR techniques, notably stayed this time until I finished, and seemingly amused by my naiveté, assured me that my chain reaction would not work because the five to three prime nuclease activity of polymerase would destroy the primers and the products.

One or two technicians were interested, and on the days when she still loved me, Jennifer thought it might work. On the increasingly numerous days when she hated me, my ideas and I suffered her scorn together.

I continued to talk about it, and by late summer had a plan to amplify a 400-bp fragment from human nerve growth factor, which Genentech had cloned and published in *Nature*. I would start from whole human placental DNA from Sigma, taking a chance that the cDNA sequence had derived from a single exon. No need for a cDNA library. No colonies, no nothing. It would be dramatic. I would shoot for the moon. Primers were easy to come by in my lab, which made oligonucleotides for the whole company. I entered the sequences I wanted into the computer and moved them to the front of the waiting list.

My friend Ron Cook, who had founded Biosearch, and produced the first successful commercial DNA synthesis machine, was the only person I remember during that summer who shared my enthusiasm for the reaction. He knew it would be good for the oligonucleotide business. Maybe that is why he believed it, or maybe he's a rational chemist with an intact brain. He's one of my best friends now, so I have to disqualify myself from claiming any really objective judgment regarding him. Perhaps I should have followed his advice, but then things would have worked out

differently and I probably would not be here on the beach in La Jolla writing this, which I enjoy. Maybe I would be rich in Tahiti. He suggested one night at his house that since no one at Cetus had taken it seriously, I should resign my job, wait a little while, make it work, write a patent, and get rich. By rich he wasn't imagining three hundred million—maybe one or two. The famous chemist Albert Hoffmann happened to be at Ron's that night. He invented LSD in 1943. At the time he did not realize what he was sitting on either. It only dawned on him slowly, and then things worked their way out over the years like no one would have ever predicted, or could have controlled by forethought and reason.

I responded weakly to Ron's suggestion. I had already described the idea at Cetus, and if it turned out to be commercially successful they would have lawyers after me forever. Ron was not sure that Cetus had rights on my ideas unless they were directly related to my duties. I was not sure about the law, but I was pretty happy working at Cetus and assumed innocently that if the reaction worked big time I would be amply rewarded by my employer.

The subject of PCR was not yet party conversation, even among biochemists, and it quickly dropped. Albert being there was much more interesting, even to me. He had given a fine talk that afternoon at Biosearch.

Anyhow, my problems with Jennifer were not getting any better. That night was no exception to the trend. I drove home alone feeling sad and unsettled, not in the mood for leaving my job, or any big change in what was left of stability in my life. PCR seemed distant and very small compared to our very empty house.

In September I did my first experiment. I like to try the easiest possibilities first. So one night I put human DNA and the nerve growth factor primers in a little screw-cap tube with an O-ring and a purple top. I boiled for a few minutes, cooled it, added about 10 units of DNA polymerase, closed the tube, and left it at 37°C. It was exactly midnight on the ninth of September. I poured a cold Becks into a 400-ml beaker and contemplated my notebook for a few minutes before heading home.

My supply of beer in the lab refrigerator had begun to attract criticism from the laboratory danger officer. The company had grown rapidly in the four years since I'd arrived. These days, for any rule that was written down somewhere you could find at least one middle manager who was willing to order at least one employee to enforce it. My beer supply, keeping company with isotopes and poisons, had survived this long because Pete Farley was still President, had an occasional thirst, was partial to Becks, and knew his way into my lab. The first and the last of these were about to change, and so was the rest of my life. The second and third are probably still true.

Driving home I figured that the primers would be extended right away, and I hoped that at some finite rate the extension products would come unwound from their templates, be primed and recopied, and so forth. I did not relish the idea of heating, cooling, adding polymerase over and over again, and held this for a last resort method of accomplishing the chain reaction. I was thinking of DNA–DNA interactions as being reversible reactions with all the ramifications thereof. I was not concerned about the absolute rate of dissociation, because I did not care how long the reaction took as long as nobody had to do anything. I assumed there would always be some finite concentration of single strands, which would be available for priming by a relatively high concentration of primer with pseudo-first-order kinetics.

For a reaction with the potential that I dreamed of for this one, especially in light of the absence of anything else that could do the same thing, time was only a very secondary consideration. Would it work at all was important. The next most important thing was, would it be easy to do? Then came time.

At noon the next day I came into the lab to take a 12-hour sample. There was no sign by ethidium bromide of any 400-bp bands. I could have waited another hundred years as I had no idea what the rates might be. But I succumbed slowly to the notion that I could not escape much longer the unpleasant prospect of cycling the reaction between single-stranded temperatures and double-stranded temperatures. This

also meant adding the thermally unstable polymerase after every cycle.

For three months I did sporadic experiments while my life at home and in the lab with Jennifer was crumbling. It was slow going. Finally I retreated from the idea of starting with human DNA; I was not even absolutely sure that the Genentech sequence from *Nature* that I was using was from a single exon. I settled on a target of more modest proportions, a short fragment from pBR322, a purified plasmid. The first successful experiment happened on December 16th. I remember the date. It was the birthday of Cynthia Gibson, my former wife from Kansas City, who had encouraged me to write fiction and bore us two fine sons. I had strayed from Cynthia eventually to spend two tumultous years with Jennifer. When I was sad for any other reason, I would also grieve for Cynthia. There is a general place in your brain, I think, reserved for "the melancholy of relationships past." It grows and prospers as life progresses, forcing you finally, against your grain, to listen to country music.

And now as December threatened Christmas, Jennifer, that crazy, wonderful woman chemist, had dramatically left our house, the lab, and even California, headed to New York and her mother for reasons that seemed to have everything to do with me but which I, of course, couldn't fathom. I was beginning to learn tragedy. It differs a great deal from pathos, which you can learn from books. Tragedy is personal. It would add strength to my character and depth someday to my writing. Just right then, I would have preferred a warm friend to cook with. Hold the tragedy lessons. December is a rotten month to be studying your love life from a distance.

In spite of my personal tragedy, I celebrated my scientific victory with Fred Faloona, a young mathematician and a wizard of many talents whom I had hired as a technician. Fred had helped me that afternoon set up this first successful PCR reaction, and I stopped by his house on the way home. As he had learned all the biochemistry he knew directly from me he was not certain whether or not to believe me when I informed him that we had just changed the rules in molecular biology big time.

"Okay, Doc, if you say so." He knew I was more concerned with my life than with those cut little purple-topped tubes. In Berkely it drizzles in the winter. Avocados ripen at odd times and the tree in Fred's front yard was wet and sagging from a load of fruit. I was sagging as I walked out to my little silver Honda Civic, which never failed to start. Neither Fred, empty Becks bottles, or the sweet smell of the dawn of the age of PCR could replace Jenny. I was lonesome.

Part III

There was no reasonable doubt in my mind, as I watched PCR develop from a spring conception to a breathing process by Christmas and then on to lurid full-page colored ads in *Science* and *Nature* that I had invented something. Al Halluin, the head of intellectual property at Cetus, had recognized immediately that it might be very important. Like Ron, Al could feel the thrill of it a little easier than people who had no vested interest, or worse, felt threatened by it.

Al's enthusiasm gave me a good solid lift early on when I really needed it. He congratulated me warmly, and assigned his assistant Janet Hasak to write the application. At the time Al was busy trying to dispose of the Cohen and Boyer patent so Cetus would not have to pay a licensing fee for cloning. It was a diversion not worth the money, because Stanford was licensing it reasonably, and he eventually dropped it. But Janet and I got on well together and chipped away at a patent application for two years. We knew for certain that we had a novel invention. It was hard to find any prior art to describe in the introductory section of the patent application.

The reception I got at Cold Spring Harbor in May 1986, when I presented PCR to a large and impressive audience of molecular biologists, was definitive. I had invented something they could use. Everyone told me that it was new and that furthermore it was a splendid contribution. I did not feel like anybody was just putting me on because they thought I needed a break. By the time 1989 rolled

around there had been about two thousand papers published using PCR and no one had publicly questioned that it had been developed in 1985 and was a surprisingly useful invention.

So I was a little surprised when I heard that DuPont was seriously going after the PCR patent on the grounds that it had been invented much earlier. Pretty quickly I discovered they weren't so much interested in the whole story, the one that had convinced me with its emotional scenes and the smell of invention all around. They were interested in whether the claims read on some prior art. As Thelma observed in *Thelma and Louise*, "Law is some tricky shit, idn' it?"

A patent claim, besides being a single, long, run-on sentence with which your worst English teacher in high school would have been unamused, and your best English teacher would have been intrigued on account of your cleverness for contriving its intricacies, is a mechanism by which you describe what you have invented and distinguish it from what may have been done similarly in the past, with the ultimate goal of claiming that you have done something that makes almost everything possible and that is exemplary of anything useful someone might want to do in the future and yet is not exemplary of anything that has been done in the past, most of which simply pointed out the need for your invention without showing the way to it.

When Janet and I were writing the application for what became US 4,683,202, Janet told me at first to leave the claims mainly to her, which suited me fine, as I was ignorant of the central importance of claims and had never appreciated their puzzling elegance. I had no idea I would someday be testifying as to their appropriateness in a federal court and that on their validity would hang a serious fraction of a billion dollars. We worked pretty well together though and as time passed so did the division of labor. The claims were as much my fault as hers.

A claim is the meat of a patent. If it is not in the claims, then you do not own it in the end, and if it is in a claim and somebody can prove to the patent office or a court that anything in your claim has already been done somewhere else in the past and published, then your patent can be invalidated.

The patent office and the federal courts arise from independent branches of government. The executive branch patent and trademark lawyers, in keeping with the general irrational nature of civilization as augmented by Thomas Jefferson et al., are constitutionally subordinate even in matters requiring their specialized skills to the plain old general practitioner type of lawyers and judges who hang around federal courts and are more skilled in the arts of murder and rape than in chemistry. It is the judicial branch, these guys, that finally decides.

Disregarding this technicality, it is fair that if something's already in the public domain, a pretender to its invention should not be allowed to have a monopoly on its use just because of greed or a misunderstanding.

If someone explained patent litigation to me while Janet and I were drafting our claims, I certainly was not paying attention. Our claims were not baroque enough to deal bruskly, when the time came, with the infidels from Wilmington.

We had a breakthrough, a pioneering invention, and we wanted broad claims that would not appear shortsighted when derivative technologies started to appear. But I did not want them to wander all over the place or diverge into triple counterpoint. I wanted them to say what they had to say in the least number of words, and get out of there. Janet was not a debater in high school, would not stoop to vitriol when logic failed, and could not type as fast as I. She is an agreeable person and friendly. As we batted sections of the draft back and forth on the computer, I prevailed in bringing a sense of my own esthetics into the document, and in my desire that the wording be lean, I naively left the patent open to attack. In a lean, logical way we covered everything, but without the benefit of comfortable near-redundant fall back positions. I'd never been in litigation. I was playing without a full deck, emulating an academic publication. Janet sensed what it might be like to have a patent challenged, but couldn't bring herself to expose me to the fact that her colleagues were not lean and logical, in fact, with exceptions, they

were fat and illogical, and somebody else was always paying for the paper, and the writing on it, and the later reading of it, by the hour.

We ended up with a number of more specific claims, but we left the real value of the patent hanging precariously on the sparsely metered syllables of the first two. It was not arrogance, it was just inexperience.

We claimed:

1. A process for amplifying at least one specific nucleic acid sequence contained in a nucleic acid or a mixture of nucleic acids wherein each nucleic acid consists of two separate complementary strands of equal or unequal length, which process comprises:

(a) treating the strands with two oligonucleotide primers, for each different specific sequence being amplified, under conditions such that for each different sequence being amplified an extension product of each primer is synthesized that is complementary to each nucleic acid strand, wherein said primers are selected so as to be sufficiently complementary to different strands of each specific sequence to hybridize therewith such that the extension product synthesized from one primer, when it is separated from its complement, can serve as a template for synthesis of the extension product of the other primer;

(b) separating the primer extension products from the templates on which they were synthesized to produce single-stranded molecules; and

(c) treating the single-stranded molecules generated from step (b) with the primers of step (a) under conditions that a primer extension product is synthesized using each of the single strands produced in step (b) as a template.

2. The process of claim 1, wherein steps (b) and (c) are repeated at least once.

So the issue that DuPont was bringing before the court then was whether or not anybody had ever been able to make any nucleic acid, using two primers and template directed polymerization, from any other nucleic acid, and to repeat the process at least once during which repetition the newly synthesized nucleic acid now also functioned as a template. In spite of the fact that all useful applications of PCR started from DNA molecules lacking the specific ends that were being generated in the product by the reaction, as all the examples in the patent demonstrated, there was no claim necessarily limited to the case where the original template would be imbedded in a larger molecule. And, very significantly, there was no claim drafted where the target was necessarily a minor part of a complex mixture. We understood that this was almost always going to be the case, and that the economic usefulness of PCR depended on it, but we did not include a set of claims specifically restricted to this situation, claims that for all practical purposes would have been functionally as broad as the claims we drafted. Such claims would have been sufficient to protect the economic value of PCR, even if the rest had fallen, and they would have been unassailable under the prior art which turned up from Khorana's lab. We could have saved Cetus several million in the short run with a few simple words, but I would not have had the pleasure of being the inventor in a big patent litigation case and Cetus in the long run may not have made so much money on the sale of PCR. When the price was being bartered, it mattered that the patent had been reexamined and court-approved in a highly publicized case.

As written, the claims read on the possibility that Kjell Kleppe, who in 1969 had a pure synthetic fragment of DNA, might want more of it. And he might try to make it with polymerase. He would need a primer for each of the two strands. He had primers and he had polymerase, and what he would do might look a lot like what our claims described.

Part IV

In many people's opinion, the evidence that PCR had really been invented in 1971 required a minor suspension of judgment. But really and legally can be two separate issues. In this case to know what really happened we have to look at the details.

By 1971 it had been known for some time, initially due to work from Arthur Kornberg's lab, that there were enzymes, which could, in the presence of a suitable DNA primer hybridized to a single-stranded DNA template, polymerase nucleotides from monomeric nucleoside triphosphates in solution. The product was a complementary, double-stranded DNA molecule consisting of the template, the primer, and the newly polymerized nucleotides. The existence of some such copying mechanism shy the biochemical details had not escaped the notice of Watson and Crick in their 1953 letter to *Nature*. By 1957 or thereabouts Kornberg had found an enzyme that he thought had the right activity to do the job. He was almost right, and over the next few years he and others described several polymerase activities, and Kornberg fell in love with his.

But in 1971 there was little detailed information available concerning the quantitative aspects of the process. In order to understand the earliest attempts at using two primers in the same tube to multiply a preexisting DNA molecule, and this is of course the sine qua non for identifying early fossils of the PCR fluorescence, it is necessary to know some of the details of what was known and what was misunderstood about single primer extensions. In the Khorana lab first at Wisconsin and then later at MIT (Kleppe et al., 1971) a typical protocol for extending a primer with polymerase would be as follows: "The reaction was carried out at 15°C. Before the addition of the enzyme the reaction mixtures were heated to 70°C for 2 min, then cooled to 15°C over a period of 1 hr and then kept at 15° for 1 hr." Three hundred units of DNA polymerase per nanomole template would then be added, and the incorporation of ^{32}P from an α-labeled dNTP would be followed for up to 4 hr.

These experiments would usually result, remarkably enough, in a hyperbolic accumulation of the label into what seemed to be DNA for 4 hours. In a laboratory at Hofmann-La Roche in New Jersey (Olson et al., 1975) the same protocol produced data indicating that the reaction was greater than 95% complete in less than 15 min, and independent of the temperature from 10 to 25°C after which the incorporated counts would drift very slowly upward for 4 or more hours. It is not clear what was happening, but temperature insensitivity in the rate of a reaction is usually taken as an indication that it is not enzymatic.

The template oligonucleotide would typically be present at micromolar concentrations and the primer at 2 μM, so the priming step would have really been over within seconds, as soon as the temperature was down to where the hybrid would be stable. It is known today that a 27-nucleotide oligomer at a concentration 1 μM in excess of a complementary target 25°C below its melting temperature will hybridize to 99% of its complement in one-seventh of a second (Bill Sutherland, Kodak, personal communication). In the early 1970s there was a lot of loose talk about "incubation" of things like oligonucleotides as if they were eggs slowly hatching. This probably spilled over from the enzyme people and hung around for awhile. Even into the 1980s people were still treating oligonucleotide hybridizations as though the oligomers were little organisms that needed a long time to solve what appeared to be a difficult puzzle.

In Kleppe's experiments, where only one oligonucleotide was being hybridized to only one single-stranded target, it was of little consequence that a great deal of ritual time was consumed, and the experiment should have proceeded as planned as soon as the enzyme was finally added. And it did proceed as planned, but there must have been something similar to the incubation theory that got incorporated into the plan that said that polymerases did not add bases to primers in experiments as fast as they added bases when their specific activity was being measured. And the data came out according to the plan. Why this happened is anybody's guess. Why, for example, would 300 units of polymerase, defined as that amount that could add 3000 nmol of nucleotide in 30 min at 37°C, take 60 min to add 1.2 nmol in a reaction that was independent of temperature from 10 to 25°C or in a separate experiment 2 hr to add 0.6 nmol. Something was really screwy and the explanation had to be more than the marginal effect, postulated by Kleppe, of running the reactions at a pH that

was not optimal for the polymerase (pH 6.9 as compared to pH 7.5 recommended today by BRL). There was something else going on. A lot of things can go on in an hour.

But when we come to understand what happened when they tried to run similar reactions with two primers and a double-stranded template, we do not need to be concerned about the enzyme at all, since by the time he got around to adding it, the complementary templates at micromolar concentrations would for all practical purposes have been completely and irreversibly reassociated with each other and any primer that had been bound to either strand would have been displaced.

Kleppe's final paragraph in the 1971 paper, which has by now probably been memorized by every high school student thinking about a career in litigation, reads as follows:

The principles for extensive synthesis of the duplexed tRNA genes which emerge from the present work are the following. The DNA duplex would be denatured to form single strands. This denaturation step would be carried out in the presence of a sufficiently large excess of the two appropriate primers. Upon cooling, one would hope to obtain two structures, each containing the full length of the template strand appropriately complexed with the primer. DNA polymerase will be added to complete the process of repair replication. Two molecules of the original duplex should result. The whole cycle could be repeated, there being added everytime a fresh dose of the enzyme. It is however, possible that upon cooling after denaturation of the DNA duplex, renaturation to form the original duplex would predominate over the template-primer complex formation. If this tendency could not be circumvented by adjusting the concentrations of the primers, clearly one would have to resort to the separation of the strands and then carry out repair replication. After every cycle of repair replication, the process of strand separation would have to be repeated. Experiments based on these lines of thought are in progress. [Kleppe et al., 1971]

He almost had it. He saw the problem, but he did not realize how fast things happen and that the template reassociation would not be reversible at low temperatures. The tendency of the templates to reassociate could have been circumvented, but not by more concentrated primers. The primers were alright, the template concentration needed to be much lower, and the enzyme needed to be put in quickly as soon as the temperature was low enough for it to survive.

But even if he had got it, Kleppe was still a long way from PCR. He was not seeing the possibility that if you do three cycles or more of two-primer extensions in the presence of a target that is contained in a larger piece of DNA, then you amplify a limited segment of the DNA with ends that are determined by the five prime ends of the oligonucleotide primers. Instead of spending 5 man years synthesizing a defined sequence of DNA and then trying to make more, Kleppe could have pulled it out of a DNA sample with just two primers as in PCR. But they were not looking for this kind of thing. After all, the synthetic methods that they were using to make defined fragments of DNA were fairly new and had just recently allowed the Khorana and Nirenberg groups to solve the genetic code. They assumed that modification of those methods would always be the way to make defined DNA sequences.

Furthermore, synthetic DNA was hard to make in quantity and therefore very precious. They kept it in a safe. It would have been hard to recognize in any particular case that one needed much less DNA, rather than much more, I suppose.

Maybe the reason we cannot do cold nuclear fusion today is because we are chemists and fusion is physics. A paradigm is enabling and at the same time, particularly when it is only implicit, a paradigm is restricting. We always have to have them, but we need also to be on the lookout for that rare moment when by the grace of the bumpiness of things we flop momentarily out of the paradigm, like a virtual particle flaming from nothing into existence, and we discover something shocking.

By 1974 the Khorana lab had done at least a few experiments with two primers and a synthetic duplex in the same tube. They had not discovered something shocking and had not published any detailed results of these experiments. They had made synthetic dsDNAs by diester synthesis and ligation of short ssDNAs, a method that, with the addition of very important improvements to the organic synthesis

methodology, would still be in use in the 1980s. Over a hundred papers chronicle the fact that many significant advances in nucleic acid chemistry were achieved during that era in that lab, but the use of DNA polymerase to make large quantities of DNA available from the tiny amounts in nature or created by organic synthesis was not one of them.

In the Introduction to a 1974 paper in the *Journal of Biological Chemistry* (Panet and Khorana 1974) it was reported that the preferred way to duplicate a DNA duplex enzymatically would be to attach single strands to an insoluble cellulose support so that the immobilized templates could be separated from newly synthesized complementary strands after being copied by polymerase. The authors describe the then current state of the art in the enzymatic duplication of DNA.

Correct extensive replication of these synthetic DNA would be crucial to ensuring their availability for future studies. . . . None of the presently known DNA polymerases evidently utilizes a linear DNA duplex with even ends as a template or brings about the de novo synthesis of new polynucleotide chains. So far, it has been only possible to bring about "repair replication" by using single-stranded deoxypolynucleotides as templates and short polynucleotides complementary to one end of the template strands as primers. [They make reference to Kleppe et al., 1971.] Even so, in this primer-dependent replication, the reaction comes to a halt when the duplex has been completed and further synthesis requires separation of the duplex and a restart in the presence of an excess of the primer. [Reference to K. Kleppe and I. J. Molineux, unpublished work.] Similarly the problem of the extensive and orderly transcription of a defined deoxyribopolynucleotide remains to be solved. [References to Terao et al., 1972; Kleppe and Khorana, 1972; Panet and Khorana, 1974.]

Now all of this sounds to me like they are saying that they have been thinking and tinkering with ways to duplicate DNA, but they aren't satisfied yet that they have found a good one. They could have just said that to justify the research effort they had put into this paper, which explored a very un-PCR-like attempted solution to the problem, but that would be underestimating the Khorana lab, which at the time was probably the foremost lab in the world dealing with these issues. They knew what they had done and what they had not.

So where did they go from there? It looks like, rereading the paper (Panet and Khorana, 1974), that they did not really do very much. They made a lot of vague remarks about what was and was not effective for replicating DNA, concluding that the particular manner in which they had attached the template to a solid support in this study was ideal and would be the method of choice. However, they really did not say much in quantitative terms about how well any of the methods they had tried could duplicate DNA, which should it seems have been at least one important criterion by which the methods were compared. The paper is notable because it contains the final mention in the literature of an attempt at two-primer-mediated DNA replication up until the mid-1980s when the discovery of PCR as we know it today was announced.

The paragraph has been examined by the shrewdest and the best patent lawyers in the world. The wording is ambiguous and tantalizing, but the message can only be reasonably interpreted as a restatement of what had been said already in this paper, and been suggested by Kleppe in 1971. Attempts at copying both strands of DNA in the same tube will be met with failure due to the reassociation of template.

In unpublished work carried out in this laboratory by Dr. I. J. Molineux, the replication of relatively short DNA duplexes containing base paired ends was investigated in the presence of deoxyribonucleotide primers corresponding to both of the constituent DNA chains. Briefly, these experiments showed that (a) indeed, replication occurred only by primer elongation, (b) to form the appropriate template primer complexes, it was necessary to add, after each cycle, fresh amounts of the primers so as to maintain the appropriate primer-template ratios. The above results seemed to place a severe limit on the extent of net synthesis that could be achieved in the above approach and the work described herein was therefore undertaken. Clearly, if each of the template strands could be attached to an insoluble polymer, the total process of replication could be much more convenient and very economical with respect to the primer. [Kleppe et al., 1971]

The remainder of the discussion summarizes the successful use of cellulose bound templates in duplicating valuable DNA.

In the Chemical Research Department of Hoffmann-La Roche in New Jersey the problem of enzymatic duplication of synthetic DNA was also being approached (Olsen et al., 1975). Responding to the same template reassociation problem as the researchers in Khorana's lab, the Roche group proposed another cumbersome solution without commenting and probably without considering the far simpler alternative of just diluting the complementary template strands sufficiently so that they would not interfere with each other's priming and extension. Water is what they needed; instead they opted for Sephadex G-75. With terminal transferase they added a string of adenosines to the south end of their template, primed it just to the north of the As, extended the primer northward with polymerase, and separated the copy from the somewhat longer template on Sephadex. It worked. So do unicycles.

In their *Nucleic Acids Research* paper, Olsen et al. acknowledged Panet and Khorana. "Very recently, an alternative method for accomplishing the objective of this paper has been described [reference to Panet and Khorana, 1974]. These authors attached the template covalently to a cellulose support and separated the product after denaturation."

For historical purposes it is reassuring that an interpretation of the Panet and Khorana paper by their contemporaries in New Jersey 20 years ago does not measurably differ from that which we would make today. Olsen et al. in reading Panet and Khorana were not led to attempt experiments along the line of those unpublished experiments of Molineux that had been at least temporarily abandoned.

How long it was after this work was completed before the scientists in Khorana's lab at MIT first became aware of the fact that in some late night delicatessen in Oahu, Herb Boyer and Stanley Cohen were exchanging nightmares about what would happen if one were to take a plasmid specifically cleaved with a restriction enzyme and an unrelated DNA molecule trimmed by the same enzyme, ligate them together, and insert the horrible recombinant plasmid back into its frightened host. It could not have been too long, because Cambridge was not a backwater country town even then.

The impact of this new lightning bolt on everything happening in every DNA lab in the world was explosive. Even the custodians pushing brooms through the labs at night could feel something of the magic of cloning.

The problem of the replication of synthetic DNA had been solved beside another body of water far from the Charles River in a totally surprising manner and one that everyone would learn. The single strands on cellulose at Cambridge and the strands extended by terminal transferase in New Jersey were stuffed in the freezer where they worked their way slowly to the rear as the memory faded.

Part V

DuPont came to Cetus in 1987 looking to license PCR, which they had decided would be essential to their entry into clinical DNA diagnostics. Kleppe's notes were yellowing peacefully in their Cambridge cabinet, quivered privately in the dark. It had been a long time. Only another year or two now before the lawyers would come and pry open the door. The subpoena that would call them back to life, the Great White Light that would flash a hundred times, the Drum that would roll under the light and form their image into Carbon and lay it onto the Clean White Sheets as they issued from the Feeder, the Stapler that would bind the Copied Ones, the Great Fed Ex that would lift them into the air and carry them in all directions throughout the world, and the Experts who would be waiting. It was coming.

Bob Fildes, who by then had been running the show at Cetus with a managerial consensus, sometimes as thin as his own uninformed suspicions, knew this time for certain, and this time he was correct, what had to happen, what DuPont had to be told. It was unfortunate, but it was true. PCR had already been spoken for by a large Swiss firm with an appetite for biotechnology. They had come some months ago

with an offer that Fildes could not refuse. The story will be written down, but not here.

The gentlemen from DuPont were not used to "no thank you." Certainly not from little California companies struggling to exist past the next annual report. They flew back to Wilmington, where it is said the DuPont river flows into a grey sea of lawyers. Godfather II was showing on the plane, but they were too busy to watch. There were things to do. Meetings had to be arranged, memos circulated and prior art had to be found.

And so it happened. Two years later, while Desert Storm was raging through Iraq, DuPont and Cetus squared off in federal court in the Northern District of California Federal Court, Her Honour Marilyn Patel presiding. Preparations had not been cursory. Witnesses came in from everywhere.

Jim Dahlberg came down from Wisconsin to explain to the jury how it was that despite testimony they had heard from Arthur Kornberg, Bruce Wallace, Ian Molineux, John Van de Sande, and Ruth Kleppe, the widow of Kjell Kleppe, the notebooks and the publications from the lab during the time PCR was supposed to have been developed there, indicated that it had not.

The things that Dahlberg testified about were well out of the range of even the most sophisticated of the jurors. He had analyzed the primary data and its interpretation by the post-docs who had generated it. He was probably more familiar with the material than anybody in Khorana's lab had been while the experiments were in progress. I was shocked when I first realized how extensively those notes had been studied. Kleppe was comfortably out of the controversy that would now play itself out. Certainly he had never imagined that the routine notes he would make on his day-to-day experiments in 1969 were going to be the subject of a trial that would employ 10 to 20 experts, some of them for months, to go over those notes with a legally inclined finetooth comb, a trial that would cost millions of dollars to stage, and would happen in a federal court in San Francisco in 1991, long after Kleppe himself had passed away. He had no idea that Dahlberg, David Gelfand, and Kevin

Kaster from Cetus and Barbara Mierke, Jim Lewis, and Lyn Pasahow from McCutchen Doyle, to mention only a few would be paid many thousands of dollars to pore over his handwritten scribbles to himself. People wearing stylish new neck ties would be sitting around fine wood tables on the top floors of Embarcadero III, peering down at sailboats under the Golden Gate, discussing and recalculating the fine points of his daily uncelebrated labor, finding minor mistakes in his numbers, omissions in his lists, being unable even with the help of scholars from far-off places to decipher some of his characters, would slowly acquire an intimate familiarity with his experiments eventually understanding every minute detail . . . experiments he probably considered mundane and of no consequence. And they would take it seriously.

The jury had no idea what was going on, but they enjoyed Dahlberg's boyish personality and they knew that this man would not lie to them.

In a big litigation like this all the "witnesses" are on one payroll or the other. No one is here for free. A thousand a day, two thousand . . . Kornberg was taking home five; it was for his research, they said. The jurors being paid by the government were getting about 30 dollars a day and I wondered how they felt about these fancy doctor/lawyer types racking it in. One of the questions the opposing council asks during cross-examination just to make sure it hasn't escaped some juror's memory that "expert witness" means "hired gun" is "Are you being compensated for your testimony? And how much would that be?"

But French Anderson wasn't getting a nickel. He was working for the government. NIH allowed him only so many paid consulting days a year, and he was over his limit, so for his trouble he could only take pleasure in the fact that he was on the dextral side of the courtroom sitting with the good guys. And that is where he belonged. French could not look crafty in a Nixon mask. His sincerity seems attached to his slender frame, and his concern about the issues in the case seemed derived from a social sense rather than a personal connection.

French Anderson explained that he had been thinking about gene transplantation almost all of his professional life, and would have been excited to find a method like PCR back in the 1970s. He had worked with Marshall Nirenberg sorting out the genetic code with oligonucleotides, had synthesized the very last codon, and made the first public presentation of the complete code. Gobind Khorana's lab at MIT had been involved in the same endeavor, and there were probably no Khorana lab secrets kept from him. He had sat in on many of their lab meetings, and nobody had ever mentioned to him that a method existed for amplifying DNA. He was aware that Kleppe had done some experiments with two primers, but nothing had ever suggested that even a purified fragment of DNA could be successfully duplicated and certainly no one was thinking in terms of an amplification that could pull a specific sequence up out of a complex background and amplify it indefinitely. If a technique had been known in the 1970s that would do anything like this, he would have had great need for it in his early gene transplantation experiments, and would have gone to great lengths to make it work.

It was only in the 1980s, from the people at Cetus, that French first learned of PCR. He did not immediately believe it, but after a meeting in California, he sent some coded samples back and was pleasantly surprised at the results.

And he was an effective witness, a dedicated MD working at the frontiers of gene replacement theory. Just by chance there had been an article about his experiments with a little girl suffering from ADA deficiency in the San Francisco Chronicle the day before he took the stand. His testimony was animated. When Lynn asked him who invented PCR he pointed at me. The jury was beginning to get the point.

French Anderson reminded me of why I had become a scientist instead of the kind of lawyer I would have likely become if I had become one. On the morning he was to testify, French awoke in the wee hours and read transcripts. Then he had a piece of toast with Lynn before heading down to the courthouse. He expected his cross-examination to be much worse than it was and seemed slightly nervous at first. I think that played nicely to the jury. It hinted at a man who in spite of his very impressive and understandable accomplishments, had a healthy respect for the court. And he was not being paid. He got their attention and told the truth. The jury, understanding what little of it they did, understood that; and that he was a sincere and honorable physician, the kind of doctor who cared about sick children, and they understood that French Anderson was grateful to this man Mullis over there on the Cetus side of the courtroom for inventing something he found invaluable in his work. And as for these other people whose unfortunate need for distorting reality had driven them to this circus of tawdry testimonials, let them go back to their eastern churches to pray for their souls.

They may not have thought all that, but the jury listened thoughtfully to French, and in the quiet you could hear the death knell ringing for DuPont. I reached into my briefcase and withdrew an 8 × 10 glossy I had prepared months before. It was a shot I had made one morning in Paris wandering in the Montparnasse Cemetary. I'd come across an ornate, overground tomb inscribed Famille DuPont. I positioned it selectively, the face to Jeff Miller, the scientist from DuPont who had sat at their counsel table parallel to me from the beginning of the trial. The edge of the photograph faced Judge Patel so as not to upset the dignity of the court. Jeff returned a weak smile. I imagined him tired, and ready to go home. There would be no celebration in Wilmington, but it would be home.

The trial had gone on for two months. Besides Dahlberg and Anderson and a number of Cetus employees, and one former employee, me, we had heard testimony from Hamilton

Smith, and sworn statement from Aaron Klug, tutorials on patent law, and so on and so on. I have only scratched the surface here. The whole story, at least the public parts of it, is preserved in many tons of documents, which occupied a room at McCutchen Doyle during the trial. A lot of it remains only in the personal notes and recollections of those involved. I'm presently writing a book.

Acknowledgments. The author thanks Academic Press Inc. for its permission to quote extensively from Kleppe et al. (1971) and The American Society for Biochemistry and Molecular Biology for permission to quote from Panet and Khorana (1974).

References

Kleppe K, Ohtsuka E, Kleppe R, Molineux I, Khorana H (1971): Studies on polynucleotides XCVI repair replication of short synthetic DNAs as catalyzed by DNA polymerases. *J Mol Biol* 56:341.

Mullis K, Faloona F, Scharf S, Saiki R, Horn G, Erlich H (1986): Specific amplification of DNA in vitro: The polymerase chain reaction. *Cold Spring Harbor Symp Quant Biol* 51:260.

Mullis K (1987): US Patent 4,683,202 Process for amplifying nucleic acid sequences.

Mullis K (1990): The unusual origin of the polymerase chain reaction. *Sci Am* 262:56.

Olsen K, Gabriel T, Michalewsky J, Harvey C (1975): Enzymatic multiplication of a chemically synthesized DNA fragment. *Nucl Acids Res* 2:43.

Panet A, Khorana HG (1974): The linkage of deoxyribopolynucleotide templates to cellulose and its use in their replication. *J Biol Chem* 24:5213.

Terao T, Dahlberg J, Khorana HG (1972): *J Biol Chem* 247:6149.

Index